Endocrine Therapy
in
Malignant Disease

Contributors

THOMAS H. ACKLAND

H. J. G. BLOOM

D. C. BODENHAM

GEORGE CRILE JR

J. D. FERGUSSON

K. FOTHERBY

BRENDAN HALE

CHARLES HUGGINS

FRANCES JAMES

ROBERT W. KISTNER

J. S. MALPAS

WALTER J. MOON

ALBERT SEGALOFF

BASIL A. STOLL

PAUL TALALAY

Endocrine Therapy
in
Malignant Disease

Edited by

BASIL A. STOLL

Radiotherapy Department,
St Thomas' Hospital, London
and Royal Free Hospital, London

1972

W. B. Saunders Company Ltd   LONDON · PHILADELPHIA · TORONTO

W. B. Saunders Company Ltd: 12 Dyott Street
London WC1A 1DB

West Washington Square
Philadelphia, Pa. 19105

1835 Yonge Street
Toronto 7, Ontario

Endocrine Therapy in Malignant Disease   ISBN 0–7216–8615–X

Text set in 10/11 pt. Monotype Baskerville 169, printed by letterpress, and bound in Great Britain at The Pitman Press, Bath.

Print No: 9   8   7   6   5   4   3   2   1

Preface

The results of the pioneering researches of Dr Charles Huggins 30 years ago led to the wide adoption of endocrine therapy in advanced prostatic cancer, and stimulated the practice of similar treatment in advanced breast cancer. In the last 10 years, endocrine therapy has established a place also in the management of cancers of the uterine body, kidney and thyroid, while steroid therapy is widely used in the treatment of the leukaemias and lymphomas. The place of endocrine therapy in the management of cancers of the cervix, ovary, testis and malignant melanoma is also being investigated.

By collating in one volume the experience of experts in the various fields, it is hoped that there will emerge a unifying concept of hormone-sensitive cancer in the human, and its rationale of treatment. To achieve this, it is essential in the first place to distinguish the clinical response to corticoid and androgenic steroids which is often observed in late cancer *of all types*. This is likely to be by a non-specific host effect, and by juxtaposing this type of response to the *specific* response of hormone-sensitive cancer to endocrine manipulation, it is hoped that our understanding of both mechanisms will be clarified.

The field of hormone therapy in malignant disease tends to involve many different specialists—endocrinologist, urologist, gynaecologist, general surgeon, general physician and radiotherapist. Because of this diversity of specialists, and because of a very extensive world literature claiming effectiveness for multiple methods of treatment and multiple new agents, it has become increasingly difficult, even for the specialist clinician, to judge the relative merits of each form of treatment. Because of these uncertainties, it is likely that different treatment will be received for the same type of lesion according to the centre where the patient has decided to take advice.

While these uncertainties cannot yet be resolved, certain guide-lines are possible in treatment. Where two methods appear to yield similar results in the palliation of a specific type of cancer, it is obviously humane to choose the method with the lesser morbidity and lesser risk. Even if a controlled trial shows one method to yield better *overall* results than another method of treatment, this does not indicate that it should be used as a routine. Our knowledge has developed to the extent that, at least in the case of prostatic and breast cancer, we can take certain aspects of the tumour-host relationship into consideration, in determining the type of treatment necessary in the individual patient. In the case of these tumours, reasonably reliable indices are available of three aspects of the tumour-host relationship: the pattern of the patient's hormonal environment, the activity of the tumour, and the sensitivity of the tumour to its hormonal environment.

To help in understanding the reasons for the choice of therapy, each section includes a discussion of factors which may have a bearing on the initiation and maintenance of that particular type of hormone-sensitive cancer. There will probably be noted some degree of overlap between some of the sections. This has purposely not been edited, as it permits the expression of different viewpoints in a field which has developed mainly by empiricism.

By the very nature of the volume, it makes no attempt to describe the surgical, radio-therapeutic or general management of the patient suffering from advanced malignant disease. Where it is appropriate, however, the choice is made clear between endocrine therapy on the one hand, and radiotherapy, cytotoxic therapy or 'masterly inactivity' on the other.

Acknowledgement is gratefully made to the management of Imperial Chemical Industries Ltd, Lederle Laboratories, Roche Products Ltd, Schering Chemicals Ltd, G. D. Searle and Co. Ltd, Upjohn Ltd, and W. B. Pharmaceuticals Ltd who provided financial assistance in various clinical trials mentioned in this book. I would also like to express my gratitude to the contributors, all of whom cooperated willingly in the general plan and in providing thoughtful and original reviews of their experience. Finally, my thanks and admiration go to Mr Michael Jackson, the Editor of W. B. Saunders Co. Ltd, and to Miss Mary Bramwell, for whom nothing was too much trouble in the aim of achieving the highest standards in the production of this book.

London, 1972

Basil A. Stoll

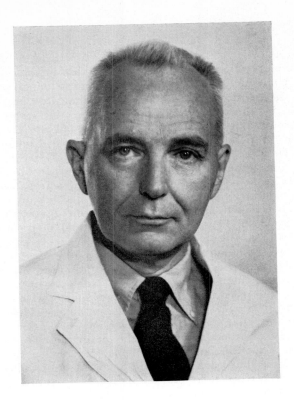

Charles Huggins

Father of the Hormonal Treatment of Human Cancer

This commemorative volume honouring Charles Huggins on the occasion of his seventieth birthday provides a further opportunity for commenting on the career of one of the truly fascinating personalities of our time. Just 10 years ago, the scientific community expressed its indebtedness to Professor Huggins for the new insight that he had brought to the cancer problem by contributing a series of papers entitled 'On Cancer and Hormones'. The surprisingly broad range of these essays bears testimony to Huggins' scientific genius and his inspiring leadership in many areas of experimental medicine.

Fortunately, several recent accounts of his scientific work have been presented by Charles Huggins himself and by his friends and colleagues on the occasion of the Lasker Award (1963), the Passano Award (1965), and the award of the Nobel Prize in Medicine or Physiology (1966), at which time the personal philosophy of the man and his career were also subjected to affectionate scrutiny.

In 1927, when Charles Huggins, fresh

from surgical training at Michigan, joined that remarkable group of founding members of the faculty of the University of Chicago School of Medicine, he seemed certainly destined for a career in clinical surgery, and he had in fact seriously but briefly considered the alternative of private surgical practice in Michigan. He was then—as he is now—young in spirit and enthusiastic, and as yet untouched by the seductive influences of scientific discovery which have engrossed his energies and have given his fertile mind little rest for nearly 45 years. Few would have predicted that Huggins was to have three outstanding careers: as a urological surgeon, as a creative scientist, and as a remarkable teacher who has left an indelible influence on so many young physicians and scientists.

It is deeply gratifying that Professor Huggins' enthusiasm and capacity for attacking scientific problems have in no way diminished with time and that each day continues to find him at his bench in the Ben May Laboratory of the University of Chicago, engaged in the business of discovery which he loves so much and which he regards as one of the most pleasant and satisfying vocations of man.

The present volume bears eloquent testimony to the far-reaching influence of Professor Huggins' discoveries on the endocrinology of cancer, yet it deals with merely one facet of his scientific career. The Nobel Prize was awarded to Huggins (jointly with Peyton Rous whom he deeply admired and revered) 'for his discoveries concerning the hormonal treatment of prostatic cancer', yet the significance of these discoveries was far broader, leading him to enunciate two new principles of medicine: '1. Cancer is not necessarily an autonomous and intrinsically self-perpetuating process, and 2. Cancer can be sustained and propagated by hormonal function which is not necessarily abnormal in kind or exaggerated in rate, but which is operating at normal or even subnormal levels.'

The remarkable first paper by Huggins and Hodges announcing the anti-androgenic treatment of human prostatic cancer, reveals clearly that these important discoveries were not a scientific longshot, but were the culmination of painstaking quantitative experimentation on the fundamentals of prostatic physiology. Moreover, in this same study Huggins demonstrated that androgens adversely influenced the disease process and thereby clarified the scientific rationale for his treatments. On this basis he stated that 'the method of proof of a proposition can sometimes be of greater interest than that which is proved'.

In addition to his monumental contributions to our understanding of prostatic cancer, four other broad fields of study have engaged Charles Huggins. In his first major scientific work in the early 1930s he observed the formation of well-developed ectopic bone when the epithelial cells of the urinary tract were transplanted to connective tissue sites. He recognised quite clearly that transitional epithelium could induce the transformation of fibroblasts into differentiated bone. This potentially extremely important discovery, which lay dormant for nearly 40 years, is currently attracting considerable scientific attention. In fact, Huggins himself has recently returned to a full-scale attack on this problem. He now finds that totally non-viable transplants of powdered, dehydrated, acid-demineralised matrix of bone and tooth are competent under certain conditions and with some species restrictions to induce self-perpetuating transformations of normal rodent fibroblasts into cartilage and bone. The nature of the chemical principles responsible for these transformations is currently Professor Huggins' consuming interest.

Pioneering studies on the biochemistry and physiology of the male urogenital tract, preparative for and concomitant with the work on human prostatic cancer, formed the scientific basis for the development of the hormonal treatment of this disease. A comprehensive series of studies on mammary cancer in man and rodents were initiated in 1951 when Professor Huggins demonstrated the remarkable beneficial effects of bilateral adrenalectomy in a substantial proportion of women with advanced metastatic carcinoma of the mammary gland. In 1956 he devised a rapid and highly reproducible method for the induction of mammary tumours that were (unlike most other rodent mammary cancers) hormonally dependent. The Huggins 7,12-dimethylbenz[a]anthracene rat mammary tumour has become an invaluable laboratory model for the study of hormone-dependent breast cancers. These studies encompassed a detailed analysis of the hormonal influences favouring growth or regression of such tumours. They also contributed considerable understanding of the process of tumour induction itself, including a most penetrating analysis of the steric and electronic features contributing to the carcinogenicity of these polycyclic hydrocarbons.

Even a cursory recounting of Professor Huggins' scientific efforts should not omit mention of his studies on serum enzyme levels which he found to be such useful indicators in the monitoring of malignant disease in man. Seeking simplified methodology, he introduced the concept and coined the term 'chromogenic substrates', for colourless compounds which on hydrolytic cleavage yielded coloured products. In searching for other means for evaluating the course of cancer in man, he was led to study the characteristics of coagulation of serum proteins, and one of the most prominent byproducts of these studies was the discovery of the sulphydryl-disulphide interchange chain reaction by Huggins and Jensen in 1948. This basic concept was subsequently to play a central role in clarifying certain oddities in the formation of the three-dimensional structure of insulin and other proteins containing cystine.

It seems only fitting to close with some few words on the scientific philosophy which has guided Charles Huggins' work and has provided insight and inspiration for so many of his students as well as his peers. We are fortunate in being able to rely not only on personal reminiscences but also on his published talk to the Markle Scholars on what Professor Huggins called 'shoptalk concerned with the craft of medical research'.

Einstein once said: 'that which is eternally incomprehensible to us in Nature is her comprehensibility', and thus he placed emphasis on the basic simplicity of the scientific principles underlying the seemingly unbelievable complex phenomena of Nature. In his own way, Charles Huggins always espoused the virtue of simplicity in the interpretation of experimental findings, and viewed complex explanations with suspicion as a possible cloak for confusion or ignorance. Although Huggins has never shunned the use of sophisticated methodology or instrumentation when necessary, much of his work has displayed the utmost simplicity in its design and economy in its execution, and has rather relied upon his extraordinary powers of observation. He has often emphasised that we are surrounded by many natural phenomena seeking to be recognised and understood. But how to experiment and to discover in the most fruitful manner requires unending practice. It is the key to success, but is an evolutionary process throughout the scientist's life. Huggins has pointed to the importance of working on noble problems which yield conceptual advances and 'influence the age by provoking activity' in others in the scientific community, always bearing in mind that medical research workers 'are the beneficiaries of the hopes and prayers of mankind for the solution of heavy problems of disease'.

At all times Charles Huggins has admonished us against the squandering of our most precious commodity—time. He has stressed the stupendous 'self-pilferage of one's time' which plagues most scientists, and has warned eloquently against the chairbound scientist engaged in administration or in needless travel, and the futility of committee work. Charles Huggins practises what he preaches, and it is a pleasure to find him at the approaching of his seventieth birthday exuberant, enthusiastic and addicted to the noble cause of medical discovery.

Paul Talalay

The Johns Hopkins University
Baltimore, USA

Contents

Section II: Breast Cancer—Endocrine Therapy

Section III: Prostatic Cancer—Endocrine Therapy

Section IV: Other Tumours—Endocrine Aspects

Section V: Prospective Considerations

Contributors

THOMAS H. ACKLAND, MD, MS, FRCS, FRACS, FACS, Clinical Instructor, University of Melbourne; Consultant Surgeon, Royal Melbourne Hospital, Australia.

H. J. G. BLOOM, MD, FRCP, FFR, FACR(Hon.), Consultant Radiotherapist, Royal Marsden Hospital, London, and Institute of Cancer Research, London, and St Peter's Group of Hospitals; Honorary Consultant Radiotherapist, St George's Hospital, St Mary Abbots Hospital, and West End Hospital for Nervous Diseases.

D. C. BODENHAM, FRCS, FRCS(Edin), Clinical Teacher in Plastic Surgery, University of Bristol; Consultant Plastic Surgeon, Frenchay and United Bristol Hospitals.

GEORGE CRILE, Jr, MD, Senior Consultant, Department of General Surgery, Cleveland Clinic, Cleveland, Ohio, U.S.A.

J. D. FERGUSSON, MD, FRCS, Director of Teaching and Research, Institute of Urology, University of London; Surgeon to the St Peter's Hospitals and Urologist to the Central Middlesex Hospital, London.

K. FOTHERBY, PhD, FRIC, Reader in Biochemistry, Royal Postgraduate Medical School, University of London.

BRENDAN HALE, DMRT, FFR, Clinical Teacher in Radiotherapy, University of Bristol; Consultant Radiotherapist, The Radiotherapy Centre, Bristol, and the Royal United Hospital, Bath.

CHARLES HUGGINS, MD, Ben May Laboratory for Cancer Research, University of Chicago; William B. Ogden, Distinguished Service Professor.

FRANCES JAMES, PhD, Research Fellow, Royal Postgraduate Medical School, University of London.

ROBERT W. KISTNER, MD, FACS, FACOG, Associate Clinical Professor, Obstetrics and Gynaecology, Harvard Medical School, Boston; Senior Gynaecologist, Boston Hospital for Women; Consultant in Gynaecology, New England Baptist Hospital, Boston, U.S.A.

J. S. MALPAS, DPhil, FRCP, Senior Lecturer in Medicine, St Bartholomew's Hospital Medical College, London; Honorary Consultant, St Bartholomew's Hospital, and Consultant Physician, St Leonard's Hospital, London.

WALTER J. MOON, MB, BS, Department of Medicine and Department of Surgery, University of Melbourne; Chairman, Consultative Clinic, Austin Hospital, Heidelberg; Consultant

Clinical Oncologist, Preston and Northcote District Hospital; Clinical Assistant, Royal Melbourne Hospital; Clinical Medical Officer, Peter MacCallum Clinic, Melbourne, Australia.

ALBERT SEGALOFF, MD, Alton Ochsner Medical Foundation, New Orleans; Professor of Clinical Medicine, Tulane University School of Medicine; Attending Physician, Ochsner Foundation Hospital; Consultant in Internal Medicine, Tulane Unit of the Charity Hospital of Louisiana, New Orleans, U.S.A.

BASIL A. STOLL, FFR, Honorary Consultant to the Radiotherapy Department, St Thomas' Hospital, and Honorary Consultant Radiotherapist, Royal Free Hospital, London; formerly Consultant to Cancer Institute of Victoria, and Honorary Consultant to the Prince Henry's Hospital, Melbourne, Australia, and Consultant to the Radium Institute, Liverpool.

PAUL TALALAY, MD, John Jacob Abel Professor, Director of the Department of Pharmacology and Experimental Therapeutics, Johns Hopkins University, Baltimore, U.S.A.

Section I

Basic Considerations

Chapter 1

Biochemistry of Steroids in Normal Subjects

K. FOTHERBY and FRANCES JAMES

In this chapter some basic facts about steroid hormone production, secretion, metabolism and mode of action are presented to provide a reference for the comparison of changes in the hormonal environment discussed in relation to carcinogenesis in Chapter 2 and the following chapters. Obviously the different aspects can only be considered briefly and for further information more detailed reviews should be consulted (see, for example, articles by Briggs and Brotherton, 1970; Hellman, Bradlow and Zumoff, 1970; Bush, 1969).

Biosynthesis of Steroids

BIOSYNTHESIS OF C-21 STEROIDS

The two major hormones produced in the adrenal cortex are cortisol and aldosterone of which the former is quantitatively the most important. Cortisol is produced in the compact cell of the zona fasciculata whereas aldosterone is formed in the zona glomerulosa.

It is now well established that cholesterol is the building block from which all of the many steroids secreted by the adrenals

3

and the gonads are derived. Furthermore, most of the cholesterol used by the adrenals for corticosteroid synthesis is obtained from that circulating in the plasma. This steroid is converted via 20α-hydroxycholesterol and 20α,22R-dihydroxycholesterol to pregneno-

Endocrine tissues contain an active enzyme, 3β-hydroxysteroid dehydrogenase, which will convert 3β-hydroxy-5-ene steroids to steroids containing the 3-oxo-4-ene structure, for example pregnenolone to progesterone.

Until the last decade progesterone was

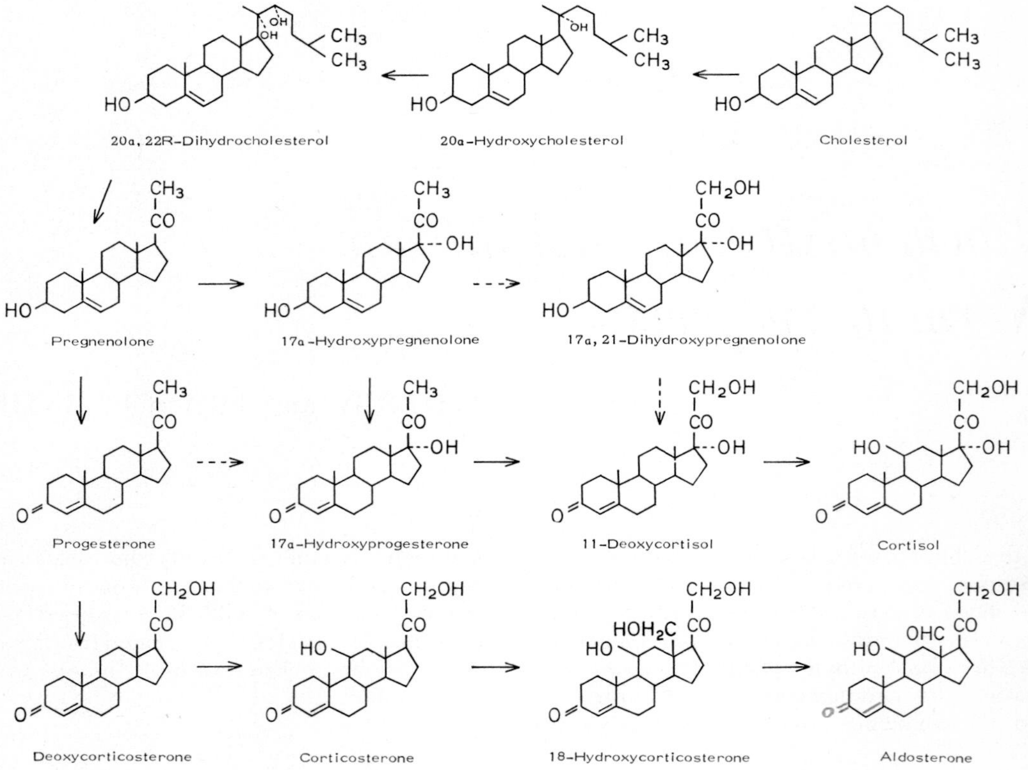

FIGURE 1.1. Biosynthesis of corticosteroids (major pathway shown in bold lines, minor pathway shown in dotted lines).

lone. It is generally assumed that this part of the pathway is of considerable importance in corticosteroid synthesis since ACTH is supposed to stimulate corticosteroid synthesis by increasing the conversion of cholesterol to pregnenolone; ACTH stimulation appears to result in increased 20α-hydroxylation of cholesterol.

The pathways for the synthesis of cortisol from cholesterol are shown in Figure 1.1.

thought to play a central role in the formation of cortisol; progesterone was thought to be formed from pregnenolone and then successively hydroxylated in a series of enzymic reactions to 17α-hydroxyprogesterone, 17α,-21-dihydroxyprogesterone and finally to cortisol by hydroxylation at the 11β-position. However, it was shown in 1961 by Mulrow and Cohn and subsequently confirmed (Mulrow, Cohn and Kuljian, 1962) that

17α-hydroxypregnenolone could be directly converted to cortisol by human adrenal tissue and it has been amply demonstrated that the human adrenal can convert pregnenolone into 17α-hydroxypregnenolone.

Thus an alternative pathway for cortisol synthesis exists which involves 17α-hydroxypregnenolone rather than progesterone as the intermediate between pregnenolone and 17α-hydroxyprogesterone. Until recently the relative importance of these two pathways has not been very clear but at the moment the evidence would suggest that the pathway involving 17α-hydroxypregnenolone is more important than that involving progesterone.

Deshpande et al (1970) perfused [³H] pregnenolone through the human adrenal gland in situ and found more radioactivity in the cortisol than in the progesterone isolated from adrenal venous blood. When [³H] 17α-hydroxypregnenolone and [¹⁴C] progesterone were perfused there was more tritium than ¹⁴C in 17α-hydroxyprogesterone and cortisol showing that 17α-hydroxypregnenolone rather than progesterone was the preferred precursor for cortisol synthesis. Only small amounts of progesterone were present in adrenocortical tissue compared to pregnenolone and cortisol.

17α-Hydroxyprogesterone may not be an obligatory intermediate in cortisol synthesis; after perfusion of [³H] 17α-hydroxypregnenolone and [¹⁴C] progesterone the ³H:¹⁴C ratio was higher in cortisol than in 17α-hydroxyprogesterone suggesting that some 17α-hydroxypregnenolone might be hydroxylated at C-21 or C-11 before oxidation of ring A to the 4-en-3-one structure. These pathways are discussed in more detail by Griffiths and Cameron (1970).

Progesterone in the adrenal cortex does appear to be important as an intermediate in the formation of corticosterone which in turn is converted via 18-hydroxycorticosterone into aldosterone. The secretion rate of cortisol (20 to 25 mg per day) is about 10 times that of corticosterone and about 100 times that of aldosterone.

BIOSYNTHESIS OF C-19 STEROIDS

The pathways for the biosynthesis of the C-19 steroids dehydroepiandrosterone, androstenedione and testosterone are shown in Figure 1.2. An enzyme, the 17,20-desmolase, is able to split off the side chain of either 17-hydroxypregnenolone or 17-hydroxyprogesterone with the formation of the C-19 steroids dehydroepiandrosterone and androstenedione respectively. These two pathways for the formation of C-19 steroids have been shown to occur both in the adrenals and the gonads but their relative importance appears to be uncertain; this topic has been discussed in detail by Eik-Nes (1970).

It would appear that the pathway from dehydroepiandrosterone to testosterone involving androstenediol is of little quantitative importance and accounts for less than 1 per cent of the testosterone secreted by the testis. In the human adrenal perfused in situ, Deshpande et al (1970) found that the major precursor of androstenedione was 17α-hydroxyprogesterone and only minor amounts were produced from dehydroepiandrosterone. In vitro and organ perfusion studies suggest that the pathways of androgen biosynthesis are qualitatively similar in the gonads and the adrenal cortex although quantitatively different, and the enzymes required to convert pregnenolone to androstenedione and testosterone are very active in the testis.

Although the adrenal is capable of forming androgens from dehydroepiandrosterone, in the adult male the plasma testosterone is derived mainly from testosterone synthesised and secreted by the interstitial cells of the testis and only a small portion is due to the peripheral conversion of precursors secreted by the adrenal cortex. However, in the female most of the testosterone and androstenedione in plasma arises from precursors secreted by the adrenal cortex; although the ovary possesses enzymes capable of converting C-21 steroids to C-19 steroids, under normal conditions the ovary appears to secrete only small amounts of androgens.

Also of importance is the secretion by the adrenal cortex of dehydroepiandrosterone

secreted in amounts up to 9 mg per day (MacDonald et al, 1965) and similar amounts of the sulphate are secreted.

The adrenal also secretes 11-oxygenated

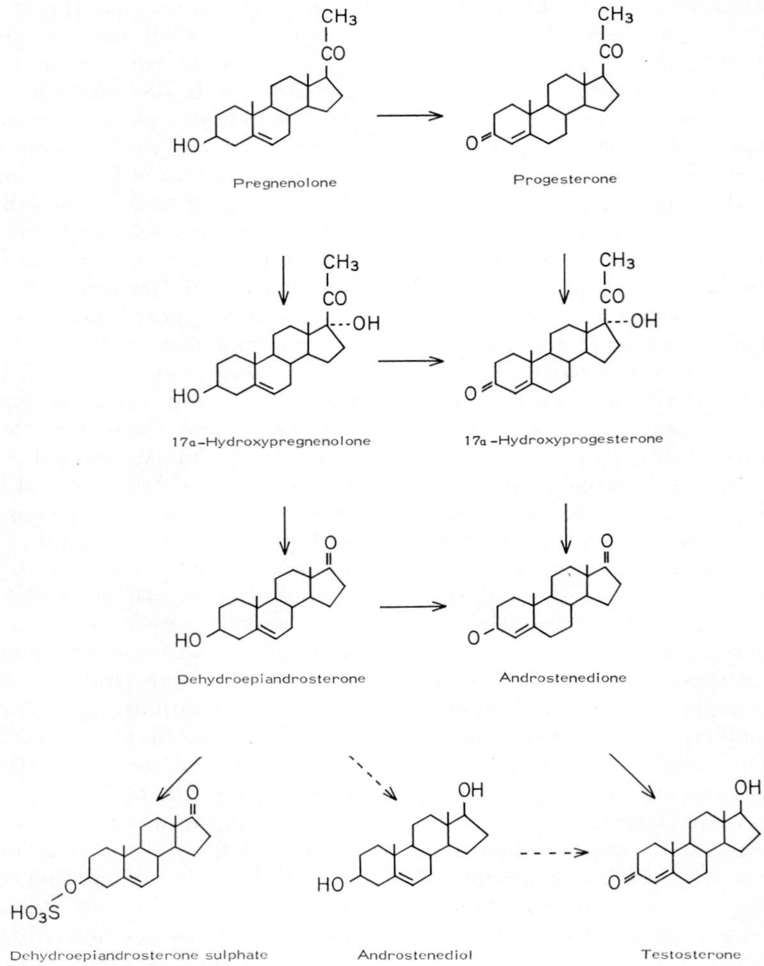

FIGURE 1.2. Biosynthesis of androgens.

sulphate which is the major precursor of the urinary 17-oxosteroids. All of the dehydro-epiandrosterone synthesised in the adrenal is produced from pregnenolone via 17α-hydroxy-pregnenolone. Dehydroepiandrosterone is

C-19 steroids, mainly 11β-hydroxyandro-stenedione, which on metabolism gives rise to the 11-oxygenated-17-oxosteroids found in urine. This steroid appears to be formed mainly from cortisol by oxidation of the side

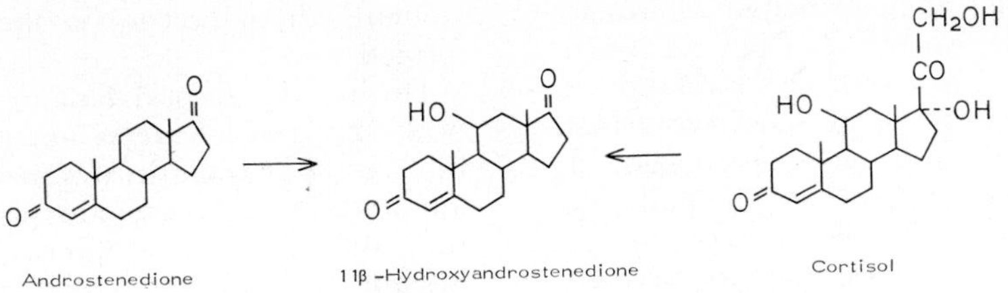

FIGURE 1.3. Biosynthesis of 11-oxygenated-17-oxosteroids.

chain and only small amounts arise by the direct 11β-hydroxylation of androstenedione (Figure 1.3).

OVARIAN STEROID BIOSYNTHESIS

The ovary produces two major types of hormone, oestrogen and progesterone, the amounts of each produced at any time being dependent on the stage of the menstrual cycle. In addition, the ovary may also produce small amounts of androgens (androstenedione) and other steroids. During the follicular phase of the cycle oestrogen biosynthesis takes place in the cells of the theca interna, although the granulosa cells may also be necessary, and involves a complex series of reactions which are illustrated in Figure 1.4.

In the follicle the pathway involving pregnenolone and 17α-hydroxypregnenolone appears to be important. Androstenedione is hydroxylated at C-19 and further enzymic reactions lead to the loss of the C-19 carbon atom; this probably occurs after oxidation of the alcohol to the aldehyde followed by the loss of formaldehyde or alternatively of formic acid. The 1β-hydrogen atom is also lost in the aromatisation process.

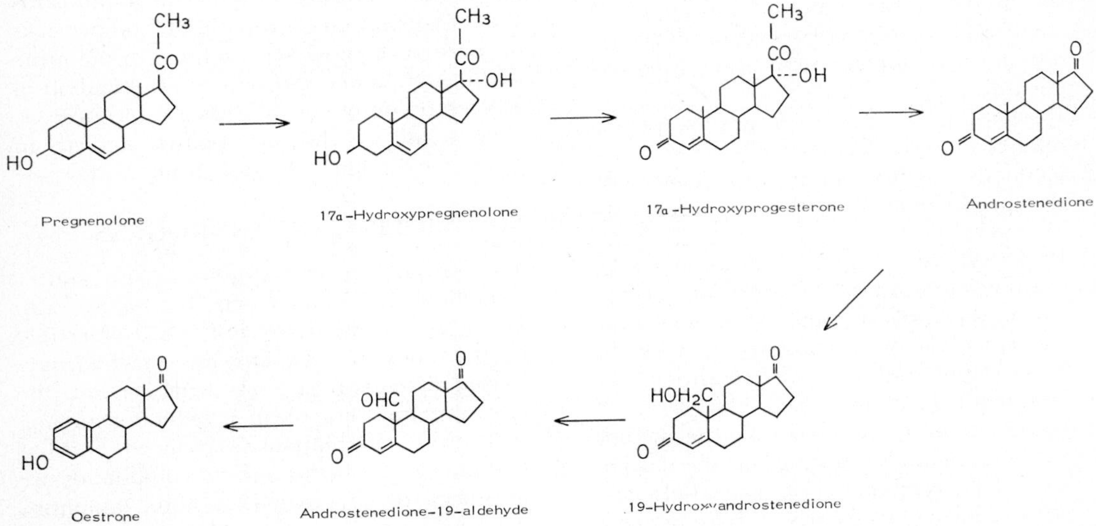

FIGURE 1.4. Biosynthesis of oestrogens.

Oestradiol is the principal hormone produced by the ovary but in plasma it is in equilibrium with oestrone, the oxidation of oestradiol to oestrone being more rapid than the reduction of oestrone to oestradiol. It should be emphasised here that the pathways involved in oestrogen biosynthesis in the ovary of the non-pregnant woman are completely different from oestrogen biosynthesis in the fetoplacental unit of the pregnant woman where oestriol is the main steroid formed.

During the second half of the menstrual cycle the ovary secretes not only oestrogens but also large quantities of progesterone. The amounts of the hormones produced at this time reflect the development of the corpus luteum (see Figure 1.12); as the corpus luteum regresses, oestrogen and progesterone secretion decreases.

Metabolism of Steroids

METABOLISM OF CORTISOL

The major pathways of cortisol metabolism are shown in Figure 1.5. Cortisol and cortisone are interconvertible by the enzyme 11β-hydroxysteroid dehydrogenase. The other changes which occur are as follows:

1. Reduction of the C-4,5 double bond in ring A, which leads mainly to the formation of 5β-reduced compounds although a small amount of 5α-reduced products are also formed, for example allotetrahydrocortisol.
2. Reduction of the 3-oxo group leading mainly to 3α-hydroxysteroids.
3. Reduction of the oxo-group at C-20 with the production of both 20α- and 20β-hydroxysteroids.
4. Hydroxylation at the C-6β position; under normal circumstances formation of 6β-hydroxycortisol accounts for less than 2 per cent of the cortisol secreted by the adrenal but under certain conditions the amounts may be increased.
5. Oxidation of the side-chain by the enzyme 17,20-desmolase resulting in the formation of 11-oxygenated-17-oxosteroids; this pathway accounts for less than 10 per cent of the cortisol secreted by the adrenal.

The 11-oxygenated 17-oxo-steroids produced are mainly of the 5β type.

As shown in Figure 1.5 the major metabolites of cortisol are tetrahydrocortisone, tetrahydrocortisol, allotetrahydrocortisol and the cortols and cortolones. Only a small amount of cortisol is excreted in the urine unchanged but this may nevertheless reflect adrenocortical function. After the administration of cortisol labelled with ^{14}C, 90 per cent or more of the dose was excreted in the urine within 48 hours showing that metabolism and excretion of cortisol was a rapid process. Nearly all of the metabolites appear in urine conjugated with glucuronic acid.

METABOLISM OF ANDROGENS

The metabolism of testosterone and androstenedione is summarised in Figure 1.6. These two compounds are interconvertible in the body by the enzyme 17β-hydroxysteroid dehydrogenase. As with cortisol, the first stage in metabolism is reduction in ring A leading to compounds reduced both at C-3 and C-5. The 5α and 5β compounds are produced in approximately equal amounts. Although some 3β-hydroxysteroids are formed, the reduction takes place mainly to

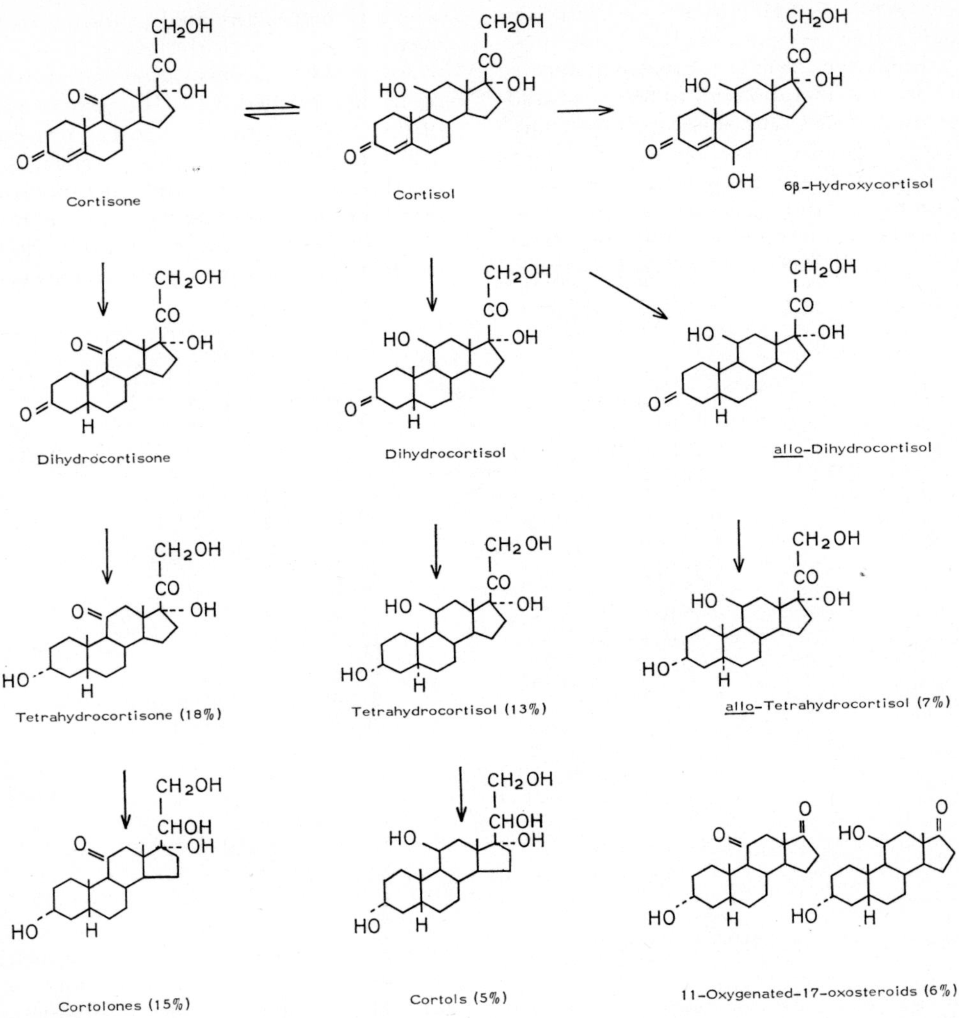

FIGURE 1.5. Metabolism of cortisol (figures in parentheses denote percentage of administered dose of cortisol recovered as urinary metabolites).

the 3α position. Some testosterone is reduced at the double bond with the formation of 5α-dihydrotestosterone which has considerable biological activity; this reaction takes place mainly in the target organs for the male sex hormone.

5α-Androstanolone (androsterone) and 5β-androstanolone (aetiocholanolone) are the major metabolites of androstenedione and testosterone. Hydroxylation of testosterone occurs at various positions and small amounts of androstenedione are reduced to epitestosterone. After the administration of testosterone labelled with ^{14}C, about 90 per cent of the dose was excreted within 48 hours. The majority of the androgen metabolites are excreted as glucuronide conjugates although some conjugates with sulphuric acid are also excreted. Dehydroepiandrosterone is also metabolised to the 5α- and 5β-androstanolones although in some subjects large amounts may be found in the urine as a sulphate conjugate. The three compounds 5α- and 5β-androstanolone and dehydroepiandrosterone, account for about 80 per cent of the total urinary 17-oxosteroids.

which is then methylated to form 2-methoxy-oestrone.

After the administration of oestrone or oestradiol labelled with ^{14}C, 50 to 80 per cent of the dose was excreted in the urine within 4 to 6 days and up to 18 per cent was found in the faeces; thus the metabolism and excretion of the oestrogens is slower than that of cortisol and the androgens probably due to the fact that enterohepatic circulation of the

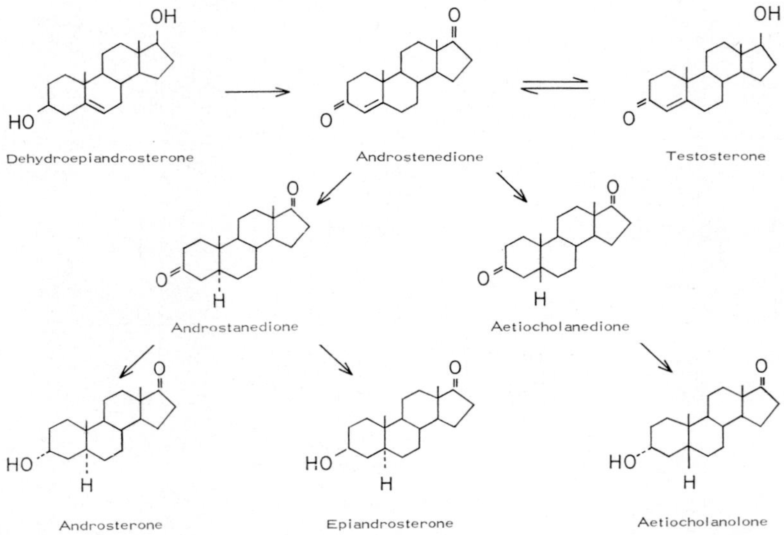

FIGURE 1.6. Metabolism of testosterone.

METABOLISM OF OESTROGENS

The metabolism of oestrogens is summarised in Figure 1.7. Although oestrone and oestradiol are interconvertible the reduction of oestrone to oestradiol appears to be less rapid than the conversion of oestradiol to oestrone and the latter probably serves as the precursor of the hydroxylated metabolites. One of the main metabolic pathways appears to be hydroxylation at C-16 leading predominantly to the production of oestriol (16α-hydroxyoestradiol). Another important pathway appears to be hydroxylation at C-2 with the formation of 2-hydroxyoestrone

oestrogens occurs. As with the androgens, the metabolites are mainly excreted as glucuronides although some sulphates occur. The amount of the dose excreted as various metabolites is shown in Figure 1.7.

METABOLISM OF PROGESTERONE

The metabolism of progesterone is shown in Figure 1.8. As with cortisol and the androgens, reduction of ring A appears to occur first with the formation mainly of the 3α-hydroxy-5β-steroid (pregnanolone). Although some pregnanolone occurs in urine, most of it is reduced to the 20α-hydroxysteroid—

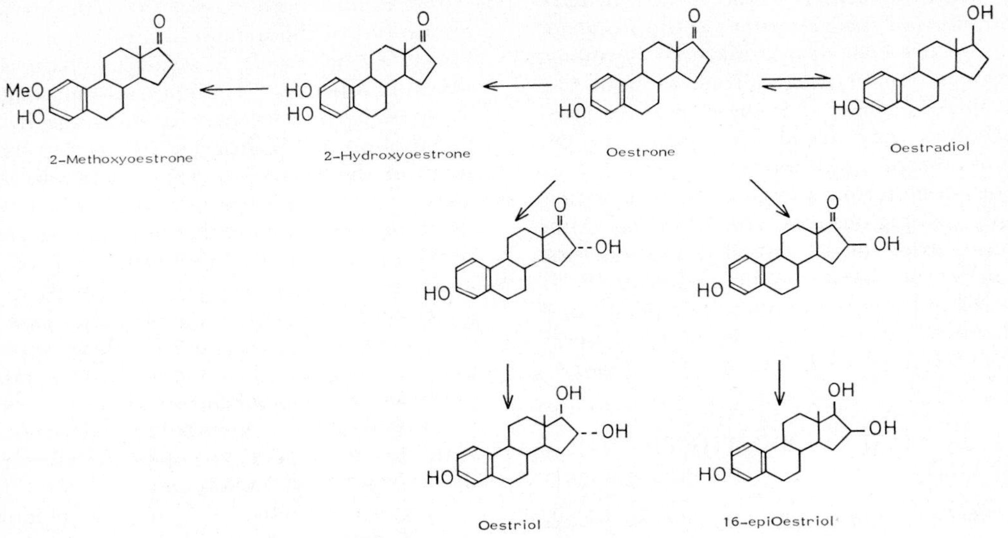
MeO
HO
2-Methoxyoestrone
HO
HO
2-Hydroxyoestrone
HO
Oestrone
OH
HO
Oestradiol
OH
HO
OH
HO
OH
OH
HO
Oestriol
OH
OH
HO
16-epiOestriol

FIGURE 1.7. Metabolism of oestrogens.

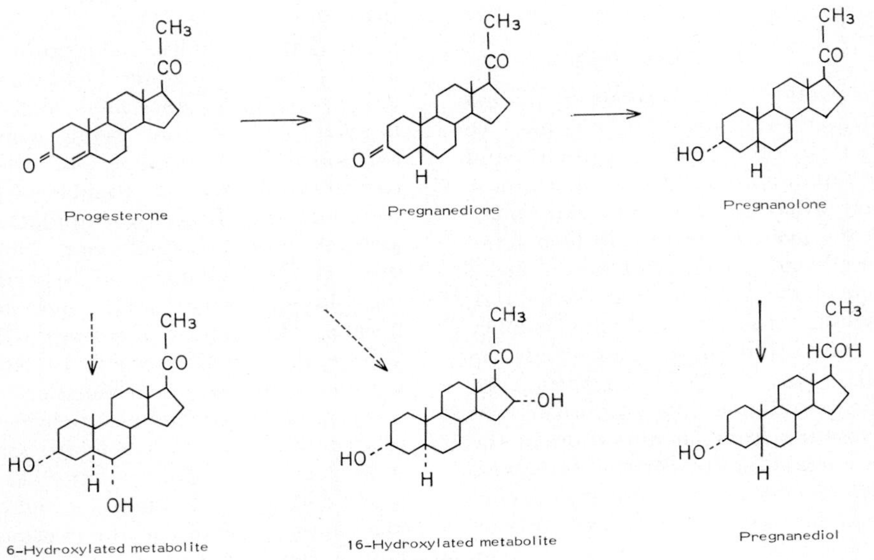
CH3
CO
O
Progesterone
CH3
CO
O
H
Pregnanedione
CH3
CO
HO
H
Pregnanolone
CH3
CO
HO
H
OH
6-Hydroxylated metabolite
CH3
CO
OH
HO
H
16-Hydroxylated metabolite
CH3
HCOH
HO
H
Pregnanediol

FIGURE 1.8. Metabolism of progesterone.

pregnanediol—which is the major urinary metabolite of progesterone accounting for up to 20 per cent of administered hormone. Hydroxylation of progesterone at both C-6 and C-16 occurs and these hydroxylated metabolites may account for about 10 per cent of administered hormone.

The progesterone metabolites in urine are mainly conjugated as glucuronides. After administration of ^{14}C-labelled progesterone about 50 per cent of the radioactivity is excreted in the urine in a five-day period and further amounts may be excreted in the faeces but this has not been extensively investigated.

METABOLISM OF SYNTHETIC STEROIDS

In general the many synthetic steroids which are used therapeutically are metabolised in a similar manner to the naturally occurring hormones. However, in many cases knowledge of the metabolism of the synthetic steroids is meagre; the available knowledge has recently been reviewed (Fotherby and James, 1972).

FACTORS AFFECTING THE METABOLISM OF STEROIDS

The concentration of a hormone in plasma and its degree of protein binding may be affected both by other body constituents and by other administered drugs. For those compounds where metabolism takes place mainly in the liver, a decrease in liver function may well lead to a decrease in the rate of metabolism of the administered compound. Zumoff et al (1967) found the urinary excretion of 17-hydroxycorticosteroids to be low in many cases of cirrhosis even though the production rate of cortisol was normal, resulting in an alteration in the peripheral metabolism of cortisol. However, in the case of oestrogens, there may sometimes be an increased urinary excretion of oestrone, oestradiol and oestriol in liver disease.

It has also been shown that considerable alterations in the metabolism of a number of hormones occurs as a result of changes in thyroid function (Hellman et al, 1970). In hypothyroidism there is a change in the metabolism of androgens which results in more of the hormones being metabolised to 5β steroids, thus causing an increase in the ratio of aetiocholanolone to androsterone; conversely, in hyperthyroidism more of the androgen precursors are metabolised to androsterone (5α-steroid). In the case of oestrogens, in hypothyroidism there appears to be a stimulation of the 16-hydroxylation pathway of metabolism so that oestriol is the major urinary metabolite; concomitant with this there is a decreased formation of the 2-oxygenated metabolites.

In hyperthyroidism the converse is found, that is an increase in the excretion of 2-oxygenated metabolites and a decrease of the 16-hydroxylated metabolites is observed. Cortisol production is increased in hyperthyroidism resulting in an increased excretion of cortisol metabolites in urine, whereas in hypothyroidism these changes are reversed. The increased cortisol secretion in hyperthyroidism results from changes in the peripheral metabolism of cortisol, since the activity of the enzyme 11β-hydroxysteroid dehydrogenase is increased and results in more of the cortisol being converted to cortisone. This decrease in the plasma cortisol level causes a stimulation of ACTH secretion and hence a stimulation of the adrenal production of more cortisol. In spite of these changes, in hyperthyroidism the plasma cortisol level tends to remain normal. The half-life of cortisol is decreased.

Several anabolic steroids are also known to affect adrenocortical function. Administration of 17α-methyltestosterone or the related compound 1-dehydro-17α-methyltestosterone (methandienone) leads to a fall in the cortisol production rate and a reduced inactivation rate of cortisol (Vermeulen and Ferin, 1962; James, Landon and Wynn, 1962). Administration of oestrogen is also known to produce widespread effects on the metabolism of cortisol as well as a number of other hormones. Oestrogen appears to act upon the production of the proteins responsible for hormone binding. After the administration of oestrogens there is an increase in the plasma level of the cortico-steroid-binding globulin which leads to an increased plasma cortisol level without an increased urinary excretion of cortisol metabolites. The half-life of cortisol in plasma is increased and there is a decrease in the metabolic clearance rate (Burke, 1970).

Administration of oestrogen also increases the excretion of 6β-hydroxycortisol without increasing the adrenal secretion rate of cortisol; phenobarbital administration has a similar effect (Burstein et al, 1967). It is now known that a large number of hydroxylation reactions occurring in the body, including many of those involved in metabolism of the steroid hormones, are mediated by NADPH-dependent enzymes in liver microsomes, the reaction being catalysed by cytochrome P 450 (for a review of these alterations see Conney, 1967). The activity of these enzymes can be stimulated by a variety of different compounds including phenylbutazone and triparanol as well as phenobarbital. The metabolism of testosterone via hydroxylation pathways can also be stimulated by phenobarbital treatment. This stimulation of the metabolism of hormones may lead to a decrease in the biological effect they are able to produce.

Age also has an effect on steroid metabolism, both cortisol and testosterone production declining with age. However, plasma levels of the steroids remain approximately constant until very late in life, suggesting that there are changes in the metabolism of the hormones. Changes in hormone excretion also occur in obesity. The cortisol secretion rate and urinary excretion of total 17-oxogenic steroids are increased in obesity but when the values are related to body weight the difference between normal and obese subjects is not significant. Similarly, obese subjects not only excrete more oestrogens than non-obese ones but excrete a larger proportion of their oestradiol production as oestriol and a smaller proportion as oestrone (Brown and Strong, 1965). The correlation of these changes in steroid production and excretion with body mass may also partly account for the decline in steroid production with age.

The effect of a number of factors on the metabolism of the synthetic steroids and the effect of these latter compounds on endogenously produced steroids has been reviewed by Fotherby and James (1971).

Steroids in Blood and Urine and their Estimation

STEROIDS IN BLOOD

Most of the steroids in blood are transported attached to proteins. About 5 per cent of cortisol is present in blood in the free state and appears to be the fraction responsible for the biological activity of the hormone, the remainder being associated with a specific binding protein (transcortin, corticosteroid-binding globulin). Cortisol levels in plasma show a diurnal variation with a peak of about 15 to 20 μg/100 ml between 6 a.m. and 9 a.m. falling to less than 8 μg/100 ml at midnight. The plasma half-life of cortisol is between 80 and 100 minutes. The half-life of some of the synthetic corticosteroids is longer and some of these appear to bind with the corticosteroid binding globulin to a much less extent than cortisol.

Only about 3 per cent of progesterone appears to be in an unbound state in plasma, the majority being bound either to albumin, to an α-glycoprotein or to the corticosteroid-binding globulin. Progesterone is turned over rapidly and its half-life is less than 20 min. During the follicular phase of the menstrual cycle, the progesterone concentration in plasma is less than 1 ng/ml; after ovulation, with the development of the corpus luteum the values increase to reach a peak of between 10 to 20 ng/ml on days 22 to 24 of the cycle when, if fertilisation does not occur, the levels begin to decrease reflecting the regression of the corpus luteum (see Figure 1.12).

About 95 per cent of the oestrogens in plasma, of which some are present as glucuronide and sulphate conjugates, are protein bound. The free oestrogens in plasma appear to have half-lives of 20 min and 70 min. The oestrogen concentration (oestrone plus oestradiol) in plasma rises from about 100 pg/ml during the early follicular phase to a peak of about 500 pg/ml at mid cycle. A second peak, reaching levels of about 300 pg/ml occurs during luteal phase (see Figure 1.12). The ratio of oestradiol to oestrone also varies during the menstrual cycle being smaller during the early follicular phase (1:1) than at the mid-cycle peak (2:1). In postmenopausal women the oestrogen concentration is about 50 pg/ml.

The androgens present a more complicated picture. The half-life of testosterone in plasma is about 20 minutes and about 2 per cent circulates in blood in the free state, the remainder being bound either to albumin, to the corticosteroid-binding globulin or to a β-globulin specific for binding testosterone. The levels of testosterone in plasma range from 0·2 to 1·7 μg/100 ml for males and 0·05 to 0·1 μg/100 ml for females. Although the production of testosterone decreases with

age, plasma levels of testosterone do not decline until very late in life.

Small amounts of androstenedione are also present in plasma but this steroid binds only weakly to the plasma globulins. In contrast to testosterone the concentration of androstenedione is lower in male plasma (less than 0·1 μg/100 ml) than in female plasma (0·1 to 0·3 μg/100 ml). However, the amounts of other 17-oxosteroids in plasma are much larger. The two major 17-oxo-steroids in plasma are dehydroepiandro-sterone and androsterone; they are present mainly as sulphates and bound to albumin. Whereas dehydroepiandrosterone levels in males (70 to 170 μg/100 ml) are higher than in females (40 to 140 μg), the levels of androsterone show no sex difference (10 to 60 μg/100 ml). These values are compared by Sommerville and Collins (1970). Andro-stenedione, and to a much lesser extent dehydroepiandrosterone, are important in females since they contribute to the greater part (60 per cent) of the blood production rate of testosterone although in males they make a negligible contribution.

The androgenic hormones in blood are also important in that they act as precursors of oestrogens. Many previous studies have shown that administration of testosterone and related steroids leads to an increased urinary excretion of oestrogens. It is possible that these conversions take place only in the liver so that the oestrogens thus produced would not necessarily contribute to the plasma levels of oestrogen. However, the work of MacDonald, Rombaut and Siiteri (1967) and Longcope, Kato and Horton (1969) has shown that the circulating androgens do give rise to circulating oestrogens. Although only a small proportion of the androgens are converted (about 1 per cent of androstenedi-one and less than 0·5 per cent of testosterone), the conversion accounts for a large proportion of the circulating oestrogens; in males about half of the plasma oestradiol arises from testosterone but in females, where the level of testosterone is much lower than in males, the contribution is insignificant. In both sexes at least 20 to 30 per cent of the blood oestrone is derived from androstenedione. Although oestrogens derived from circulating androgens may be of minor quantitative importance compared to the ovarian production of oestrogens in premenopausal women, they are of considerable importance in castrated or postmenopausal women where, as in males, the major amount of circulating oestrogen arises from conversion of blood androgens.

The peripheral conversion of androgens of adrenocortical and testicular origin makes it uncertain how much, if any, oestrogen is produced and secreted directly by the adrenal cortex and testes. Oestrogens have been detected in both of these tissues, which are known from in vitro studies to be capable of synthesising oestrogens and the recent work of Baird, Uno and Melby (1969) would suggest that small amounts of oestrone are secreted by the adrenal.

ESTIMATION OF STEROIDS IN PLASMA

For details regarding the limitations and advantages of methods for estimating the individual groups of steroids the monographs by Loraine and Bell (1971) and Gray and Bacharach (1967) should be consulted. There is little doubt at the moment that competitive protein-binding assays (saturation analysis) offer a simple and sensitive method for the estimation of many of those steroids which will either combine with a specific binding protein or will affect the binding of another steroid to such a binding protein. Thus cortisol, testosterone and progesterone can readily be estimated in blood using the binding proteins present in plasma, and the oestrogens can be measured either by utilising the plasma proteins or the cytosol fraction prepared from the uteri of rabbits. Competitive protein-binding methods have been discussed in detail by Murphy (1967) and also at a recent symposium (Diczfalusy, 1970). Estimation of cortisol

by such a technique is relatively rapid and the binding assay can be carried out on a methylene dichloride extract of plasma.

Similarly, simple methods have been described for the estimation of progesterone and testosterone. Although the simple methods for these two hormones are satisfactory for most clinical purposes, if specific estimates of the two hormones are required, then a chromatographic separation is necessary to separate the hormone from other substances present in the plasma extract which are likely to interfere in the reaction.

Another technique which is now coming into widespread use is the radio-immunoassay of steroids; in these methods the steroid to be measured is bound to a protein and an antibody raised to the protein-bound steroid in animals to which it is injected. This procedure is analagous to the estimation of protein hormones by radioimmunoassay and the relevant literature has been reviewed by Caldwell (1971).

Another technique which has been widely used for estimating steroids in blood because of its sensitivity and specificity is gas-liquid chromatography. In addition to measuring the hormones themselves by this technique, one can also measure many of the metabolites which might be present in blood. Thus it offers wider scope than methods based upon protein binding. Numerous methods involving gas-liquid chromatography have been devised and monographs such as those by Eik-Nes and Horning (1968), Grant (1967) or Lipsett (1965) should be consulted for details.

Since the level of cortisol in plasma is very much higher than that of the other hormones, other techniques can be used for the estimation of this hormone. Two of these have found widespread use in clinical laboratories:

1. Estimation by fluorimetry (Mattingly, 1962): cortisol and some similar steroids fluoresce when shaken with ethanolic sulphuric acid and the intensity of fluorescence produced with a methylene

chloride extract of plasma shows a correlation with the plasma cortisol level.

2. The Porter–Silber colour reaction: an extract of plasma is allowed to react with phenylhydrazine in sulphuric acid when steroids such as cortisol, containing the dihydroxyacetone side-chain, give rise to a yellow colour.

ESTIMATION OF STEROIDS IN URINE

Most of the methods referred to above (for example, competitive protein binding assay,

and hence are not measured. Only about 25 per cent of the cortisol metabolites are measured by this reaction.

A much better and more widely used method is that devised by Norymberski (see Gray et al, 1969), to overcome the instability of the corticosteroid glucuronides present in urine when they are hydrolysed by acid prior to extraction. In this method sodium borohydride is added to the urine to reduce those steroids containing an oxo group at C-20 to the C-20 hydroxysteroid, and at the same time the 17-oxosteroids in urine are reduced to 17β-hydroxysteroids.

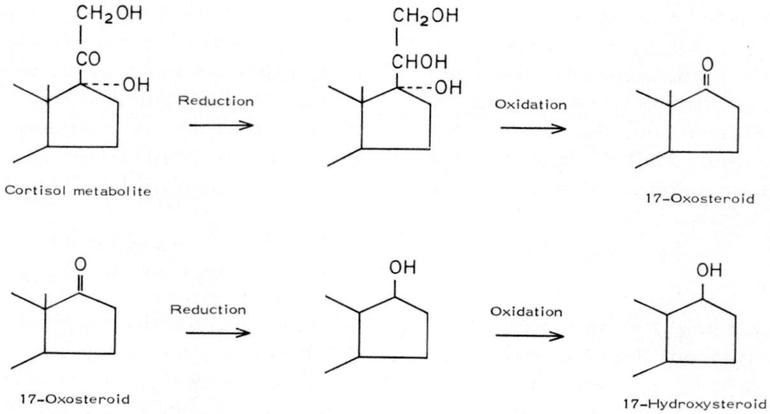

FIGURE 1.9. Estimation of 17-oxogenic steroids.

radioimmunoassay and methods involving gas-liquid chromatography) for the estimation of steroids in blood have also been applied to the estimation of steroids in urine.

In spite of the small amount of cortisol present in urine, its estimation provides a good index of adrenocortical function (see Burke, 1970) and shows a good correlation with the estimates of total 17-oxogenic steroids. Although in the past the Porter–Silber reaction has been used for estimating corticosteroid metabolites in urine, it suffers from the disadvantages that it is very susceptible to interference from non-steroidal substances and many of the cortisol metabolites do not retain the dihydroxyacetone side-chain

The urine is then oxidised with an oxidising agent, either sodium bismuthate or sodium metaperiodate which is specific for the oxidation of glycols so that the reduced corticosteroid metabolites are oxidised to 17-oxosteroids (see Figure 1.9) and can be estimated by the Zimmermann colour reaction. The 17β-hydroxysteroids produced by reduction of the 17-oxosteroids originally present in urine are not oxidised and therefore do not interfere in the estimation. Values for the normal excretion of 17-oxogenic steroids by males and females are shown in Figure 1.10; it can be seen that excretion reaches a peak in the late twenties and then declines steadily.

Similar changes with age also occur in respect of total 17-oxosteroid excretion. Although the total 17-oxosteroids are relatively easy to determine in urine, the estimation provides information which is of very little value since it measures both 11-oxygenated and 11-deoxy-17-oxosteroids, the former arising from the metabolism of cortisol or from 11β-hydroxyandrostenedione secreted by the adrenal whereas the latter arise from precursors secreted by either the gonads or the adrenals.

simple column chromatographic technique (Goldzieher and Axelrod, 1962; Fotherby, Selwood and Burn, 1970). The range of normal values for the 11-deoxysteroids in urine is wide but typical values would be androsterone 0·5 to 3·7 mg/24 h, aetiocholanolone 0·7 to 3·5 mg/24 h and dehydroepiandrosterone 0·2 to 4·2 mg/24 h. The values tend to be lower in females than in male subjects.

The estimation of oestrogens in urine, particularly in urine from non-pregnant subjects, is a more difficult problem. The

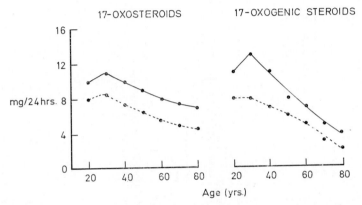

FIGURE 1.10. Some mean values for the excretion of 17-oxosteroids and total 17-oxogenic steroids by males and females at various ages.

Excretion of total 17-oxosteroids does not appear to be affected by ovariectomy or the menopause. More information is obtained by estimating the individual 17-oxosteroids; the estimation of two in particular (androsterone and aetiocholanolone) has assumed some importance in the investigation of patients with cancer (see Chapter 2). Various procedures have been described for fractionating the 17-oxosteroids in urine. These depend upon either a chromatographic separation of the individual steroids by paper (Brooks, 1958), thin-layer (Chambers, Reis Valle and Fotherby, 1967) or gas-liquid chromatography (Thomas and Bulbrook, 1964) or in some procedures the 11-deoxysteroids or androsterone and aetiocholanolone are estimated together by a

quantity of oestrogen present is small and the amount of interfering material large. The 'standard' method in use is that devised by Brown (Brown, 1955; Brown, Bulbrook and Greenwood, 1957). The sensitivity, however, of this method as originally described was such that at levels below 5 μg of each oestrogen per 24-hour urine sample, the loss of specificity was sufficient to throw considerable doubt on the validity of the results obtained.

This raised considerable difficulties in estimating the oestrogen production in women, for example, with breast cancer since these women were usually either post-menopausal or ovariectomised and values obtained were consequently at or below the limit of sensitivity of the method. Values obtained during the menstrual cycle are shown in Figure 1.11; values for total oestrogens (the sum of oestrone, oestradiol and oestriol) for postmenopausal women and men were 2·5 to 14 μg/24 h and 7 to 19 μg/24 h respectively.

levels of oestrogen excretion although in the near future the method may be superseded by radioimmunoassay procedures. The values obtained by the fluorimetric method agree fairly well with those of the previous method. The number of metabolites of the oestrogens

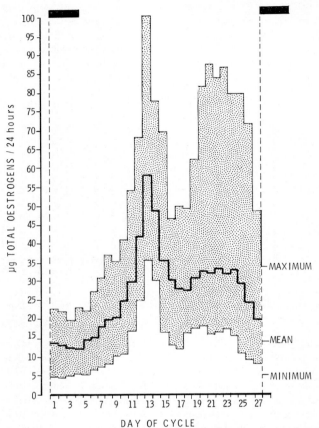

FIGURE 1.11. Mean, maximum and minimum levels of total oestrogen excretion during the menstrual cycle. ▬ = menstruation. (From Brown, 1960, Advances in Clinical Chemistry, **3**, pp. 157–233, by permission of the Academic Press.)

A less laborious method for the estimation of oestrogens in urine is one recently described by Brown et al (1968) which estimates by fluorimetry total oestrogens (oestrone, oestradiol, oestriol and other minor oestrogens but not 2-hydroxy or 2-methoxy oestrogens) in urine. At present this method would be the one of choice for the investigation of low

in urine is very large and no method capable of measuring all of them is available that can be applied to a large number of samples.

HORMONE PRODUCTION RATES

Under normal circumstances the blood level of a hormone is a satisfactory indicator of the exposure of the tissues to the hormone.

TABLE 1.1. *Values for the production rate of steroids*

Steroid		Production rate	
Cortisol		8–25	mg/day
Aldosterone		70–300	μg/day
Dehydroepiandrosterone		6–17	mg/day
Dehydroepiandrosterone sulphate		7–23	mg/day
Testosterone:	males	6–7	mg/day
	females	0·2–0·5	mg/day
Androstenedione:	males	1·4—3	mg/day
	females	2·5–3·5	mg/day
Oestrogens	females luteal phase	0·3–0·6	mg/day
	ovulatory peak	0·6–1·5	mg/day
	postmenopausal women	50–280	μg/day
	males	100–300	μg/day
Progesterone:	luteal phase	up to 30 mg/day	

The concentration in blood will depend on the production rate of the hormone and the rate of removal of the hormone from the circulation either by distribution throughout the body tissues or by metabolism and excretion. The production rate is the amount of hormone secreted by the endocrine gland in a given time (the hormone secretion rate) plus the amount produced as a result of conversion from circulating precursors. The hormone production rate will equal the secretion rate in those cases where none of the circulating hormone is derived from circulating precursors. The blood concentration (c) is proportional to the production rate (PR) and the two are related by the following equation:

$$PR = MCR \, (c)$$

where MCR is metabolic clearance rate, the volume of plasma from which the steroid is 'cleared' in unit time. For a more detailed discussion of the determination of hormone production rates, the articles by Hellman et al (1970) and Gurpide and Gandy (1971) should be consulted.

Determination of the production rate is the only way of knowing the absolute amount of hormone produced within a given period, but this type of determination cannot be considered suitable as a routine procedure since it also involves the administration of a radioactive steroid, it is often technically complicated, and furthermore the interpretation of the results may be difficult. Even determination of the production rate only gives an approximate idea of the amount of hormone available to the target tissues. Table 1.1 shows values for the production rate of various steroid hormones.

Control of Steroid Secretion

It has long been recognised that the level of activity of the steroid-producing tissues depends on an interplay of the secretion of the tissue with that of the hypophysis and the hypothalamus. Possibly the simplest case is the control of cortisol secretion. An increase in the plasma cortisol level leads to a decreased secretion of ACTH from the pituitary and

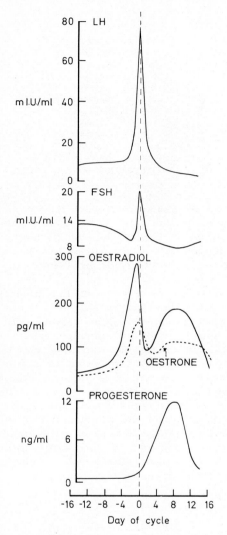

FIGURE 1.12. Plasma levels of gonadotrophins and ovarian steroids during a menstrual cycle. (Day 0 is the day on which the level of luteinising hormone reaches a peak.)

hence a reduced stimulus to the adrenal cortex. The effect on the pituitary is brought about by cortisol acting on the hypothalamus

producing an inhibition of corticotrophin-releasing factor from the median eminence and hence a decreased secretion of ACTH from the pituitary. Connections to the hypothalamus make it possible for impulses from the other higher centres of the brain to modify the activity of the pituitary-adrenal axis. The above pathways for the regulation of adrenal activity have become known as the 'long-feedback' mechanism.

In addition, a 'short-feedback' mechanism may also be involved; the levels of ACTH itself in blood may also act on receptors in the median eminence and hence affect the secretion of corticotrophin-releasing factor. The investigation of pituitary-adrenal function is considered at length in the monograph of James and Landon (1968). There is still considerable uncertainty about what controls the secretion of androgens by the adrenal. Although the secretion of these compounds is increased by ACTH adminis-tration, it has been suggested (Mills, 1968) that they may also be controlled by an addi-tional pituitary hormone.

Similar long and short feedback mechan-isms have been proposed for the regulation of steroid production in the ovary by gona-dotrophin, although in this case the picture is complicated by the fact that there is an interplay of two gonadotrophic hormones, follicle-stimulating hormone (FSH) and luteinising hormone (LH, interstitial cell stimulating hormone). Levels of FSH in blood are high at the beginning of the menstrual cycle but during the follicular phase show a decrease which is ascribed to the increasing concentration in plasma of oestrogens from the developing follicle. At about mid-cycle there is a sharp burst of secretion of LH and also of FSH, both poss-ibly in response to the increased oestrogen concentration in plasma (see Figure 1.12). After the mid-cycle peak, levels of both LH and FSH are low during the luteal phase. These interrelationships are considered in detail by Ross et al (1970).

It is not clear at present what controls

either the development of the corpus luteum and its secretion of oestrogens and progesterone, or the regression of the corpus luteum if fertilisation of the ovum does not occur. Although there is evidence for the presence in some animal species of a uterine factor, luteolysin, which causes the corpus luteum to regress there is no evidence that a similar substance exists in the human uterus. In the male, FSH stimulates spermatogenesis and LH is necessary for the development and maintenance of function of the Leydig cells which under LH stimulation secrete testosterone.

Mechanism of Action of Steroid Hormones

After administration of the sex hormones one of the earliest detectable biochemical events occurring in the cells of the target organs is the stimulation of the production of nuclear RNA and RNA polymerase activity which in turn is followed by protein synthesis. Following the definition of Roberts and Szego, the target organs could be defined as those tissues which are acutely responsive under normal conditions to a particular hormone.

It has been postulated that the hormone reacts with a receptor (most likely protein) in the target tissue in some manner which elicits the tissue's response. Experimental support of this concept has been provided by the demonstration of a specific uptake of certain hormones by the target tissues but not by the tissues in general. One of the most clearly defined examples of this is the uptake of oestradiol by the uterus and vagina of the rat reported by Jensen and Jacobson (1962). In these studies the uterus took up more of a dose of tritiated oestradiol and retained it for a longer period of time than other tissues investigated.

Breast tissue also behaves as a target organ for oestradiol and similar studies have been performed with labelled testosterone and the rat ventral prostate. The amount of hormone taken up by the target tissues and hence necessary for producing a biological effect, is very small (approximately 0·1 per cent of an administered dose of hormone). These studies have been extended by various investigators and specific oestrogen or androgen-binding proteins have been isolated from homogenates of uteri or ventral prostate respectively.

It has also been assumed that similar tissues in human subjects also contain specific receptors which interact with the steroid hormones in a similar manner, but further evidence for their existence in humans is desirable. If they do exist they would obviously be of great importance in regulating cell metabolism and might also be involved in either the induction or the suppression of malignant changes. The hormone appears to interact initially with the protein receptor in the cytoplasm of the cell and the steroid-protein complex is transported to the nucleus and initiates the chain of biochemical events.

Although the hypothesis put forward is an attractive one, further evidence is needed to show that the specific oestrogen or androgen-binding proteins in the target tissues have a function beyond that of acting as a transport mechanism for the passage of the hormone from the intercellular fluid to the cell nucleus. The retention of the steroid hormones by the nucleus of the cell and interaction with nuclear chromatin of the target cells is circumstantial evidence in favour of the view that the steroid hormones and their receptors act directly on the gene surface to regulate RNA synthesis. The interaction of the sex hormones with target tissues has been reviewed by James and Fotherby (1970) and this article should be consulted for further information.

References

Baird, D. T., Uno, A. & Melby, J. C. (1969) Adrenal secretion of androgens and oestrogens. *Journal of Endocrinology*, **45**, 135–136.

Briggs, M. H. & Brotherton, J. (1970) *Steroid Biochemistry and Pharmacology*. London: Academic Press.

Brooks, R. V. (1958) A method for the quantitative fractionation of urinary 17-oxo steroids. *Biochemical Journal*, **68**, 50–57.

Brown, J. B. (1955) A chemical method for the determination of oestriol, oestrone and oestradiol in human urine. *Biochemical Journal*, **60**, 185–193.

Brown, J. B., Bulbrook, R. D. & Greenwood, F. C. (1957) An additional purification step for a method for estimating oestriol, oestrone and oestradiol in human urine. *Journal of Endocrinology*, **16**, 49–56.

Brown, J. B., MacLeod, S. C., Macnaughtan, C., Smith, M. A. & Smyth, B. (1968) A rapid method for estimating oestrogens in urine using a semi-automatic extractor. *Journal of Endocrinology*, **42**, 5–15.

Brown, J. B. and Strong, J. A. (1965) The effect of nutritional status and thyroid function on the metabolism of oestradiol. *Journal of Endocrinology*, **32**, 107–115.

Burke, C. W. (1970) Effect of oral contraceptives on cortisol metabolism. *Journal of Clinical Pathology*, **23**, Suppl. 3, 11–18.

Burstein, S., Kimball, H. L., Klaiber, E. L. & Gut, M. (1967) Metabolism of 2α and 6β-hydroxy-cortisol in man: Determination of production rates of 6β-hydroxycortisol with and without phenobarbital administration. *Journal of Clinical Endocrinology*, **27**, 491–499.

Bush, I. E. (1969) Determination of oestrogens, androgens, progesterone and related steroids in plasma and urine. *Advances in Clinical Chemistry*, **12**, 57–139.

Caldwell, B. V. (1971) Antibodies to steroids. *Bibliography of Reproduction*, **17**, 1–5.

Chambers, R., Reis Valle, A. dos & Fotherby, K. (1967) Method for the estimation of 11-deoxy-17-oxosteroids in urine. *Clinica chimica acta*, **17**, 135–137.

Conney, A. H. (1967) Pharmacological implications of microsomal enzyme induction. *Pharmacological Reviews*, **19**, 317–366.

Deshpande, N., Jensen, V., Carson, P., Bulbrook, R. D. & Doouss, T. W. (1970) Adrenal function in breast cancer; biogenesis of androgens and cortisol by the human adrenal gland *in vivo*. *Journal of Endocrinology*, **47**, 231–242.

Diczfalusy, E. (1970) Steroid Assay by Protein Binding. *Acta endocrinologica*. (København), Suppl. 147.

Eik-Nes, K. B. (1970) *The Androgens of the Testis*. New York: Marcel Dekker.

Eik-Nes, K. B. and Horning, E. C. (1968) *Gas Phase Chromatography of Steroids*. Berlin: Springer.

Fotherby, K. & James, F. (1972) Metabolism of synthetic steroids. *Advances in Steroid Biochemistry*, **3**. In press.

Fotherby, K., Sellwood, R. A. & Burn, J. I. (1970) Urinary steroid excretion in patients with advanced breast cancer. *British Journal of Surgery*, **57**, 859.

Goldzieher, J. W. & Axelrod, L. R. (1962) A study of methods for the determination of total, grouped and individual urinary 17-ketosteroids. *Journal of Clinical Endocrinology*, **22**, 1234–1241.

Grant, J. K. (1967) *Gas Liquid Chromatography of Steroids*. Mem. Soc. Endocr., No. 16. Cambridge: University Press.

Gray, C. H. & Bacharach, A. L. (1967) *Hormones in Blood*. New York: Academic Press.

Gray, C. H., Baron, D. N., Brooks, R. V. & James, V. H. T. (1969) A critical appraisal of a method of estimating urinary 17-oxosteroids and total 17-oxygenic steroids. *Lancet*, **4**, 124–127.

Griffiths, K. & Cameron, E. H. D. (1970) Steroid biosynthetic pathways in the human adrenal. *Advances in Steroid Biochemistry*, **2**, 223–265.

Gurpide, E. & Gandy, H. M. (1971) Dynamics of hormone production and metabolism. In *Endocrinology of Pregnancy* (ed. Fuchs, F. & Klopper, A.). New York: Harper & Row.

Hellman, L., Bradlow, H. L. & Zumoff, B. (1970) Recent advances in human steroid metabolism. *Advances in Clinical Chemistry*, **13**, 1–35.

James, F. & Fotherby, K. (1970) Interaction of sex hormones with target tissues. *Advances in Steroid Biochemistry*, **2**, 315–372.

James, V. H. T. & Landon, J. (1968) *The Investigation of Hypothalamic-Pituitary-Adrenal Function*. Memoirs of the Society of Endocrinology, No. 17, Cambridge: University Press.

James, V. H. T., Landon, J. & Wynn, V. (1962) Effect of an anabolic steroid (methandienone) on the metabolism of cortisol in the human. *Journal of Endocrinology*, **25**, 211–220.

Jensen, E. V. & Jacobson, H. I. (1962) Basic guides to the mechanism of estrogen action. *Recent Progress in Hormone Research*, **18**, 387–414.

Lipsett, M. B. (1965) *Gas Chromatography of Steroids in Biological Fluids*. New York: Plenum Press.

Longcope, C., Kato, T. & Horton, R. (1969) Conversion of blood androgens to estrogens in normal adult men and women. *Journal of Clinical Investigation*, **48**, 2191–2201.

Loraine, J. A. & Bell, E. T. (1971) *Hormone Assays and Their Clinical Application*. Edinburgh: Livingstone.

MacDonald, P. C., Chapdelaine, A., Gonzalez, O., Gurpide, E., Van de Wiele, R. L. & Lieberman, S. (1965) Studies on the secretion and interconversion of the androgens. *Journal of Clinical Endocrinology*, **25**, 1557–1568.

MacDonald, P. C., Rombaut, R. P. & Siiteri, P. K. (1967) Plasma precursors of estrogens. I. Extent of conversion of plasma Δ^4-androstenedione to estrone in normal males and nonpregnant normal, castrate and adrenalectomized females. *Journal of Clinical Endocrinology*, **27**, 1103–1111.

Mattingly, D. (1962) A simple fluorimetric method for the estimation of free 11-hydroxycorticoids in human plasma. *Journal of Clinical Pathology*, **15**, 374–379.

Mills, I. H. (1968) The control of the adrenal precursors of 17-oxosteroids. In *The Investigation of Hypothalamic-Pituitary-Adrenal-Function*. Memoirs of the Society of Endocrinology, No. 17, 83–101.

Mulrow, P. J. & Cohn, G. L. (1961) Corticosteroid release and synthesis *in vitro* by adrenal slices from patients with Cushing's Syndrome. *Journal of Clinical Investigation*, **40**, 1250–1262.

Mulrow, P. J., Cohn, G. L. & Kuljian, A. (1962) Conversion of 17-hydroxypregnenolone to cortisol by normal and hyperplastic human adrenal slices. *Journal of Clinical Investigation*, **41**, 1584–1590.

Murphy, B. E. P. (1967) Some studies of the protein-binding of steroids. *Journal of Clinical Endocrinology*, **27**, 973–990.

Ross, G. T., Cargille, C. M., Lipsett, M. B., Rayford, P. L., Marshall, J. R., Strott, C. A. & Rodbard, D. (1970) Pituitary and gonadal hormones in women during spontaneous and induced ovulatory cycles. *Recent Progress in Hormone Research*, **26**, 1–62.

Sommerville, I. F. & Collins, W. P. (1970) Indices of androgen production in women. *Advances in Steroid Biochemistry*, **2**, 267–314.

Thomas, B. S. & Bulbrook, R. D. (1964) In *Androgens*, p. 49, ed. Vermeulen, A. Amsterdam: Excerpta Medica.

Vermeulen, A. & Ferin, J. (1962) The influence of 17α-methyl-19-nortestosterone on the metabolism of cortisol. *Acta endocrinologica (København)*, **39**, 22–31.

Zumoff, B., Bradlow, H. L., Gallagher, T. F. & Hellman, L. (1967) Cortisol metabolism in cirrhosis. *Journal of Clinical Investigation*, **46**, 1735–1743.

Chapter 2

Biochemistry of Steroids in Subjects with Cancer

K. FOTHERBY and FRANCES JAMES

From their investigation of the effect of orchiectomy in patients with prostatic carcinoma, Huggins and Hodges (1941) suggested that some cancers in man might be hormone dependent. At about the same time, Lipschutz and his colleagues (Lipschutz, Murillo and Vargas, 1939; Lipschutz and Maas, 1944) showed that progesterone administration could cause regression of oestrogen-induced uterine fibroids in guinea pigs. These studies, following the pioneer work of Beatson, gave rise to the concept that many tumours, particularly those of tissues which were subject to direct hormonal stimulation, might not only be dependent on particular hormones for their continued growth but might also regress on administration of various hormones or compounds related to them.

Although in general the rationale for ablation of endocrine tissue or administration of steroids is not clear and the results often disappointing, the concepts have stimulated a large number of investigations aimed at either distinguishing differences in hormonal production and interaction between normal subjects and those with cancer, or attempting to determine which patients are likely to respond to a particular form of therapy. This chapter summarises the results of many of these investigations, mainly as applied to cancer in humans.

Breast Cancer

STEROID HORMONE PRODUCTION IN SUBJECTS WITH BREAST CANCER

DISCRIMINANT RATIOS

During the past decade a considerable amount of energy has been devoted to studying the excretion of urinary total 17-oxogenic steroids and 11-deoxy-17-oxo-steroids (particularly aetiocholanolone), and their relationship either to the treatment or prognosis of patients with breast cancer. This subject has been extensively reviewed (see Bulbrook, 1970; Forrest and Kunkler, 1968; Bulbrook and Strong, 1958). Much of this work stems from the early report of Allen, Hayward and Merivale (1957) which was subsequently examined in greater detail by Bulbrook, Hayward and their colleagues.

Their first report (Bulbrook, Greenwood and Hayward, 1960) showed that by measuring the urinary excretion of aetiocholanolone and 17-oxogenic steroids (17-OGS), it was possible to derive a 'discriminant function' calculated from the formula

$$80–80 \ [17–OGS \ mg/24h] + aetiocholanolone \ (\mu g/24h)$$

which gave a better distinction between those patients with advanced breast cancer likely to respond to treatment by hypophysectomy or adrenalectomy and those less likely to respond, than did either the measurement of total 17-oxogenic steroids or aetiocholanolone excretion separately.

Out of a total of 59 patients studied, 14 had an objective remission of whom 13 had a positive value for the discriminant function; of 27 patients who failed to respond to treatment 21 had negative discriminants. The 6 patients in the latter group, where the discriminant function did not give a good prediction, had all been treated by adrenalectomy, and the authors suggested therefore

that the discriminant function might be more useful for predicting the response to hypophysectomy than to adrenalectomy. Eighteen patients were classified as an intermediate group in their response; of these patients 6 had positive and 12 had negative discriminants.

The same correlations were apparent if the 'mean clinical value' assessed at three months after operation was used as the index of response, rather than objective remission alone. Thus women with advanced breast cancer who failed to respond to treatment by adrenalectomy or hypophysectomy excreted smaller amounts of 11-deoxy-17-oxosteroids in their urine than patients who responded to treatment; in a further publication it was shown that these values were significantly lower than those excreted by normal women.

Comparison of steroid excretion by different patients is complicated by the marked decrease in the excretion of 17-oxosteroids (including aetiocholanolone and androsterone) and 17-oxogenic steroids which occurs with increasing age in both normal subjects and patients with cancer. Bulbrook et al (1962a) found that the correlation of steroid excretion with age in the patients who responded to treatment was similar to that observed in normal women, whereas the excretion of these steroids by unresponsive patients did not show a significant correlation with age. Because of these changes in steroid excretion with age, the discriminant function also correlated with age and the value falls as age increases; so much, in fact, that the value of the discriminant as a prognostic tool in general loses its validity when patients reach their early sixties.

In a study of 30 patients with early breast cancer, Bulbrook et al (1962b) collected urine samples either just prior to or after mastectomy. About two thirds of the women excreted subnormal amounts of 11-deoxy-17-oxosteroids and had negative discriminants. It was found that the incidence of recurrence and the death rate at either 12 months or 36 months was less in patients who had a positive discriminant at mastectomy than in those who had a negative discriminant.

It seemed probable therefore on this basis that the clinical course of the disease was highly correlated with some aspects of steroid production. Patients with negative discriminants may have a relatively rapid recurrence of the disease after mastectomy, and cannot usefully be treated by endocrine ablation. These earlier results were confirmed in a subsequent publication and the survival of the two groups of patients compared. Eight years after mastectomy three times more patients had died in the group with a negative discriminant than in that with a positive one.

In view of the relationship of the discriminant to the course of the disease both in early and advanced breast cancer, it was thought possible that the changes in steroid excretion might precede the clinical appearance of the disease. In order to test this hypothesis a prospective study was set up and urine was collected from about 5000 women in Guernsey (Bulbrook, 1970). To date 21 of these women have developed breast cancer. It was claimed that the majority of these 21 women showed deviations from the normal in their excretion of 17-oxogenic steroids and 11-deoxy-17-oxosteroids. This abnormality in steroid excretion has been termed a 'multi-directional' one, since some women showed a high excretion of both groups of steroids, some a low excretion of both and some high of one and low of the other. However, it is clear from the figure published by Bulbrook and colleagues that *almost half* of those patients developing breast cancer excreted amounts of steroids which were well within the limits excreted by normal subjects.

Sisters of the women in this trial who developed breast cancer also tended to show abnormalities in their steroid excretion pattern, a finding which is of interest in view of the fact that sisters of women with breast cancer have an increased incidence of the disease.

Since determination of the discriminant function involving the specific estimation of aetiocholanolone is a laborious procedure, a number of groups of investigators have shown that estimations either of the 11-deoxy-17-oxosteroids, or of androsterone and aetiocholanolone together, provide a simpler and satisfactory alternative. When the values obtained from this type of estimation are expressed as a ratio with the total urinary 17-oxogenic steroids, the figures obtained for the ratio show a good correlation with values for the discriminant function.

Support in various degrees and of varying kinds for the findings of Bulbrook and his colleagues has come from the work of a number of other groups. Juret (1968) studied 121 patients treated by implantation of yttrium-90 into the pituitary and found that objective remission was significantly higher in those patients in whom the excretion of androsterone and aetiocholanolone was greatest, with a remission rate of about 50 per cent in patients who had a combined steroid excretion greater than 1·2 mg/day. When the values for steroid excretion were considered in relation to the free interval, a better prognostic value was obtained than with either of the indices separately. Surprisingly, Juret also claims that the blood cholesterol level had a prognostic value in these patients.

Gutierrez and Williams (1968) studied only *eight* premenopausal women who had undergone mastectomy for breast cancer and claimed that their excretion of a number of steroids—androsterone, aetiocholanolone, 11-hydroxy-aetiocholanolone and 11-oxo-aetiocholanolone—was significantly lower than that of 10 women of comparable age who had not developed breast cancer.

Kumaoka et al (1968) found a significant difference in urinary 17-oxosteroid excretion between responsive and unresponsive cases. In addition, the excretion of aetiocholanolone, androsterone and dehydroepiandrosterone in patients of various ages who responded to treatment was similar to that found in healthy subjects, whereas the excretion of steroids in young unresponsive cases was lower and resembled the excretion seen in older healthy subjects. Furthermore, the urinary excretion of total 17-oxosteroids by patients with advanced cancer before adrenalectomy was correlated with the length of survival after adrenalectomy. Those patients excreting more than 4 mg per day of urinary 17-oxosteroids showed a median survival of 23 months, while that of subjects excreting less than 4 mg per day was less than 10 months. The value of 4 mg per day for urinary total 17-oxo-steroid excretion would discriminate about 85 per cent of responsive cases from un-responsive ones. These authors found that their methods were not satisfactory for patients over 50 years of age.

Marmorston et al (1965a) found that premenopausal patients with breast cancer excreted significantly lower levels of andro-sterone, aetiocholanolone and 11-oxy-17-oxosteroids than patients with benign breast disease, sick control or well control patients. Urinary excretion of the same steroids by similar groups of postmenopausal patients did not show significant differences. The number of patients in each group was small and the conclusions must be accepted tenta-tively.

Wilson and Moore (1968) used a different discriminant factor which involved measuring the increase in the excretion of 17-hydroxy-corticosteroids and 17-oxosteroids produced in response to ACTH; the value of this dis-criminant was significantly different in those patients who responded to adrenalectomy and those who did not. The predictive value of the discriminant factor was increased by taking the free interval into consideration.

Fotherby, Sellwood and Burn (1970) studied 110 patients with advanced breast cancer. Although there was a significant difference in the incidence of response to treatment between patients with a positive and negative discriminant factor calculated according to Bulbrook's formula, a better distinction was obtained by using the ratio of total 17-oxogenic steroids to 11-deoxy-17-oxosteroids measured by a simple column chromatographic procedure. The lower this ratio (that is the higher the 11-deoxy-17-oxosteroid excretion) the greater the likeli-hood of a favourable response to treatment. Of 47 patients with a ratio greater than nine, only 6 responded to treatment compared to 24 of 63 patients with a ratio less than nine. There was also a significant difference in the survival curve for the two groups of patients. The percentage survival for the group with a ratio of less than nine was significantly higher than that of the patients with a ratio greater than nine.

SIGNIFICANCE OF DISCRIMINANT RATIOS

These claims regarding the discriminant have not, however, been substantiated by all investigators. In early studies no correlation was found between the steroid excretion pattern in the pretreatment stage and the response of the patients to treatment (Hob-kirk and Forrest, 1957; Plantin et al, 1958). Schweppe, Jungman and Lewin (1967) measured the urinary excretion of 17-oxosteroids, oestrogens and pregnanediol in normal postmenopausal subjects and in patients with mammary carcinoma and found the steroid excretion to vary widely between individuals. There were no signi-ficant differences between steroid excretion in the two groups under basal conditions nor after ACTH stimulation or dexamethasone suppression.

Wade et al (1969) found no significant difference in the discriminant value between normal women, women with early breast cancer and women who did not have breast cancer but were admitted to hospital for other operations. They found a lower propor-tion of negative discriminants in their early breast cancer cases than was found by

Bulbrook, and they conclude that the discriminant may not be specifically affected in any way in early breast cancer. The value of the discriminant was not affected by operation; a finding in agreement with that of Ahlquist et al (1968) and Fotherby et al (1971) who found the value for the ratio to be constant over a period of time which included admission to hospital and operation.

Ahlquist et al (1968) also found only a small proportion of patients with early breast cancer to have a negative discriminant and concluded that the discriminant gave no useful prognostic indication with regard to individual patients either for early breast cancer cases treated by surgery or radiotherapy, or in late cases treated by radiotherapy, hormone therapy or chemotherapy.

The relationship of the discriminant function to the prediction of response in breast cancer and its use in identifying patients at risk from this disease has been dealt with in some detail, but without disparaging the importance of the work of Bulbrook, Hayward and their colleagues (which represents a major advance in this field), it should be stated that the widely held view of its usefulness appears to be an exaggerated one.

There can be no doubt that the findings of the three subsequent investigations (Wade et al, 1969; Ahlquist et al, 1968; Fotherby et al, 1970, 1971), involving a sufficient number of patients and based on methodology showing a close correlation with that used by workers at the Imperial Cancer Research Fund, indicates that the accuracy of prediction of response to treatment by the use of the discriminant function is not as good as was indicated by the highly encouraging first reports. A substantial proportion of patients with negative discriminants can be expected to have a favourable response to treatment. Similarly, although the results of the Guernsey prospective trial are claimed to show that the deviation in steroid excretion is a 'multi-directional' one, the results are not as convincing at the moment as one would like them to be.

A number of groups have now suggested that the degree of discrimination between responsive and unresponsive patients can be improved by taking into account clinical factors such as the free interval, menopausal status of the patient and stage of the disease (Armitage, McPherson and Copas, 1969). An interesting extension of the work of Bulbrook and his colleagues has been reported by Gleave (1969) who measured the excretion of 17-oxogenic steroids and 11-deoxy-17-oxosteroids by 63 patients with benign disease of the breast, 30 patients with primary breast cancer and 64 with advanced breast cancer and compared the values with those obtained from 21 control subjects. Although there was no significant difference between the various groups in the excretion of 17-oxogenic steroids, the excretion of aetiocholanolone was significantly lower in the advanced cases than in the other three groups studied.

The lower level of excretion of aetiocholanolone in the group of patients with advanced disease was caused primarily by a sub-group with advanced local disease in which the excretion was particularly low; in patients with advanced general disease the level of aetiocholanolone was not significantly different from that of the control subjects. There was also a correlation with the prognosis since the patients with advanced local disease showed a lower proportion of remissions from treatment and a shorter survival compared with the patients with generalised disease.

Because of the above facts a few investigations have been carried out to ascertain what factors might affect the value of the discriminant function. Undoubtedly age is one of the important factors. From the early reports of Bulbrook and colleagues it was obvious that for the majority of patients the discriminant begins to lose its predictive value once the patient was about 60. Miller and Durant (1969) found that in patients aged 50 years or more, negative discriminants occurred with equal frequency in the normal women and those with breast cancer.

The suggestion that negative discriminants should be expected in women with advanced breast cancer because of the associated debility causing a rise in 17-oxogenic steroid excretion has not been substantiated. Miller and Durant (1969) found the majority of negative discriminants were due to a fall in androgen excretion rather than to an increase in 17-oxogenic steroids. Many of the responsive patients who appear to be critically ill have a normal pattern of steroid excretion and many patients at the early stage of the disease have a subnormal excretion of 11-deoxy-17-oxosteroids and a negative discriminant.

These findings are supported by the investigations of Werk, MacGee and Sholiton (1964) who found that the ratio of 6β-hydroxycortisol to 17-hydroxycorticosteroids (measured by the Porter–Silber reaction) in urine was greater than one in patients with advanced cancer whereas this ratio was elevated to a much lesser degree in other patients in the terminal stages of severe illness. Miller and Durant also found that liver disease with jaundice was usually associated with a negative discriminant, again due mainly to decreased androgen excretion. Surgical stress itself did not alter the discriminant.

Sneddon, Steel and Strong (1968) found that the discriminant function was not altered in obese subjects but that changes occurred in patients with thyroid dysfunction. Whereas the 17-oxogenic steroid excretion was increased in hyperthyroidism and there was an increase also in the ratio of androsterone to aetiocholanolone in urine, the value for the discriminant was reduced; in hypothyroidism 17-oxogenic steroid excretion was lower than normal, the androsterone to aetiocholanolone ratio was much reduced, but the discriminant was still lower than in normal subjects. They also found that 20 subjects with early breast cancer had a significantly lower discriminant than 20 normal subjects.

It is likely that a large number of patients included in the trials will be taking various drugs and these may well affect values obtained for the discriminant. Women taking oral contraceptives excreted smaller amounts of 17-oxogenic steroids and androsterone and aetiocholanolone in urine than women not using them. The 11-deoxy-17-oxosteroids tended to show a slightly larger decrease than the 17-oxogenic steroids and this would most likely lead to a more negative value for the discriminant (Bulbrook and Hayward, 1969).

ANDROGEN AND CORTICOSTEROID PRODUCTION

The excretion in urine of a metabolite of dehydroepiandrosterone, androst-5-ene-3β, 16α, 17β-triol, was found by Adams and Wong (1968) to be increased in patients with breast cancer or benign breast disease. When values for the excretion of this steroid were expressed as a ratio to dehydroepiandrosterone excretion, there was a significant difference in the values for the ratio from control subjects. These investigators also found that an ovariectomised adrenalectomised woman with carcinoma of the breast excreted dehydroepiandrosterone, 16α-hydroxydehydroepiandrosterone and 16-oxo-androstenediol in the urine. The amounts of all of these steroids in urine were increased after the infusion of dehydroepiandrosterone sulphate and it was suggested that these compounds were formed from dehydroepiandrosterone sulphate by breast tumour tissue.

It is unlikely, however, that breast tumour tissue is responsible for the metabolism of *all* the dehydroepiandrosterone to these compounds since it is known that 16α-hydroxylation of dehydroepiandrosterone in vivo can be carried out in liver tissue (Fotherby et al, 1957). The finding that tumour tissue is capable of synthesising and metabolising steroids is of obvious importance and may help to explain the excretion of steroids in the urine of ovariectomised adrenalectomised patients as well as the increased excretion of oestrogens in ovariec-tomised adrenalectomised women after the administration of androgens. The role of the liver in these transformations is likely to be far more important than that of the tumour tissue and it is unlikely that tumour produc-tion of steroids or metabolism of circulating steroids will account for the abnormal pattern of steroids found in urine.

From the finding that measurements of urinary 11-deoxy-17-oxosteroids and 17-oxogenic steroids might be of use in the investigation of patients with breast cancer, it was a logical step to see whether measure-ments of cortisol and some of the androgenic hormones in plasma might not be more suitable. This, however, has not proved to be the case.

The production rate of cortisol appears to be higher in patients with advanced breast cancer than it is in either healthy subjects or in patients with early breast cancer and this leads to an increased level of 17-hydroxy-corticosteroids in plasma. Deshpande et al (1969) found that in some patients different values for the production rate were obtained depending upon which urinary metabolite was used in the calculation of this value, and they suggest that there may be other pre-cursors secreted by the adrenal which give rise to urinary compounds measured as metabolites of cortisol. There appeared to be no correlation between the cortisol production rate and the urinary total 17-oxogenic steroid excretion.

The levels of total plasma 11-deoxy-17-oxosteroids (dehydroepiandrosterone and androsterone) did not show any significant differences between normal women and women with either early or advanced breast cancer, although the levels in the patients with cancer tended to be low. Again, when dehydroepiandrosterone sulphate and andro-sterone sulphate were measured separately in plasma there was no difference between normal women and women with early or advanced disease. There does, however, appear to be a correlation between the plasma levels of dehydroepiandrosterone sulphate and androsterone sulphate and the ratio in urine of 11-deoxy-17-oxosteroids to 17-oxogenic steroids. The relevance of plasma androgens in breast cancer has been reviewed by Wang (1969) but it is obvious that much more work is required before the plasma levels of these various androgenic steroids can be related to the course of the disease.

A number of other aspects of plasma steroids have been investigated but none appear to show significant differences. Plasma levels of unconjugated dehydroepiandro-sterone, aetiocholanolone and androsterone were extremely low and there was no dif-ference between the values found in women with benign breast disease and those with early or advanced breast cancer. The meta-bolic clearance rate of dehydroepiandro-sterone appears to be the same in normal women and in those with breast cancer; and there does not appear to be any dif-ference between normal women, women with benign breast disease and patients with either early or advanced breast cancer in the binding by plasma of a number of other steroids including cortisol, oestradiol, oestriol dehydroepiandrosterone, androsterone, aetio-cholanolone, testosterone, androstenedione, progesterone and the sulphates of dehydro-epiandrosterone and androsterone.

OESTROGEN PRODUCTION

Since it has been assumed for a long time that there is a relationship between oestrogen production and either the cause or the course of breast cancer, much effort has been expended in trying to determine this rela-tionship, but with little success. Much of the early work has been reviewed by Brown (1960), Bulbrook and Strong (1958) and Bulbrook (1970). The failure to find a rela-tionship may partly be due to technical difficulties in the measurement of oestrogens. In the premenopausal subject, oestrogen excretion shows wide and cyclical variations. In the postmenopausal, ovariectomised or adrenalectomised subject, oestrogen excretion is at the lower limit of sensitivity of most methods in use. In addition, it must be born in mind that the excretion of the three classical oestrogens, oestrone, oestradiol and oestriol, represents only a small part, less than 20 per cent of the total oestrogen production.

Oestrogen excretion has been variously reported to be low, normal or high and there appears to be no correlation with the response to various types of treatment. There does, however, appear to be a substantial amount of evidence suggesting that oestriol excretion is raised. Brown (1960) administered small doses of oestradiol to postmenopausal patients with cancer of the breast and to control subjects. The mean percentage of the dose recovered in the urine as oestrone, oestradiol and oestriol was the same in the two groups but the subjects with cancer excreted a higher proportion of the total as oestriol, suggesting there was a change in the metabolism of oestradiol. However, this change does not appear to be specific to breast cancer for it is also seen in other conditions.

Similar investigations have been carried out by Crowley et al (1965) using [4-14C] oestradiol; this steroid was administered to 38 postmenopausal women with advanced breast cancer prior to endocrine therapy and to five postmenopausal women with benign mammary dysplasia. These workers suggested that some of the postmenopausal women with advanced cancer converted oestradiol more rapidly to oestrone and then to oestrial. In this respect there was no difference between those patients who responded to treatment and those who did not. Most authors are agreed that measurement of oestrogens in urine is unhelpful in predicting the response of a patient to treatment.

Lemon et al (1966) expressed their values for the excretion of the three oestrogens by means of the following ratio:

oestriol (μg/24 h)/oestrone + oestradiol (μg/24 h).

This ratio was lower in patients with breast cancer than in normal controls and no change occurred in this ratio at the menopause. They observed no remissions in 12 patients whose ratio remained unchanged or decreased, while objective remissions were observed in patients whose ratio rose towards or exceeded one during therapy. However, since these changes could only be observed after therapy was started they were of little value in predicting the response to treatment.

Barlow, Emerson and Saxena (1969) showed that the postmenopausal ovary made no contribution to oestrogen production. Oestradiol production rates were determined prior to, and on the fifth day after, bilateral ovariectomy in both premenopausal and postmenopausal patients stimulated with ACTH to achieve comparable levels of adrenocortical activity. Although a marked reduction in the oestradiol production rate occurred in premenopausal patients after ovariectomy, no change occurred in the postmenopausal subjects.

Gallagher et al (1966) found that there were changes in oestrogen metabolism in men with breast cancer. They studied oestrogen metabolism in five men with this condition. Compared with normal men, the men with breast cancer produced smaller amounts of 2-hydroxyoestrone and 2-methoxyoestrone from administered radioactive oestradiol; oestrone production was only about half that of normal males but an increased amount of oestriol was produced. In one subject with breast cancer it was found that orchiectomy caused no change in the pattern of oestrogen metabolism. In a control series of older men who had cancer unrelated to the endocrine system, the excretion of 2-hydroxyoestrone and 2-methoxyoestrone after administration of labelled oestradiol was similar to that in normal subjects and thus was higher than in men with breast cancer.

UPTAKE AND METABOLISM OF STEROIDS BY BREAST TUMOUR TISSUE

The uptake of steroids, particularly oestrogens, by breast tumour tissue has been studied with a view to determining whether or not the local concentration of a hormone is related in any way to the responsiveness of the tumour to endocrine therapy. This aspect has received particular attention recently in view of the demonstration (see Chapter 1) that target tissues for the sex hormones, including breast tissue, have the ability specifically to take up oestrogen from the circulation. Since the chemical methods available are not sufficiently sensitive for the measurement of the minute amounts of steroids in most tissues, all investigators interested in such determinations have in fact measured the relative amounts of radioactivity in various tissues after administration of radioactively labelled compounds.

The earliest study was carried out by Folca et al (1961) who injected tritiated hexoestrol intravenously 6 hours prior to mastectomy into 10 patients with breast cancer. They found that in four patients who subsequently responded to adrenalectomy, the ratio of radioactivity in the tumour relative to that in plasma was much higher than the muscle to plasma ratio, whereas in the six subjects who failed to respond the ratios were similar. The authors suggested therefore that determination of the relative oestradiol concentrations in tumour tissue might prove useful in predicting the response of a patient to adrenalectomy.

Although this suggestion has not been substantiated, subsequent studies have confirmed that human breast tumour tissue may contain a higher concentration of radioactivity after the administration of labelled oestradiol (but not of oestrone) than is found in other tissues studied which have included adipose tissue, muscle, normal breast tissue (in so far as a breast which contains a carcinoma may contain normal tissue) and plasma. This appears to be so whether the steroid is injected intravenously (Demetriou et al, 1964; Deshpande, 1967) or given by a constant intravenous infusion over a period of time in order to achieve steady state conditions (Pearlman et al,

1969; Braunsberg, Irvine and James, 1967; Braunsberg et al, 1970).

Braunsberg and colleagues administered tritiated oestradiol to 14 patients with tumours of other tissues or with non-malignant growths in the breast. Further patients with breast cancer were treated either with testosterone or drostanolone propionate. Normal breast tissue and other normal tissue studied (with the exception of liver) did not concentrate oestrogen. A number of the breast tumours concentrated oestrogen but none of the other tumours studied (including tumours of the colon, rectum, stomach, bladder and ovary) nor non-malignant tissues from the breast (fibroadenomas, cysts, lymphoadenomas) did so.

There was no correlation between the ability of the tumour to concentrate oestrogen and the stage of the disease. The uptake of oestrogen by the breast tumour was not influenced by previous treatment with testosterone propionate or drostanolone propionate. This finding is in contrast to that of Deshpande (1967) who reported that drostanolone propionate when injected 100 to 300 minutes before operation, reduced the amount of oestradiol taken up by the tumour but had no effect on the uptake of labelled oestradiol by normal mammary tissue.

Although androgens will cause a regression of the disease in a number of cases of mammary carcinoma there is no evidence at the moment that either human breast tumours or dimethylbenzanthracene-induced tumours in rats specifically take up and retain either testosterone or 17α-methyltestosterone in vivo (for details see James and Fotherby, 1970). Nor do human tumours appear to show a specific uptake of progesterone.

Because of the difficulties of carrying out hormone uptake experiments in vivo, the feasibility of performing the measurements on tumour tissue removed at operation and incubated in vitro has been investigated. In rats dimethylbenzanthracene-induced mammary tumours, which were subsequently shown to be hormone responsive, concentrated oestradiol to a greater extent than did un-responsive tumours on incubation in vitro (Mobbs, 1966; Sander and Attramadal, 1968). Administration of progesterone did not affect the uptake of oestradiol by breast tumours in animals, which is of interest since adminis-tration of progesterone increases the inci-dence and growth rate of mammary tumours induced by dimethylbenzanthracene.

Tumour tissue from humans has also been investigated in vitro to see whether any dif-ference could be found between responsive and non-responsive tumours. The uptake of [3H] oestradiol by breast tumour slices in vitro was found to be very variable (Sander, 1968; Johansson, Terenius and Thoren, 1970; James et al, 1971) and there appears to be no correlation between hormone up-take and histological classification of the tumours. However, the number of patients which have been investigated by these techniques so far are too few to evaluate the usefulness of this type of study in predicting the response of patients to treatment.

Until fairly recently it was thought that the metabolism of steroids took place mainly, if not only, in the liver. Although the con-version of steroids by peripheral tissues is now recognised, the importance of these conversions relative to that in the liver is still not known. However, even though the con-version of a steroid in tissues other than liver may represent metabolism of only a small fraction of the total amount of steroid available for metabolism, it could be im-portant in that it might provide a sufficient local concentration of an active metabolite to influence biochemical reactions in that tissue. Such metabolites might be detected only with difficulty by examination of blood or urine specimens.

The metabolism of steroids by malignant tissues has been studied, both with a view to determining the rate of inactivation of compounds which are used therapeutically and also to see whether the tissue is capable of converting one steroid to another which might affect the carcinogenic process. Although

breast tumour tissue appears specifically to take up oestradiol, it appears to have little ability to metabolise this steroid; the predominant steroid found in tumour tissue after administration of labelled oestradiol in vivo was the administered steroid itself.

An interesting finding by Adams and Wong (1969) was that human breast tissue contains all the enzymes capable of converting chole-sterol to pregnenolone, progesterone, 17α-hydroxyprogesterone, then to dehydroepi-androsterone, androstenedione, testosterone and finally to oestriol. Oestriol appears to be formed by the 16α-hydroxylation of testo-sterone or androstenedione. This is the first report of the occurrence of enzymes capable of carrying out these conversions in tissues other than those of the endocrine organs.

In addition, breast carcinoma tissue con-tains not only steroid sulphatase activity but also steroid sulphokinases. These enzymes are capable of sulphating steroids with the formation of steroid sulphates which may act as intermediates in some of the trans-formations described. However, some of the results obtained by Adams and Wong have been criticised. Jones et al (1970) incubated human breast tumour tissue with a number of steroid substrates and confirmed the occur-rence of many of the reactions described above, for example hydrolysis of dehydro-epiandrosterone sulphate, and conversion of dehydroepiandrosterone to androstene-dione and testosterone; 16α-hydroxylating activity was not as great as that found by Adams and Wong. There was also no evi-dence for oestriol formation but oestrone may have been present when adrostenedione was used as substrate.

Testosterone was converted into 5α-di-hydrotestosterone in large yields and this steroid was also isolated when dehydro-epiandrosterone sulphate or androstenedione were perfused in vivo through breast tumours at mastectomy. This reaction has also been demonstrated in rat mammary tumour tissues and 5α-dihydrotestosterone will inhibit the growth of the oestrogen-dependent rat mammary fibroadenoma.

Forchielli et al (1967) also showed that testosterone could be metabolised to androstenedione and 5α-dihydrotestosterone and, although there was a wide variation in activity between various samples of tissue, tumour tissue tended to be more active in metabolism of testosterone than was normal tissue obtained from the same patient. Human breast tumour tissue will also metabolise cortisol and corticosterone (Haley, Dimick and Williamson, 1966) and again tumour tissue may be more active than normal tissue.

Dao (1969) has shown that breast tumour tissue, normal mammary tissue, normal liver tissue and liver metastases contain enzyme systems that are capable of forming sulphate conjugates of various steroids when these steroids are incubated with the tissue homogenate. The ability of the tissue to sulphate steroids varied with the different steroid substrates. It was also claimed that the sulphating activity of the tumour was related to the response of the patient to adrenalectomy; patients in whom the sulphokinase activity in respect of dehydroepiandrosterone relative to that of oestradiol was greater than one tended to respond to adrenalectomy whereas those in which this ratio was less than one did not respond. This interesting finding obviously needs further investigation.

Prostatic Cancer

STEROID HORMONE PRODUCTION IN PATIENTS WITH PROSTATIC CANCER

Although the prostate is known to be under androgenic control, the role of androgens in the aetiology of carcinoma of the prostate or of benign prostatic hypertrophy is not clear. Although some of the early reports suggested a decreased excretion of 17-oxosteroids in patients with prostatic cancer, most authors are now agreed there is no difference in urinary 17-oxosteroid excretion between patients with carcinoma of the prostate and subjects of similar age in whom there is no clinical evidence of cancer (for references to earlier work see Marmorston et al, 1965b, and Isurugi, 1967). This is not surprising since, as shown in Chapter 1, measurement of 17-oxosteroid excretion is a poor index of androgenic function.

Robinson and Goulden (1949) found that the excretion of dehydroepiandrosterone, androsterone and 11β-hydroxyandrosterone was low in patients with prostatic carcinoma and was subnormally raised by the administration of ACTH. Stern et al (1964) by measuring gonadotrophins and a number of steroid metabolites in urine (androsterone, aetiocholanolone, 11-oxygenated-17-oxosteroids, 17-oxogenic steroids, pregnanediol, oestrone, oestradiol or oestriol) were able to derive a discriminant index which distinguished between patients with prostatic cancer and normal subjects although it is doubtful whether this index is of use in distinguishing patients who are likely to respond to treatment.

In a subsequent publication (Marmorston et al, 1965b) these investigators found that there was no significant difference between the amount of androsterone excreted by patients with prostatic carcinoma and those with benign hypertrophy, but that in both conditions the levels were lower than those found in normal subjects. Excretion of androsterone tended to be decreased more than that of aetiocholanolone resulting in a significantly lower androsterone to aetiocholanolone ratio.

In an extension of this work Weiner et al (1966) compared the excretion of a number of steroid metabolites by 21 men with prostatic carcinoma and 17 with benign prostatic hypertrophy. Of the various metabolites that they measured the only one to show a significant difference between the two groups was oestriol, which tended to be higher in cases of carcinoma than in benign prostatic hypertrophy. They were able to use five of their measurements to derive a linear discriminant function which gave significantly different scores for carcinoma and benign hypertrophy. Although this function distinguishes between these two conditions it does not appear to have been used in assessing the most suitable form of therapy.

Gallagher et al (1963) carried out a detailed analysis of urinary steroids before and after orchiectomy in 15 patients with prostatic cancer. They found a decreased excretion of androgen metabolites after operation and also observed a decrease in the excretion of metabolites of cortisol. There was no correlation between the preoperative steroid levels or the decrease in androgens after operation, and remission in response to the treatment.

There appears to be no difference between urinary oestrogen excretion by normal men and by those with untreated prostatic cancer. After castration of patients with prostatic cancer there was a fall in the level of oestrogen excretion which was accompanied by regression of the tumour. About six months later oestrogen output started to rise and this was accompanied by renewed growth of the tumour. In patients treated with synthetic oestrogens and surviving five years or more, oestrogen excretion remained low even when there was renewed activity of the tumour (Bulbrook, Franks and Greenwood, 1959). It was suggested that there was a correlation between the growth of the tumour and the

output of urinary oestrogens, although these results need confirming using a larger number of patients.

In addition, Marmorston et al (1965c) found that there was no difference in the excretion of oestrone, oestradiol and oestriol by the patients with prostatic cancer, benign hypertrophy or normal subjects; these findings are in agreement with the earlier work of a number of other investigators.

In summary, therefore, determination of the urinary steroid excretion has not proved useful in distinguishing a steroid pattern characteristic of prostatic carcinoma or benign hypertrophy nor does it correlate with the appearance or recurrence of the disease.

In view of this, many investigators turned their attention to the measurement of testosterone levels in plasma and testosterone production rate, but as yet there is no evidence for an overproduction of testosterone in subjects with cancer of the prostate. Kent and Young (1964) found the testosterone levels in blood to be within the normal range in 13 patients with cancer, so it would appear that increased androgen production is not one of the aetiological factors involved in these disorders.

However, Farnsworth (1971) measured testosterone, androstenedione and dehydroepiandrosterone in plasma of 10 subjects with benign prostatic hypertrophy and found that the levels of testosterone and dehydroepiandrosterone were lower than those found in normal males of similar ages. Isurugi (1967) found that the testosterone production rates in five patients with carcinoma of the prostate and three patients with benign hypertrophy were reduced compared to normal subjects; this reduction was due mainly to a decrease in the metabolic clearance rate of the hormone and a tendency for the plasma concentration of the hormone to be slightly low.

In a later study (Young and Kent, 1968) of 28 patients with Stage 3 or 4 prostatic carcinoma, the pretreatment values observed in patients with Stage 3 carcinoma did not differ significantly from those of normal men but those with the Stage 4 disease had a statistically significant lower level of plasma testosterone. Orchiectomy markedly lowered plasma testosterone levels in most cases as did treatment with stilboestrol. There was no correlation between the plasma level of testosterone and the response of the patient to therapy and failure to benefit from treatment was not attributable to inadequate lowering of plasma testosterone levels.

Low levels of plasma testosterone were also found in patients with other malignancies and with chronic diseases. Alder et al (1968) found no difference in the plasma concentrations of luteinising hormone and testosterone between subjects with carcinoma and normal subjects. Oestrogen treatment caused a fall of at least 50 per cent in both hormones after two to three weeks, but the suppression was incomplete and it was not sustained in all cases on continuation of the treatment. From their results the authors suggest that oestrogen, in addition to exerting an effect on testosterone production via the pituitary, also had a direct effect on the testis.

A similar dual mechanism has been postulated by Geller et al (1969) for the effects produced after administering the anti-androgenic compound cyproterone acetate to patients with carcinoma of the prostate. During treatment with this compound the urinary excretion of testosterone glucuronide decreased but there was no change in the plasma levels or urinary excretion of luteinising hormone. Recovery of injected testosterone propionate as urinary testosterone glucuronide was not affected by administration of the anti-androgen, and administration of HCG increased testosterone excretion in subjects not treated with cyproterone acetate, but not in patients who were receiving treatment.

It was suggested therefore that the anti-androgen inhibited the rise in luteinising hormone that would follow from a decrease in testosterone production and that the compound also had a direct inhibitory effect on the synthesis of testosterone. In a previous study (Geller et al, 1968) in which 11 patients with advanced carcinoma of the prostate were treated with cyproterone acetate there was a decrease in plasma testosterone levels to about one third of the control values, but no significant change in the excretion of total 17-oxosteroids, 17-oxogenic steroids or gonadotrophins.

UPTAKE AND METABOLISM OF STEROIDS BY PROSTATIC TUMOUR TISSUE

In considering the uptake of hormones by the prostate, whether normal or cancerous, the question of zonation and homogeneity of the tissue samples used is important. Although in the rat the different parts are clearly distinguishable, there still appears to be a controversy regarding the extent to which the human prostate can be divided into distinct zones. For details regarding the morphology and pathology of the prostate the articles by McNeal (1968, 1969) and Franks (1969) should be consulted. The inner part of the gland surrounding the urethra appears to give rise to benign hyperplasia whereas carcinoma usually appears to begin in the outer part. Whether these parts show different sensitivities to oestrogens and androgens remains to be made clear.

In experimental animals a number of investigators (see the review by James and Fotherby, 1970) have shown that the cytoplasm and nuclei of the rat prostate contain receptor proteins which will interact with and bind testosterone. In dogs in which tritium-labelled testosterone was infused intravenously for two hours in order to obtain steady state conditions (Kowarski, Shalf and Migeon, 1969), it was found that the prostate had the highest concentration both of testosterone and dihydrotestosterone, the concentration of dihydrotestosterone in plasma being below the sensitivity of the method.

Farnsworth (1971) found that the concentrations of testosterone, androstenedione, and dehydroepiandrosterone in mixed tissue obtained at prostatectomy or in the nodules and stromal tissue examined separately were 4·6 to 10 times higher than the concentrations found in plasma. However, there appear to be no reports so far which show that the human prostate has the ability to take up and specifically retain testosterone in vivo, although it might be expected to do so; any conclusions based upon the interaction of testosterone with human prostatic tissue must therefore be regarded as tentative.

Following in vitro experiments Braunsberg and James (1967) reported that human prostatic tissue did not appear to concentrate testosterone. In a more recent paper (Jonsson, 1969) it was found that slices from the lateral lobe of the prostate of subjects with benign hypertrophy took up radioactive testosterone, but this uptake of testosterone was not blocked by preincubation of the slices in a medium containing either oestradiol or cyproterone. Similar experiments in the author's laboratory (Ghanadian and Fotherby, 1971) have also shown that human prostatic slices will take up labelled testosterone but the ability of the human prostate to do so is much less than that of rat prostatic tissue.

Rather more work has been concerned with the metabolism of compounds in the prostate. For details of this work and an account of the influence of hormones on the structure and the function of both the normal and neoplastic prostate the review by Ofner (1968) should be consulted. The human prostate has been shown to convert testosterone to 5α-dihydrotestosterone (Farnsworth and Brown, 1963; Wilson and Gloyna, 1970) and it appears to be the latter metabolite of testosterone which is mainly concentrated by the prostatic nuclei.

Chamberlain, Jagarinec and Ofner (1966) showed in prostatic tissue from humans with benign hypertrophy of the prostate, the presence of a large number of enzymes metabolising steroids, including 3α-, 3β- and 17β-hydroxysteroid dehydrogenases, 5α- and 5β-reductases and some hydroxylases. Testosterone was metabolised to at least 10 different products on incubation in vitro (metabolites identified included androstenedione, 5α- and 5β-androstanedione, 5α- and 5β-dihydrotestosterone, 5α- and 5β-androstane-3,17-diols and androsterone).

Siiteri and Wilson (1970) found that there was no significant difference in the content of androstenedione and testosterone between 15 samples of normal prostatic tissue and 10 samples from hypertrophic prostates. However, the content of dihydrotestosterone was significantly greater in hypertrophic tissue than in the normal glands and, moreover, the dihydrotestosterone content was two to three times greater in the periurethral area than in the outer regions of the gland.

That the prostate metabolises testosterone to 5α compounds in vivo as well as in vitro was shown by the work of Morfin et al (1970). These authors infused physiological amounts of [^{14}C] testosterone into the arterial supply to the prostate and bladder in five adult dogs for 9 min until the animals were killed. Recovery of the radioactivity in the prostate and bladder accounted for 1 to 5 per cent and 1 to 3 per cent of the administered dose respectively. Almost all the metabolites in the prostate were reduced to the 5α configuration and half of the radioactivity was associated with 5α-dihydrotestosterone and 5α-androstane-3β,17β-diol. In the bladder the metabolism of testosterone underwent a different pathway, the main product being androstenedione with small amounts of 5α-androstane-3,17-dione.

Pike et al (1970) infused tritiated testosterone into men with benign prostatic hypertrophy 20 minutes before prostatectomy. Investigation of the steroid content of the prostatic tissue showed that 5α-dihydrotestosterone was the main product present. The conversion of testosterone into the 5α reduced metabolites appeared to be a rapid reaction. Since 5α-dihydrotestosterone appears to be the compound responsible for androgenic activity in the target organs, the conversion of testosterone to this metabolite is obviously of great importance and may well be related to the development of the carcinogenic process.

In addition, the conversion of testosterone to these metabolites is of interest in view of the work of Baulieu, Lasnitzki and Robel (1969) who showed that in explants of rat prostate maintained in organ culture, 5α-dihydrotestosterone stimulated cell division whereas 5α-androstane-3β,17β-diol maintained epithelial height and stimulated secretory activity but did not provoke cell division; 5α-androstane-3α,17β-diol was much less active. Testosterone was active in each respect but this may well have been due to metabolism to the other compounds.

The metabolism of oestrone, androstenedione and progesterone by human prostatic tissue from patients with benign hypertrophy or carcinoma was studied by Acevedo and Goldzieher (1965) who showed the presence in the tissue of a number of enzymes capable of metabolising these steroids. There appeared to be no difference between the metabolic patterns of the hypertrophic and malignant tissue. Reduction of oestrone to oestradiol occurred, oestriol was formed by 16α-hydroxylation,

and there was hydroxylation and subsequent methylation of oestrone with the formation of 2-hydroxyoestrone and 2-methoxyoestrone. Androstenedione was converted to testosterone and to 5α-androstane-3, 17-dione.

There was also evidence for the presence of 2β-hydroxylase, 6β-hydroxylase and 17β-hydroxy dehydrogenase activities. Metabolism of progesterone occurred to a much lesser extent than that of the C-18 or C-19 steroids. The relevance of these findings to the metabolism of steroids in the normal prostate in vivo or to the development of carcinogenesis or hyperplasia remains uncertain. Mabin, McMahon and Thomas (1970) have also shown interconversion of oestrone and oestradiol in benign prostatic hyperplastic tissue of human origin maintained in organ culture.

Oestrogens have a direct effect on the metabolism of testosterone by the prostate (Farnsworth, 1969). When slices of benign hypertrophic glands were incubated with testosterone in vitro, addition of a number of oestrogens (the most active were oestrone, oestradiol and stilboestrol) diminished the metabolism of testosterone. This inhibition of metabolism appears also to involve the 5α-reductase enzyme and so reduces the conversion of testosterone to 5α-dihydrotestosterone.

Cancer of the Endometrium and Cervix

STEROID HORMONE PRODUCTION IN PATIENTS WITH CANCER OF THE ENDOMETRIUM OR CERVIX

De Waard et al (1968) studied 27 women who had recently undergone operation on account of endometrial cancer. Urine samples were collected on the ninth postoperative day and

the excretion of oestrone, oestradiol, oestriol, dehydroepiandrosterone, aetiocholanolone, androsterone, total 17-oxosteroids and total 17-oxogenic steroids was measured. It was found that the ratio of aetiocholanolone to 17-oxogenic steroid excretion and the ratio of aetiocholanolone to oestriol excretion were decreased compared to normal postmenopausal patients. However, there was still a considerable overlap between patients with cancer and the normal subjects.

Prior to operation for endometrial carcinoma, Charles et al (1965) found that in nine patients the excretion of oestrone, oestradiol and oestriol was within the normal range for postmenopausal women. They made the interesting observation that, in spite of this, only one patient had an atrophic vaginal smear, the remainder having high cornification indices, a finding reported also by other workers, so that in this condition vaginal smears would appear to be an unreliable index of oestrogenic activity. There appears to be no biochemical data showing that high oestrogen production is a factor in the cause of the disease, nor is there any substantial evidence that subjects with cancer metabolise oestrogens differently from normal postmenopausal women.

This aspect has been studied by Hausknecht and Gusberg (1969) who were unable to find any significant difference between oestrogen metabolism in 17 normal post-menopausal females and 34 postmenopausal women with endometrial carcinoma. After the administration of labelled oestradiol the percentage recovery of radioactivity in the oestrone, oestradiol and oestriol fractions was the same in both groups. However, the difference between the specific activity of oestrone and oestriol was significantly less in patients with endometrial carcinoma than it was in the normal women.

Since there was no apparent difference in the metabolism of injected tritiated oestradiol in these two groups of patients, it was suggested that the results could be explained by postulating a diminished production of oestriol precursors, other than oestrone or oestradiol, in the women with cancer. Since in postmenopausal women almost all the oestrogen arises as a result of conversion of C-19 steroids produced by the adrenal cortex, this finding might suggest that the adrenal production of these steroids was decreased.

This finding would certainly fit in with the finding of de Waard et al (1968) of a lowered aetiocholanolone excretion, assuming that no changes in metabolism of the C-19 steroids occurs in this condition. Whether these changes are caused by the presence of the cancerous tissue or whether they result from changes in the metabolic state of the patient remains to be determined.

The amount of oestrogen excreted by women with cervical carcinoma has been variously reported as being normal, increased or decreased (Fraser et al, 1967). Another article quoted by these authors indicates a high oestradiol excretion with a decreased oestriol excretion in premenopausal women with cervical cancer. Fraser et al themselves studied nine patients with cervical carcinoma and compared oestrogen production by these patients with 12 control subjects. There was no significant difference in the total excretion of oestrone, oestradiol and oestriol between the two groups of subjects nor in the percentage of radioactivity recovered in each of these fractions after the administration of tritium-labelled oestradiol.

However, the ratio of both oestrone and oestradiol to oestriol was lower in the carcinoma group than in the control group, whether calculated on the basis of endogenously produced oestrogens or on the amount of radioactivity recovered in the fractions after the administration of isotopically labelled oestradiol, showing that the patients with carcinoma tended to excrete more oestriol. The oestradiol production rate of the carcinoma group tended to be higher than that of the controls although the difference was not statistically significant. These abnormalities in oestrogen metabolism were present in patients in the early stage of cervical carcinoma.

UPTAKE AND METABOLISM OF STEROIDS BY ENDOMETRIUM

Davis et al (1963) administered tritiated oestradiol intramuscularly to one non-pregnant woman and to four pregnant women.

In the non-pregnant patient, endometrium and myometrium contained two to five times the concentration of tritium in blood at the time of hysterectomy two to three hours later. Moreover the concentration of radioactivity appeared to vary with the different parts of the uterus. Similar experiments have also been carried out by Brush et al (1968) who have extended their studies to measure the uptake of tritiated oestradiol by human endometrial carcinoma tissue. Twelve postmenopausal patients were injected with tritiated oestradiol and hysterectomy was carried out one to two hours later; the uptake did not appear to differ significantly from that of normal endometrium. Milgrom and Baulieu (1968) have suggested that the uterus contains a specific binding protein for progesterone.

Endometrial tissue has the ability to metabolise steroids (see Collins et al, 1969; Sweat and Bryson, 1970). Progesterone was reduced both by human endometrial and myometrial tissue primarily to 5α-pregnane derivatives in contrast to the production of 5β-pregnane derivatives by the liver. 17-Hydroxylase activity was low but the presence of a 17β-hydroxysteroid dehydrogenase was shown by the interconvertibility of oestrone and oestradiol and of androstenedione and testosterone, with the equilibrium favouring the formation of the 17-oxosteroid in each case.

Miscellaneous Cancers

NASOPHARYNGEAL CANCER

Clifford and Bulbrook (1966) studied the urinary excretion of oestrogens, androgen and cortisol metabolites in African males with nasopharyngeal cancer. This cancer shows a sex distribution of about 5 to 1 in favour of males. Total oestrogen excretion was slightly higher in the patients with cancer and it was mainly due to an increase in oestriol excretion. Although the excretion of aetiocholanolone was the same in the subjects with cancer and in the control subjects, the latter excreted higher amounts of androsterone and dehydroepiandrosterone than the subjects with cancer. There was no significant difference between the two groups in the excretion of 17-oxogenic steroids.

In plasma, levels of dehydroepiandrosterone sulphate tended to be lower in patients with cancer than in control subjects but there was no difference in regard to androsterone sulphate (Wang, Bulbrook and Clifford, 1968). The extent to which the steroid production by the subjects with cancer deviates from that of normal subjects and whether such deviations play a role in the genesis of this type of cancer remains to be further investigated.

LUNG CANCER

Surprisingly, steroid excretion patterns may be changed in subjects with carcinoma of the lung and these deviations may be sufficient to suggest that measurement of certain steroids may help in predicting the response of the patients to treatment. From the following discussion are excluded those cancers of the lung which produce conspicuous endocrine abnormalities due usually to production of trophic hormones by the tumour, and the studies are concerned only with patients with lung cancer who show no clinically apparent endocrine disease.

Marmorston et al (1966) have reviewed the earlier literature dealing with endocrine abnormalities in lung cancer and have carried out analyses of a number of hormonal metabolites in 55 patients with lung cancer, 45 patients with emphysema, and 59 control subjects. By using a linear discriminant function they were able to show a difference in the pattern of metabolites between the patients and the controls.

A detailed study of steroid excretion in patients with lung cancer has been carried out by Rao (1970). One hundred and forty-two male patients with cancer of the lung were compared with 100 normal subjects and 52 subjects in hospital with chest diseases other than lung cancer. Patients with inoperable lung cancer excreted less androsterone and more 17-oxogenic steroids than control subjects.

The androsterone and aetiocholanolone ratio was also significantly different between subjects with lung cancer and the controls, and when values for the excretion of these steroids were combined with the values for the excretion of 17-oxosteroids and 17-oxogenic steroids it was possible to derive a discriminant function which gave an error of misclassification of less than 10 per cent. The formula for this discriminant function is

$$(5.285 \times A/E) - (0.089 \times KS/A) - (0.190 \times OGS/E) - 2.279$$

where A, E, KS and OGS are the excretion in mg/24 h of androsterone, aetiocholanolone, 17-oxosteroids and 17-oxogenic steroids respectively. This discriminant gave a negative value in 75 out of 84 inoperable lung cancer patients and a positive value in 92 out of 100 healthy control subjects. The low androsterone to aetiocholanolone ratio in subjects with lung carcinoma was not affected by removal of the tumour.

In a group of 23 subjects who had had their tumours removed 1 to 15 years previously, although the mean androsterone to aetiocholanolone ratio was higher than in the inoperable cases, it was still significantly lower than in the control subjects. Interestingly, Rao found that the ratio of 17-oxogenic steroids to aetiocholanolone excretion showed a highly significant difference between patients with lung cancer and healthy controls but not between patients with lung cancer and hospitalised control subjects. From these results it would appear that the preoperative level of steroid excretion may be of some value in predicting the prognosis of the patient.

Although there appears to be no difference in the excretion of 17-oxogenic steroids by patients with lung cancer and hospitalised control subjects, Sholiton, Werk and Marnell (1961) showed that the free plasma 17-hydroxycorticosteroids in ambulatory patients with lung cancer exhibited a less marked diurnal change and were generally higher than in chronically ill patients; in advanced lung cancer patients the diurnal rhythm was completely absent. These findings were confirmed by McNamara et al (1968) and Kawai et al (1969). The metabolism of cortisol by pulmonary tumour tissue from 14 patients was studied by Kemeny et al (1968). Cortisone was produced to a varying extent by 10 of these samples, an unidentified polar metabolite in 1 and a non-polar metabolite in 4. The amount of cortisone produced was highest in undifferentiated tumours.

LEUKAEMIA

In five male patients with chronic lymphatic leukaemia Dobriner, Kappas and Gallagher (1954) found that the urinary excretion of 17-oxosteroids was markedly lower than that of normal males of comparable age. Corticosteroid metabolism in male and female patients with chronic lymphatic leukaemia was also studied by Gallagher et al (1962). They found that the leukaemic patients produced more tetrahydrocortisol than tetrahydrocortisone, which was the reverse of the situation found in normal subjects. Men with leukaemia showed a relatively low excretion of androsterone plus aetiocholanolone compared with the excretion of these compounds by men with prostatic carcinoma.

Cells originating from a murine lymphosarcoma were found by Dougherty, Berliner and Berliner (1961) to oxidise cortisol to cortisone, to reduce cortisol and cortisone to the C-20 hydroxysteroid, and to remove the side chain with the formation of 11β-hydroxyandrostenedione. These cells were apparently unable to reduce the double bond in cortisol to form dihydro- and tetrahydro-compounds. Malignant lymphocytes had a greater activity with respect to reduction of C-20 and side-chain oxidation than either mature or immature lymphocytes but, in contrast, a reduced ability to convert cortisol to cortisone.

Forker et al (1963) showed that human leucocytes could also metabolise cortisol, although the metabolites were not completely characterised. In untreated chronic lymphatic leukaemia, the conversion of cortisol to an unidentified polar metabolite was similar to that by the leucocytes of non-leukaemic subjects and only one half of that by leucocytes from patients with acute leukaemia.

The metabolism of cortisol in vitro by white cells from 20 patients suffering from various forms of leukaemia was studied by Jenkins and Kemp (1969) and compared with the metabolism by normal leucocytes. Cells from acute lymphatic and myeloid leukaemia were four times as active as normal leucocytes in reducing cortisol to the C-20 hydroxysteroid and twice as active in reduction of ring A; cells from patients with chronic leukaemia were intermediate in their degree of metabolic activity. The equal facility with which lymphatic and myeloid leukaemic cells transformed cortisol makes it unlikely that a change in metabolism of steroids is involved in the therapeutic response of leukaemia to the administration of cortisol.

Forker et al (1963) found that administration of corticosteroids to patients with chronic

lymphatic leukaemia decreased the conversion of cortisol to the more polar metabolite (see above) by about 66 per cent, but in patients with acute leukaemia the formation of the polar metabolite was unaffected by steroid administration. Burton (1964) was also unsuccessful in demonstrating any difference in the metabolism of cortisol by steroid-sensitive and steroid-resistant cell lines of mouse lymphatic leukaemia and mouse lymphosarcoma.

The development of resistance to the growth-inhibiting effect of steroids was investigated by Berliner (1965) who studied the growth of mouse fibroblasts in vitro in media containing various concentrations of cortisol, tetrahydrocortisol, 11-deoxycortisol, dexamethasone and fluocinolone acetonide. It was found that the initial growth depression evoked by dexamethasone, cortisol and prednisolone was generally overcome within three to five days. Cell lines were isolated which could grow in the presence of increased amounts of cortisol or fluocinolone acetonide.

It was found (Grosser et al, 1962) that a cell line which was resistant to cortisol at a concentration of 25 μg/ml medium could metabolise this hormone twice as effectively as the cortisol-sensitive strain. The steroid-resistant cells were then subcultured in media devoid of steroid and found to grow at the same rate as in the presence of the steroid. After approximately 10 subcultures in medium without steroid over a period of eight weeks, the cells were replaced in medium containing the steroid and were found to continue to grow at the same rate; that is, their growth rate had become independent of the presence or absence of steroid. Although this work is interesting it is difficult to assess its relevance to the development of steroid resistance in vivo.

Cell suspensions of lymphoid tissue from steroid-sensitive and steroid-resistant animal tumour lines were found by Burton (1964) to bind [^{14}C] cortisol to the same extent. He concluded that the development of resistance to corticosteroids in tumours could not be attributed to differences in the binding or metabolism of cortisol since no correlation between these processes and the response of the tissue to cortisol in vivo could be demonstrated.

Role of Steroids in Production and Remission of Cancer

In general this discussion is limited to topics which are applicable to cancer developing in any of the target organs for sex hormones rather than a consideration of specific factors relevant to cancer in any one particular tissue. It has been suggested repeatedly in the past that increases in the production of the sex hormones are important in the development of cancer of the sex hormone target organs, oestrogens in the case of cancer of the breast and endometrium and testosterone in the case of cancer of the prostate. This view must be reconsidered since from the investigations carried out so far, many of which have been reviewed in this Chapter, there is little evidence in favour of such a hypothesis which rests mainly upon evidence derived from animal studies.

It is now becoming increasingly clear that studies of this type in animals may have very little relevance to the human situation. Not only do the different strains of animals and different species vary considerably in their susceptibility to the induction of cancer (Bischoff, 1969), but it is also clear that there are very large species differences in their endocrinological environment which may greatly influence the carcinogenic process and, in addition, make the relevance of these results to human cancer impossible to assess.

The role of steroid hormones in the aetiology and pathogenesis of cancer has been reviewed recently by Hertz (1967) and Bischoff (1969). Although a large number of experiments have shown the capacity of steroid hormones to induce cancer at numerous tissue sites in animals, the evidence suggesting that the same phenomenon occurs in humans is slender. Bischoff concludes that 'the most important factor in carcinogenesis is the genetic one and the cancer incidence for any particular type in humans is always lower than the significant incidence induced by steroids in groups of experimental animals.'

It should be recognised, as stressed by Hertz (1967), that properly designed studies to ascertain the true state of affairs in humans have not yet been carried out. However, it would appear from a review of all the evidence that *the steroid hormones in humans do not play any major role in carcinogenesis*. Possibly as far as humans are concerned, evidence in relation to this will only come from large scale epidemiological studies or from prospective endocrinological and biochemical studies of the type being carried out in Guernsey (Bulbrook, 1970). These studies would need to be well designed and controlled, are likely to be long term, technically complex, at times frustrating, and certainly costly.

MacMahon and Cole (1969) and Cole and MacMahon (1969) have discussed some of the aspects of the endocrinology and epidemiology of breast cancer and considered many of the aspects which suggest that oestrogen, particularly that produced during the early years of reproductive life, may be an important factor determining the risk of developing breast cancer, but many of their conclusions must be accepted with caution. In view of the above facts one of their statements, namely 'the information now available clearly identifies the ovary as the prime target for aetiologic investigations', would appear to be untenable and the evidence on which they base their statement and their further suggestions that oestrogens are one of the prime causes of breast cancer must be accepted with considerable reserve.

Their hypothesis has been criticised by Smith and Smith (1970) on the ground that it does not take into account the role played by the anterior pituitary. Again, not all of the conclusions in Smith and Smith's articles can be accepted but one interesting finding in relation to their suggestions is that of Adamopoulos, Loraine and Dove (1971) who showed that LH levels are approximately seven times higher and FSH levels approximately three times higher in women approaching the menopause than they are in normal women studied earlier in reproductive life.

However, the role of the adrenal would also appear to be important. Although with the onset of puberty in the early teens the ovary begins to produce increased amounts of oestrogens, from shortly before this time and for about the next decade the activity of the adrenal also increases dramatically; this in turn, because of the mechanisms discussed above, will also contribute to the total production of oestrogens. In addition to this, the exposure of the body to the range of other hormones produced by the adrenal will also occur.

The work of Bulbrook and Hayward already referred to shows that compounds which are either androgenic themselves or related to the androgens may be important. Bulbrook et al, among others, have suggested that the excretion of the 11-deoxy-17-oxosteroids may give some indication of the degree of androgenic stimulation in these patients and that the androgenic precursors of the 11-deoxy-17-oxosteroids may be exerting an anti-oestrogen effect. They also suggested that a defect in androgen production (that is, a decrease in anti-oestrogen effect) in patients with a normal range of oestrogen production may be as important in the aetiology of breast cancer as an over-production of oestrogens.

Moreover, the role of progesterone should also surely be taken into consideration. This compound is known to be antitumourogenic in some species although at other times it may also act synergistically with oestrogens and other carcinogens. It will certainly interact with oestrogens in the control of breast and endometrial function, and possibly also modify hormonal effects on the prostate. In studies carried out so far there has been no correlation between the excretion of the main metabolite of progesterone, pregnanediol, and any of the other factors studied. But it must be born in mind that pregnanediol accounts for only a small proportion of the secreted progesterone and it may not be an accurate reflection of the endocrinological activity of the hormone.

Undoubtedly, particularly in breast cancer, the pituitary hormones other than the gonadotrophins may play an important part, as will also other hormones in the extent to which they act as modifiers of steroid hormone action. Discussions of which endocrine glands might be most relevant to the carcinogenic process are useless since, as explained in Chapter 1, each endocrine gland has the ability to produce and secrete a large number of different compounds and these compounds undergo a series of complex metabolic interactions after secretion.

Even in considering the oestrogens themselves, the situation is not a straightforward one. Although oestrone and oestradiol are classified as being carcinogenic since they are powerful carcinogens in experimental animals, oestriol does not appear to be at all carcinogenic and, moreover, the latter steroid often inhibits the growth-promoting effect of oestrone and oestradiol. The role of oestriol and other 'impeded' oestrogens in the carcinogenic process has been considered by Lemon (1970) who suggests that oestriol plays a significant anticarcinogenic role in humans, and also by Wotiz et al (1968).

The work of Lemon et al (1966), concerned

with the ratio of oestriol to oestrone and oestradiol excretion in subjects with breast cancer, has already been referred to, and the protective effects of pregnancy against breast cancer in humans may be due to the large increase in oestriol secretion which occurs at this time. Wotiz et al (1968) have shown that oestriol will interfere with oestradiol binding in the uterus and may in this way influence the interaction of oestradiol with the tissue receptors. However, before this view can be accepted it must be shown that the concentration of oestriol in plasma is sufficient to exert an inhibitory effect.

The mode of action of steroids in inducing remission of cancer is not known. Three postulates have been proposed:

1. *A general metabolic action:* It has been proposed that the various forms of treatment, whether hormone administration or ablation of hormone-producing tissues, produce a general metabolic effect which in some cases may be so deleterious to the tumour that it begins to regress.

2. *A pituitary-mediated action:* This postulates that the effect of treatment is mediated through the pituitary; administration of therapeutic agents inhibits the pituitary production of trophic hormones required for the maintenance of the steroid-producing glands so that the production of compounds presumed to have a carcinogenic effect is reduced or obliterated. Although at one time there was thought to be a correlation between the clinical effectiveness of any particular compound and its ability to inhibit the pituitary, other steroids have been developed which cause regression of the tumour but are claimed not to depress gonadotrophin excretion and presumably therefore do not have any marked inhibitory effect on the pituitary.

In general, even for those compounds which do have pituitary-inhibiting activity, the doses used are much higher than those required to produce inhibition and if this were the sole means of action much lower doses should suffice. The concept that gonadotrophin inhibition accounts for the remission of tumours in all cases is not tenable, since in many young women with breast cancer ovariectomy or irradiation of the ovaries is beneficial although each results in an increase in gonadotrophin production and remissions have been observed in hypophysectomised patients. This has led to the suggestion that other pituitary factors might be involved in the support of tumour growth and the secretion of prolactin has been invoked on many occasions.

3. A *direct (local) action:* In support of a direct effect of the steroid on the tumour cells, both Kaiser (1959) and Sherman (1966) showed that administration of synthetic progestogens depressed mitosis in uterine cancer cells. Ofner (1968) has reviewed the evidence for a local effect of hormones on the prostate. Administration of oestradiol alone to rats caused a decrease in prostatic weight and an atrophy of epithelial tissue, whereas rats treated with testosterone showed hyperplasia of the glandular epithelium and an increase in prostatic weight. When the oestrogen and androgen were administered in the ratio of 2 to 1 no significant difference occurred in prostatic weight or histology between treated and control animals, and a similar effect was seen when the hormones were administered in the same ratio to intact orchiectomised, adrenalectomised or hypophysectomised animals, showing that influences on the other endocrine glands could be eliminated.

In regard to a local tissue effect, the concept of receptor proteins in the tissues which bind the hormone provides a feasible hypothesis for the explanation of the remissions produced by administration of therapeutic agents. Such a theory would presuppose that the administered compound prevents binding by the tumour of the appropriate sex hormone thus preventing the sex hormone from exerting a biological effect. There are now numerous examples of these interactions at the in vitro level (see review by James and Fotherby, 1970). This theory would further presuppose that tumours with a high content of the receptor protein, and which are therefore capable of binding increased amounts of the sex hormones, are the ones that would respond to treatment by the therapeutic agent.

However, there is little evidence at present to support such a hypothesis, nor have the type of interactions which have been clearly shown in in vitro experiments been confirmed as a result of in vivo experiments. Although, as referred to earlier, Deshpande (1967) suggested that drostanolone propionate prevented oestradiol binding in breast tumours, a repetition of these experiments when drostanolone or testosterone propionate were administered to patients being infused with oestradiol (Braunsberg et al, 1970) did not confirm this finding, and the latter authors suggested that the drostanolone may have been altering the clearance rate of oestradiol from plasma.

In most cases it is likely to be a combination of these three effects which produces any remission which is obtained, and the task of separating one effect from another in the case of steroid compounds may well be a difficult one since most of the steroid hormones show a multitude of biological activities. Pincus (1965) has listed some of the properties which may be associated with the steroid molecule; anabolic, androgenic, antiandrogenic, oestrogenic, antioestrogenic, progestogenic, antiprogestogenic, antigonadotrophic, active on the circulatory and haematopoietic systems among others. Although any one particular steroid does not have all of these biological activities, many of them have a considerable number.

The ability of steroids to produce cancer in animals and the finding that some of the tumours produced were 'hormone dependent' suggested that some of the tumours arising in humans might also be hormone dependent although the existence of hormone-dependent tumours in humans has not been documented. Although remissions of cancer may be produced by hormone therapy or ablation of endocrine glands, such remissions are rarely permanent. Very much more remains to be done concerning the biochemical changes associated with these remissions and particularly why these so often last for only short periods.

References

Acevedo, H. F. & Goldzieher, J. W. (1965) The metabolism of [4-^{14}C] progesterone by hypertrophic and carcinomatous human prostate tissue. *Biochimica et biophysica acta*, **111**, 294–298.

Adamopoulos, D. A., Loraine, J. A. & Dove, G. A. (1971) Endocrinological studies in women approaching the menopause. *Journal of Obstetrics and Gynaecology of the British Commonwealth*, **78**, 62–79.

Adams, J. B. & Wong, M. S. F. (1968) A correlation between urinary steroid metabolites and pathways of steroidogenesis in human breast tumour tissue. *Lancet*, **ii**, 1163–1166.

Adams, J. B. & Wong, M. S. F. (1969) Desmolase activity of normal and malignant human breast tissue. *Journal of Endocrinology*, **44**, 69–77.

Ahlquist, K. A., Jackson, A. W. & Stewart, J. G. (1968) Urinary steroid values as a guide to prognosis in breast cancer. *British Medical Journal*, **1**, 217–221.

Alder, A., Burger, H., Davis, J., Dulmanis, A., Hudson, B., Sarfaty, G. & Straffon, W. (1968) Carcinoma of prostate: Response of plasma luteinizing hormone and testosterone to oestrogen therapy. *British Medical Journal*, **1**, 28–30.

Allen, B. J., Hayward, J. L. & Merivale, W. H. H. (1957) The excretion of 17-ketosteroids in the urine of patients with generalised carcinomatosis secondary to carcinoma of the breast. *Lancet*, **272**, 496–499.

Armitage, P., McPherson, C. K. & Copas, J. C. (1969) Statistical studies of prognosis in advanced breast cancer. *Journal of Chronic Diseases*, **22**, 343–360.

Barlow, J. J., Emerson, K. & Saxena, B. N. (1969)

Estradiol production after ovariectomy for carcinoma of the breast. *New England Journal of Medicine*, **280**, 633–637.

Baulieu, E.-E., Lasnitzki, I. & Robel, P. (1969) Testosterone metabolism in rat prostate grown in organ culture and hormone action. Advances in the Biosciences, **3**, 169–174.

Berliner, D. L. (1965) Studies of the mechanisms by which cells become resistant to corticosteroids. *Cancer Research*, **25**, 1085–1095.

Bischoff, F. (1969) Carcinogenic effects of steroids. *Advances in Lipid Research*, **7**, 165–244.

Braunsberg, H., Irvine, W. T. & James, V. H. T. (1967) A comparison of steroid hormone concentrations in human tissues including breast cancer. *British Journal of Cancer*, **21**, 714–729.

Braunsberg, H. & James, V. H. T. (1967) Observations on the binding of testosterone to malignant mammary tumours and other tissues *in vitro*. *British Journal of Cancer*, **21**, 703–713.

Braunsberg, H., James, V. H. T., Irvine, W. T. & Carter, A. E. (1970) Relative oestrogen concentrations in human tumours. *Hormones*, **1**, 73–79.

Brown, J. B. (1960) The determination and significance of the natural estrogens. *Advances in Clinical Chemistry*, **3**, 157–233.

Brush, M. G., Taylor, R. W., King, R. J. B. & Kalinga, A. A. (1968) The uptake and metabolism of [6,7-^{3}H] oestradiol by human endometrial carcinoma tissue *in vivo* and *in vitro*. *Journal of Endocrinology*, **41**, xii–xiii.

Bulbrook, R. D. (1970) Prognostic value of steroid assays in human breast cancer. *Advances in Steroid Biochemistry*, **1**, 387–417.

Bulbrook, R. D., Franks, L. M. & Greenwood, F. C. (1959) Hormone excretion in prostatic cancer; an attempt to correlate urinary hormone excretion and clinical state. *British Journal of Cancer*, **13**, 45–58.

Bulbrook, R. D., Greenwood, F. C. & Hayward, J. L. (1960) Selection of breast-cancer patients for adrenalectomy or hypophysectomy by determination of urinary 17-hydroxycorticosteroids and aetiocholanolone. *Lancet*, **i**, 1154–1157.

Bulbrook, R. D. & Hayward, J. L. (1969) Excretion of urinary 17-hydroxycorticosteroids and 11-deoxy-17-oxosteroids by women using steroidal contraceptives. *Lancet*, **ii**, 1033–1035.

Bulbrook, R. D., Hayward, J. L. & Thomas, B. S. (1964) The relation between the urinary 17-hydroxycorticosteroids and 11-deoxy-17-oxo-steroids and the fate of patients after mastectomy. *Lancet*, **i**, 945–947.

Bulbrook, R. D., Hayward, J. L., Spicer, C. C. & Thomas, B. S. (1962a) A comparison between the urinary steroid excretion of normal women and women with advanced breast cancer. *Lancet*, **ii**, 1235–1237.

Bulbrook, R. D., Hayward, J. L., Spicer, C. C. & Thomas, B. S. (1962b) Abnormal excretion of urinary steroids by women with early breast cancer. *Lancet*, **ii**, 1238–1239.

Bulbrook, R. D. & Strong, J. A. (1958) Hormone studies in breast cancer. In *Cancer*, ed. Raven, R. W., Vol. 6, pp. 215–251. London: Butterworths.

Burton, A. F. (1964) The binding and metabolism of cortisol-4-C^{14} by lymphatic tissue and tumors of rats and mice. *Cancer Research*, **24**, 470–474.

Chamberlain, J., Jagarinec, N. & Ofner, P. (1966) Catabolism of [4-^{14}C] testosterone by subcellular fractions of human prostate. *Biochemistry Journal*, **99**, 610–616.

Charles, D., Bell, E. T., Loraine, J. A. & Harkness, R. A. (1965) Endometrial carcinoma-endocrinological and clinical studies. *American Journal of Obstetrics and Gynecology* **91**, 1050–1059.

Clifford, P. and Bulbrook, R. D. (1966) Endocrine studies in African males with nasopharyngeal cancer. *Lancet*, **i**, 1228–1231.

Cole, P. & MacMahon, B. (1969) Oestrogen fractions during early reproductive life in the aetiology of breast cancer. *Lancet*, **i**, 604–606.

Collins, W. P., Mansfield, M. D., Bridges, C. E. & Sommerville, I. F. (1969) Studies on steroid metabolism in human endometrial tissue. *Biochemical Journal*, **113**, 399–407.

Crowley, L. G., Demetriou, J. A., Kotin, P., Donovan, A. J. & Kushinsky, S. (1965) Excretion patterns of urinary metabolites of estradiol-4-C^{14} in post-menopausal women with benign and malignant disease of the breast. *Cancer Research*, **25**, 371–376.

Dao, T. L. (1969) Studies on the mechanism of regression of mammary cancer after adrenalectomy. In *The Human Adrenal Gland and its Relation to Breast Cancer*, pp. 99–103. Cardiff: First Tenovus Workshop.

Davis, M. E., Wiener, M., Jacobson, H. I. & Jensen, E. V. (1963) Estradiol metabolism in pregnant and non pregnant women. *American Journal of Obstetrics and Gynecology*, **87**, 979–990.

Demetriou, J. A., Crowley, L. G., Kushinsky, S., Donovan, A. J., Kotin, P. & MacDonald, I. (1964) Radioactive estrogens in tissues of post-menopausal women with breast neoplasms. *Cancer Research*, **24**, 926–934.

Deshpande, N. (1967) Uptake of steroid hormones by human breast tissue. In *The Treatment of Carcinoma of the Breast*, ed. Jarrett, A. S., pp. 45–55. Amsterdam: Excerpta Medica Foundation.

Deshpande, N., Jensen, V., Carson, P., Bulbrook, R. D. & Lewis, A. A. (1969) Some aspects of the measurement of cortisol production in patients with breast cancer. *Journal of Endocrinology*, **45**, 571–578.

Dobriner, K., Kappas, A. & Gallagher, T. F. (1954) Studies in steroid metabolism. XXVI Steroid isolation studies in human leukaemia. *Journal of Clinical Investigation*, **33**, 1481–1486.

Dougherty, T. F., Berliner, D. L. & Berliner, M. L.

(1961) Corticosteroid tissue interactions. *Metabolism*, **10**, 966–989.

Farnsworth, W. E. (1969) A direct effect of estrogens on prostatic metabolism of testosterone. *Investigative Urology*, **6**, 423–427.

Farnsworth, W. E. (1971) Uptake of plasma androgens by human benign hypertrophic prostate. *Investigative Urology*, **8**, 367–372.

Farnsworth, W. E. & Brown, J. R. (1963) Metabolism of testosterone by the human prostate. *Journal of the American Medical Association*, **183**, 436–439.

Forchielli, E., Thomas, P. Z., Freymann, J. G., Parsons, D. & Dorfman, R. I. (1967) *Current Concepts in Breast Cancer*, ed. Segaloff, A., Meyer, K. K. and DeBakey, S. Baltimore: Williams and Wilkins.

Folca, P. J., Glascock, R. F. & Irvine, W. T. (1961) Studies with tritium labelled hexestrol in advanced breast cancer. Comparison of tissue accumulation of hexestrol with response to bilateral adrenalectomy and oophorectomy. *Lancet*, **ii**, 796–798.

Forker, A. D., Bolinger, R. E., Morris, J. H. I. & Larson, W. E. (1963) Metabolism of cortisol-C^{14} by human peripheral leukocyte cultures from leukemic patients. *Metabolism*, **12**, 751–759.

Forrest, A. P. M. & Kunkler, P. B. (1968) *Prognostic Factors in Breast Cancer*. Edinburgh and London: Livingstone.

Fotherby, K., Colas, A., Atherden, S. M. & Marrian, G. F. (1957) The isolation of 16α-hydroxydehydroepiandrosterone from the urine of normal men. *Biochemical Journal*, **66**, 664–669.

Fotherby, K., Sellwood, R. A. & Burn, J. I. (1970) Urinary steroid excretion in patients with advanced breast cancer. *British Journal of Surgery*, **57**, 859.

Fotherby, K., Sellwood, R. A. & Burn, J. I. (1971) Unpublished.

Franks, L. M. (1969) The pathology of prostatic tumours. *British Journal of Hospital Medicine*, **2**, 575–583.

Fraser, R. C., Cudmore, D. C., Melanson, J. & Morse, W. I. (1967) The metabolism and production rate of estradiol-17β in premenopausal women with cervical carcinoma. *American Journal of Obstetrics and Gynecology*, **98**, 509–515.

Gallagher, T. F., Bradlow, H. L., Miller, D. G., Zumoff, B. & Hellman, L. (1962) Steroid hormone metabolism in chronic lymphatic leukemia. *Journal of Clinical Endocrinology*, **22**, 1049–1056.

Gallagher, T. F., Fukushima, D. K., Noguchi, S., Fishman, J., Bradlow, H. L., Cassouto, J., Zumoff, B. & Hellman, L. (1966) Recent studies in steroid hormone metabolism in man. *Recent Progress in Hormone Research*, **22**, 283–303.

Gallagher, T. F., Whitmore, W. F., Zumoff, B. & Hellman, L. (1963) Steroid hormone metabolites before and after orchiectomy for prostatic cancer. *Journal of Clinical Endocrinology*, **23**, 523–532.

Geller, J., Baron, A., Warburton, V. & Loh, A. (1969) The effect of progestational agents on male gonadal and pituitary function. *Annals of Internal Medicine*, **70**, 1062.

Geller, J., Vazakas, G., Fruchtman, B., Newman, H., Nakao, K. & Loh, A. (1968) The effect of cyproterone acetate on advanced carcinoma of the prostate. *Surgery, Gynecology and Obstetrics*, **127**, 748–758.

Ghanadian, R. & Fotherby, K. (1971) Unpublished.

Gleave, E. N. (1969) Primary and advanced breast cancer in South Wales. A study of urinary steroids. In *The Human Adrenal Gland and its Relation to Breast Cancer*, pp. 86–90. Cardiff: First Tenovus Workshop.

Grosser, B. I., Sweat, M. L., Berliner, D. L. & Dougherty, T. F. (1962) Comparison of cortisol metabolism by two variants of cultured fibroblasts. *Archives of Biochemistry and Biophysics*, **96**, 259–264.

Gutierrez, R. M. & Williams, R. J. (1968) Excretion of ketosteroids and proneness to breast cancer. *Proceedings of the National Academy of Science*, **59**, 938–943.

Haley, H. B., Dimick, D. F. & Williamson, M. B. (1966) Corticosteroid metabolism by human breast tumour tissue. *Surgery, Gynecology and Obstetrics*, **123**, 812–818.

Hausknecht, R. U. & Gusberg, S. B. (1969) Estrogen metabolism in patients at high risk for endometrial carcinoma. *American Journal of Obstetrics and Gynecology*, **105**, 1161–1167.

Hertz, R. (1967) The role of steroid hormones in the etiology and pathogenesis of cancer. *American Journal of Obstetrics and Gynecology*, **98**, 1013–1019.

Hobkirk, R. & Forrest, A. P. M. (1957) Urinary steroid patterns in breast cancer. *Lancet*, **272**, 637.

Huggins, C. & Hodges, C. V. (1941) Studies on prostatic cancer. 1. The effect of castration, of estrogen and of androgen injection on serum phosphatases in metastatic carcinoma of the prostate. *Cancer Research*, **1**, 293–297.

Isurugi, K. (1967) Plasma testosterone production rates in patients with prostatic cancer and benign prostatic hypertrophy. *Journal of Urology*, **97**, 903–908.

James, F. & Fotherby, K. (1970) Interaction of sex hormones with target tissues. *Advances in Steroid Biochemistry*, **2**, 315–372.

James, F., James, V. H. T., Carter, A. E. & Irvine, W. T. (1971) A comparison of *in vivo* and *in vitro* uptake of oestradiol by human breast tumours and the relationship to steroid excretion. *Cancer Research*. **31**, 1268–1272.

Jenkins, J. S. & Kemp, N. H. (1969) Metabolism of cortisol by human leukemic cells. *Journal of Clinical Endocrinology*, **29**, 1217–1221.

Johansson, H., Terenius, L. & Thoren, L. (1970) The binding of estradiol-17β to human breast cancers and other tissues *in vitro*. *Cancer Research*, **30**, 692–698.

Jones, D., Cameron, E. H. D. & Griffiths, K., Gleave, E. N. & Forrest, A. P. M. (1970) Steroid metabolism by human breast tumours. *Biochemical Journal*, **116**, 919–921.

Jonsson, C-E. (1969) *In Vitro* uptake of tritiated testosterone and oestradiol by the lateral lobe of the hypertrophied human prostate and the accessory sex glands of the rat. *Acta endocrinologica (København)*, **61**, 25–32.

Juret, P. (1968) Urinary androgen excretion as prognostic factor before hypophysectomy. In *Prognostic Factors in Breast Cancer*, ed. Forrest, A. P. M. and Kunkler, P. B., pp. 393–398. Edinburgh and London: Livingstone.

Kaiser, R. (1959) The action of progestogens on carcinoma of the corpus uteri. *Archiv für Gynäkologie*, **193**, 195.

Kawai, A., Tamura, M., Tanimoto, S., Honma, H. and Kuzuya, N. (1969) Studies on adrenal cortical function in patients with lung cancer. *Metabolism*, **18**, 609–619.

Kemény, V., Farkas, K., Körösi, A. & Szarvas, T. (1968) The cortisol metabolism of human pulmonary tumour tissue. *Experientia*, **24**, 611–613.

Kent, J. R. & Young, H. H. (1964) Plasma testosterone levels in patients with prostatic carcinoma. *Surgical Forum*, **15**, 485–486.

Kowarski, A., Shalf, J. & Migeon, C. J. (1969) Concentration of testosterone and dihydrotestosterone in subcellular fractions of liver, kidney, prostate, and muscle in the male dog. *Journal of Biological Chemistry*, **244**, 5269–5272.

Kumaoka, S., Sakauchi, N., Abe, O., Kusama, M. & Takatani, O. (1968) Urinary 17-ketosteroid excretion of women with advanced breast cancer. *Journal of Clinical Endocrinology*, **28**, 667–672.

Lemon, H. M. (1970) Abnormal estrogen metabolism and tissue estrogen receptor proteins in breast cancer. *Cancer*, **25**, 423–435.

Lemon, H. M., Wotiz, H. H., Parsons, L. & Mozden, P. J. (1966) Reduced estriol excretion in patients with breast cancer prior to endocrine therapy. *Journal of the American Medical Association*, **196**, 1128–1136.

Lipschutz, A. & Maas, M. (1944) Progesterone treatment of uterine and other abdominal fibroids induced in the guinea pig by estradiol. *Cancer Research*, **4**, 18–23.

Lipschutz, A., Murillo, R. & Vargas, L. (1939) Antitumorigenic action of progesterone. *Lancet*, **ii**, 420–421.

Mabin, T. A., McMahon, M. J. & Thomas, G. H. (1970) The interconversion of oestrone and oestradiol by human endometrium and human benign prostatic hyperplasia in organ culture. *Biochemical Journal*, **118**, 8–9.

MacMahon, B. & Cole, P. (1969) Endocrinology and epidemiology of breast cancer. *Cancer*, **24**, 1146–1150.

Marmorston, J., Crowley, L. G., Myers, S. M., Stern, E. & Hopkins, C. E. (1965a) I. Urinary excretion of neutral 17-ketosteroids and pregnanediol by patients with breast cancer and benign breast disease. *American Journal of Obstetrics and Gynecology*, **92**, 447–459.

Marmorston, J., Lombardo, L. J., Myers, S. M., Gierson, H., Stern, E. & Hopkins, C. E. (1965b) Urinary excretion of neutral 17-ketosteroids and pregnanediol by patients with prostatic cancer and benign prostatic hypertrophy. *Journal of Urology*, **93**, 276–286.

Marmorston, J., Lombardo, L. J., Myers, S. M., Gierson, H., Stern, E. & Hopkins, C. E. (1965c) Urinary excretion of oestrone, oestradiol and oestriol by patients with prostatic cancer and benign prostatic hypertrophy. *Journal of Urology*, **93**, 287–295.

Marmorston, J., Weiner, J. M., Hopkins, C. E. & Stern, E. (1966) Abnormalities in urinary hormone patterns in lung cancer and emphysema. *Cancer*, **19**, 985–995.

McNamara, J. J., Varon, H. H., Paulson, D. L., Shah, I. & Urschel, H. C. (1968) Steroid hormone abnormalities in patients with carcinoma of the lung. *Journal of Thoracic and Cardiovascular Surgery* **56**, 371–377.

McNeal, J. E. (1968) Regional morphology and pathology of the prostate. *American Journal of Clinical Pathology*, **49**, 347–357.

McNeal, J. E. (1969) Origin and development of carcinoma in the prostate. *Cancer*, **23**, 24–34.

Milgrom, E. & Baulieu, E. E. (1968) *Comptes rendus hebdomadaires des séances de l' Academie des sciences (Paris)*, **267**, 2005–2007.

Miller, H. & Durant, J. A. (1969) Discriminants and breast cancer. *Lancet*, **i**, 1313–1314.

Mobbs, B. G. (1966) The uptake of tritiated oestradiol by dimethylbenzanthracene-induced mammary tumours of the rat. *Journal of Endocrinology*, **36**, 409–414.

Morfin, R. F., Aliapoulios, M. A., Chamberlain, J. & Ofner, P. (1970) Metabolism of testosterone-4-^{14}C by the canine prostate and urinary bladder *in vivo*. *Endocrinology*, **87**, 394–405.

Ofner, P. (1968) Effects and metabolism of hormones in normal and neoplastic prostate tissue. *Vitamins and Hormones*, **26**, 237–291.

Pearlman, W. H., de Hertogh, R., Laumas, K. R. & Pearlman, M. R. J. (1969) Metabolism and tissue uptake of estrogen in women with advanced carcinoma of the breast. *Journal of Clinical Endocrinology*, **29**, 707–720.

Pike, A., Peeling, W. B., Harper, M. E., Pierrepoint, C. G. & Griffiths, K. (1970) Testosterone metabolism *in vivo* by human prostatic tissue. *Biochemical Journal*, **120**, 443–445.

Pincus, G. (1965) *The Control of Fertility*. New York: Academic Press.

Plantin, L-O., Birke, G., Diczfalusy, E., Franksson, C., Hellstrom, J., Hultberg, S. & Westman, A. (1958) In *Endocrine Aspects of Breast Cancer*, p. 244. Edinburgh: Livingstone.

Rao, L. G. S. (1970) Discriminant function based on steroid abnormalities in patients with lung cancer. *Lancet*, **ii**, 441–445.

Robinson, A. M. & Goulden, F. (1949) A qualitative study of urinary 17-ketosteroids in normal males and in men with prostatic disease. *British Journal of Cancer*, **3**, 62–71.

Sander, S. (1968) The *in vitro* uptake of oestradiol in biopsies from twenty-five breast cancer patients. *Acta pathologica et microbiologica Scandinavica*, **74**, 301–302.

Sander, S. & Attramadal, A. (1968) An autoradiographic study of oestradiol incorporation in the breast tissue of female rats. *Acta endocrinologica (København)*, **58**, 235–242.

Schweppe, J. S., Jungman, R. A. & Lewin, I. (1967) Urine steroid excretion in postmenopausal cancer of the breast. *Cancer*, **20**, 155–163.

Scott, W. W. & Wade, J. C. (1969) Medical treatment of benign nodular prostatic hyperplasia with cyproterone acetate. *Journal of Urology*, **101**, 81–85.

Sherman, A. I. (1966) Progesterone caproate in the treatment of endometrial cancer. *Obstetrics and Gynecology*, **28**, 309–314.

Sholiton, L. J., Werk, E. E. & Marnell, R. T. (1961) Diurnal variation of adrenocortical function in non-endocrine disease states. *Metabolism*, **10**, 632–646.

Siiteri, P. K. & Wilson, J. D. (1970) Dihydrotestosterone in prostatic hypertrophy. 1. The formation and content of dihydrotestosterone in the hypertrophic prostate of man. *Journal of Clinical Investigation*, **49**, 1737–1745.

Smith, O. W. & Smith, G. V. (1970) Urinary oestrogen profiles and aetiology of breast cancer. *Lancet*, **i**, 1152–1155.

Sneddon, A., Steel, J. M. & Strong, J. A. (1968) Effect of thyroid function and of obesity on discriminant function for mammary carcinoma. *Lancet*, **ii**, 892–894.

Stern, E., Hopkins, C. E., Weiner, J. M. & Marmorston, J. (1964) Hormone excretion patterns in breast and prostate cancer are abnormal. *Science*, **145**, 716–719.

Sweat, M. L. & Bryson, M. J. (1970) Comparative metabolism of progesterone in proliferative human endometrium and myometrium. *American Journal of Obstetrics and Gynecology*, **106**, 193–201.

de Waard, F., Thyssen, J. H. H., Veeman, W. & Sander, P. C. (1968) Steroid hormone excretion pattern in women with endometrial carcinoma. *Cancer*, **22**, 988–993.

Wade, A. P., Davis, J. C., Tweedie, M. C. K., Clarke, C. A. & Haggart, B. (1969) The discriminant function in early carcinoma of the breast. *Lancet*, **i**, 853–857.

Wang, D. Y. (1969) Plasma androgens in breast cancer. In *The Human Adrenal Gland and its Relation to Breast Cancer*, pp. 71–79. Cardiff: First Tenovus Workshop.

Wang, D. Y., Bulbrook, R. D. & Clifford, P. (1968) Plasma levels of the sulphate esters of dehydroepiandrosterone and androsterone in Kenyan men and their relation to cancer of the nasopharynx. *Lancet*, **i**, 1003–1004.

Weiner, J. M., Marmorston, J., Stern, E. & Hopkins, C. E. (1966) Urinary hormone metabolites in cancer and benign hyperplasia of the prostate. *Annals of the New York Academy of Science*, **125**, 974–983.

Werk, E. E., MacGee, J. & Sholiton, L. J. (1964) Altered cortisol metabolism in advanced cancer and other terminal illnesses: excretion of 6-hydroxycortisol. *Metabolism*, **13**, 1425–1438.

Wilson, R. E. & Moore, F. D. (1968) Biochemical and clinical factors in the selection of patients for endocrine surgery. In *Prognostic Factors in Breast Cancer*, ed. Forrest, A. P. M. and Kunkler, P. B., pp. 399–408. Edinburgh and London: Livingstone.

Wilson, J. D. & Gloyna, R. E. (1970) The intranuclear metabolism of testosterone in the accessory organs of reproduction. *Recent Progress in Hormone Research*, **26**, 309–336.

Wotiz, H. H., Shane, J. A., Vigersky, R. & Brecher, P. I. (1968) The regulatory role of oestriol in the proliferative action of oestradiol. In *Prognostic Factors in Breast Cancer*, ed. Forrest, A. P. M. and Kunkler, P. B., pp. 368–382. Edinburgh and London: Livingstone.

Young, H. H. & Kent, J. R. (1968) Plasma testosterone levels in patients with prostatic carcinoma before and after treatment. *Journal of Urology*, **99**, 788–792.

Chapter 3

Endocrine-Induced Regression of Cancers[*]

CHARLES HUGGINS

The natural course can be utterly different in various sorts of malignant disease. Some tumours grow without any apparent restraint whatever. When man harbours a neoplasm of this kind, an increase in the size of the cancer is readily evident from day to day and death ensues in, say six weeks. Conversely, some malignant growths disappear spontaneously. Both of these antipodal effects are rare. Mostly, man with cancer lives one year or a little longer after the neoplasm becomes manifest, and it would appear that some inhibition of growth of the tumour takes place to produce this protracted course.

The net increment of mass of a cancer is a function of the interaction of the tumour and its soil. Self-control of cancers results from a highly advantageous competition of host with his tumour. There are multiple factors which restrain cancer—enzymatic, nutritional, immunologic, the genotype and others. Prominent among them is the endocrine status, both of tumour and host—the subjects of this discourse.

In hormone-responsive cancers, appropriate endocrine modification results in catastrophic effects on cancers of several kinds (Table 3.1) in man and animals, even in those in the terminal stages of the disease. Of course, there ensues pari passu improvement in the host's condition. The results are often spectacular. The benefit can be evident within a few hours after the intervention. The improvement can persist throughout the remainder of the life of the organism; in man regressions lasting more than a decade are not uncommon. There can be complete disappearance of the lesions. But worthwhile benefit ensues only when all or much of the cancer is hormone-responsive and only a small proportion of cancers possess this functional characteristic in pronounced degree.

The therapeutic system of endocrine-restraint of cancer came from the efforts of many workers. I was never alone in my

TABLE 3.1. *Eight hormone-responsive cancers of man and animals*

Type of cancer	Species	References
Carcinoma of breast	Human: female	Beatson, 1896
	male	Farrow & Adair, 1942
	Rat	Huggins, Briziarelli & Sutton, 1959
Carcinoma of prostate	Human	Huggins & Hodges, 1941
Carcinoma of thyroid	Human	Balme, 1954; Crile, 1966
Lymphosarcoma, leukaemia	Mouse	Heilman & Kendall, 1944
	Human	Pearson et al, 1949
Carcinoma of kidney	Hamster	Kirkman, 1959
	Human	Bloom, Dukes & Mitchley, 1963
Carcinoma of endometrium	Human	Kelley & Baker, 1961
Carcinoma of seminal vesicle	Human	Rodriguez Kees, 1964
Carcinoma of scent-glands	Hamster	Kirkman & Algard, 1964
	Dog	Nielsen & Aftsomis, 1964

studies in which one or two students always participated as colleagues. It is a privilege to thank the scores of young men and women who sustained our work.

Lacassagne (1932) was the first to indicate that a correlation probably exists between hormones and the *development* of cancer since injections of oestrone evoked mammary cancer in each of three males of a special strain of mice; carcinoma of the breast had never been observed previously in animals in this category. The proof that hormones can influence the *growth* of cancer was derived from tumours of the prostate of the dog and, later, of man.

The second quarter of our century found the biological sciences much preoccupied with two noble topics: (i) chemistry and physiology of steroids and (ii) biochemistry of organo-phosphorus compounds. The key to the puzzle of the steroid hormones in cancer was the isolation of crystalline oestrone by Doisy, Veler and Thayer (1929) from extracts of urine of pregnant women. In the phosphorus field there were magnificent findings of hexose phosphates, nucleotides, coenzymes and high energy phosphate intermediates. These wonderful discoveries provided the Zeitgeist for our work.

Through the portal of phosphorus metabolism we entered on a series of interconnected observations in steroid endocrinology. A programme was not prepared in advance for this basic physiologic study. The work was fascinating and informative so that it provided its own momentum and served as an end in itself. There were blind alleys but eventually the labyrinth of the experimental series was traversed and we were somewhat amazed to find ourselves studying the effects of hormonal status on advanced cancers of people.

PHOSPHORUS METABOLISM IN THE GENITAL TRACT

The fluid of spermatocele contains spermatozoa which become motile upon exposure to air. It was observed (Huggins and Johnson, 1933) that, remarkably, spermatocele fluid is devoid of acid-soluble phosphorus and free hexoses, whereas human semen contains very large amounts of inorganic phosphorus and a monosaccharide identified as fructose by Mann (1964). At the time of ejaculation in the human male, the environment of spermatozoa is altered by a sharp rise in its content of fructose and acid-soluble phosphorus. We found (Huggins and Johnson, 1933) that the seminal vesicle in man is the chief source of these components in semen.

It was somewhat difficult to obtain unmixed secretions from the various accessory sex glands of man, so a simple technique (Huggins et al, 1939) was devised to collect the prostatic secretion (Figure 3.1) of dogs

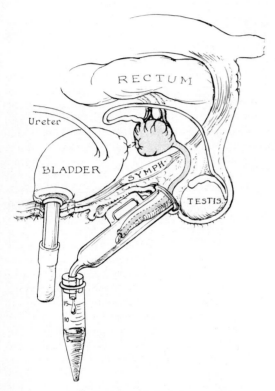

FIGURE 3.1. The prostatic isolation operation.

quantitatively at frequent intervals for years. Often the prostatic fluid of normal adult dogs is secreted for many months with little variation in its quantity or chemical characteristics. This steady state is noteworthy since secretion of the prostate is the end product of a chain of antecedent events involving synthesis of steroids and protein hormones.

Following orchiectomy, the prostate shrinks, the oxidative phase of carbohydrate metabolism declines (Barron and Huggins, 1944), and secretion stops. Testosterone corrects these defects. The cycle of growth and atrophy created by alternately providing and then withholding testosterone was induced repeatedly in the course of the life of the castrate dog. The prostatic cell does not die in the absence of testosterone, it merely shrivels. But the hormone-dependent cancer cell is entirely different. It grows in the presence of supporting hormones but it dies in their absence and for this reason it cannot participate in growth cycles.

A remarkable effect of testosterone is the promotion of growth of its target cells during complete deprival of food. Androstane derivatives conferred on the prostate of puppies a selective nutritional advantage (Pazos and Huggins, 1945) during starvation of three weeks, whereby abundant growth of this gland occurred while there was serious cell breakdown in most of the tissues of the body. It is useless growth since it does not mitigate the ordeal of starvation. It is reminiscent of a nutritional advantage for growth which some malignant tumours possess in undernourished hosts. Starvation does not cure cancer.

HORMONAL CONTROL OF PROSTATE CANCER

It was good fortune that some of our metabolic experiments had been carried out on dogs since this is the only species of laboratory animal in which tumours of the prostate occur. As in man, it is very common to find spontaneous neoplasms of prostate in aged dogs. Among the signs of great age in this species are cataracts and worn teeth. When testes are present in dogs with these stigmata a prostatic tumour is likely; if, in addition, the dog had an interstitial cell tumour of the testis (this was common) a prostatic neoplasm was always found. Most of the canine prostatic tumours are benign growths with much hyperplasia of epithelium and many cysts; carcinoma is usually detected only by histological examination.

At first it was vexatious to encounter a dog with a prostatic tumour during a metabolic study but before long such dogs were sought. It was soon observed (Huggins and Clark, 1940) that orchiectomy or the administration of restricted amounts of phenolic oestrogens caused a rapid shrinkage of canine prostatic tumours.

The experiments on canine neoplasia proved relevant to human prostate cancer; there had been no earlier reports indicating any relationship of hormones to this malignant growth.

Measurement of phosphatases in blood serum furnished the proof that cancer of the prostate in man is hormone-responsive. The methodology is simple and the results are unequivocal. Kutscher and Wolbergs (1940) discovered that acid phosphatase is rich in concentration in the prostate of adult human males. Gutman and Gutman (1938) found that many patients with metastatic prostate cancer have significant increases of acid phosphatase in their blood serum. Cancer of the prostate frequently metastasises to bone, where it flourishes and usually evokes proliferation of osteoblasts. In the school of Robert Robison, Kay (1929) found that brisk osteoblastic activity gives rise to increased alkaline phosphatase levels in serum.

Human prostate cancer which had metastasised to bone was studied at first. The activities of acid and alkaline phosphatases in the blood were measured concurrently at frequent intervals. The methods are reproducible and not costly in time or materials; both enzymes were measured in duplicate in a small quantity (0·5 ml) of serum. The level of acid phosphatase indicated activity of the disseminated cancer cells in all metastatic loci. The titre of alkaline phosphatase revealed the function of the osteoblasts as influenced by the presence of the prostatic cancer cells that were their near neighbours.

By periodic measurement of the two enzymes one obtains a view of overall activity of the cancer and the reaction of non-malignant cells of the host to the presence of that cancer. Thereby the great but opposing influences of, respectively, the administration or deprival of androgenic hormones upon prostate cancer cells were revealed with precision and simplicity. Orchiectomy or the administration of phenolic oestrogens resulted in regression of cancer of the human prostate (Huggins and Hodges, 1941) whereas, in untreated cases, testosterone enhanced the rate of growth of the neoplasm.

Results consistent with the foregoing were obtained by studying another enzyme of the prostate, fibrinolysin, in blood of patients with disseminated prostate cancer. In our metabolic studies it had been found that human prostatic fluid contained large amounts of many proteolytic enzymes (Huggins and Neal, 1942) and especially one which was highly active against fibrin as a substrate. Prostatic fibrinolysin differs from plasmin and trypsin.

Subsequently Tagnon, Whitmore and Shulman (1952) observed that the blood of some patients who have metastases of cancer of the prostate becomes incoagulable because of its concentration of prostatic fibrinolysin. The content of this proteolytic enzyme in serum is reduced or eliminated by the administration of oestrogenic substances or by gonadectomy; orchiectomy is hazardous when the blood is incoagulable but, fortunately, the pills of diethylstilboestrol are effective therapy. Testosterone causes fibrinolysin to reappear in such patients. The entry of prostatic fibrinolysin into the blood is similar to that of acid phosphatase; each enzyme enters the plasma but only from metastasis and not from the primary neoplasm. The antiandrogenic measures restore the coagulability of the blood.

The control of activity of cancer by excision of endocrine glands is physiologic surgery wherein removal of a normal structure can cause healing of distant disease.

Stilboestrol, which had been discovered in 1938 by E. C. Dodds et al (1939), was the first synthetic substance to control cancer; hence the study of the prostate cancers was the start of chemotherapy of malignant disease.

The first series of patients with prostatic cancer treated by orchiectomy (Huggins, Stevens and Hodges, 1941) comprised 21 patients with far advanced metastases; only four of them survived for more than 12 years. Despite regressions of great magnitude, it is obvious that there were many failures of endocrine therapy to control the disease but, on the whole, the life span had been extended by the novel treatments and there had been a decrease of man-pain hours.

CLINICAL MAMMARY CANCER

The first indication that advanced cancer can be induced to regress was the beneficial effect of oophorectomy on cancer of the breast of two women. This empirical observation of Beatson in 1896 was remarkable since it was made before the concept of hormones had been developed. The beneficial action of removal of ovaries was not understood until steroid hormones had been isolated four decades later.

But why does breast cancer thrive in folks who do not possess ovarian function—in men, old women, and females who have had oophorectomy? Farrow and Adair (1942) observed that benefits of great magnitude frequently follow orchiectomy in mammary cancer in the human male. Thereby, they established that testis function can sustain mammary cancer.

A half century after the classic invention of Beatson it was found out that adrenal function can maintain and promote growth of human mammary cancer. The adrenal factor supporting growth of cancer was identified (Huggins and Bergenstal, 1952) when it was shown that bilateral adrenalectomy (with glucocorticoids as substitution therapy) can result in profound and prolonged regression of mammary carcinoma in men and women who do not possess gonadal function. In developing the idea of adrenalectomy for treatment of advanced cancer in man we were considerably influenced by the discovery of Woolley, Fekete and Little (1939) that adrenals can evoke cancer of the breast in the mouse. Regression of great magnitude of human mammary cancer also can be brought about by hypophysectomy (Luft, Olivecrona and Sjögren, 1952) as well as by adrenalectomy.

Haddow, Watkinson and Paterson (1944) found that phenolic oestrogens can have an ameliorative effect in human mammary cancer. A paradox seemed to be involved since, in some circumstances, oestrogenic compounds are activating agents for cancer of the breast. In one room the surgeons were removing sources of oestrogenic hormones, while nearby the physicians were prescribing oestrogens for mammary cancer; both groups were achieving therapeutic triumphs in some cases. Emerson said, "The ambitious soul sits down before each refractory fact". The vexatious paradox was resolved by experimental studies.

EXPERIMENTAL MAMMARY CANCER

Many of the early investigations in this area were carried out on mice and admirable discoveries had been made; chiefly, these concerned the aetiology of mammary cancer. But there was a serious disadvantage in use of the mouse—mammary cancers in this species are seldom hormone-responsive. True, in some strains breast cancer diminished somewhat during lactation (Haddow, 1938; Bielschowsky, 1947; Foulds, 1949) and increased in size during pregnancy. But Mühlbock (1958) found that in most strains of mice mammary cancers are hormone-independent when the tumours have reached palpable size. Yet the thing about cancers is to cure them.

Studies of the rat altered the course of research on breast cancer because this species has a remarkable propensity to develop mammary carcinoma after exposure to aromatics or, to a lesser extent, irradiation. Further, many of the cancers of rat evoked by these methods are completely hormone-dependent and so can be extinguished by endocrine methods.

Compared with mouse and other rodents, rat is extremely vulnerable (Huggins, Ford and Jensen, 1965) to polynuclear aromatic hydrocarbons. In the rat, small amounts of carcinogenic aromatics exert the following effects:

(i) profound depression of incorporation (Huggins, Ford and Jensen, 1965) of thymidine in DNA;

(ii) augmented production of messenger RNA (Loeb and Gelboin, 1964);

(iii) induction of synthesis of a soluble enzyme, menadione reductase (Williams-Ashman and Huggins, 1961) and of microsome-bound enzymes and other proteins (Arcos, Conney and Buu-Hoi, 1961);

(iv) cause cancer or kill the recipient (Huggins and Fukunishi, 1964).

Maisin and Coolen (1936) repeatedly painted mice with 3-methylcholanthrene (3-MC) and observed that, in addition to cancer of the skin, mammary cancer developed in a small but significant percentage of the animals after seven months. Shay et al (1949) fed rats a small dose of 3-MC each day for many months and observed a high incidence of mammary cancer; the tumours were first detected after four months. We found that, under conditions which are highly restricted but easily satisfied, a single massive but tolerable dose of any of a large number (Huggins and Yang, 1962) of polynuclear aromatic hydrocarbons or aromatic amines rapidly and selectively induced breast cancers which were palpable within one month. It is a method of extreme simplicity. Two carcinogenic aromatics, 7,12-trimethyl- and 7,12-

dimethyl-benz(a)anthracene (7,12-DMBA), are more efficient than all others by 10 times.

Whereas a single feeding of a solution of 7,12-DMBA always induces breast tumours (Huggins, Grand and Brillantes, 1961), intravenous injection of a concentrated lipid emulsion (Geyer et al, 1953; Huggins, Morii and Grand, 1961) of the aromatic is more efficacious and has an additional advantage—it introduces the compounds suddenly into the blood as a pulse-dose. When three pulse-doses of 7,12-DMBA were given to Sprague-Dawley female rats, at age 50, 53 and 56 days, mammary tumours were evoked in all animals and large numbers of breast cancers (Huggins, Grand and Fukunishi, 1964) were palpable within four weeks. The superficial location of rat's mammary glands readily permits detection of the cancers by palpation and the end point is sharp because the cancers are firm in consistency and discrete. A tumour weighing 8 to 10 mg can be detected with ease. The earliest mammary cancer was found by histological search on day 11 and by palpation on day 20 after the pulse-dose. This is somewhat comparable to a famous experiment of Rous (1911) who injected a cell-free filtrate of chicken sarcoma I into other fowls and observed the first palpable tumour 10 to 21 days thereafter. In contradistinction to the Rous virus, aromatic hydrocarbons elicit benign tumours of the breast in addition to the cancers.

The mammary cancers of the rat seldom metastasise but kill the host by attaining great size and invading adjacent tissues. Metastases can be produced readily; in the experiments of Dao (1964) injection of mammary cancer cells in portal vein caused multiple cancers in the liver. The respiration values (Rees and Huggins, 1960) of the mammary cancers are similar to those of normal lactating mammary gland. The high rate of glycolysis, which Warburg (1930) found to be distinctive of the metabolism of cancer, prevailed in the induced carcinomas.

Rats are also rather susceptible to the development of mammary cancer after exposure to a big dose of ionising radiation (Hamilton, Durbin and Parrott, 1954; Shellabarger et al, 1957). 7,12-DMBA (Ford and Huggins, 1963) and radiation (Regaud and Blanc, 1906) possess in common the ability to inflict selective lesions of identical sort in rat's testis. With both agents the prime targets are those germinal cells which multiply by mitosis and hence synthesise DNA; in contrast those cells of testis which proliferate by meiosis and do not synthesise DNA are spared from injury by 7,12-DMBA.

HORMONE-DEPRIVAL IN CONTROL OF CANCER

Mammary cancers induced in the male rat by aromatics were not influenced by orchiectomy and hypophysectomy (Huggins and Grand, 1966); by definition, these neoplasms are hormone-independent. In contrast to male rat, most mammary cancers of men wither impressively after deprival of supporting hormones.

The hormone-responsiveness of established mammary cancers induced in female rat by aromatics (Huggins, Briziarelli and Sutton, 1959) or ionising radiation (Huggins and Fukunishi, 1963) is identical; it was a newly recognised property of experimental breast cancers. Prior to this finding, clinical study of patients with mammary cancer was the only material available for investigation of hormonal-restraint of neoplasms of the breast.

In female rat, growth of the mammary cancers was accelerated in pregnancy and by progestational compounds (Huggins, Moon and Morii, 1962). We have not found any dosage of oestradiol-17β which markedly enhanced the growth of these tumours.

In female rat, many but far from all of the induced mammary cancers vanished after removal of ovaries or the pituitary. In our experiments hypophysectomy was the most efficient of all methods to cure rat's mammary cancer. Malignant cells which succumb to hormone-deprival, by definition, are hormone-dependent. The quality of hormone-dependence resides in the tumour cells whereas their growth is determined by the host's endocrine status. Both man and the animals can have some of their cancer cells which are hormone-dependent while other neoplastic cells in the same organism are not endocrine responsive.

The cure of a cancer after hormone-deprival results from death of the cancer cells whereas their normal analogues in the same animal shrivel but survive. It is a basic proposition in endocrine-restraint of malignant disease that cancer cells can differ in a crucial way from ancestral normal cells in response to modification of the hormonal milieu intérieur of the body.

HORMONE-INTERFERENCE IN CANCER CONTROL

It was unexpected to find that mammary cancers can be extinguished by providing excessive amounts of ovarian steroids; this effect is cancer control by hormone-interference.

We induced mammary carcinoma in rats which were then treated for a limited time with large amounts of oestradiol plus progesterone (Huggins et al, 1962). This combination of hormones excited such exuberant growth of normal mammary cells that the breasts resembled those of rats late in pregnancy. Nevertheless, many of the mammary cancers were completely eliminated and 52 per cent of the rats were free from cancer (Huggins and Yang, 1962) six months after steroids had been discontinued. These rats had been cured of cancer because the tumours did not reappear during subsequent pregnancy. The heavy hormonal burden of pregnancy upon mammary cancer had not reactivated dormant cancer cells if any had been present.

In patients, the combination of huge

amounts of progesterone and of oestradiol injected intramuscularly induced measurable and worthwhile improvement (Landau, Ehrlich and Huggins, 1962; Crowley and Macdonald, 1965; Kennedy, 1965) in patients with far advanced disseminated mammary cancer, both in women and men. Moreover, benefit was obtained in patients in whom other forms of endocrine therapy such as adrenalectomy and oophorectomy had previously promoted tumour regression followed by recrudescence.

In another type of hormone-interference, cancer cells are exterminated in parallel with normal cells of similar kind. Glucocorticoids will cause a remission of some lymphogenous tumours and leukaemia. Heilman and Kendall administered large amounts of cortisone to mice bearing a transplanted lymphosarcoma: 'Although dramatic and apparently complete cures are produced, they are only temporary in a majority of animals (Heilman and Kendall, 1944)'. In contrast to the beneficial effects of cortisone, adrenalectomy enhances growth of lymphomas in mouse (Murphy and Sturm, 1943). Pearson et al (1949) found that corticotropin (ACTH) or cortisone caused dramatic if temporary regression in certain cases of human leukaemia and Hodgkin's disease.

Dougherty and White (1943) found that administration of pituitary ACTH to the mouse causes a regression of lymph nodes and thymus. Regression of lymphomas brought about by glucocorticoids does not differ in principle from the effect of corticosteroids on the lymphocytes of normal animals and man.

CONCLUSIONS

Cancer is not necessarily autonomous and intrinsically self-perpetuating. Its growth can be sustained and propagated by hormonal function in the host which is not unusual in kind or exaggerated in rate but which is operating at normal or even subnormal levels.

Hormones, or synthetic substances inducing physiologic effects similar thereto, are of crucial significance for survival of several kinds of hormone-responsive cancers of man and animals. Opposite sorts of change of the hormonal status can induce regression and, in some instances, cure of such cancers. These modifications are deprivation of essential hormones, and hormone interference by giving large amounts of critical compounds.

The control of cancer by endocrine methods can be described in three propositions: (1) Some types of cancer cells differ in a cardinal way from the cells from which they arose in their response to change in their hormonal environment. (2) Certain cancers are hormone-dependent and these cells die when supporting hormones are eliminated. (3) Certain cancers succumb when large amounts of hormones are administered.

References

Arcos, J. C., Conney, A. H. & Buu-Hoi, N. P. (1961) *Journal of Biological Chemistry*, **236**, 1291.

Balme, H. W. (1954) *Lancet*, **i**, 812.

Barron, E. S. G. & Huggins, C. (1944) *Journal of Urology*, **51**, 630.

Beatson, G. T. (1896) *Lancet*, **ii**, 104, 162.

Bielschowsky, F. (1947) *British Medical Bulletin*, **4**, 382.

Bloom, H. J. G., Dukes, C. E. & Mitchley, B. C. V. (1963) *British Journal of Cancer*, **17**, 611.

Crile, G. Jr (1966) *Journal of the American Medical Association*, **195**, 721.

Crowley, L. G. & Macdonald, I. (1965) *Cancer*, **18**, 436.

Dao, T. L. (1964) *Progress in Experimental Tumour Research*, **5**, 157.

Dodds, E. C., Golberg, L., Lawson, W. & Robinson, R. (1939) *Proceedings of the Royal Society, Series B*, **127**, 140.

Doisy, E. A., Veler, C. D. & Thayer, S. (1929) *American Journal of Physiology*, **90**, 329.

Dougherty, T. F. & White, A. (1943) *Proceedings of the Society for Experimental Biology and Medicine*, **55**, 132.

Farrow, J. H. & Adair, F. E. (1942) *Science*, **95**, 654.

Ford, E. & Huggins, C. (1963) *Journal of Experimental Medicine*, **118**, 27.

Foulds, L. (1949) *British Journal of Cancer*, **3**, 345.

Geyer, R. P., Bryant, J. E., Bleisch, V. R., Peirce, E. M. & Stare, F. J. (1953) *Cancer Research*, **13**, 503.

Gutman, A. B. & Gutman, E. B. (1938) *Journal of Clinical Investigation*, **17**, 473.

Haddow, A. (1938) *Journal of Pathology and Bacteriology*, **47**, 553.

Haddow, A., Watkinson, J. M. & Paterson, E. (1944) *British Medical Journal*, **ii**, 393.

Hamilton, J. G., Durbin, P. W. & Parrott, M. (1954) *Journal of Clinical Endocrinology and Metabolism*, **14**, 1161.

Heilman, F. R. & Kendall, E. C. (1944) *Endocrinology*, **34**, 416.

Huggins, C. & Bergenstal, D. M. (1952) *Cancer Research*, **12**, 134.

Huggins, C., Briziarelli, G. & Sutton, H. Jr (1959) *Journal of Experimental Medicine*, **109**, 25.

Huggins, C. & Clark, P. J. (1940) *Journal of Experimental Medicine*, **72**, 747.

Huggins, C. & Ford, E. & Jensen, E. V. (1965) *Science*, **147**, 1153.

Huggins, C. & Fukunishi, R. (1963) *Radiation Research*, **20**, 493.

Huggins, C. & Fukunishi, R. (1964) *Journal of Experimental Medicine*, **119**, 923.

Huggins, C. & Grand, L. C. (1966) *Cancer Research*, **26**, 2255.

Huggins, C., Grand, L. C. & Brillantes, F. P. (1961) *Nature*, **189**, 204.

Huggins, C., Grand, L. & Fukunishi, R. (1964) *Proceedings of the National Academy of Sciences of the United States of America*, **51**, 737.

Huggins, C. & Hodges, C. V. (1941) *Cancer Research*, **1**, 293.

Huggins, C. & Johnson, A. A. (1933) *American Journal of Physiology*, **103**, 574.

Huggins, C., Masina, M. H., Eichelberger, L. & Wharton, J. D. (1939) *Journal of Experimental Medicine*, **70**, 543.

Huggins, C., Moon, R. C. & Morii, S. (1962) *Proceedings of the National Academy of Sciences of the United States of America*, **48**, 379.

Huggins, C., Morii, S. & Grand, L. C. (1961) *Annals of Surgery Supplement*, **154**, 315.

Huggins, C. & Neal, W. (1942) *Journal of Experimental Medicine*, **76**, 527.

Huggins, C., Stevens, R. E. Jr & Hodges, C. V. (1941) *Archives of Surgery*, **43**, 209.

Huggins, C. & Yang, N. C. (1962) *Science*, **137**, 257.

Kay, H. D. (1929) *British Journal of Experimental Pathology*, **10**, 253.

Kelley, R. M. & Baker, W. H. (1961) *New England Journal of Medicine*, **264**, 216.

Kennedy, B. J. (1965) *Cancer*, **18**, 1551.

Kirkman, H. (1959) *National Cancer Institute Monograph*, **1**, 1–58.

Kirkman, H. & Algard, F. T. (1964) *Cancer Research*, **24**, 1569.

Kutscher, W. & Wolbergs, H. (1940) *Zeitschrift für Physiologische Chemie*, **236**, 237.

Lacassagne, A. (1932) *Comptes Rendus Hebdomadaires des Séances de l'Académie des Sciences*, **195**, 630.

Landau, R. L., Ehrlich, E. N. & Huggins, C. (1962) *Journal of the American Medical Association*, **182**, 632.

Loeb, L. A. & Gelboin, H. V. (1964) *Proceedings of the National Academy of Sciences of the United States of America*, **52**, 1219.

Luft, R., Olivecrona, H. & Sjögren, B. (1952) *Nordisk Medicin*, **47**, 351.

Maisin, J. & Coolen, M.-L. (1936) *Comptes Rendus des Séances de la Société de Biologie et de ses Filiales*, **123**, 159.

Mann, T. (1964) *Biochemistry of Semen and of the Male Reproductive Tract*. London: Methuen.

Mühlbock, O. (1958) In *Endocrine Aspects of Breast Cancer*, ed. Currie, A. R., p. 291. Edinburgh: Livingstone.

Murphy, J. B. & Sturm, E. (1943) *Science*, **98**, 568.

Nielsen, S. W. & Aftsomis, J. (1964) *Journal of the American Veterinary Medical Association*, **144**, 127.

Pazos, R. Jr & Huggins, C. (1945) *Endocrinology*, **36**, 416.

Pearson, O. H., Eliel, L. P., Rawson, R. W., Dobriner, K. & Rhoads, C. P. (1949) *Cancer*, **2**, 943.

Rees, E. D. & Huggins, C. (1960) *Cancer Research*, **20**, 963.

Regaud, C. & Blanc, J. (1906) *Comptes Rendus des Séances de la Société de Biologie et de ses Filiales*, **58**, 163.

Rodriguez Kees, O. S.(1964)*Journal of Urology*, **91**, 665.

Rous, P. (1911) *Journal of Experimental Medicine*, **13**, 397.

Shay, H., Aegerter, E. A., Gruenstein, M. & Komarov, S. A. (1949) *Journal of the National Cancer Institute*, **10**, 255.

Shellabarger, C. J., Cronkite, E. P., Bond, V. P. & Lippincott, S. W. (1957) *Radiation Research*, **6**, 501.

Tagnon, H. J., Whitmore, W. F. Jr & Shulman, N. R. (1952) *Cancer*, **5**, 9.

Warburg, O. (1930) *Metabolism of Tumours*. London: Constable.

Williams-Ashman, H. G. & Huggins, C. (1961) *Medicina Experimentalis*, **4**, 223.

Woolley, G. W., Fekete, E. & Little, C. C. (1939) *Proceedings of the National Academy of Sciences of the United States of America*, **25**, 277.

Chapter 4

Steroid Effects upon the Host and his Tumour

WALTER J. MOON

In this chapter we consider the use of steroid therapy in the treatment of tumours not generally regarded as hormone sensitive. These responses represent non-specific host effects of the steroids as opposed to the specific tumour effects by steroids which are being elucidated in other chapters. The sum of the two responses is that usually reported in the patient with a hormone-dependent tumour regressing on therapy. By breaking it into its components, we may learn more about the mechanism of response in hormone-dependent tumours.

Whenever any hormone is being considered for the treatment of malignant neoplastic disease, the clinician weighs up the anticipated tumour effect and the secondary beneficial host effects against any likely unwanted effects that will determine the selection of the drug, its dose and duration of therapy. At best, only a percentage of hormone-dependent tumours will show regression under steroid therapy, but all hosts will react to administered hormones in a dose-determined manner. This reaction may be either beneficial or deleterious and it may be either objective or subjective.

When reporting a favourable subjective response, the therapist tends to downgrade it in much the same fashion as a family apologises for an elderly relative or mentally retarded child. Not so the patient, who is more impressed by subjective improvement, whether or not accompanied by objective tumour control, than he is by a tumour control which does not result in subjective improvement. This illustrates the distinction between 'palliation' and 'tumour response' which has befogged and bedevilled the evaluation of steroid therapy in the treatment of advanced malignant disease.

Corticosteroids and their Synthetic Analogues

EFFECT ON CEREBRAL LESIONS

The presence of either a primary or a metastatic tumour of the brain is associated with cerebral oedema (Scheinberg et al, 1969). The degree of oedema is said to be related more to the rate of growth than to the histological type of tumour (Russell and Rubinstein, 1959). The symptoms produced by the cerebral tumour and the oedema may be focal or may be confined to mental disturbances such as confusion, lethargy, impairment of memory and personality or behavioural changes. In some cases, the presence of a cerebral lesion may be unsuspected and, in the series of Lesse and Netsky (1954), 32 per cent of the patients had 'asymptomatic' tumours in the central nervous system. Nevertheless, it is highly likely that such cerebral lesions do produce effects which are not recognised in the general symptomatology of late cancer. Response to corticosteroids in such cases may be regarded as 'general' improvement and the brightening of the patient's outlook categorised as euphoria.

The anti-oedema effect of the corticoids is used in association with cerebral surgery when the synthetic analogues, betamethasone and dexamethasone, are commonly prescribed. French (1966) has shown by means of cerebral biopsies, that dexamethasone appeared partially to reverse all the changes in oedematous brain tissue, short of necrosis. Although Millburn, Hibbs and Hendrickson (1968) point out that acute oedema developing from radiotherapy has not been documented, corticoids are often used to 'cover' this possibility during a course of cerebral radiotherapy and may be responsible for a significant part of the early improvement.

In clinical practice, corticoid therapy is instituted if symptoms persist after surgery and/or radiotherapy, particularly if they are associated with a neurological deficit sufficient to interfere with function. Corticoid therapy is my initial choice if the diagnosis of cerebral metastasis is made in the presence of active malignant disease elsewhere. Radiotherapy is reserved either for those cases with an incomplete response to corticoid therapy or for those in whom it is considered that survival may be prolonged and the dose of the drug required is likely to produce complications during the anticipated survival of the patient.

All synthetic glucocorticoids share this anti-oedema effect, so the choice of drug is not important. The dose, although empirical, is all important because the response is not 'all or none', but a function of the dose used (King, Moon and Brown, 1965). Reductions of the dose from the optimum for 'that patient at that time' will result in a deterioration which may appear in a few hours or be delayed a week or so, depending on how rapidly the oedema recurs. Increases in the dose, of the order of 50–100 per cent, may be required from time to time to maintain the improved neurological state.

During the initial therapy, the daily amount must be given in four equally divided doses at six-hourly intervals, otherwise considerable fluctuation in clinical state will occur. Once the clinical state is stable and satisfactory, adequate control may be achieved with eight-hourly doses. I have never been satisfied with the results of intermittent therapy or alternate-day therapy, because of clinical fluctuation, despite the attraction of a possible reduction in complications by this means.

A commencing dose of 60 mg of predniso-lone per day, or its equivalent in other analogues, is recommended in most cases. Thereafter, clinical assessments, which are mainly orientated to mental and physical function, level of communication, ambulation, self help and relief of symptoms, are made at 48-hourly intervals. If the clinical state is still less than satisfactory at later assessments, then the dose is increased 50–100 per cent (up to a limit of 500 mg of prednisolone per day) for the ensuing 48 hours. If, at this maximum dose level, the patient's state is still unsatisfactory, the corticoid is gradually withdrawn and radiotherapy or cytotoxic chemotherapy is considered. Sudden reduction in dosage, especially on prolonged therapy, may cause headaches and intracranial hypertension with papilloedema (*Lancet*, 1964).

When the dose level for a satisfactory response is established, it is maintained for seven days, after which it is gradually reduced at 48-hourly intervals until a deterioration is appreciated. The dose is then increased to regain lost ground and becomes the lowest effective dose. When this has been deter-mined, the situation is reviewed and judge-ment made on the following aspects. Has the response been sufficient to justify con-tinuing on the lowest effective dose, relative to the unwanted effects and complications of this dose? Does the overall prognosis warrant added radiotherapy or cytotoxic chemotherapy in the hope that these will further reduce or replace the need for corti-coids? As more experience is gained by the clinician, there is a tendency to accept the unwanted effects of long-term treatment with a higher corticoid dose and to use this as the sole treatment.

EFFECT ON SPINAL CORD COMPRESSION

Spinal cord compression occurring during the course of any neoplastic disease is an emergency situation. The nervous tissue of the spinal cord does not seem to be able to accommodate to compression in the same way as the brain and the critical period be-fore the damage is permanent is much shorter. Recovery of spinal cord function is only possible while the blood supply remains intact and this blood supply seems to be vulnerable both to the acuteness and dura-tion of the compression.

The treatment of spinal cord compression depends on the underlying pathological condition. Extradural compression, due to the lymphomas, usually responds to radio-therapy and systemic chemotherapy, including the corticosteroids for their anti-tumour effect (Williams et al, 1959). But com-pression due to vertebral collapse, secondary to lymphomatous infiltration, or from any cause associated with a solid tumour, is best treated by decompression laminectomy with postoperative radiotherapy.

Corticosteroid therapy is often given in association with spinal cord decompression by laminectomy and continued during sub-sequent radiotherapy, presumably to reduce initial oedema and to prevent the develop-ment of oedema consequent on operative interference and later radiotherapy.

I am unaware of any evidence which, at present, supports the use of corticosteroids in this condition. The variation in the rate and completeness of recovery of spinal cord function after these treatments would make such evidence extraordinarily difficult to obtain.

EFFECT ON RADIATION MYELITIS

There are considerable differences of opinion amongst radiotherapists on the value of corticosteroid therapy in radiation myelitis due, no doubt, to the variation in the natural history of this condition. Because the sub-jective phenomena may be as distressing to the patient as any objective neurological change, I believe that the patient is the best judge of response in any individual case.

Prednisolone in doses of 40–60 mg per day, in divided doses, is given for a period of two weeks and then withdrawn over a further two weeks. If the patient believes he is better on the drug, particularly if he can appreciate any deterioration during its withdrawal, then the prednisolone is resumed at the lowest dose level which gives relief of symptoms.

EFFECT ON PERIPHERAL NERVES

The pain which results from tumour infiltration of peripheral nerves, such as the brachial plexus or the intercostal nerves, may be difficult to relieve with analgesics alone. Not infrequently, the corticosteroids will be of value in controlling this pain, especially if given early. Their effect seems to be reduced if they are given later when, in addition to pain, there are associated paraesthesiae.

EFFECT ON ADVANCED HEAD AND NECK MALIGNANCY

There is a place for corticosteroid therapy in the management of both acute and chronic problems associated with advanced cancer of the head and neck. Loeb and McQuarrie (1968) report simultaneous bilateral neck dissection carried out in six cases without major complications, whereas cerebral oedema and marked venous congestion with facial oedema have frequently attended this procedure in the past. In addition to detailing certain operative precautions, they state: 'the most effective item has been the administration of short-term anti-inflammatory steroids in the operating room and postoperatively for 48 to 72 hours'. In a controlled trial involving the surgical removal of impacted third molar teeth, Hooley and Francis (1969) reported that betamethasone cover reduced the subsequent oedema to one sixth of that of a control group.

A more chronic problem exists in recurrent or inoperable cases of head and neck malignancy in which there is often oedema and brawny induration surrounding the tumour and the treated areas. This oedema may result partly from the presence of the tumour, partly from the effect of previous surgery and/or radiotherapy by interference with vascular and lymphatic supply, and partly from the effect of secondary infection. I have found that the use of diuretics alone is not rewarding at an early stage, but corticosteroids and antibiotics may reduce the oedema sufficiently to bring about worthwhile palliation of pain and an improvement in ability to swallow. The subsequent addition of diuretics, given on alternate days, may still further improve the oedema.

It is usually found that the chronic oedema is worse in the morning, apparently accumulating in the hours of the night when the patient is relatively motionless. For this reason, I have tended to give half the daily dose of prednisolone at 6 a.m., with two further doses at six-hourly intervals. Commencing with a daily dose of 40 mg of prednisolone, this may be increased in two increments until the morning dose is 60 mg and the total daily dose is 120 mg. I have not exceeded 120 mg as a total daily dose and do not exceed 40 mg as maintenance therapy.

EFFECT ON SUPERIOR VENACAVAL BLOCK

Corticosteroids reduce, often partially but rarely completely, the oedema of face, neck and arms associated with the superior venacaval block syndrome and should be combined with diuretics and urgent antitumour therapy, either by chemotherapy or irradiation. When thrombosis is superimposed on the extravascular tumour compression, the corticosteroids will contribute more to the relief of oedema than either radiotherapy or chemotherapy. In the presence of thrombosis, the corticosteroids should be given on a long-term basis combined with anticoagulants.

EFFECT ON LUNG METASTASES

Lymphangitis carcinomatosis is the term applied to diffuse permeation by tumour of the pulmonary lymphatics. In the case of metastatic permeation, the primary cancer frequently arises in the stomach, breast, lung, prostate, pancreas, occasionally in the ovary and sometimes may be one of the lymphomas, but many other sites have been recorded. A series of 154 cases reviewed by Harold (1952) showed a survival of only a few months with progressively increasing dyspnoea, cough, cyanosis and general physical deterioration. I have seen this clinical picture develop acutely in a matter of days. All such patients have survived only for a very short time and, at autopsy, both the lungs and heart have shown hundreds of small tumour emboli. This acute condition is resistant to therapy.

Early in lymphangitis carcinomatosis, a prompt symptomatic relief can often be obtained with corticosteroids with supporting chest physiotherapy, elimination of infection and bronchial dilators. This relief is presumably due to the reduction of oedema and inflammatory reaction which appear to be evoked in the region surrounding the permeation, and relief frequently occurs in the absence of objective clinical or radiological change. By these means, it may be possible to delay the time when the patient requires increasing periods of oxygen therapy.

The dose of prednisolone employed is 60–100 mg per day in divided doses, but this dose frequently has to be increased to maintain relief as progressive disease puts more and more lung out of action.

More discrete pulmonary metastases may also be surrounded by a zone of reaction which increases their effective size, causing dyspnoea and a cough of a lesser degree than in lymphangitis carcinomatosis. Corticosteroids frequently palliate these symptoms.

Objective regression of lymphangitis carcinomatosis is rarely seen, but may sometimes be achieved by corticoids combined with cytotoxic chemotherapy or by specific hormone therapy appropriate to the primary cancer. Schwarz et al (1969) report the case of a 60-year-old male patient with a primary adenocarcinoma of the prostate who developed lymphangitis carcinomatosis while on stilboestrol. All manifestations, including the pulmonary infiltration, regressed following orchidectomy and this control was still present thirteen months later when the case was reported. Emirgil, Zsoldos and Heinemann (1964) reported a short-lived response, with both symptomatic relief and improvement in pulmonary function studies, in a patient with lymphangitic pulmonary infiltration from a carcinoma of the breast treated with prednisone. The patient survived for ten months and finally died with liver metastases and hepatic coma.

When large volumes of lung are irradiated, as in the tangential technique for breast irradiation, the delayed radiation effect on the lung is associated with oedema and fibrosis which may cause dyspnoea, cough and a wheeze, with fine crepitations in the area of lung involved. Corticosteroids will produce a symptomatic improvement quite rapidly and it is possible that their prolonged use may reduce the ultimate fibrosis.

Gracey and Divertie (1970) have reported a biopsy proven case of diffuse interstitial pulmonary fibrosis in which prednisolone in high doses (60 mg a day) brought about both symptomatic improvement and an almost complete return to normal lung architecture on later biopsy.

EFFECT ON LIVER METASTASES

Reference is made by Sherlock (1970) to a trial by Cook, Mulligan and Sherlock (1970) using prednisolone in patients with active chronic hepatitis, which was concluded after six years when the results so greatly favoured the prednisolone treated group that it became unjustifiable to continue further. The authors considered that, aside from any possible beneficial effect in suppressing immune responses, the prednisolone had a marked effect on parameters which are apparently specific measures of hepatocellular function.

There is experimental evidence (John and

Miller, 1969) and observations in man (Cain, Mayer and Jones, 1970) quoted by Sherlock (1970), that prednisolone therapy is associated with significant increases in the plasma concentration and rate of synthesis of albumen. The above evidence suggests the possibility that prednisolone might have a direct effect on hepatocellular function. Added to this, there is some evidence (Pack and Molander, 1960) that cortisone enhances liver regeneration and has a protective effect against liver injury (Hall and Bieri, 1953; Olson, 1959).

In patients with long-continued high serum bilirubin, corticosteroids may cause a sharp fall in serum bilirubin level (Mills, 1964). This steroid 'whitewash' (Shaldon and Sherlock, 1957) occurs in both hepatocellular and obstructive jaundice and this mitigates against its value in differentiating between the two conditions (Chalmers et al, 1956). There is usually no significant rise in faecal pigment and there is a fall in urinary bilirubin. There is no evidence that the half life of red cells is changed by the steroid, but it seems that the serum bilirubin is reduced by increasing its excretion by a metabolic pathway other than by the pigments normally measured in the excreta.

Taylor, Perlia and Kofman (1958), reporting on the effects of corticosteroids in breast cancer, state, 'painful hepatomegaly, due to metastatic disease, was reduced in several', but such a response was frequently associated with the appearance of new metastatic lesions or the growth of old ones.

Stoll (1969) writes of corticosteroid therapy: 'pain arising from metastases . . . in the liver is usually markedly reduced. Nevertheless, in the majority of cases in which such subjective benefit results, there is little or no associated objective evidence of tumour regression.' Similar effects can be seen where the liver metastases arise from primary neoplasms which are not themselves responsive to hormones.

The benefit to the patient resulting from the corticosteroids may be the disappearance or reduction of jaundice, with relief of nausea, vomiting, anorexia and lethargy. Although some authors report decrease in size of the liver, I have not found this to be a frequent occurrence with corticosteroids alone. In the absence of a reduction in liver size and weight, there may be no relief from the heavy, dull and dragging feeling in the upper abdomen so often complained of in hepatomegaly. Such relief may, however, be obtained by radiotherapy or appropriate cytotoxic chemotherapy.

In cases of pain, often severe, due to metastases invading the liver capsule, the corticosteroids will frequently reduce the pain quite dramatically and allow both analgesics and radiotherapy to be deferred or withheld, especially in ill patients.

Thus it would appear that the effects of the corticosteroids on metastatic liver disease, in the absence of tumour control, indeed with growth of active tumour elsewhere, must be due to a host effect.

EFFECT ON HYPERCALCAEMIA

Most cancer patients with hypercalcaemia have osseous metastases, indicated by radiological or isotope scanning evidence or suspected because of pain. In these cases of demonstrable bone destruction, it is easy to believe that this local bone dissolution results in an upset in the blood-bone equilibrium, with more calcium coming from bone than is being deposited in bone. This concept is strengthened by reports of minimal gastrointestinal absorption of calcium and enhanced urinary calcium excretion in patients with widespread osteolytic metastases (Lazlo et al, 1952; Pearson et al, 1952; Lazor, Rosenberg and Carbone, 1963; Watson, 1964). If, in addition, the bony lesions are painful, the resultant inactivity will increase the calcium being mobilised from the bones (David, Verner and Engel, 1962; Jowsey, 1966).

In order to explain hypercalcaemia in the absence of bone metastases, the suggestion had been made by Albright that some malignancies might produce a hormone factor. Evidence for the elaboration by certain tumours of a substance biologically and immunologically similar to parathyroid peptide was reviewed by Bower and Gordan (1965), Munson, Tashjian and Levine (1965) and Watson (1966), and extended by Berson and Yalow (1966), and Sherwood et al (1967).

In addition, osteolytic sterols have been identified in the plasma and tumour extracts of patients with breast cancer, both local and disseminated, and in nursing mothers, but not in the plasma of normal non-lactating women or in normal breast tissue (Gordan, Fitzpatrick and Lubich, 1967). So far, it has not been determined whether the sterols arise from tumour synthesis or from the diet. While it has been shown that human breast cancer tissue can lyse bone in rats (Gordan et al, 1962), presumably because of its osteolytic sterol content, the relationship between these sterols and hypercalcaemia can only be assumed. The osteolytic sterols have been shown to be qualitatively present in more cases of mammary cancer than exhibit hypercalcaemia, and also at times other than during episodes of hypercalcaemia (Gordan, 1967).

Should the osteolytic sterols arise from synthesis by neoplastic cells, it is interesting to speculate whether one action of the steroids in the hypercalcaemia of breast cancer may be to affect the production, release, distribution or excretion of the osteolytic sterols. The hypercalcaemia sometimes provoked by the sex hormones may result from increased sterol production or release, whereas the corticosteroids may have the opposite effect. These actions, both of the corticosteroids and the sex steroids on the suggested sterol production by the tumour, may be independent of their ability beneficially to influence tumour growth, because the corticoids can control hypercalcaemia in the absence of tumour control, and Hall, Dederick and Nevinny (1963) found clinical evidence of

tumour healing on persisting with androgen therapy in patients with androgen-induced hypercalcaemia.

There may be some benefit in 'covering' with corticoids the initial period of administration of the sex hormones. It may help to reduce the incidence of induced hypercalcaemia in patients with either widespread bony metastases, a serum calcium level at the upper limit of normal or increased urinary calcium excretion.

The correction of hypercalcaemia by corticosteroid therapy was originally observed in sarcoidosis (Shulman, Schoenrich and Harvey, 1952; Dent, Flynn and Naborro, 1953). Since then, many authors have reported on the effectiveness of corticosteroids in reducing the concentration of serum calcium in some, but not all patients with hypercalcaemia of non-parathyroid origin (Connor et al, 1956; Myers, 1958; Merigan and Hayes, 1961; Watson, 1964). In the case of hypercalcaemia associated with cancer, Watson (1966) reports that it is only in far advanced disease that corticosteroids will fail to cause a fall in elevated serum calcium levels. Gardner (1969) considers that 70 per cent of hypercalcaemic patients with breast cancer will respond to fluid and corticoid administration. Thyrocalcitonin has not been shown to be effective in hypercalcaemia associated with malignant disease.

Corticosteroids reduce the serum calcium level by their action on the kidneys. This action is to increase the renal blood flow and glomerular filtration rate (McMahon et al, 1960), to increase calcium clearance due to a fall in the tubular reabsorption of calcium (Laake, 1960; Gardner and Gordon, 1962). Corticosteroids may possibly antagonise antidiuretic hormone at the tubular level (Ahmed et al, 1967), or inhibit antidiuretic hormone release from the posterior pituitary (Davis et al, 1969).

Within normal ranges of serum calcium concentration, increasing the urinary volume would not be expected to increase urinary calcium excretion, since there is an efficient tubular reabsorption mechanism for this ion. Once hypercalcaemia exists, the maximum tubular absorption capacity for calcium is exceeded and the rate of urinary calcium excretion becomes a function of the rate of urine flow. The critical serum calcium level is approximately 12 mg/100 ml, and above this level the maximum tubular reabsorption rate is exceeded and an increased urinary output increases urinary calcium loss.

The details of treatment of hypercalcaemia are covered in other chapters.

EFFECT ON IMMUNE RESPONSE

The importance of corticosteroid depression of the immune response will only become apparent in the future when the part played by immunity in the control of cancer is more fully understood. Green (1954), Burnet (1957) and later Thomas (1959) suggested that an immunosurveillance mechanism might operate in the control of cancer. Sir Gordon Gordon-Taylor (1959) expressed the perplexity which has been felt by many clinicians faced with examples of long free interval, slow growth and even apparent spontaneous regression of cancer.

IMMUNOSURVEILLANCE AND CANCER

The unpredictable resistance of the individual to cancer invasion is reviewed by Keast (1970) who presents the evidence for a system of immunosurveillance. Doll and Kinlen (1970) elaborate the evidence based on human observation. If such a system exists, its degree and duration may determine, firstly, whether a malignant transformation develops, and, secondly, the rate and extent of local and metastatic spread.

If immunological competence can be stimulated, this should achieve some degree of tumour control and, on this point, Mathé (1969) indicated that, although approaches to cancer control by immunological means were still at the experimental level, some had

progressed to the stage of early clinical trials. Some temporary effects upon malignant melanoma have been reported from the injection of irradiated tumour cells (Ikonopisov et al, 1970).

On the other hand, suppression of immunity should result in loss of tumour control. Doll and Kinlen (1970) review the literature on the appearance of primary malignant tumours following immunosuppression for organ transplants. There appears to be a fifty-fold increase in the incidence of the reticuloses in such cases and over forty primary malignant neoplasms have been recorded in the literature. Of particular interest are seven reports of malignant transplantation coincidentally when kidneys, apparently clear of tumour, were used from donors dying of malignancy. In one such case (Wilson et al, 1968), the recipient of a kidney from a donor with bronchogenic carcinoma developed an abdominal tumour. This was partially excised and cessation of immuno-suppressive measures was followed by total disappearance of the neoplastic tissue, confirmed at later laparotomy. Zukoski et al (1970) reported the development of pulmonary metastases in a similar case, the metastases disappearing on withdrawal of immunosuppressive measures.

Studies in animals have demonstrated that a number of factors, some of which are immunosuppressants, enhance the tendency of tumours to metastasise. These factors include, firstly, the size, rate and duration of tumour growth, secondly, various hormonal factors—ACTH, corticosteroids and growth hormone—and thirdly, treatment by irradiation or cytotoxic chemotherapy.

Sherlock and Hartman (1962) reported a significant difference in the distribution of metastases from breast cancer between a control group and a group treated with corticosteroids in pharmacological doses. The treated group had an increased incidence of metastases to the opposite breast, the gastrointestinal tract, spleen and brain. Patients to whom the corticosteroids were given at replacement levels, showed only an increased incidence of metastases of the spleen.

The occasional observation in breast cancer patients of reactivation of local tumour, confined for some considerable time to the field of irradiation, is suspicious of a breakdown of local immunity. Moreover, the shortened survival of patients with carcinoma of the lung treated with corticoids (Wolf et al, 1960) may be the result of immunosuppression on the tumour or of reduced resistance to bacterial infection.

In the presence of widespread human cancer, there is evidence of a depression of immune response to tetanus toxoid (Lytton, Hughes and Fulthorpe, 1964) and to skin tuberculin testing (Hughes and Mackay, 1965). This applies also to tetanus toxoid in the reticuloses (Barr and Fairley, 1961). However, early in the course of these diseases, immune responses are normal. It has not yet been determined at what stage the immune response fails in the course of human neoplastic disease.

The concept of immunosurveillance would imply critical periods in the course of tumour growth, firstly when it is established locally, and again when it metastasises. Immunosuppression would occur at each site of metastasis and, finally, when the tumour becomes widespread, there is a general suppression of immune response. Whatever causes the induction of malignant transformation, the establishment of metastases may depend on local immunosuppression, either by immunologic paralysis or by hormone action, so metastases may occur early or late, and be many or few.

This concept of immunosurveillance may mean that the cancer is widespread because the immune response is reduced, and treatment should be directed towards supporting the immune response, or at least not further suppressing it by corticoids or chemotherapeutic immunosuppressants. It is known that the cancer cell produces a variety of hormonally active substances. Some of these,

for example the parathyroid-like hormones and the osteolytic sterols, may be active in preparing bone for the development of metastases (Segaloff, 1963; Bower and Gordan, 1965). Other hormones are known to enhance metastases in animals, for example ACTH and growth hormone, and local secretion of these hormones by the tumour may provide one explanation of the local or metastatic spread of the tumour in man. Another possibility is that the increasing tumour mass may produce such an amount of antigen as to cause immunologic paralysis, resulting both in tumour spread and loss of general immune competence.

While Denoix (1970) accepts the ability of corticoids to suppress the BCG reaction, he also states that there is no evidence that these drugs affect the body defences against human breast cancer. When the disease is widespread, any further damage to the immune status of the patient by corticoids or other immunosuppressive agents may not be relevant. Despite this, it is probably wise, in early cancer, to be cautious in the prolonged and continuous use of immunosuppressive drugs, such as corticoids or cytotoxic agents.

In early cancer, the clinical end result of anti-tumour therapy which is also immunosuppressive, may reflect the difference between the benefits of tumour cell damage (with a reduction in either the amount of tumour antigen or immunosuppressive hormone produced by the tumour cells) and the ill effects of the immunosuppression produced by the therapy. In early cancer, it is important that immunosuppressive anti-tumour therapy should be given only for disease that is actively progressing. It is equally important to be able to assess tumour response to therapy as early as possible, so as not to persist in a therapy which may be more than just not beneficial, but may be harmful. If, in addition to early tumour assessment, some simple test could be used to determine progressively the degree of immunological competence in each individual patient, then immunosuppressive anti-tumour therapy might be used rationally. At present, we can only assess the benefit which accrues from such therapy. Are the ill-effects concealed in the manifestations of non-responding disease?

SEX HORMONES AND THE RETICULO-ENDOTHELIAL SYSTEM

Natural oestrogens of high potency are also potent stimulators of the reticulo-endothelial system. So also are the highly potent synthetic oestrogens, diethyl stilboestrol and oestradiol monobenzoate. However, the two properties do not always parallel in synthetic oestrogens. The other sex hormones, testosterone and progesterone, have little effect on phagocytic activity (Stuart, 1970).

Small doses of cortisone stimulate granulopoietic function while larger doses cause dissolution of lymphoid tissue and acute atrophy of the thymus. Large doses reduce the resistance of man to bacteria, viruses and fungi (Stuart, 1970). Further references to this subject are made in Chapter 5 and 21.

THE PLACE OF SUPPORTIVE CORTICOSTEROID THERAPY

The corticosteroids are of proven value for their anti-oedema and anti-inflammatory effects in cerebral metastases and neoplastic infiltration of peripheral nerves, for the oedema of both advanced head and neck malignancy and superior venacaval block, and in pulmonary infiltration.

The symptoms of both liver metastases and hypercalcaemia may improve because of the host effect of the corticosteroids, along with improvement in the biochemical abnormalities associated with these conditions.

The beneficial effect of corticosteroids in spinal cord compression and any effect,

either good or bad, mediated through immune mechanisms remain unproven. The benefits of this therapy in radiation myelitis are mainly subjective.

SUBJECTIVE EFFECTS OF CORTICOSTEROIDS

Whether he denies his diagnosis and prognosis or not, the patient with advanced cancer is still left with the daily burden of living with his disease. Some contend with, some are crushed by, but none can ignore this burden. The corticosteroids, by their neuropsychic reaction, may enable this burden to be more easily carried. The patient finds strength, often physical, but more often mental, to regain as much of normal life as the disease will allow and his attendants permit. Appetite frequently returns and may be enhanced even in the presence of continuing weight loss. Sometimes these drugs create such an abnormal feeling of vigour and spurious good health that even the clinician may begin to doubt his former estimates of prognosis.

HAZARDS OF CORTICOSTEROID THERAPY

The hazards of corticoid therapy are well known and are related to the selected drug, dose and duration of therapy. At any particular stage of the disease, it is a matter of precise clinical judgement whether the hazards outweigh the benefits which may be produced by corticoid therapy. In late cancer, this is not always easy to do. As Philip Massinger says, too often are we 'driven into a desperate strait and cannot steer a middle course'. For some clinicians, corticosteroids are to be used like Drake's Drum, 'when your powder's runnin' low' (Newbolt), for others 'in vain, with lavish kindness' (Heber).

Androgens

The male sex hormones have two main actions which may be designated androgenic or virilising, and anabolic. In cancer therapy, the virilising effects are usually unwanted and are acceptable only when, in addition, tumour control can be established and maintained.

ANABOLIC EFFECTS

The anabolic effects of androgens are brought about by the conversion of ribonucleic-acid-amino-acid conjugates to microsomal nucleo-protein, which results in nitrogen retention and the synthesis of new body protein, mainly in muscles. Although the sexual target tissues are more responsive, testosterone exerts an anabolic effect on all tissues. The so-called anabolic steroids stimulate protein anabolism in general, without a selective action upon the sexual tissues. On the other hand, the anabolism of the oestrogens is mainly confined to the female sexual tissues and does not significantly affect general protein metabolism.

The therapeutic index is the anabolic-androgenic ratio and, for the more efficient anabolic steroids, is between 2 and 3. This index is reduced the longer the drug is administered, with concurrent corticosteroid administration, and in hypogonadal adults, so that, in these circumstances, the so-called anabolic steroids will virilise with a potency approaching that of testosterone.

In addition to the anabolic effect of either endogenous or exogenous androgenic hormones, adequate calories, proteins and other nutrients are required for protein anabolism. While the non-specific effects of the anabolic steroids in increasing appetite and promoting a feeling of wellbeing frequently ensure the satisfaction of the nutritional needs, it is only rarely in late cancer that these anabolic steroids actually succeed in building up body protein. At best, there may occasionally be a reduction in rate of weight loss with a subjective increase in energy.

SEX HORMONES IN OSTEOPOROSIS

The problem of osteoporosis may arise during the course of cancer, firstly, as a diagnostic problem in the radiology of bones in a patient with potential bony metastases, particularly if pain is also present; secondly, during long-term corticosteroid therapy; and lastly, in the management of the elderly patient.

The evidence that osteoporosis is a condition towards which all people gradually progress after the age of 20 is reviewed by Rose (1966). Among other things, this process can be accelerated by corticosteroids given in excess of replacement needs, excess being defined as anything above 7 mg daily of prednisone or its equivalent (*British Medical Journal*, 1967).

The effects of androgens, oestrogens and the synthetic anabolic agents on the adult skeleton appear to be qualitatively similar (Harris and Heaney, 1969). In acute studies, these hormones depress bone resorption with little or no effect on formation. With continued treatment, resorption remains at the depressed level, but bone formation is found to be decreased rather than increased and the skeletal balance returns to equilibrium without any increase in bone mass. Repeated kinetic studies in the same patients reported by Harris and Heaney (1969) show a reduction in bone formation beginning some time after the sixth month of therapy with sex steroids. They considered that the hormone therapy had reduced resorption, but that

the body had responded by reducing formation to match, positive balance being confined
to the interval when the one was catching up
with the other.

The osteoporosis induced by the corticosteroids cannot be prevented by the use of
anabolic steroids (Jackson, 1967). Using both
isotope and balance studies, Dymling,
Isaaksson and Sjogren (1962) could demonstrate no significant changes in calcium
metabolism and osteoporosis in humans
treated with anabolic hormones.

The evidence so far produced for the
value of oestrogens in female osteoporosis is
unconvincing (Seventeenth Rheumatism
Review, 1966; Raisz, 1970). Placebos have
been found to be as effective as the sex
hormones in relieving bone pain (Solomon,
Dickerson and Ei nberg, 1960).

ORAL ANABOLIC STEROID EFFECT ON GLUCOCORTICOID METABOLISM

The orally active anabolic steroids increase
the half life of cortisol by interfering with the
reduction of the cortisol to dihydrocortisol
in the liver (Wynn, 1967). Given to patients
after ablation of the pituitary or adrenal
glands, the oral anabolic steroids may
prolong the half life of the replacement
corticosteroids so that the combination has
an effect at a level above replacement needs.
This action of the oral anabolic steroids
on the synthetic glucocorticoids is variable.
The effect on some patients is similar to that
described for cortisol, but in most, the biological activity of the synthetic glucocorticoids
is not altered. The parenterally administered
anabolic agents do not have this effect
(Wynn, 1967).

ANDROGENS AND ERYTHROPOIESIS

The effects of hormones on erythropoiesis
have been studied in both animals and man
and, in the latter, many authors report
stimulation of erythropoiesis by androgens
(Brodsky and Kahn, 1967; Brodsky et al,
1965; Gardner and Pringle, 1961a, b);
Kennedy, 1962). However, Greenwald (1967)
suggested that, because of the lack of well
designed, controlled studies, there is still
considerable doubt as to the usefulness of
the androgens as marrow stimulants.

Many reports need to be reconciled.
Gurney and Fried (1965) showed that 48
hours after the second of two daily subcutaneous injections of 2·5 mg testosterone
propionate, the plasma of female mice
contained an elevated level of erythropoietic
stimulating factor. Clinical experience in
man shows that the increased erythropoiesis
resulting from androgens comes on after
two and, more frequently, three months of
treatment (Kennedy, 1965a, b); Sanchez-
Medal et al, 1964; Sanchez-Medal, Gomez-
Leal and Duarte-Zapata, 1966; Allen et al,
1968; Alexanian, 1969).

Evidence in rodents suggests that the action
of testosterone on erythropoiesis is mediated
through erythropoietin (Mirand, Gordon and
Wenig, 1965) and, in addition, it has been
shown that erythropoietin antibodies suppress the enhancement of erythropoiesis
induced by testosterone (Schooley, 1966).
But in patients with aplastic anaemia, the
level of erythropoietin may be high initially,
yet fall even while erythropoiesis is showing
stimulation as a result of androgen therapy.
It is presumed that the erythropoietin level
falls as the stimulus of the anaemia is reduced
and the bone marrow erythroid-precursor
pool expands (Gardner and Nathan, 1966).
These authors suggest that, for successful
androgen therapy in man, a minimum
number of erythroid precursors must be
present in the spleen or the bone marrow and
that these erythroid precursors are stimulated directly by androgens to repopulate
the marrow. This mechanism is independent
of erythropoietin production.

Kennedy (1962) reported that a slight
decrease in the haemoglobin level occurred
during the first month of androgen therapy

and regarded this as a dilutional effect due to the increase in plasma volume from the sodium and fluid retaining effects of the hormone. But Verwilghen et al (1966) claim that the later rise in haemoglobin level following the administration of anabolic androgens is predominantly due to haemo-concentration.

Brown, Altschuler and Cooper (1963) considered that large doses of testosterone in man could alter the lipid content of the erythrocytes, resulting in haemolysis which stimulated erythropoiesis. The addition of corticosteroids could be expected to reduce haemolysis (Gardner and Pringle, 1961b). Allen et al (1968) combined oxymetholone with doses of prednisone from 15–60 mg per day and obtained a satisfactory bone marrow response in aplastic anaemia. Kennedy (1965a) also suggested that the addition of corticosteroid therapy improves results. The combination of androgens and corticoids is not always necessary because a haemo-poietic response is common in patients receiving only an androgenic hormone (Sanchez-Medal et al, 1964).

Hormones, other than androgens, have been shown, under certain conditions, to have an effect on erythropoiesis. Cortico-steroids intensify the effects of erythropoietin in hypophysectomised rats (Mirand et al, 1965). On the other hand, both natural and synthetic oestrogens overcome the stimulating effect of hypoxia on erythropoiesis and the stimulation of red cell formation by erythro-poietin in mole rats can be reversed by the administration of oestrogen. The inhibitory effect of oestrogen can be partly overcome by the amount of erythropoietin used (Dukes and Goldwasser, 1961).

Growth hormone may also be a factor in erythropoiesis. Jepson and McGarry (1968) found that pituitary dwarfs on maintenance doses of thyroid hormone and adrenal steroids had a red cell mass level which was 50–75 per cent of normal. The addition of human growth hormone raised the level to within the normal female range, and the

further addition of testosterone increased the level to the normal male range.

In spite of the confusion as to the mechan-ism of action, there is no doubt as to the efficiency of androgen therapy in some cases. However, the effective dose of androgens is large. It should be stressed that in order to achieve a satisfactory erythropoietic response in females, the risk of moderate to severe virilisation must be accepted by the patient. For the clinician, certain guidance can be given. Dosage of testosterone propionate is 100 mg intramuscularly three times a week; of testosterone enanthate 400–1600 mg IMI once a week (Kennedy, 1965b); and of oral oxymetholone 3–4 mg/kg/day (Allen et al, 1968). The daily oral dose of fluoxyme-sterone is 10 mg/m² for hypogonadal males and anaemic females, but a dose of 40 mg/m² is required for anaemic males (Alexanian, 1969).

Prolonged treatment is necessary and the initial response may take two to four months to appear. If the patient is iron deficient or develops relative iron lack during the res-ponse, the red cell mass will not be augmented. The response in any one patient is unpredict-able, but Sanchez-Medal et al (1966) report a remission rate in aplastic anaemia of 70 per cent of those treated for over two months (oxymetholone) and Alexanian (1969) re-ports that, of patients treated for at least three months, two thirds developed an eleva-tion in red cell volume of in excess of 15 per cent (fluoxymesterone).

THE PLACE OF SUPPORTIVE ANDROGEN THERAPY

Despite their popularity, based on clinical impressions, the androgens are not effective in building up body protein or in reducing osteoporosis in the patient with advanced cancer. The erythropoietic effect of the androgens is bought at the price of gross virilisation in the female and a delay of at least two months from the onset of therapy in both male and female. There is no good evidence that the androgens protect against the side effects of cytotoxic therapy as is discussed below.

ANDROGENIC EFFECT AND LIBIDO

Both the crisis of primary cancer diagnosis and treatment, and the stress of persistent cancer place emotional, physical and intellectual burdens on husband and wife, no matter which one is the patient. There is no need to emphasise the enormous importance of psychological and emotional influences on the act of sexual intercourse. Frequently, the cancer or its treatment leads to a disturbance of the techniques and aesthetics of intercourse, resulting in an unnecessary cessation of the sex life of the patient. Continence may be indicated for part of, but not necessarily for all the course of fatal cancer. Unnecessary abstinence may add further burdens to the relationships of a married couple. For example, courteous abstinence by her husband may only confirm her loss of femininity in the eyes of a woman with a mastectomy, ovarian ablation or hysterectomy. For a man with a colostomy, his wife's abstinence may be interpreted as revulsion.

Where normal relationships are not physically disturbed, they may be intellectually and emotionally desired, but psychologically inhibited. In this situation, a short course of androgens, such as fluoxymesterone 2·5–5 mg per day for one to two months may increase libido sufficiently to overcome this inhibition. Equally, it is well to remember that, for the single woman or the widow, androgens in the larger doses used in therapy, may be an intolerable trial to her sexual composure.

Protection against the Side-effects of Cytotoxic Drugs

The common belief that steroids can protect against the side effects of cytotoxic agents rests more on clinical impressions than on controlled trials. In most reports in the literature, the absence of a control group, the smallness of patient numbers and the range of variables, all combine to cast doubt on the conclusions. Nevertheless the administration of steroids may have other beneficial effects.

An example of the problem is in reports on the combination of androgens and thiotepa in the treatment of breast cancer. Watson and Turner (1959) (23 patients) and Cree (1960) (11 patients) suggested that androgens protected the marrow, but not the tumour, against thiotepa. However, Rider (1960) (11 patients), Stoll and Matar (1961) (9 patients) and Lyons and Edelstyn (1962) (46 patients) failed to confirm such protection.

Carbone (1963), Kennedy (1965a, b), Brodsky and Kahn (1967) and Brodsky, Denis and Kahn (1964) have reported beneficial effects in cancer chemotherapy from androgens on the bone marrow, not confined to erythropoiesis. Condit (1960), however, mentioned testosterone administration (along with renal failure and previous marrow damage) as decreasing the tolerance to methotrexate. This effect of androgen therapy was also noted by Vogler, Huguley and Kerr (1965).

Greenwald (1967), in his monograph on cancer chemotherapy, regards the suggestion of marrow protection by steroids as not proven, and in a similar monograph, Boesen and Davis (1969) do not mention the use of steroids in marrow protection. Perry (1969), in a paper entitled 'Reduction of Toxicity in Cancer Chemotherapy', refers only obliquely to corticoids in dealing with the problem of incompatibility in platelet transfusion.

In malignant disease, agranulocytosis can result from the production of autoantibodies (Killman, 1960). It can also result from the effect of some drugs which may cause leucocyte agglutination. Videbaek (1969) states that little is known of the true value of corticosteroids in immune agranulocytosis. Antigens may appear in blood cells after treatment by alkylating agents or ionising radiation so that an immunologic response may increase the acute tissue injury from these agents. Some protection from this immunologic response has been conferred by immunosuppressive therapy (Harrington, Pugh and Pochron, 1967).

If corticosteroids cause an increase in the circulating leucocyte level, the increased count does not necessarily represent increased production or increased availability at a tissue level. In the presence of marrow hypoplasia, the so-called capillary tightening effect of the corticosteroids may block the egress of leucocytes from the blood vessels into the tissues. In addition to this reduced migration from the vessels, there is a mobilisa-tion of neutrophils from the marginal granulocyte pool.

It is possible that, in the future, marrow damage will be minimised by administering corticoids at a scheduled time before the cytotoxic agent. Decreased toxicity in mice by scheduling the administration of cortisone and the cycle-orientated drug 6-thioguanine was reported by LePage and Kaneko (1969). These authors investigated the effect of cortisone in protecting the marrow by de-pression of DNA synthesis at a time when high levels of 6-thioguanine were present. However, for such a principle to be applied in man, we would need to be certain that the tumour cells are not similarly protected by cortisone. It is obvious that such a technique can be applied only to cycle-orientated cytotoxic agents.

To sum up, while at present the best evidence for steroid protection of the marrow is limited to the use of androgens for stimula-tion of erythropoiesis, controlled trials, especially with the scheduling of drugs, may usefully extend our application of the pre-sently available drugs and indicate the desiderata for future agents.

Oestrogens

There are those who advocate the continuous use of oestrogens for the duration of life in a postmenopausal woman to reduce the inci-dence of adverse cardiovascular effects in the ageing woman, as well as osteoporosis and some other aspects of ageing. Kupperman (1967) goes so far as to say that this continu-ous use of oestrogens 'is no longer in the realm of the investigator'. In addition, it is well known that symptoms of the female climac-teric may persist for some considerable time and some of these symptoms respond to oestro-gens. It is essential to distinguish between these effects and true tumour growth control in assessing the benefits of oestrogen treatment of advanced carcinoma of the breast.

Tumour-Host Relationships

TUMOUR IMMUNITY AND HOST IMMUNITY

Most hormones exhibit multiple actions on normal tissues, such as regulating growth, development and a variety of metabolic functions. It is not known whether the hormones produce these different effects by their action at a single site or whether there are multiple sites of action, with a different site for each major effect (Tata, 1969). Equally, we do not know whether the anti-tumour activity of the hormones results from any of the mechanisms by which they act on normal tissues or from unrelated actions.

According to our present criteria, only a percentage of potentially sensitive tumours respond favourably to hormone therapy. Inherent in our concepts of remission are elements both of time and of degree, so that the control of the tumour by the hormone must persist for a period long enough to be useful for the patient and be of such a degree that it can be measured by objective means. A period of quiescence induced by therapy is regarded as arrested disease and such a patient is relegated to the group of non-responders.

Within fairly well defined limits, the physiological and pharmacological actions of the hormones are predictable on all sensitive normal tissues. Similarly, it may be possible that all potentially sensitive tumours respond to the appropriate hormones, the difference between clinical responders and non-responders being one of time and degree of response.

Whereas normal target tissues retain their sensitivity to the action of hormones, and other tissues may acquire sensitivity to the sex hormones, much as an artificial vagina, there is some mechanism by which tumours become resistant. If such resistance was to develop before our crude methods of assessment could recognise a remission, the tumour would be considered a non-responder, but in reality it might be an occult responder.

Both the results of clinical trials and usage by clinicians would seem to indicate that the members of any particular hormone group, for example the various oestrogens in breast cancer, vary not so much in their anti-tumour effect as in their side effects. Allowing for variations in assessment, in cancer of the breast there is an overall uniformity in the responses to a large variety of natural and synthetic hormones. This uniformity in remission rate may not be an expression of the ability of each hormone manipulation to control the tumour initially, but may be related to the ability of the tumour to escape from control. In the latter case, future hormonal agents might not be expected to give better results than already achieved with our present hormones. When it is possible to block the mechanism by which resistance develops, we may be able to prolong remissions, not only in the tumours which respond objectively at present, but also in the occult responders, with a considerable increase in remission rate.

On the other hand, the tumours at present objectively responding to hormone therapy may represent all those in whom the hormones exercise any control. Non-responding tumours could then represent those tumours in which the hormone had no effect. This 'all or none' concept correlates with the fact that some normal tissues are sensitive to hormones, but others are not. It does not explain how either a hormone-sensitive or a hormone-resistant tumour can develop from a normal tissue which is itself sensitive to hormones.

The sensitivity of normal tissues to hormones is not lost with the passage of time, but all tumours eventually become resistant to hormone control. This would imply that the anti-tumour activity of the hormones may be unrelated to the usual hormone actions, and there may be no increased benefit from agents with a greater hormone effect, the more androgenic androgen, or the more oestrogenic oestrogen suggested by Segaloff (1967). If the anti-tumour activity of the hormones is related to their usual hormone actions, then, for androgens in breast cancer, the response rate should parallel the androgenic effects, such as virilisation, and be a function of dose and duration of therapy. This does not appear to be the case. If the anti-tumour and hormone effects are unrelated, non-hormonal agents with only a specific mechanism, similar to the anti-tumour action of the present hormones, may be developed in the future, but these agents would still control only a proportion of tumours.

RECURRENCE-FREE INTERVAL AND THE HOST DEFENCE

Carcinoma of the breast is a disease which proceeds, not in measured cadence, but by fits and starts (Segaloff, 1967). If this is true of clinical breast cancer, it is probably true of the subclinical disease which exists both before primary diagnosis and during the period between mastectomy and recurrence, the so-called free interval.

There is a difference in response to treatment between those tumours with a free interval of less than two years and those with a free interval in excess of two years. If the growth of the tumour was continuous, we might be able to use the free interval to assess the rate of growth. Despite the value of the free interval in predicting response to treatment, I do not believe that it does so by separating tumours according to their inherent rates of growth. I am not aware that breast carcinomas which have a very long free interval of 10 to 30 years, behave any differently from those with a free interval of two years once they have advanced to a stage of clinical recognition.

A long free interval may mean that the tumour is a slow grower, in which case its subsequent rate of growth will be observed to be slow. Equally, it may mean that the tumour may be 'slow to get growing' or unable to maintain uninterrupted growth in its host environment. This host environment may include both hormonal and immunological elements. By the time clinical disease is present, the latter may be only of minor importance.

Equally, a short free interval may be more apparent than real. The standard of preoperative assessment varies considerably and an inappropriate mastectomy may precede, by only a very short period, the discovery of metastatic disease. Such a 'free interval' may not necessarily reflect the rate of growth, but rather the extent of preoperative disease.

The great need for improvement in the assessment, both of the extent of the tumour and its behaviour during treatment, has been stressed by Hayward (1970). I believe that this assessment should be directed to the status both of the tumour and of the host defences during the subclinical stage of the disease, the so-called free interval. If immunosurveillance plays a part in the natural history of cancer, the host defences have most chance of controlling tumours when they are small and produce small amounts of antigen.

Koldovsky (1966) has drawn attention to some of the potential difficulties of cancer immunotherapy such as the inadequacy of the host response to weak, although specific antigens, immune paralysis by mass antigen effect, and the danger of tumour enhancement by coating the tumour cells with antibodies, thereby reducing their immunosensitivity. Presumably, these are also the same difficulties faced by the natural defences in their attempt to confine the tumour growth.

For these reasons, it is unjustifiable, at present, to consider active immunotherapy during the free interval. But equally, until we can assess the host defences, it is important to reduce the damage caused to these defences by irradiation or drugs (*British Medical Journal*, 1966).

The attraction of confining the disease in a subclinical stage has led to a variety of prophylactic procedures in breast cancer. Hayward (1970) refers to the dilemma produced in considering prophylactic therapy because of our inability to predict the patients in whom the chosen therapy will be beneficial. This dilemma exists in the treatment of established disease. The suggestion is

made by Hayward that not only the hormone environment has to be taken into account in deciding on prophylactic therapy but also the reaction of the tumour to this environment. The effects of prophylactic therapy on the host defences may be equally important.

We must ensure that what we achieve by way of endocrine therapy in cancer is not bought at too high a price by the patient, a price which includes the known effects on the patient, the unknown effects on the immune reaction and on the tendency of the tumour to metastasise. For this price, the patient is entitled to expect symptomatic relief and, at times, objective tumour regression.

References

Ahmed, A. B. J., George, B. C., Gonzales-Auvert, C. & Dingman, J. F. (1967) Increased plasma arginine vasopressin in clinical adrenocorticol insufficiency and its inhibition by glucocorticoids. *Journal of Clinical Investigation*, **46**, 111–124.

Alexanian, R. (1969) Erythropoietin and erythropoiesis in anaemic man following androgens. *Blood*, **33**, 4, 564.

Allen, D. M., Fine, M. K., Necheles, T. F. & Dameshek, W. (1968) Oxymetholone therapy in aplastic anaemia. *Blood*, **32**, 1, 83.

Barr, M. & Fairley, G. H. (1961) Circulating antibodies in reticuloses. *Lancet*, **i**, 1305.

Berson, S. & Yalow, R. (1966) Parathyroid hormone in plasma in adenomatous hyperparathyroidism, uremia and bronchogenic carcinoma. *Science*, **154**, 907.

Boesen, E. & Davis, W. (1969) *Cytotoxic Drugs in the Treatment of Cancer*. London: Arnold.

Bower, B. F. & Gordan, G. S. (1965) Hormonal effects of non-endocrine tumors. *Annual Review of Medicine*, **16**, 83.

British Medical Journal (1966) Immunotherapy of cancer. *British Medical Journal*, **iii**, 185.

British Medical Journal (1967) **ii**, 258.

Brodsky, I., Dennis, L. H., DeCastro, N. A., Brady, L. & Kahn, S. B. (1965) Effect of testosterone enanthate and alkylating agents on multiple myeloma. *Journal of the American Medical Association*, **193**, 874.

Brodsky, I. & Kahn, S. B. (1967) The effect of androgens on cancer chemotherapy. In *Cancer Chemotherapy, Basic and Clinical Applications*, ed. Brodsky, I., Kahn, S. B. and Moyer, P. New York: Grune and Stratton.

Brodsky, I., Dennis, L. H. & Kahn, S. B. (1964) Testosterone enanthate as a bone marrow stimulant during cancer chemotherapy, Preliminary Report. *Cancer Chemotherapy Reports*, **34**, 59.

Brown, J. R., Altschuler, N. A. & Cooper, J. (1963) Erythropoietic effect of red cell components and heme-related compounds. *Proceedings of the Society for Experimental Biology and Medicine*, **112**, 840–843.

Burnet, M. (1957) Cancer—a biological approach. *British Medical Journal*, **i**, 785.

Cain, G. D., Mayer, G. & Jones, E. A. (1970) Augmentation of albumen but not fibrinogen synthesis by corticosteroids in patients with hepatocellular disease. *Gastroenterology*. Quoted by Sherlock, S. (1970).

Carbone, P. R. (1963) Neoplastic plasma cell: combined clinical staff conference at the National Institutes of Health. *Annals of Internal Medicine*, **58**, 1029.

Chalmers, T. C., Gill, R. J., Jernigan, T. P., Svec, F. A., Jordan, R. S., Waldstein, S. S. & Knowlton, M. (1956) *Gastroenterology*. **30**, 894.

Condit, P. T. (1960) Studies on the folic acid vitamins. II The acute toxicity of amethopterin in man. *Cancer*, **13**, 222.

Connor, T. B., Hopkins, T. R., Thomas, W. C. Jr,

Carey, R. A. & Howard, J. E. (1956) Use of cortisone and ACTH in hypercalcemic states. *Journal of Clinical Endocrinology and Metabolism*, **16**, 945.

Cook, G. C., Mulligan, R. A. & Sherlock, S. (1970) A controlled trial of prednisolone therapy in active chronic hepatitis. In preparation, quoted by Sherlock, S. (1970).

Cree, I. C. (1960) Toxic marrow failure after treatment of carcinoma with cytotoxic drugs. *British Medical Journal*, **ii**, 1499.

David, N. J., Verner, J. V. & Engel, F. L. (1962) The diagnostic spectrum of hypercalcemia. *American Journal of Medicine*, **33**, 88.

Davis, D. B., Bloom, M. E., Fields, J. B. & Mintz, D. H. (1969) Hyponatremia in pituitary insufficiency. *Metabolism*, **18**, 821–832.

Denoix, P. (1970) *Recent Results in Cancer Research. Treatment of Malignant Breast Disease*, p. 48. London: Heinemann.

Dent, C. E., Flynn, F. V. & Naborro, J. N. D. (1953) Hypercalcemia and impairment of renal function in generalised sarcoidosis. *British Medical Journal*, **ii**, 808.

Doll, R. & Kinlen, L. (1970) Immunosurveillance and cancer, Epidermiological evidence. *British Medical Journal*, **ii**, 420.

Dukes, P. P. & Goldwasser, E. (1961) Inhibition of erythropoiesis by oestrogens. *Endocrinology*, **19**, 21.

Dymling, J. F., Isaaksson, B. & Sjogren, B. (1962) *Protein Metabolism, Influence of Growth Hormones, Anabolic Steroids and Nutrition in Health and Disease*, ed. Gross, F., Berlin.

Emirgil, C., Zsoldos, S., Heinemann, H. O. (1964) Effect of metastatic carcinoma to the lung on pulmonary function in man. *American Journal of Medicine*, **36**, 382.

French, L. A. (1966) The use of steroids in the treatment of cerebral edema. *Bulletin of the New York Academy of Medicine*, **42**, (4) 301–311.

Gardner, B. (1969) The Relation between serum calcium and tumour metastases. *Surgery Gynecology and Obstetrics*, **128**, 369.

Gardner, B. & Gordan, G. S. (1962) Does urinary calcium excretion reflect growth or regression of disseminated breast cancer. *Journal of Clinical Endocrinology and Metabolism*, **22**, 627.

Gardner, F. H. & Nathan, D. G. (1966) Androgens and erythropoiesis. *New England Journal of Medicine*, **274**, 420.

Gardner, F. H. & Pringle, J. C. (1961a) Androgens and erythropoiesis. *New England Journal of Medicine*, **264**, 103.

Gardner, F. H. & Pringle, J. C. (1961b) Androgens and erythropoiesis. *Archives of Internal Medicine*, **107**, 846.

Gordan, G. S., Fitzpatrick, M. E. & Lubich, W. P. (1967) Identification of osteolytic sterols in human breast cancer. *Transactions of the Association of American Physicians*, **80**, 183.

Gordan, G. S., Eisenberg, E., Loken, H. F., Gardner, B. & Hayashida, T. (1962) Clinical endocrinology of parathyroid hormone excess. *Recent Progress in Hormone Research*, **18**, 297.

Gordon-Taylor, Sir Gordon (1959) The incomputable factor in cancer prognosis. *British Medical Journal*, **i**, 455.

Gordan, G. S. (1967) Hormonal effects of non-endocrine tumors with special reference to the hypercalcaemia of breast cancer. In *Current concepts in Breast Cancer*, ed. Segaloff, A., Meyer, K. K. & DeBakey, S. Baltimore: Williams & Wilkins.

Gracey, D. R. & Divertie, M. B. (1970) Cortisone treatment of diffuse interstitial pulmonary fibrosis. *Journal of the American Medical Association*, **211**, (3) 495–497.

Green, H. N. (1954) An immunological concept of cancer: a preliminary report. *British Medical Journal*, **ii**, 1374.

Greenwald, E. S. (1967) *Cancer Chemotherapy, Medical Outline Series*, p. 162. London: Heinemann.

Gurney, C. W. & Fried, W. (1965) The mechanism of action of androgens on erythropoiesis. *Journal of Clinical Investigation*, **44**, 1057.

Hall, C. E. & Bieri, J. G. (1953) Modification of the choline deficiency syndrome in the rat by somatrophin and hydrocortisone. *Endocrinology*, **53**, 661.

Hall, T. C., Dederick, M. M. & Nevinny, H. B. (1963) Prognostic value of hormonally induced hypercalcemia in breast cancer. *Cancer Chemotherapy Reports*, **30**, 21.

Harold, J. T. (1952) Lymphangitis carcinomatosa of the lungs. *Quarterly Journal of Medicine*, **21**, 353.

Harrington, W. J., Pugh, R. P. & Pochron, S. P. (1967) Selective haemolysis of erythrocytes following alkylating agents. *Blood*, Abstract, **30**, 869.

Harris, W. H. & Heaney, R. P. (1969) Skeletal renewal and metabolic bone disease. *New England Journal of Medicine*, **280**, 193.

Hayward, J. (1970) *Hormones and Human Breast Cancer—Recent Results in Cancer Research*. London: Heinemann.

Heber, Bishop Reginald (1783–1826) *Hymns, Brightest and Best. The Concise Oxford Dictionary of Quotations*, p. 101. Oxford University Press.

Hooley, J. R. & Francis, F. H. (1969) Betamethasone in traumatic oral surgery. *Journal of Oral Surgery*, **26**, (6) 398.

Hughes, L. E. & Mackay, W. D. (1965) Suppression of tuberculin response in malignant disease. *British Medical Journal*, **ii**, 1346.

Ikonopisov, R. L., Lewis, M. G., Hunter-Craig, I. D., Bodenham, D. C., Phillips, T. M., Cooling, C. I., Proctor, J., Fairley, G. H. & Alexander, P. (1970) Autoimmunisation with irradiated tumor cells in human malignant melanoma. *British Medical Journal*, **ii**, 752.

Jackson, W. P. O. (1967) *Calcium Metabolism and Bone Disease*, p. 109. London: Arnold.

Jepson, J. H. & McGarry, E. E. (1968) Effect of

growth hormone and other hormones on erythro-poiesis and erythropoietin excretion of pituitary dwarfs. *Annals of Internal Medicine*, **68**, 1169.

John, D. W. & Miller, L. L. (1969) Regulation of net biosynthesis of serum albumen and acute phase plasma proteins. *Journal of Biological Chemistry*, **244**, 6134–6142.

Jowsey, J. (1966) Quantitative microradiography. A new approach in the evaluation of the metabolism of bone. *American Journal of Medicine*, **40**, 485–491.

Koldovsky, P. (1966) Dangers and limitations of the immunological treatment of cancer. *Lancet*, **i**, 654.

Keast, D. (1970) Immunosurveillance and cancer. *Lancet*, **ii**, 710–712.

Kennedy, B. J. (1962) Stimulation of erythropoiesis by androgenic hormones. *Annals of Internal Medicine*, **57**, 917.

Kennedy, B. J. (1965a) Androgenic hormone therapy in lymphatic leukaemia. *Journal of the American Medical Association*, **190**, 104.

Kennedy, B. J. (1965b) Stimulation of haematopoiesis by androgenic hormones. *Geriatrics*, **20**, 808–815.

Killman, S. A. (1960) *Leukocyte Agglutinins*. Thesis. Oxford: Blackwell. (Quoted by Videbaek, A. 1969.) Glucocorticoids in haematology. *Acta Medica Scandinavica*, supplement. Supp. **500**, 35–41.

King, D. F., Moon, W. M. & Brown, N. (1965) Corticosteroid drugs in the management of primary and secondary malignant cerebral tumours. *Medical Journal of Australia*, **2**, 878.

Koldovsky, P. (1966) Dangers and limitations of the immunological treatment of cancer. *Lancet*, **i**, 654.

Kupperman, H. S. (1967) Drugs in endocrine function. In *Drugs of Choice* 1968–69, ed. Modell, St Louis: Mosby.

Laake, H. (1960) The activity of corticosteroids and the renal reabsorption of calcium. *Acta Endocrinologica*, **34**, 60.

Lancet (1964) Intracranial hypertension and steroids. *Lancet*, **ii**, 1052.

Lazlo, D., Schulman, C. A., Bellin, J., Gottesman, E. D. and Schilling, A. (1952) Mineral and protein metabolism in osteolytic metastases. *Journal of the American Medical Association*, **148**, 1027.

Lazor, M. Z., Rosenberg, L. & Carbone, E. P. (1963) Studies of calcium metabolism in multiple myeloma with Ca^{47} and metabolic balance techniques. *Journal of Clinical Investigation*, **42**, 1238.

LePage, G. A. & Kaneko, T. (1969) Effective means of reducing toxicity without concomitant sacrifice of efficiency in carcinostatic therapy. *Cancer Research*, **29**, 2314.

Lesse, S. & Netsky, M. G. (1954) Metastases of neoplasms to the central nervous system and meninges. *Archives of Neurology and Psychiatry*, **72**, 133.

Loeb, M. & McQuarrie, D. G. (1968) Management of simultaneous bilateral neck dissection. *Surgery, Gynecology and Obstetrics*, **127**, 1322–1323.

Lyons, A. & Edelstyn, G. (1962) Thiotepa in treatment of advanced breast cancer. *British Medical Journal*, **ii**, 1280.

Lytton, B., Hughes, L. E. & Fulthorpe, A. J. (1964) Circulating antibody response in malignant disease. *Lancet*, **ii**, 69.

McMahon, F. G., Gordon, E. S., Kenover, W. C. & Keil, P. (1960) Renal and pituitary inhibiting effects of exogenous corticosteroids in normal subjects. *Metabolism*, **9**, 511.

Massinger, Philip (1583–1640) *Great Duke of Florence*, III, 1. *British Drama*, Vol. 1. Vizetelly, London: 1887.

Mathé, G. (1969) Approaches to the immunological treatment of cancer in man. *British Medical Journal*, **iv**, 7.

Merigan, T. C. Jr & Hayes, R. E. (1961) Treatment of hypercalcemia in multiple myeloma. *Archives of Internal Medicine*, **107**, 389.

Millburn, L., Hibbs, G. G. & Hendrickson, F. R. (1968) Treatment of spinal cord compression from metastatic carcinoma. *Cancer*, **21**, 447–452.

Mills, T. H. (1964) *Clinical Aspects of Adrenal Function*, p. 210. Oxford: Blackwell.

Mirand, E. A., Gordon, A. S. & Wenig, J. (1965) Mechanism of testosterone action in erythropoiesis. *Nature*, **206**, 270.

Munson, P. L., Tashjian, A. H. & Levine, L. (1965) Evidence for parathyroid hormone in non-parathyroid tumors associated with hypercalcemia. *Cancer Research*, **25**, 1062.

Myers, W. P. L. (1958) Cortisone in the treatment of hypercalcemia in neoplastic disease. *Cancer*, **11**, 83.

Newbolt, Sir Henry J. (1862–1938) *The Island Race. Drake's Drum. The Concise Oxford Dictionary of Quotations*. Oxford University Press, 1964.

Olson, R. E. (1959) Nutrition. *Annual Revue of Biochemistry*, **28**, 467.

Pack, G. T. & Molander, D. W. (1960) Metabolism before and after hepatic lobectomy for cancer; studies on 23 patients. *Archives of Surgery*, **80**, 685.

Pearson, O. H., West, C. D., Hollander, V. P. & Escher, G. C. (1952) Alterations in calcium metabolism in patients with osteolytic tumors. *Journal of Clinical Endocrinology*, **12**, 926.

Perry, S. (1969) Reduction of toxicity in cancer chemotherapy. *Cancer Research*, **29**, 2319.

Raisz, L. G. (1970) Estrogens and bone resorption. *New England Journal of Medicine*, **282**, 1376.

Rider, W. D. (1960) Bradford approach to breast cancer. *British Medical Journal*, **i**, 1501.

Rose, G. A. (1967) Some thoughts osteoporosis and osteomalacia. *Scientific Basis of Medicine—Annual Review*, 1966, p. 252.

Russell, D. S. & Rubinstein, L. J. (1959) *The Pathology of Tumors of the Nervous System*. London: Arnold.

Sanchez-Medal, L., Gomez-Leal, A. & Duarte-Zapata, L. (1966) *Blood*, Abstract, **28**, 974.

Sanchez-Medal, L., Pizzuto, J., Torre-Lopez, E. &

Derbez, R. (1964) Effect of oxymetholone in refractory anaemia. *Archives of Internal Medicine*, **113**, 721.

Scheinberg, L. C., Herzog, I., Taylor, J. M. & Katzman, R. (1969) Cerebral oedema in brain tumors: ultrastructure and biochemical studies. *Annals of the New York Academy of Sciences*, **159**, (2), 509–532.

Schooley, J. C. (1966) Inhibition of erythropoietic stimulation by testosterone in polycythemic mice receiving anti-erythropoietin. *Proceedings of the Society of Experimental Biology and Medicine*, **122**, 402.

Schwarz, M. I., Waddell, L. C., Dombeck, D. H., Weill, H. & Ziskind, M. M. (1969) Prolonged survival in lymphangitic carcinomatosis. *Annals of Internal Medicine*, **71**, 779–783.

Segaloff, A. (1963) The endocrinologic effects of tumors. *Journal of Chronic Diseases*, **16**, 727.

Segaloff, A. S. (1967) *Treatment of Breast Cancer*, ed. Jarrett, A. S. Published for Syntex Pharmaceuticals by Excerpta Medica Foundation.

Seventeenth Rheumatism Review (1966) *Arthritis and Rheumatism*, **9**, 181.

Shaldon, S. & Sherlock, S. (1957) Virus hepatitis with features of prolonged bile retention. *British Medical Journal*, **ii**, 734.

Sherlock, S. (1970) Causes and effects of acute liver damage. *Scandinavian Journal of Gastroenterology*. Supplement 6, 187–202.

Sherlock, P. & Hartman, W. H. (1962) Adrenal steroids and the pattern of metastases of breast cancer. *Journal of the American Medical Association*, **181**, 313–7.

Sherwood, L. M., O'Riordan, J. L. H., Aurbach, G. D. & Potts, J. T. Jr (1967) Production of parathyroid hormone by non-parathyroid tumors. *Journal of Clinical Endocrinology*, **27**, 140.

Shulman, L. E., Schoenrich, E. H. & Harvey, A. M. (1952) The effects of adrenocorticotrophic hormone (A.C.T.H.) and cortisone on sarcoidosis. *Bulletin of the Johns Hopkins Hospital*, **91**, 371–415.

Solomon, G. F., Dickerson, W. J. & Eisenberg, E. (1960) *Geriatrics*, **15**, 46.

Stoll, B. A. (1969) *Hormonal Management of Breast Cancer*, p. 74. London: Pitman.

Stoll, B. A. & Matar, J. (1961). Cyclophosphamide in advanced breast cancer. A clinical and haematological appraisal. *British Medical Journal*, **ii**, 283.

Stuart, A. E. (1970) The Reticulo-Endothelial System. Edinburgh: Livingstone.

Tata, J. R. (1969) Hormonal Control of Protein Synthesis. *Scientific Basis of Medicine, Annual Review 1969*, p. 112.

Taylor, S. G. III, Perlia, C. P. & Kofman, S. (1958) Cortical steroids in the treatment of disseminated breast cancer. In *Breast Cancer*, ed. Segaloff, A., p. 219 St Louis: Mosby.

Thomas, L. (1959) In *Cellular and Humoral Aspects of the Hypersensitive State*, ed. Lawrence, H. S., p. 529. London: Hoeber.

Verwilghen, R., Louwagie, A., Waes, J. & Vandenbroucke, J. (1966) Anabolic agents and relative polycythemia. *British Journal of Haematology*, **12**, 712–716.

Videbaek, A. (1969) Glucocorticoids in haematology. *Acta Medica Scandinavica*. Suppl **500**, 35–41.

Vogler, W., Huguley, C. Jr & Kerr, W. (1965) Toxicity and anti-tumor effect of divided doses of methotrexate. *Archives of Internal Medicine*, **115**, 285.

Watson, G. W. & Turner, R. L. (1959) Breast cancer. A new approach to therapy. *British Medical Journal*, **i**, 1315.

Watson, L. (1964) Hypercalcemia and cancer. *Quarterly Journal of Medicine*, **33**, 525.

Watson, L. (1966) Calcium metabolism and cancer. *Australasian Annals of Medicine*, **15**, 359.

Williams, H. M., Diamond, H. D., Craver, L. F. & Parsons, H. (1959) *Neurologic Complications of Lymphoma and Leukaemias*. Springfield, Illinois: Thomas.

Wilson, R. E., Hager, E. B., Hampers, C. L., Corson, J. M., Merrill, J. P. & Murray, J. E. (1968) Immunologic rejection of human cancer transplanted with a renal allograft. *New England Journal of Medicine*, **278**, 479.

Wolf, J., Spear, P., Yesner, R. & Patno, M. E. (1960) Nitrogen mustard and the steroid hormones in the treatment of inoperable bronchogenic carcinoma. *American Journal of Medicine*, **29**, 1008.

Wynn, V. (1967) Anabolic steroids and protein metabolism. In *Modern Trends in Endocrinology*, *3*, ed. Gardiner-Hill, H. London: Butterworth.

Zukoski, C. F., Killen, D. A., Ginn, E. & Matter, B. (1970) Transplanted carcinoma in an immunosuppressed patient. *Transplantation*, **9**, 71.

Chapter 5

Assessment of Tumour-Host Relationship

BASIL A. STOLL

In order to select *rational* endocrine treatment for the patient with a hormone-responsive cancer, we need knowledge of the tumour-host relationship in that patient: the factors in the tumour's environment which are maintaining its growth. Our knowledge and ability to measure such factors are developing, but are still uncertain for the majority of tumours. Subsequently, in order to assess the response of the tumour to the selected therapy, we require both clinical and laboratory criteria which will measure the activity of the tumour and the degree of its response to treatment. There is little unanimity on such criteria.

The first part of this chapter attempts to establish clinical criteria of response which can be applied to all types of hormonally treated cancer. The subsequent section on laboratory criteria which measure tumour-host relationship and tumour response, is applied particularly to breast cancer (a field where considerable attempts at rationalisation have been made in recent years) but similar criteria for cancer of the prostate are considered in Chapter 14.

Clinical Criteria of Response

The length of survival is the logical choice of index for assessing the results of a radical form of treatment in cancer. It can also be used to compare the benefit of different methods of palliative endocrine therapy, although it is uncertain whether to measure survival from the onset of the disease, or from the first attempt at curative treatment, or from the beginning of palliative therapy. However, length of survival by itself offers no measurement of the quality of life provided by a treatment, or of the morbidity resulting from its use. Therefore, in comparing two methods of palliative endocrine therapy, simple standard criteria are required to reflect not only the degree of palliation, but also the quality of life and morbidity resulting from each method.

In order to demonstrate benefit in endocrine-treated cancer patients over untreated patients, length of survival is unsuitable as a criterion. It is now generally accepted that slowly growing tumours with a long free interval, are, as a group, more likely to respond to endocrine therapy. Prolonged survival alone does not therefore necessarily indicate the beneficial results of treatment, and it becomes necessary to use a direct index such as tumour response. A major reason for the confusion as to the value of endocrine therapy in late cancer is the disagreement on criteria of tumour response (Hayward and Bulbrook, 1966). Reports of the same technique or agent in different hands yield vastly differing response rates.

The writer has summarised the following difficulties in assessment as the cause of the widely divergent results in the literature of endocrine therapy in cancer (Stoll, 1969).

PROBLEMS IN ASSESSMENT

In recurrent or metastatic cancer it is not uncommon to see soft tissue tumour which, without any therapy, barely changes in size over a period of several months. To avoid a false impression of having achieved endocrine control in tumours of low activity, it is important that tumours should have shown measurable progression over a period of at least two months, before instituting a trial of endocrine therapy (Segaloff, 1960). In this respect, it is advisable to judge progressing growth on the basis of new

metastatic lesions appearing, rather than by a change in existing lesions (Brennan, 1966). The growth rate of a tumour tends to be slower with increasing size of the lesion, and the development of necrosis in larger lesions may sometimes be misinterpreted as progression.

In the absence of tumour exacerbation, it is essential to give at least three months' trial of additive endocrine therapy before regarding it as a failure. Clinical evidence of regression often takes this length of time to manifest, and may take even longer in the case of slowly growing tumour. Similarly, unless there are urgent manifestations of advancing disease, six months should be allowed after radiation castration, and at least two months after surgical castration, before considering such therapy to have failed. Otherwise a delayed response occurring at that stage may be credited to a subsequent treatment which is then uselessly continued. A 'withdrawal' response occurring when additive hormone therapy is stopped in breast cancer may also be credited to a subsequent treatment, and new therapy should therefore be delayed two months for this reason.

Patients who die or who discontinue medication within one month of beginning a course of additive hormone therapy are obviously failures of palliation. They are not necessarily failures of a treatment method because clinical trial has not been adequate (see Chapter 18). Similarly, early postoperative deaths after surgical or radiation endocrine ablation are failures of palliation, but whether also failures of a treatment method is a matter of argument. Different interpretation of the category in both groups mentioned can lead to considerable differences in remission rates between two series of advanced cancer patients.

EQUIVOCAL RESPONSE

It may not be universally known that evidence of tumour remission from endocrine therapy does not follow the 'all or none' law, either qualitatively or quantitatively. Many observers have introduced a category of 'partial' or 'equivocal' response as a third grouping, apart from success and failure of response. It is important to stress that failure to achieve an acceptable degree of tumour regression is not necessarily a sign of hormone independence by its cells. Even an agent which completely stops cell division in a tumour will not reduce the size of a tumour unless spontaneous cell loss is taking place at the same time, or unless death of adult cells is being caused.

A major source of confusion is the disagreement on the minimum percentage decrease in size of a lesion which is acceptable as a remission. A recent critical analysis of tumour response to chemotherapy in 253 cancer patients could quote either a 7 per cent tumour remission rate or a 48 per cent tumour remission rate, according to whether the criterion was a 50 per cent decrease or a 10 per cent decrease in size of the observed lesion (Rimm, Ahlstrom and Bross, 1966).

There is also disagreement as to the minimum duration of tumour regression following endocrine therapy to justify the term 'remission'. Practically all authorities now insist on a minimum period of three months, although the widely quoted report of the AMA Committee on Research (1960) did not stipulate this. Some insist on at least six months' duration of regression, while others may accept lesser periods than three months so long as the tumour regression can be regarded as 'useful' palliation.

There is no unanimity as to whether lesions remaining unchanged in size after endocrine treatment (while previously advancing) should be regarded as an equivocal response or as a remission or as non-responding. This difficulty applies also to the case of bone metastases where, associated with relief of pain, it is common for the radiographic appearance to remain 'arrested' over months of steroid therapy, whereas it was showing progression before treatment.

A systemic endocrine change which inhibits tumour growth might be expected to cause regression of metastases in *all* systems, yet it is quite common to see soft-tissue metastases from a cancer regressing under treatment while existing bone or visceral metastases are progressing. The reverse also occurs, but is much less common.

For the recording of response in such cases the 'mean clinical value' has been suggested (Walpole and Paterson, 1949), and adopted in some clinics. Each individual lesion is measured at every attendance and given a rating according to its progress. The mean value of all the ratings is then quoted as an index of response. Such an index is indeed a measure of 'average' tumour inhibition but not necessarily of palliation, because regression of symptomless nodules or nodes is given the same 'weighting' as regression of more serious visceral or bone metastases.

TUMOUR INHIBITION AND PALLIATION

In the endocrine therapy of late cancer, we are aiming at prolongation of life, even if only for a few months. But these months of extra life must be useful and pain free, and we are therefore looking for evidence of *palliation* as well as evidence of *tumour inhibition*. They do not always proceed together, and this is the reason for much of the disagreement on response rates in the literature.

Obvious palliation of symptoms results in about two thirds of cancer patients in whom objective evidence of tumour inhibition occurs. In the remaining one-third of cases, there are no symptoms to palliate, but visible evidence of hormonal sensitivity (even if limited in extent) implies to the clinician a possible control also of occult metastases, and therefore prolongation of survival. A common example is the regression of subcutaneous nodules in breast cancer or submucous vaginal nodules in endometrial cancer.

On the other hand, there are patients with no objective evidence of tumour inhibition in observable lesions but who nevertheless achieve palliation of symptoms following endocrine therapy. This form of palliation due to steroidal mechanisms acting on the host does not imply control of tumour growth. It is non-specific, as it may occur also in patients bearing types of tumour which are not generally regarded as hormonally dependent (see Chapter 4).

Pain relief is sometimes quoted as an indicator of response to endocrine therapy in late cancer (Neal, 1966), but while it undoubtedly represents desirable clinical palliation, it does not necessarily signify tumour inhibition which could lead to prolongation of survival. It is a common observation that the pain of bone metastases is relieved by additive endocrine therapy or by ablative endocrine therapy while, at the same time, there is concurrent objective evidence of progressing bone destruction. Such pain relief probably involves a steroidal effect on the host tissues, but does not indicate inhibition of tumour growth (see Chapter 21).

Included among the criteria of benefit in some reports of endocrine therapy in cancer are increase in weight, increase in exercise tolerance or increase in 'performance status' (Karnofsky and Burchenal, 1949). These criteria also represent desirable palliation and improved quality of life, but do not necessarily indicate evidence of a biological response to hormone therapy in the tumour.

Decrease in the signs of raised intracranial pressure or decrease in frequency of paracentesis during endocrine therapy may involve a steroidal mechanism acting on the host tissue, but are not necessarily evidence of tumour inhibition. Nor does improvement in erythrocyte sedimentation rate, haemoglobin or serum calcium level, or urinary calcium excretion necessarily signify inhibition of tumour activity.

RECORDING BENEFIT FROM ENDOCRINE THERAPY

In order to avoid some of the confusion discussed above, the writer advises that

subjective and objective signs of palliation and evidence of tumour inhibition should be distinguished in the *individual* in the following way:

Palliation (which may or may not result from response in the tumour) including :
Improvement in appetite, performance status and well-being,
Relief of pain, cough, dyspnoea,
Improvement in exercise tolerance, decrease in frequency of paracentesis, increase in weight,
Decrease in indirect effect of lesion, for example neurological signs of pressure,
Improvement in non-specific laboratory criteria, for example blood urea, liver function tests, serum calcium, haemoglobin.

Tumour inhibition (which may or may not cause palliation):
Decrease in size of tumour lesions,
Accompanying change in laboratory criteria indicating tumour inhibition, for example specific serum enzyme levels or the histological picture.

A report on the incidence of benefit from endocrine therapy in a *group* of patients will also be specified in the same way:

Palliation—as above.

Tumour inhibition—defined as above, but qualified as follows:

(a) *Overall remission rate:* indicating minimum acceptable criteria.
(b) *Extent of remission:* indicating average and maximum extent.
(c) *Duration of remission:* indicating average and maximum duration.
(d) *Site selectivity:* indicating whether soft tissue, bone or visceral metastases are most affected.

When the benefits from therapy in a group of patients are presented in this way, specification of the average and maximum extent, the duration, and the site selectivity of the response, will define also the *degree of palliation* in the group. For comparison of methods of treatment the writer prefers this way of recording the quality of response to the use of systems such as the Mean Clinical Value, which give no indication of the degree of palliation resulting from treatment.

PROTOCOL FOR ASSESSMENT OF TUMOUR REMISSION

To the writer, the minimum acceptable degree of significant tumour remission is a 50 per cent decrease in the bulk of the tumour. This is manifested by a 25 per cent decrease in the diameter of measurable lesions. In addition, all other manifestations of the disease must remain static and no new lesions appear. Such a response might be expected to be associated with *significant* prolongation of survival.

The criteria of remission in specific areas are as follows (Stoll, 1963, 1964a):

Osseous: Radiological sclerosis in lytic areas not previously treated by radiotherapy. Reduction of a raised serum calcium level is *not* accepted as a criterion of response.

Local: Significant decrease in size of primary tumour or ulcer, nodules, or regional nodes, measured by a caliper, recorded in diagrams and confirmed wherever demonstrable by photographs. 'Arrested' disease is *not* included.

Intrathoracic: Significant decrease in size of radiological opacities in the lungs or of mediastinal nodes, or decrease in the size of cytologically proven pleural or peritoneal effusion without paracentesis. Gross decrease in the rate of reaccumulation of a serous effusion is recorded, but *not* counted as tumour remission.

Visceral: Significant decrease in the size of hepatic or cerebral metastases, confirmed by scintigraphy.

The protocol for a hormonal trial insists that in all cases the diagnosis is established histologically and new treatment is instituted only if there are unequivocal objective signs of progressing lesions. Patients who have received irradiation to the part under observation within the previous two months or who are receiving cytotoxic therapy are excluded from hormone trial. Nevertheless, blood transfusions, paracentesis, and symptomatic treatment are carried out as necessary, and in all cases of inadequate nutrition attempts are made to correct this by suitable diet.

Laboratory Criteria of Tumour-Host Relationship

Hormonal therapy in breast cancer must be selected in a rational manner and, to do this, the writer has stressed the importance of relating the activity of the tumour to its hormonal environment in each individual (Stoll, 1969).

The laboratory criteria which have been used for this purpose can be classified in the following categories:

INDICES OF HORMONAL ENVIRONMENT OF TUMOUR

Urinary oestrogen excretion
Assay of vaginal or urethral cytology
Gonadotropin, prolactin and growth hormone excretion
Urinary 'discriminant' ratio or function
Tumour sex chromatin

BIOCHEMICAL INDICES OF TUMOUR
ACTIVITY

Serum calcium and urinary calcium excretion
Serum alkaline phosphatase
Hydroxyproline excretion
Serum phosphohexose isomerase and lactic
    dehydrogenase
Serum glycoproteins

INDICES USED TO ASSESS TUMOUR
RESPONSIVENESS TO HORMONES

Overlying skin temperature measurement
Tumour uptake of radioactive phosphorus
Tumour uptake and metabolism of steroids
In-vitro assay of steroid effects
Serial tumour biopsy

The division between the categories is not absolute. Thus, it is claimed that some indices of the hormonal environment of the tumour, such as the urinary 'discriminant' ratio, and tumour sex chromatin, may predict tumour responsiveness to endocrine therapy. In addition, biochemical indices of tumour activity at the outset of treatment can be used for assessing responsiveness to subsequent endocrine therapy.

INDICES OF TUMOUR'S HORMONAL ENVIRONMENT

URINARY OESTROGEN EXCRETION

On the basis of the oestrogen dependence theory, it might be expected that a very low preoperative oestrogen excretion level would indicate a lesser likelihood of response to endocrine ablation in breast cancer. Some authors have indeed noted that if oestrogen excretion levels are very low before bilateral adrenalectomy, the operation is less likely to be successful (Dao and Huggins, 1955; Block et al, 1959), but others could not confirm this observation (Birke et al, 1958; Irvine et al, 1961).

Again, on the basis of this theory one might expect a favourable tumour response to endocrine therapy to be associated with a fall in the oestrogen excretion level. Following the publication of an accurate method for the measurement of urinary excretion of oestrone, oestradiol-17β, and oestriol (Brown, 1955; Bauld, 1956), there followed numerous reports investigating this relationship (Strong et al, 1956; Bulbrook et al, 1958; Gordon and Segaloff, 1958; Scowen, 1958; Hiisi-Brummer et al, 1960; McAllister et al, 1960; Irvine et al, 1961; Swyer, Lee and Masterton, 1961; Hortling, Hiisi-Brummer and Af Bjorkesten, 1962; Palmer and Hellstrom, 1962; Jull, Shucksmith and Bonser, 1963). All reports agree that after oophorectomy, bilateral adrenalectomy or hypophysectomy, oestrogens may continue to be excreted by some patients. Their persistence and concentration bear no relationship to the likelihood of favourable clinical response by the tumour.

Such investigations may need to be repeated, as the methods of oestrogen assay used are said to yield unreliable results at the low levels being measured after endocrine ablation therapy, and this applies particularly in the presence of the metabolites of hormone replacement therapy. A more sensitive method of oestrogen determination has been developed (Brown et al, 1968) and by its use it is claimed to distinguish persistent oestrogen secretion by the ovary after the menopause from that of the adrenal cortex. Ovarian oestrogen secretion by the postmenopausal woman shows a monthly cyclical variation in level.

The source of the oestrogen which persists after combined bilateral adrenalectomy and oophorectomy is not clear. It may reflect secretion arising in aberrant adrenal tissue overlooked at operation (Bulbrook, Greenwood and Williams, 1960b), but others disagree with this assumption as the steroid levels do not rise with ACTH stimulation (Strong et al, 1956; Sim et al, 1961). An alternative explanation for the persistence of oestrogens after adrenalectomy is their origin in food or from conversion of androgens. Furthermore a proportion of breast cancers contain enzymes capable of metabolising steroids such as pregnenolone, testosterone and corticosterone, and are capable of synthesising oestrogens from other steroids (Adams and Wong, 1968).

The level of urinary oestrogen excretion has been measured in association with biopsies from the remaining breast, in patients with recurrence or metastasis after mastectomy for breast cancer (Bonser, Dossett and Jull, 1961). By assessing evidence of prolactin stimulation in the breast tissue together with the level of oestrogen excretion, it is claimed that a choice can be advised between bilateral adrenalectomy, hypophysectomy, and no endocrine ablation surgery. Unfortunately, the histological interpretation of prolactin-induced changes in normal breast tissue is difficult.

ASSAY OF VAGINAL OR URETHRAL CYTOLOGY

In the postmenopausal female, the vaginal smear pattern is a resultant of the various circulating hormone effects. Atrophic, intermediate and keratinised (or cornified) patterns are recognised, and there is a correlation between the level of oestrogen excretion measured chemically and the degree of keratinisation in the vaginal smear (Young, Bulbrook and Greenwood, 1957). The relative frequency of an oestrogenised pattern in postmenopausal patients with breast cancer, is said to be no different from that of a control group of the same age distribution (Struthers, 1956; Liu, 1957).

It has been suggested that the pretreatment vaginal smear should indicate a suitable method of hormonal therapy in breast cancer, i.e. an oestrogenised smear requires suppression of oestrogen production and an atrophic smear requires oestrogen therapy (Green, 1961). However, neither for oestrogen therapy nor for androgen therapy can the pretreatment vaginal smear pattern be correlated in this way with the likelihood of tumour growth remission (Liu, 1957; Stoll, 1967). Only in the case of progestin therapy is

there a correlation between vaginal smear pattern and the clinical response. The writer has shown that the presence of an atrophic pattern before treatment (signifying the complete absence of steroidal stimulation) is associated with a significantly lower tumour remission rate than is the presence of an intermediate or oestrogenised pattern (Stoll, 1967).

During an oral course of oestrogen therapy in breast cancer the vaginal smear pattern is useful to reflect the patient's metabolism of administered oestrogens, the regularity of their administration and the degree of absorption from the bowel. Furthermore, although the degree of oestrogen-induced cornification of the smear may be interfered with by endogenous androgen or progesterone (Pundel, 1958), there is nevertheless a correlation between the degree of cornification resulting from oestrogen therapy and the likelihood of tumour regression in breast cancer (Liu, 1957; Stoll, 1967) (Figure 5.1). It may be necessary progressively to increase the oestrogen dose at intervals in order to maintain the degree of vaginal cornification during a course of therapy (Stoll, 1967).

The degree of vaginal cornification may be reflected by the electrovaginal potential. It has been reported that after endocrine ablation or additive hormone therapy the degree of shift in electrovaginal potential can be correlated with the likelihood of tumour regression in breast cancer patients (Mozden and Parsons, 1965). This has not been confirmed (Dederick et al, 1966), and the method appears to have no advantage over the examination of the vaginal cytology.

The urethral mocosa also reflects the effect of steroid administration. It is claimed that examination of the cytological sediment of an early morning specimen of urine in the postmenopausal patient will not only reflect the presence of endogenous oestrogen but differentiate ovarian from adrenal oestrogen (Castellanos and Sturgis, 1958). The oestrogen excretion of postmenopausal women with breast cancer is being investigated by this method (de Waard et al, 1964). Administration of ACTH will *increase* the oestrogen effect on the urethra, if the oestrogen originates in the adrenal cortex, while dexamethasone administration will *decrease* the effect of adrenal oestrogen (Castellanos et al, 1963).

been suggested by Lazarev (1960) on theoretical grounds that gonadotropin is more likely to stimulate rather than to depress the growth of breast cancer in premenopausal patients.

Gonadotropin levels are normally high in the postmenopausal patient. In this age group, the presence of a higher level is

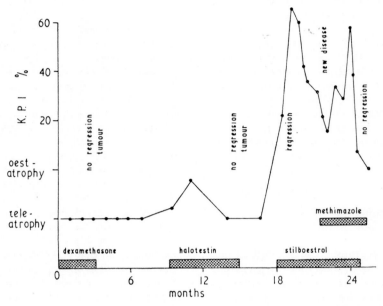

FIGURE 5.1. Clinical response by breast cancer in relation to the vaginal smear pattern, following the successive administration of dexamethasone 6·4 mg daily, fluoxymesterone (Halotestin) 40 mg daily, stilboestrol 15 mg daily, and added methimazole 30 mg daily. (Figure reproduced from Stoll, 1967, by permission of the Editor of *Cancer*, Philadelphia.)

GONADOTROPIN, PROLACTIN AND GROWTH HORMONE EXCRETION

There are conflicting reports in the literature on the correlation between gonadotropin secretion and tumour activity. The fall in oestrogen levels which follows oophorectomy and adrenalectomy in premenopausal women is associated with a rise in gonadotropin secretion, and it is suggested that the higher the gonadotropin level, the greater the likelihood of tumour regression in breast cancer patients (Douglas et al, 1961; Pommatau et al, 1963). Nevertheless, it has

said to predict a poor response by breast cancer to oestrogen therapy (Loraine, Strong and Douglas, 1957), as does also a high gonadotropin level persisting after oestrogen therapy (Stewart, Skinner and O'Connor, 1965). Attempts to correlate pretreatment gonadotropin levels with the response to *other* forms of endocrine therapy in postmenopausal patients have proved inconclusive (Segaloff et al, 1954; Hayward, Bulbrook and Greenwood, 1961; Martin, 1964).

All available preparations of human gonadotropin contain large amounts of LH, and response by breast cancer may depend on the ratio of FSH to LH in the preparation used. Nevertheless, a trial of gonadotropin administration after hypophysectomy would help to clarify the relationship between gonadotropin level and breast cancer activity both in premenopausal and postmenopausal patients (Stoll, 1964b).

It has been claimed that breast cancer patients showing tumour regression following hypophyseal ablation include a high proportion with marked fall in gonadotropin excretion (Boyland et al, 1958), but this is not confirmed by Beck et al (1966). The fall in gonadotropin levels is claimed to be a most sensitive indicator of completeness of ablation (McCullagh et al, 1965), but surprisingly, measurements of the pituitary hormone levels show no correlation between the likelihood of tumour regression after hypophyseal ablation, and the physiological completeness of ablation (see Chapter 9).

The evidence correlating hormone level and cancer activity in experimental mammary cancer is most conclusive in the case of prolactin. A radioimmunoassay for prolactin has been established in the human, and may prove to be the most useful index in predicting the likelihood of response to endocrine therapy. Decrease of prolactin secretion is likely to be a factor in the benefit from oestrogen therapy in postmenopausal patients and a fall in the urinary prolactin level after oestrogen therapy was reported to be correlated with tumour regression (Segaloff et al, 1954). Soon after, it was reported that response to hypophysectomy was associated with abolition of urinary prolactin excretion (Hadfield, 1957), then that administration of prolactin to patients after hypophysectomy may cause reactivation in controlled breast cancer (Pearson, 1957). Finally, it has been claimed that an increase in calcium excretion in patients with bone metastases following provocative injections of ovine prolactin, predicts a greater likelihood of tumour response to hypophysectomy (McCalister and Welbourn, 1962).

Human growth hormone is very similar to prolactin chemically, immunologically, and in its metabolic effects, and there is considerable difficulty in establishing their separate identity (Ferguson and Wallace, 1961; Barrett, Friesen and Astwood, 1961). Based on pain and calcium excretion as indices (Pearson and Ray, 1959), it has been suggested that human growth hormone stimulates breast cancer growth but this is not confirmed (Lipsett and Bergenstal, 1960).

URINARY DISCRIMINANT FUNCTION AND RATIO

It is suggested that the likelihood of response by breast cancer to major endocrine ablation can be predicted by the proportion of androgenic to corticoid metabolites in the urine before operation (Bulbrook, Greenwood and Hayward, 1960a). The 'discriminant function' is categorised as negative in patients with an abnormally low level of aetiocholanolone excretion relative to the 17-hydroxycorticosteroid excretion. Patients with a negative discriminant show response to major ablation therapy in only 11 per cent of cases, whereas those with a positive discriminant show response in 38 per cent of cases (Atkins et al, 1968). The likelihood of remission from major ablation therapy was found to fall as low as 5 per cent in negative discriminant cases if the recurrence-free period was less than two years, or if the patients were within six years after the menopause.

A probability curve based on the discriminant level, can be drawn to assess each individual's likelihood of response to major endocrine ablation (Sarafaty and Tallis, 1970), but as a negative discriminant is increasingly common with advancing age, the index is less useful in the older patient. To be useful in predicting response, it must reflect the *existing* hormonal environment of the tumour. It should therefore be estimated shortly before the operation, and all steroid therapy must be ceased for at least two months before the estimation. A recent report suggests that the discriminant correlates better with the results of hypophy-sectomy than with adrenalectomy (Atkins et al, 1968).

The urinary androgen excretion has also been found useful by other groups in predict-ing response to hypophyseal ablation by radioactive yttrium implant (Juret, Hayem and Flaisler, 1964) and to adrenalectomy (Wilson et al, 1967; Kumaoka et al, 1968). More recently it has been suggested that instead of aetiocholanolone, the total 11-deoxy-17-oxosteroids may be more simply measured (Miller et al, 1967; Ahlquist, Jackson and Stewart, 1968), and such an estimation can be carried out in any labora-tory with facilities for steroid measurement. The predictive value of the discriminant may apply also to additive hormonal therapy (Fotherby, Sellwood and Burn, 1968).

The cause of an abnormal discriminant is uncertain. A negative discriminant may be associated with enzymatic abnormality in the adrenal which may have a genetic basis (Deshpande et al, 1967). A negative dis-criminant is claimed to be more common in patients with breast cancer than in the nor-mal population (Bulbrook and Hayward, 1962), but this finding is not confirmed by others in *early* breast cancer (Wade et al, 1969; Cameron et al, 1970). This suggests that it is more likely to be a result of the tumour's presence, rather than a cause. In this respect it is interesting that steroid metabolism by the tumour could cause the abnormality found in patients with negative discriminants (Adams and Wong, 1968).

The level of circulating corticoids and androgens, and the proportion of their con-stituents, are related also to the level of thyroid hormone in the circulation (Hellman et al, 1961; Goldenberg, Blodinger and Grumman, 1966; Sneddon, Steel and Strong, 1968; Bruce et al, 1969), and it may be relevant that abnormal thyroid function has been noted in patients with active breast cancer (Strong, 1963; Stoll, 1965). Finally, adrenal androgen and corticosteroid secre-tion are affected by factors such as anxiety,

stress, surgical operation and chronic illness (Nabarro, 1960).

The steroid abnormality underlying a negative discriminant may therefore be due in part to abnormal adrenal secretion, steroid metabolism by the tumour, the effect of abnormal thyroid function or the effect of general illness.

TUMOUR SEX CHROMATIN

Various authors have suggested that the presence or absence of 'sex chromatin' in the breast cancer cells of women can be used to predict response of patients to endocrine therapy. Sex chromatin is believed to repre-sent the second X chromosome in the female somatic cell, and its presence in less than 5 per cent of cell nuclei is regarded as abnor-mally low (male karyotype). Its presence in over 15 per cent of nuclei is regarded as normal (female karyotype), and a proportion between 5 and 15 per cent is categorised as intermediate in type. Between 60 and 70 per cent of breast cancers in women have normal sex chromatin counts, and about 20 to 25 per cent have abnormally low sex chromatin counts, the remainder being unclassifiable.

It has been reported that an abnormally low sex chromatin count is associated with a below normal oestrogen excretion, and the normal karyotype with a normal oestrogen excretion (Regele and Vagacs, 1962). Fur-thermore, several authors have suggested that tumours with low sex chromatin counts respond poorly to endocrine therapy (Kimel, 1957; Regele, Kaufmann and Wasl, 1964; Bohle, 1965; Ehlers, Hochberg and Nuri, 1966). The presence of sex chromatin in over 45 per cent of all tumour cells is an unusually *high* proportion and, according to one author, this also is associated with a poor response to endocrine therapy (Shirley, 1967). More information is needed before sex chromatin counts can be used to predict the outcome of hormonal therapy.

Sex chromatin is less easily recognised in

poorly differentiated tumour cells, and this may account for the worse prognosis and greater likelihood of metastasis noted by some authors in patients with a low sex chromatin content in the tumour (Bohle, 1965; Wacker and Miles, 1966). According to Moore and Barr (1957) and Meier-Ruge (1966), a low proportion of cells with sex chromatin is associated with an anaplastic tumour, but Atkin (1967) does not agree.

course of diethylstilboestrol, but such a test has a limited application because provocation of tumour activity may cause a danger of hypercalcaemia. A suppression test by cortisone was suggested by the same authors, as an alternative, but in the experience of the writer, suppression of calcium excretion by cortisone in breast cancer is not a sign of sex hormone sensitivity (Stoll, 1963). Suppression by corticosteroid therapy of high

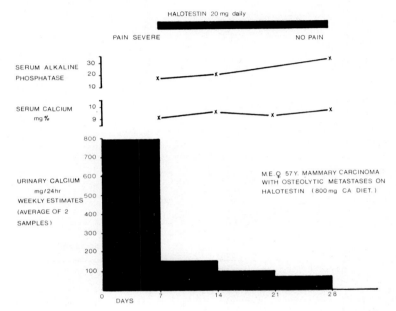

FIGURE 5.2. The effect of fluoxymesterone (Halotestin) 20 mg daily on the urinary calcium excretion, and on the serum calcium and alkaline phosphatase levels in a patient with bone metastases from breast cancer. (Figure reproduced from Stoll, 1959, by permission of the Editor, *Medical Journal of Australia.*)

INDICES OF TUMOUR ACTIVITY

SERUM CALCIUM AND URINARY CALCIUM EXCRETION

The use of serial assays of the urinary calcium excretion has been suggested for selecting breast cancer patients for therapeutic castration in the presence of osteolytic bone metastases (Pearson et al, 1952; Emerson and Jessiman, 1956). A *rise* in the urinary calcium excretion is watched for after a provocative

calcium excretion has been noted also in various tumours not regarded as sex hormone dependent (Plimpton and Gellhorn, 1956).

The writer has shown that a fall in urinary calcium excretion may precede pain relief from oestrogen or androgen therapy in postmenopausal women with bone metastases from breast cancer (Stoll, 1959) (Figure 5.2) but it does not *necessarily* predict objective evidence of remission in the disease (Gardner and Gordon, 1962). Either oestrogen or androgen administration may lead to a calcium-retaining effect in post-menopausal women *without* breast cancer (Gerbrandy and Hellendorn, 1957).

For these reasons, urinary calcium estimations are now rarely carried out in the management of breast cancer. Early prediction of pain relief from additive hormone therapy in the presence of osteolytic bone metastases may often be obtained from a fall in serum calcium levels (Figure 5.3). A fall

a sign of tumour stimulation (Figure 5.4). In some of these patients persistence with steroid therapy is followed by healing of tumour deposits (Hall, Dederick and Nevinny, 1963a).

SERUM ALKALINE PHOSPHATASE

The presence of bone metastases from breast cancer is usually associated with a rise in the

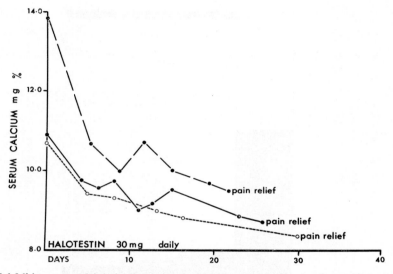

FIGURE 5.3. Serial fall in serum calcium level associated with pain relief, in three patients with bone metastases from breast cancer, receiving fluoxymesterone (Halotestin) 30 mg daily. (Figure reproduced from Stoll, 1969, by permission of Pitman Medical.)

of 1 mg/100 ml in the serum calcium level is said to correspond to a fall of approximately 100 mg calcium in the daily urinary excretion (Gerbrandy and Hellendorn, 1957).

Hypercalcaemia may occur in other forms of cancer, even in the absence of bone metastases (Plimpton and Gellhorn, 1956), but in the case of breast cancer it is associated with obvious or latent bone metastases. It should be pointed out that a rise in the serum calcium to hypercalcaemic levels immediately after the initiation of androgen or oestrogen administration indicates sensitivity of the tumour to steroids, but is not necessarily

serum alkaline phosphatase level. The enzyme level reflects osteoblastic activity in the normal bone surrounding the metastasis which, if successful, will lead to bone repair. A high enzyme level (in the absence of liver metastases) presumably reflects an effective stromal response to the presence of slowly growing tumour, and an initially high alkaline phosphatase level tends to be associated with a greater likelihood of remission from endocrine therapy (Kennedy, 1965).

Bone metastases with a slower rate of growth permit a healing response and this is manifested radiologically in a sclerotic appearance in bone metastases. This is seen most frequently in patients whose disease spans the natural menopause, and reflects the slowing-up of tumour growth which may occur at times of hormonal change.

An initial 'flare' in the serum alkaline phosphatase level often follows any attempt at endocrine therapy in the presence of bone metastases from breast cancer. The 'flare' is not correlated with later objective evidence of response to treatment, and may recur

returns to normal. Changes in serial alkaline phosphatase levels cannot be used by themselves for early prediction of response by bone metastases, but are best assessed in conjunction with changes in serial serum phosphohexose isomerase and serum calcium levels.

HYDROXYPROLINE EXCRETION

Hydroxyproline excretion reflects collagen metabolism, the majority of which is located

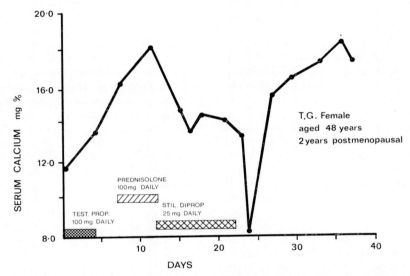

FIGURE 5.4. Serial serum calcium estimations in a patient with bone metastases from breast cancer associated with hypercalcaemia following consecutive courses of therapy of testosterone propionate 100 mg daily, prednisolone 100 mg daily and stilboestrol dipropionate 25 mg daily. (Figure reproduced from Stoll, 1969, by permission of Pitman Medical.)

when additive hormone therapy is discontinued. It reflects an attempt at repair of bone metastases during a period of hormonal change (Woodard, Escher and Farrow, 1954), and demonstrates that biological response to endocrine therapy is much more frequent in breast cancer than clinical remission rates would lead one to believe.

The serum alkaline phosphatase level tends to fall subsequently whether or not bone repair follows endocrine therapy, but if recalcification of bone metastases finally occurs, the alkaline phosphatase level usually

in bone tissue. The hydroxyproline/creatine ratio tends to be correlated with the serum alkaline phosphatase level in the presence of bone metastases, and the ratio was found raised in 76 per cent of patients with bone metastases from breast cancer (Guzzo et al, 1969). Although the hydroxyproline excretion was found more sensitive than the calcium excretion level or the serum alkaline phosphatase level in the *diagnosis* of bone metastases from breast cancer, it has not been found reliable as an index of response to endocrine therapy.

SERUM PHOSPHOHEXOSE ISOMERASE AND LACTIC DEHYDROGENASE

The level of phosphohexose isomerase in the serum is found to be raised in 85 per cent of patients with disseminate breast cancer (Joplin and Jegatheesan, 1962), the highest levels being in the presence of extensive bone or liver metastases. The enzyme level is high in rapidly growing breast cancer (Smith et al, 1970), but normal serum levels have been shown by the writer in the presence of only a small volume of actively growing tumour (Stoll, 1969).

A good clinical response by breast cancer to hypophysectomy is associated with a fall in an abnormally high serum phosphohexose isomerase level (Joplin and Jegatheesan, 1962; Beck et al, 1966). A fall in the enzyme level is also associated with evidence of breast cancer regression following oestrogen or androgen therapy, while a rise is associated with evidence of tumour reactivation (Griffith and Beck, 1963). It is of especial interest that a change in the enzyme level usually antedates clinical evidence of change in the tumour by days or even by weeks (Myers and Bodansky, 1957; Griffith and Beck, 1963).

A provocation test for assessing hormone sensitivity in breast cancer, is suggested by the experience of Beck et al (1966). They noted a rise in the enzyme level in some patients within only four to five days of beginning the administration of oestrogens or androgens, the level falling again when hormone therapy was stopped. The change appears to be independent of the site of metastasis and can be used to supplement evidence from serum calcium and alkaline phosphatase estimations in the case of bone metastases.

The serum level of phosphohexose isomerase is said to be more reliable in demonstrating changes in activity of bone metastases than is the urinary calcium excretion level (Myers and Bodansky, 1957). Ingestion of food may cause temporary change in the serum phosphohexose isomerase level, and it is therefore essential that all serial blood specimens be taken in the morning with the patient in a fasting state.

Lactic dehydrogenase is found in higher concentration in malignant tissue than in adjacent normal tissue, and the excess enzyme overflows into the bloodstream (Hill and Levi, 1954). Good correlation has been shown in patients with advanced cancer of various types, between progressive increase in the serum enzyme level and observed increase in the size of the tumour (Brindley and Francis, 1963). Conversely, decrease in serum lactic dehydrogenase levels can be correlated with the degree of tumour shrinkage after treatment by radiotherapy or by cytotoxic agents (Hall et al, 1963b).

In the assessment of tumour activity it is better to use a battery of tests (as one does with liver function tests) rather than rely on a single test. As an index of tumour activity in breast cancer, the serum lactic dehydrogenase level is less reliable than the phosphohexose isomerase level (Joplin and Jegatheesan, 1962; Beck et al, 1966). In the writer's experience, both are liable to sudden changes in level which are not obviously related to clinical changes in the tumour activity.

SERUM GLYCOPROTEINS

The serum glycoprotein level has been suggested as a means of selecting patients with breast cancer who are likely to respond favourably to endocrine therapy (Burnett, McAllister and Shields, 1963). The mean preoperative level in cases showing favourable response to radioactive yttrium ablation of the pituitary was found to be appreciably lower than in non-responding cases.

It has been suggested that the test can be simplified by estimating only the seromucoid-bound carbohydrate and seromucoid-bound tyrosine level (Bennett and Harris, 1966). Like the enzymes discussed above, the level is raised only in the presence of large tumours, but it is claimed that the serum glycoprotein level is better correlated with the persistence of tumour after surgical excision than either the phosphohexose isomerase or the lactic dehydrogenase levels (Harshman et al, 1967).

INDICES OF TUMOUR RESPONSIVENESS TO HORMONES

OVERLYING SKIN TEMPERATURE MEASUREMENT

The temperature within a tumour depends on the activity of its cellular metabolism and its by a probe inserted directly into the tumour have been shown to parallel changes in the skin temperature overlying the tumour (Mansfield et al, 1968). The writer has therefore investigated the use of serial measurements of the skin thermoprofile in an attempt to provide early indication of the response of breast cancer to additive hormone therapy (Stoll, 1971) (Figure 5.5).

Continuous recording of the skin temperature over breast cancer shows in some cases a cyclical diurnal pattern and this is most marked in tumours showing a response to

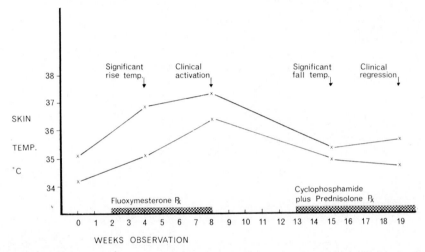

FIGURE 5.5. Clinical response in breast cancer in relation to the maximum and minimum skin temperature overlying the tumour following the successive administration of fluoxymesterone 30 mg daily, and of cyclophosphamide 100 mg daily in combination with prednisolone 30 mg daily.

effect upon the tumour vasculature. The latter is probably the major factor affecting the overlying skin temperature, and a differential of up to 2°C compared to normal skin, is commonly seen over soft-tissue lesions of breast cancer. Large temperature differentials are usually associated with a more rapidly growing tumour.

Following the administration of androgen or oestrogen, the skin temperature over breast cancer may show increase or decrease (Lloyd Williams, 1964; Mansfield et al, 1968). Observations of the tumour temperature hormonal manipulation (Mansfield et al, 1968). This pattern has been shown by the writer to run parallel to the diurnal pattern of the radioactive phosphorus uptake in the underlying breast cancer (Stoll and Burch, 1968), which again is most marked in tumours showing hormonal sensitivity (Hale, 1961). A cyclical diurnal pattern in temperature or in radioactive phosphorus uptake may reflect a tumour still sensitive to endogenous hormonal influences (Figure 5.6).

Temperature observation by probes implanted in the tumour are suitable only for

investigational purposes, while skin temperature measurement requires further investigation before it is suitable for routine clinical
use in the prediction of hormone sensitivity.

TUMOUR UPTAKE OF RADIOACTIVE
PHOSPHORUS

The uptake of radioactive phosphorus is
relatively high in breast cancer tissue, and it

Continuous recording by Geiger counters
implanted in breast cancer shows a cyclical
fluctuation in the radioactive phosphorus
uptake of some of the tumours (Hale, 1961),
and this has been confirmed (Bleehen and
Bryant, 1967; Taylor et al, 1968; Wooley-
Hart et al, 1968). The writer (Stoll and
Burch, 1968) demonstrated that the cyclical
frequency noted by surface counting was
actually diurnal and probably related to
adrenocortical secretion (Figure 5.7). The

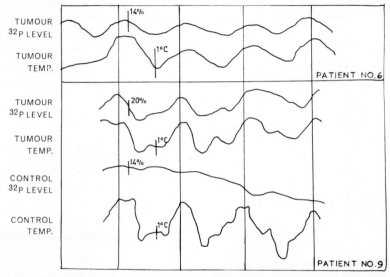

FIGURE 5.6. Recordings from two patients with breast cancer showing the relationship between the uptake of radioactive phosphorus and the adjacent skin temperature. The tumorous breast shows coincident diurnal periodicity in
both, while the lower tracings show periodicity in the temperature over the normal breast, but no periodicity in the
radioactive phosphorus uptake. (Scale is indicated on each curve.) (Figure reproduced from Stoll and Burch, 1968,
by permission of the Editor of *Cancer*, Philadelphia.)

was suggested some years ago that a change
in the uptake might be useful as an indicator
of tumour response to endocrine therapy
(Low-Beer and Green, 1952). The ^{32}P
uptake has been measured before and after
hormonal therapy, both in serial biopsy
specimens of breast cancer and by surface
counting methods (Nevinny and Hall, 1963).
A correlation is reported between clinical
response to oestrogen therapy and a change
in the level of ^{32}P uptake by the tumour
during therapy (Taylor et al, 1968).

presence in a tumour of cyclical fluctuation
in ^{32}P uptake is said to be associated with
the likelihood of clinical response to subsequent steroid therapy (Hale, 1961). When
administration of oestrogens or androgens
causes changes in the cyclical pattern, this
again is associated with a likelihood of
clinical response later (Bleehen and Bryant,
1967).

These methods of predicting hormonal
sensitivity require further investigation before
being suitable for routine clinical use.

TUMOUR UPTAKE AND METABOLISM OF STEROIDS

Hormone-dependent breast cancer may show a striking affinity for oestradiol, and a selectively higher uptake of radioactively labelled oestrogen has been shown in vivo in some cases of human breast cancer (Lewison et al, 1951; Folca, Glascock and Irvine, 1961; Crowley et al, 1962; Braunsberg, Irvine and James, 1967; Ellis et al, 1969). There is no

1969; Mobbs, 1970). The investigations to date on the selective uptake and the blocking capacity of androgens and anti-oestrogens have little bearing on the selection of agents for clinical cancer therapy.

Measurement of steroid uptake by breast cancer maintained in organ culture has been suggested to avoid the injection of radio-active materials into the patient and subsequent biopsy (Jensen, Desombre and Jungblut, 1967; Braunsberg and James, 1967).

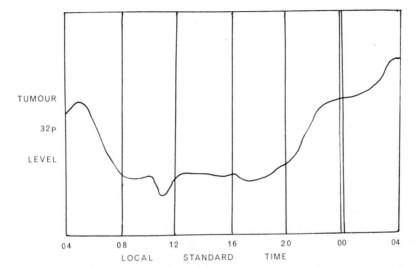

FIGURE 5.7. Diurnal periodicity in the radioactive phosphorus uptake of breast cancer. A composite curve derived by additive superposition of the individual curves from five patients. Note changes in curve at the time of waking and retiring. (Figure reproduced from Stoll and Burch, 1968, by permission of the Editor of *Cancer*, Philadelphia.)

evidence that the hormone dependence of breast cancer reflects its capacity to bind circulating oestrogen. Although higher uptake of radioactively labelled oestrogen was shown in a few patients responding favourably to subsequent adrenalectomy (Folca et al, 1961), this work has not been repeated.

Measurement of the selective uptake of androgens by breast cancer and their capacity to block oestradiol uptake in this tissue has yielded conflicting results (Deshpande, Bulbrook and Ellis, 1963; Braunsberg et al, 1967; Quincy and Gray, 1966; Ellis et al,

It has the added advantage that it is possible to correlate the quantitative uptake of a steroid with biochemical changes in the target tissue. The blocking power of steroids with anti-oestrogenic properties has been demonstrated by this method (Jensen et al, 1967; James and Braunsberg, 1969).

A proportion of human breast cancers incubated in-vitro have been shown to contain enzymes capable of metabolising steroids such as pregnenolone, testosterone, oestradiol and corticosterone (Adams, 1964). It has been shown that testosterone may be converted to oestradiol by the tumour, and this may be one source of persistent oestrogen excretion after adrenalectomy and oophorectomy (Adams and Wong, 1968). Metabolism of androgens by breast cancer tissue might also be responsible for the abnormal androgen excretion pattern noted in some of these patients (Bulbrook et al, 1960a).

A recent report notes that patients with tumours containing enzymes which metabolise androgen more effectively than oestrogen show a greater likelihood of beneficial response to bilateral adrenalectomy (Dao and Libby, 1969). This property may be more important in determining the hormonal sensitivity of breast cancer than the tumour's capacity to bind circulating oestrogen.

IN-VITRO ASSAY OF STEROID EFFECTS

An organ culture of the patient's tumour incubated with a steroid may show evidence of growth inhibition or stimulation, and thus may provide an individualised bio-assay of responsiveness to steroids. Unfortunately, this will not necessarily predict the effect of the steroid clinically, as the method excludes the influence on the tumour of the steroid metabolites and of other endogenous hormones present in the body. It also excludes any indirect action that the steroid might have on endogenous hormone secretion.

An oestrogen-sensitive dehydrogenase has been shown in some human breast cancer specimens in tissue culture, and an attempt was made to correlate the enzymatic activity of the specimen with the clinical response to subsequent endocrine ablation (Hollander, Jonas and Smith, 1958; Hollander, Smith and Adamson, 1959). The effect of androgen or oestrogen has also been reported on respiration and protein synthesis in tissue cultures of breast cancer (Rienits, 1959; Heuson and Legros, 1963).

Apart from these biochemical effects, histological evidence of growth *inhibition* has been shown from the action of androgen, oestrogen or progesterone incubated with

monolayer or organ cultures of mammary carcinoma (Kellner and Turcic, 1962; Rivera et al, 1963; Flaxel and Wellings, 1963; Altmann and Chayen, 1967; Mioduszewska, 1968; Tchao et al, 1968). On the other hand, evidence of growth *stimulation* has also been shown from pharmacological concentrations of oestrogen in a proportion of organ cultures of breast cancer tissue (Stoll, 1970; Chayen, Altmann and Bitensky, 1970). As has been mentioned previously, it is possible that every breast cancer may have an optimal level of oestrogen requirement for growth stimulation, and either higher or lower concentrations may depress its activity (Segaloff, 1967).

SERIAL TUMOUR BIOPSY

In the hope of predicting a response to hormonal therapy before clinical evidence of response becomes obvious, microscopic examination has been made of serial tumour biopsies. Progressive decrease in the proportion of mitotic cells in breast cancer biopsies has been shown in the majority of patients responding favourably to oestrogen therapy (Wolff, 1957). It is surprising that a similar observation was not evident after major ablation therapy.

An attempt has been made to correlate changes in lysosomal activity in the cell in serial biopsies with the effect of steroid administration (Emerson et al, 1953; Emerson, Kennedy and Taft, 1960). A similar attempt has been made for changes in radioactive phosphorus uptake in successive biopsy specimens (Nevinny and Hall, 1963). The heterogenous histology of breast cancer has so far prevented effective biochemical comparisons of serial biopsies, more especially because areas of spontaneous degeneration are common in the tumour.

CONCLUSION

Whatever the endocrine method of palliation used in advanced cancer, we must assess the benefit both quantitatively in terms of prolongation of survival, and qualitatively in terms of the increased well-being enjoyed by the patient during the remaining lifespan. Although only a small proportion of tumours will show sensitivity to endocrine manipulation, and then only for a limited period, we must aim to select the method of treatment most likely to be beneficial in *both* these respects to the patient.

To select the most suitable type of endocrine therapy on this basis, we must differentiate clearly between its ability to inhibit tumour growth and its ability to palliate symptoms. The former may reasonably be expected to result in prolongation of survival because of the effect on both visible and occult metastases, whereas evidence of palliation does not necessarily do so.

In order to select endocrine therapy for each individual in a scientific manner, it is essential to relate the activity of the tumour to the hormonal environment in that patient. There are three major aspects to this tumour-host relationship, and it has recently become possible to provide reasonably reliable indices of each. The aspects comprise the activity of the tumour itself, the patient's hormonal status which provides the existing environment for this activity, and the sensitivity of the tumour to change in the hormonal environment.

The division between the three categories is not absolute. It is claimed that some indices of the patient's hormonal status, such as the urinary discriminant ratio, may predict responsiveness to endocrine therapy in breast cancer. In addition, some indices of tumour activity, such as phosphohexose isomerase, can be included in a test system and used for assessing responsiveness to endocrine therapy.

References

Adams, J. B. (1964) Enzymic synthesis of steroid sulphates. II. Presence of steroid sulfokinase in human carcinoma extracts. *Journal of Clinical Endocrinology and Metabolism*, **24**, 988.

Adams, J. B. & Wong, M. S. F. (1968) Paraendocrine behaviour of human breast carcinoma. *In vitro* transformation of steroids to physiologically active hormones. *Journal of Endocrinology*, **41**, 41.

Ahlquist, K. A., Jackson, A. W. & Stewart, J. C. (1968) Urinary steroid values as a guide to prognosis in breast cancer. *British Medical Journal*, **1**, 217.

Altmann, F. P. & Chayen, J. (1967) A study of breast cancer by techniques of cellular biology and multiphase biochemistry. In *Cambridge Symposium on the Treatment of Carcinoma of the Breast*, p. 56, ed. Jarrett, A. S. Excerpta Medica Foundation.

A.M.A. Committee on Research (1960) Androgens and estrogens in the treatment of disseminated mammary carcinoma. *Journal of the American Association*, **172**, 1271.

Atkin, N. B. (1967) Sex chromatin in female breast cancer. *Lancet*, **ii**, 1145.

Atkins, H., Bulbrook, R. D., Falconer, M. A., Hayward, J. L., MacLean, K. S. & Schurr, P. H. (1968) Ten years experience of steroid assays in the management of breast cancer. *Lancet*, **ii**, 1255.

Barrett, R. J., Friesen, H. & Astwood, E. B. (1961) Electrophoresis of pituitary hormones in starch gel. *Federation Proceedings*, **20**, 183.

Bauld, W. S. (1956) A method for the determination of estriol, estrone, and estradiol-17β in human urine by partition chromatography and colorimetric estimation. *Biochemical Journal*, **63**, 488.

Beck, J. C., Blair, A. J., Griffiths, M. M., Rosenfeld, M. W. & McGarry, E. E. (1966) In search of hormonal factors as an aid in predicting the outcome of breast carcinoma. *Canadian Cancer Conference*, **6**, 3.

Bennett, R. C. & Harris, J. D. (1966) Pituitary ablation by implantations of Yttrium[90] seeds. *Medical Journal of Australia*, **2**, 673.

Birke, G., Diczfalusy, E., Franksson, C., Hellstrom, J., Hultberg, S., Plantin, L. & Westman, A. (1958) On the correlation between steroid excretion and clinical response to oophorectomy plus adrenalectomy in breast cancer. In *Endocrine Aspects of Breast Cancer*, p. 213, ed. Currie, A. R. and Illingsworth, C. F. W. Edinburgh: Livingstone.

Bleehen, N. M. & Bryant, T. H. E. (1967) *In vivo* studies of radioactive phosphorus in malignant tumours. *Clinical Radiology*, **18**, 237.

Block, G. E., Vial, A. B., McCarthy, J. D., Porter, C. W. & Coller, F. A. (1959) Adrenalectomy in advanced mammary cancer. *Surgery, Gynecology and Obstetrics*, **108**, 651.

Bohle, A. (1965) Significance of Barr bodies in mammary carcinoma. *Medizinische Welt* (Berlin), **23**, 1266. English abstract in *Cancer Chemotherapy Reports*, **6**, 252.

Bonser, G. M., Dossett, J. A. & Jull, J. W. (1961) Selection of patients for hypophysectomy or adrenalectomy. In *Human and Experimental Breast Cancer*, p. 450. Springfield: Charles C. Thomas.

Boyland, E., Godsmark, B., Greening, W. P., Rigby-Jones, P., Stevenson, J. J. & Abul Fadl, M. A. M. (1958) The effect of irradiation of the pituitary on gonadotropin excretion in women with advanced mammary cancer. In *Endocrine Aspects of Breast Cancer*, p. 170, ed. Currie, A. R. and Illingsworth, C. F. W. Edinburgh: Livingstone.

Braunsberg, H., Irvine, W. T. & James, V. H. T. (1967) A comparison of steroid hormone concentrations in human tissues including breast cancer. *British Journal of Cancer*, **21**, 714.

Braunsberg, H. & James, V. H. T. (1967) Observations on the binding of testosterone to malignant mammary tumours and other tissues in vitro. *British Journal of Cancer*, **21**, 703.

Brennan, M. J. (1966) Indices of response to breast cancer therapy. In *Clinical Evaluation in Breast Cancer*, p. 141, ed. Hayward, J. L. and Bulbrook, R. D. London: Academic Press.

Brindley, C. O. & Francis, F. L. (1963) Serum lactic dehydrogenase and glutamic-oxalacetic transaminase correlations with measurements of tumour masses during therapy. *Cancer Research*, **23**, 112.

Brown, J. B. (1955) A chemical method for the determination of oestriol, oestrone and oestradiol in human urine. *Biochemical Journal*, **60**, 185.

Brown, J. B., MacLeod, S. C., Macnaughten C., Smith, M. A. & Smyth, B. (1968) A rapid method for estimating oestrogens in urine using a semiautomatic extractor. *Journal of Endocrinology*, **42**, 5.

Bruce, J., Hamilton, T., Sneddon, A. & Smyth, B. J. (1969) Endocrine aspects of breast cancer. *British Empire Campaign, Annual Report*, 435.

Bulbrook, R. D., Greenwood, F. C., Hadfield, G. J. & Scowen, E. F. (1958) Oophorectomy in breast cancer. An attempt to correlate clinical results with oestrogen production. *British Medical Journal*, **ii**, 7.

Bulbrook, R. D., Greenwood, F. C. & Hayward, J. L. (1960a) Selection of breast cancer patients for adrenalectomy or hypophysectomy by determination of urinary 17 hydroxycorticosteroids and aetiocholanolone. *Lancet*, **i**, 1154.

Bulbrook, R. D., Greenwood, F. C. & Williams, P. C. (1960b) Comparison of biological and chemical estimations of urinary oestrogens: II Urine from patients with breast cancer maintained on cortisone after oophorectomy, adrenalectomy, or hypophysectomy. *Journal of Endocrinology*, **20**, 220.

Bulbrook, R. D. & Hayward, J. L. (1962) Steroid hormones and prognosis in human breast cancer. *Acta Unio internationalis contra cancrum*, **18**, 893.

Burnett, W., McAllister, R. A. & Shields, R. (1963) The use of serum glycoprotein levels in the selection of patients with advanced breast cancer for endocrine surgery. *Scottish Medical Journal*, **8**, 197.

Cameron, E. H. D., Griffiths, K., Cleave, E. N., Stewart, H. J., Forrest, A. P. M. & Campbell, H. (1970) Benign and malignant breast disease in South Wales: a study of urinary steroids. *British Medical Journal*, **iv**, 768.

Castellanos, H., Fairgrieve, J., O'Morchoe, P. J. & Moore, F. D. (1963) Corticotropin stimulation of urethral cornification. *Journal of the American Medical Association*, **184**, 295.

Castellanos, H. & Sturgis, S. H. (1958) Cytology of human urinary sediment. Diagnostic value of the non nucleated cell. *Journal of Clinical Endocrinology*, **18**, 1369.

Chayen, P., Altmann, F. P. & Bitensky, L. (1970) Response of human breast cancer tissue to steroid hormones *in vitro*. *Lancet*, **i**, 869.

Crowley, L. G., Demetriou, J. A., McDonald, I., Kotin, P., Kushinsky, S. & Donovan, A. J. (1962) Levels of exogenous estrogens in tissues in human mammary carcinoma. *Surgical Forum*, **13**, 103.

Dao, T. L. Y. & Huggins, C. (1955) Bilateral adrenalectomy in the treatment of cancer of the breast. *Archives of Surgery*, **71**, 645.

Dao, T. L. & Libby, P. R. (1969) Conjugation of hormones by breast cancer tissue and selection of patients for adrenalectomy. *Surgery* (*Baltimore*), **66**, 162.

Dederick, M. M., Hall, T. C., Yatsuhashi, J. W. & Nevinny, H. B. (1966) Electrovaginal potentials, vaginal cytology and hormone therapy. *Surgery Gynecology and Obstetrics*, **123**, 751.

Deshpande, N., Bulbrook, R. D. & Ellis, F. G. (1963) An apparent selective accumulation of testosterone in human breast tissue. *Journal of Endocrinology*, **25**, 555.

Deshpande, N., Jensen, V., Bulbrook, R. D. & Doouss, T. W. (1967) In vivo steroidogenesis by the human adrenal gland. *Steroids*, **9**, 393.

De Waard, F., Baanders-van Halewijn, E. A. & Huizinga, J. (1964) The bimodal age distribution of patients with mammary carcinoma. *Cancer* (*Philadelphia*), **17**, 141.

Douglas, M., Falconer, C. W. A., Strong, J. A. & Loraine, J. A. (1961) Urinary excretion of gonadotropins in relation to treatment of mammary carcinoma by bilateral adrenalectomy and oophorectomy. In *Human Pituitary Gonadotropins*, p. 249, ed. Albert, A. Springfield: Charles C. Thomas.

Ehlers, P. N., Hochberg, K. & Nuri, M. (1966) Hormonal treatment of mammary carcinoma and demonstration of Barr bodies in cellular nuclei. *Cancer Chemotherapy Abstracts*, **7**, 288.

Ellis, F. G., Berne, T. U., Deshpande, N., Belzer, F. O. & Bulbrook, R. D. (1969) The uptake of tritiated steroids by human breast carcinoma. *Surgery, Gynecology and Obstetrics*, **128**, 975.

Emerson, K. & Jessiman, A. G. (1956) Hormonal influences on the growth and progression of cancer: Tests for hormone dependency in mammary and prostate cancer. *New England Journal of Medicine*, **254**, 252.

Emerson, W. J., Kennedy, B. J., Graham, J. N. & Nathanson, I. T. (1953) Pathology of primary and recurrent carcinoma of the human breast after administration of steroid hormones. *Cancer (Philadelphia)*, **6**, 641.

Emerson, W. J., Kennedy, B. J. & Taft, E. B. (1960) Correlation of histological alterations in breast cancer with response to hormone therapy. *Cancer (Philadelphia)*, **13**, 1047.

Ferguson, K. A. & Wallace, A. L. C. (1961) Starch gel electrophoresis of anterior pituitary hormones. *Nature (London)*, **190**, 629.

Flaxel, J. & Wellings, S. R. (1963) Toxic effects of testosterone on organ cultures of mammary carcinoma cells of C3H/CRGL mice. *Federation Proceedings*, **22**, 331.

Folca, P. J., Glascock, R. F. & Irvine, W. T. (1961) Studies with tritium labelled hexoestrol in advanced breast cancer. *Lancet*, **ii**, 796.

Fotherby, K., Sellwood, R. A. & Burn, J. I. (1968) Urinary steroid excretion in patients with advanced breast cancer. *British Journal of Surgery*, **55**, 868.

Gardner, B. & Gordon, G. S. (1962) Does urinary calcium excretion reflect the growth or regression of disseminated breast cancer? *Journal of Clinical Endocrinology*, **22**, 627.

Gerbrandy, J. & Hellendorn, H. B. A. (1957) The diagnostic value of calciuria during hormonal treatment of metastasised mammary carcinoma. *Acta Endocrinologica (København)* Supplement, **31**, 275.

Goldenberg, I. S., Blodinger, P. H. & Grumman, R. A. (1966) Some observations on thyroid and adreno-cortical relationships. *Surgery*, **59**, 522.

Gordon, D. L. & Segaloff, A. (1958) Castration as a palliative therapy for advanced breast cancer. In *Breast Cancer*, p. 187, ed. Segaloff, A. St. Louis: C. V. Mosby.

Green, A. (1961) Hormone control of breast cancer. *Lancet*, **ii**, 828.

Griffith, M. M. & Beck, J. C. (1963) The value of serum phosphohexose isomerase as an index of metastatic breast carcinoma activity. *Cancer (Philadelphia)*, **16**, 1032.

Guzzo, C. E., Pachas, W. N., Pinals, R. S. & Krant, M. J. (1969) Urinary hydroxyproline excretion in patients with cancer. *Cancer (Philadelphia)*, **24**, 382.

Hadfield, G. (1957) The nature and origin of the mammotropic agent present in human female urine. *Lancet*, **i**, 1058.

Hale, B. T. (1961). A technique for studying human tumour growth *in vivo*. *Lancet*, **ii**, 345.

Hall, T. C., Dederick, M. M. & Nevinny, H. B. (1963a) Prognostic value of hormonally induced hypercalcemia in breast cancer. *Cancer Chemotherapy Reports*, **30**, 21.

Hall, T. C., Dederick, M. M., Nevinny, H. B. & Muench, H. (1963b) Prognostic value of response of patients with breast cancer to therapeutic castration. *Cancer Chemotherapy Reports*, **31**, 47.

Harshman, S., Patikas, T. P., Dayani, K. & Reynolds, V. H. (1967) Serum mucoid levels in patients with cancer and the effect of surgical treatment. *Cancer Research*, **27**, 1286.

Hayward, J. L. & Bulbrook, R. D. (1966) *Clinical Evaluation in Breast Cancer*. London: Academic Press.

Hayward, J. L., Bulbrook, R. D. & Greenwood, F. C. (1961) Hormone assays and prognosis in breast cancer. *Memoirs of the Society of Endocrinology*, **10**, 144.

Hellman, L., Bradlow, H. L., Zumoff, B. & Gallagher, T. F. (1961) The influence of thyroid hormone on hydrocortisone production and metabolism. *Journal of Clinical Endocrinology*, **21**, 1231.

Heuson, J. C. & Legros, N. (1963) *In vitro* effect of testosterone and 17β-Estradiol on L-leucine ^{14}C incorporation into human breast cancer. *Cancer (Philadelphia)*, **16**, 404.

Hiisi-Brummer, L., Hortling, H., Malmio, K. & Af Bjorkesten, G. (1960) The effect of hypophysectomy on the oestrogen effect in the body as measured by the vaginal smear technique in metastasising mammary cancer. *Acta Endocrinologica (København)*, **33**, 81.

Hill, B. R. & Levi, C. (1954) Elevation of a serum component in neoplastic disease. *Cancer Research*, **14**, 513.

Hollander, V. P., Jonas, H. & Smith, D. E. (1958) Estradiol-sensitive isocitric dehydrogenase in non-cancerous and cancerous human breast tissue. *Cancer (Philadelphia)*, **11**, 803.

Hollander, V. P., Smith, D. E. & Adamson, T. E. (1959) Studies on estrogen-sensitive transhydrogenase: the effect of estradiol 17β on α-ketoglutarate production in non-cancerous and cancerous human breast tissue. *Cancer (Philadelphia)*, **12**, 135.

Hortling, H., Hiisi-Brummer, L. & Af Bjorkesten, G. A. (1962) Endocrine therapy of metastasising breast cancer. *Acta Medica Scandinavica*, **172**, Supplement 385.

Irvine, W. T., Aitken, E. H., Rendleman, D. L. & Folca, P. J. (1961) Urinary oestrogen measurements after oophorectomy and adrenalectomy for advanced breast cancer. *Lancet*, **ii**, 791.

James, V. H. T. & Braunsberg, H. (1969) Disposition of steroid hormones in body tissue with special reference to human breast cancer. *British Empire Cancer Campaign, Annual Report*, 212.

Jensen, E. V., Desombre, E. R. & Jungblut, P. W. (1967) Estrogen receptors in hormone responsive tissues and tumour. In *Endogenous Factors Influencing Host-tumour Balance*, ed. Wissler, R. W., Dao, T. and Wood, S. Jr. Chicago: University of Chicago Press.

Joplin, G. F. & Jegatheesan, K. A. (1962) Serum glycolytic enzymes and acid phosphatas in mammary carcinomatosis. *British Medical Journal*, **i**, 827.

Jull, J. W., Shucksmith, H. S. & Bonser, G. M. (1963) A study of urinary estrogen excretion in relation to breast cancer. *Journal of Clinical Endocrinology*, **23**, 433.

Juret, P., Hayem, M. & Flaisler, A. (1964) Quoted in *Endocrine Surgery in Human Cancers*, p. 215, by Juret, P. Springfield: Charles C. Thomas, 1966.

Karnofsky, D. A. & Burchenal, J. H. (1949) Clinical evaluation of chemotherapeutic agents in cancer. In *Evaluation of Chemotherapeutic Agents*, p. 101, ed. McLeod, C. M. New York: Columbia University Press.

Kellner, G. & Turcic, G. (1962) The importance of tissue culture for hormonal therapy of mammary carcinoma. *Klinische Medizin (Wien)*, **17**, 83.

Kennedy, B. J. (1965) Hormonal control of breast cancer. *Annals of Internal Medicine*, **63**, 329.

Kimel, V. M. (1957) Clinical cytological correlations of mammary carcinoma based upon sex chromatin counts. *Cancer (Philadelphia)*, **10**, 922.

Kumaoka, S., Sakauchi, N., Abe, O., Kusama, M. & Takatani, O. (1968) Urinary 17-ketosteroid excretion of women with advanced breast cancer. *Journal of Endocrinology and Metabolism*, **28**, 667.

Lazarev, N. J. (1960) New developments in the hormone therapy of malignant tumours. In *Cancer Progress 1960*, p. 204, ed. Raven, R. W. London: Butterworth.

Lewison, E. F., Levi, J. E., Jones, G. S., Jones, H. W. & Silberstein, H. E. (1951) Tracer studies of radioactive sodium estrone sulfate in cases of advanced breast cancer. *Cancer (Philadelphia)*, **4**, 537.

Lipsett, M. B. & Bergenstal, D. M. (1960) Lack of effect of human growth hormone and ovine prolactin on cancer in man. *Cancer Research*, **20**, 1172.

Liu, W. (1957) Vaginal cytology in breast cancer patients. *Surgery, Gynecology and Obstetrics*, **105**, 421.

Lloyd Williams, K. (1964) Temperature measurement in breast cancer. *Annals of the New York Academy of Science*, **121**, 272.

Loraine, J. A., Strong, J. A. & Douglas, M. (1957) The value of pituitary gonadotrophin assays in patients with mammary carcinoma. *Lancet*, **ii**, 575.

Low-Beer, B. V. A. & Green, R. B. (1952) Radiophosphorus studies in breast tumours. *Cardiologia*, **21**, 497.

McAllister, R. A., Sim, A. W., Hobkirk, R., Stewart, H., Blair, D. W. & Forrest, A. P. M. (1960) Urinary oestrogens after endocrine ablation. *Lancet*, **i**, 1102.

McCalister, A. & Welbourn, R. B. (1962) Stimulation of mammary cancer by prolactin and the clinical response to hypophysectomy. *British Medical Journal*, **i**, 1669.

McCullagh, E. P., Feldstein, M. A., Tweed, D. C. & Dohn, D. F. (1965) A study of pituitary function after intrasellar implantation of ^{90}Yt. *Journal of Clinical Endocrinology*, **25**, 832.

Mansfield, C. M., Dodd, G. D., Wallace, J. D., Kramer, S. & Curley, R. F. (1968) Use of heat sensing devices in cancer therapy. *Radiology*, **91**, 673.

Martin, F. I. R. (1964) Urinary gonadotropins in postmenopaused women with breast cancer. *British Medical Journal*, **ii**, 351.

Meier-Ruge, W. (1966) Diagnostic significance of sex chromatin content in relationship to enzyme histochemistry, DNA content and mitotic index in breast carcinoma. *Cancer Chemotherapy Abstracts*, **7**, 467.

Miller, H., Durant, J. A., Jacobs, A. G. & Allison, J. F. (1967) Alternative discriminating function for determining hormone dependency of breast cancer. *British Medical Journal*, **i**, 147.

Mioduszewska, O. (1968) In *Prognostic Factors in Breast Cancer*, p. 347, ed. Forrest, A. P. M. and Kunkler, P. B. Edinburgh: Livingstone.

Mobbs, B. G. (1970) The effect of testosterone treatment on the uptake of oestradiol 17β by DMBA induced rat mammary tumours. *Journal of Endocrinology*, **48**, 293.

Moore, K. & Barr, M. (1957) The sex chromatin in human malignant tissues. *British Journal of Cancer*, **11**, 384.

Mozden, P. J. & Parsons, L. (1965) Patients with breast cancer using electrovaginography. *Surgical Forum*, **16**, 120.

Myers, W. P. L. & Bodansky, O. (1957) Comparison of serum phosphohexose isomerase activity and urinary calcium excretion in patients with metastatic mammary carcinoma. *American Journal of Medicine*, **28**, 804.

Nabarro, J. D. N. (1960) Selection of breast cancer patients for adrenalectomy or hypophysectomy. *Lancet*, **i**, 1293.

Neal, F. E. (1966) The choice of hormones in the treatment of advanced carcinoma of the breast. In *The Value of Cytotoxic Agents and Anabolic Steroids in the Treatment of Advanced Malignant Disease*, p. 38, ed. Abrahamson, M. London: Parcener Press.

Nevinny, H. B. & Hall, T. C. (1963) *In situ* determination of the anti-tumour effect of chemotherapeutic compounds. *2nd International Symposium on Chemotherapy, Naples*, **3**, 219.

Palmer, J. D. & Hellstrom, J. (1962) The use of urinary estrogen estimations as a means of predicting response to oophorectomy and adrenalectomy in breast cancer. *Canadian Journal of Surgery*, **5**, 180.

Pearson, O. H. (1957) Observations on the role of androgens and estrogens in body balance. *Archives of Internal Medicine*, **100**, 724.

Pearson, O. H. & Ray, B. S. (1959) Results of hypophysectomy in the treatment of metastatic mammary carcinoma. *Cancer (Philadelphia)*, **12**, 85.

Pearson, O. H., West, C. D., Hollander, V. P. & Escher, G. C. (1952) Alterations in calcium metabolism in patients with osteolytic tumours. *Journal of Clinical Endocrinology*, **12**, 926.

Plimpton, C. H. & Gellhorn, A. (1956) Hypercalcemia in malignant disease without evidence of bone destruction. *American Journal of Medicine*, **21**, 750.

Pommatau, E., Poulain, S., Dargent, M. & Mayer, M. (1963) FSH levels in the postmenopausal or castrated woman with advanced mammary cancer. Effect of adrenalectomy. English abstract in *Cancer Chemotherapy Abstracts*, **4**, 249.

Pundel, J. P. (1958) Does one need to gradually increase the dosage of administered estrogens in patients under long term estrogen therapy in order to maintain high proliferation? *Acta Cytologica*, **2**, 377.

Quincey, R. V. & Gray, G. H. (1966) Uptake of 17α-methyltestosterone by breast carcinoma and other tissues of human subjects. *British Journal of Cancer*, **20**, 271.

Regele, H., Kaufmann, F. & Wasl, H. (1964) The problem of sex chromatin in tumors. English abstract in *Cancer Chemotherapy Abstracts*, **5**, 630.

Regele, H. & Vagacs, H. (1962) Hormone dependency in malignant tumours of the breast. English abstract in *Cancer Chemotherapy Abstracts*, **3**, 828.

Rienits, K. G. (1959) The effects of estrone and testosterone on respiration of human mammary cancer *in vitro*. *Cancer (Philadelphia)*, **21**, 958.

Rimm, A. A., Ahlstrom, J. K. & Bross, I. D. J. (1966) What is objective response? *Proceedings of the American Association for Cancer Research*, **7**, 59.

Rivera, E. M., Elias, J. J., Bern, H. A., Napalkov, N. P. & Pitelka, D. R. (1963) Toxic effects of steroid hormones on organ cultures of mouse mammary tumours. *Journal of the National Cancer Institute*, **31**, 671.

Sarfaty, G. & Tallis, M. (1970) Probability of a woman with advanced breast cancer responding to adrenalectomy or hypophysectomy. *Lancet*, **ii**, 685.

Scowen, E. F. (1958) Oestrogen excretion after hypophysectomy in breast cancer. In *Endocrine Aspects of Breast Cancer*, p. 208, ed. Currie, A. R. and Illingsworth, C. F. Edinburgh: Livingstone.

Segaloff, A. (1960) Testosterone propionate therapy of breast cancer—a report from the Co-operative breast cancer group. In *Biological Activities of Steroids in Relation to Cancer*, p. 355, ed. Pincus, G. and Vollmer, E. P. New York: Academic Press.

Segaloff, A. (1967) Pituitary hormones influencing breast cancer. In *Current Concepts in Breast Cancer*, p. 94, ed. Segaloff, A., Meyer, K. K. and Debakey, S. Baltimore: Williams & Wilkins.

Segaloff, A., Gordon, D., Carabasi, R. A., Horwitt, B. N., Schlosser, J. V. & Murison, P. J. (1954) Hormonal therapy in cancer of the breast; VII Effect of conjugated estrogens (equine) on clinical course and hormonal excretion. *Cancer (Philadelphia)*, **7**, 758.

Shirley, R. L. (1967) The nuclear sex of breast cancer. *Surgery, Gynecology and Obstetrics*, **125**, 737.

Sim, A. W., Hobkirk, R., Blair, D. W., Stewart, H. J. & Forrest, A. P. M. (1961) Accessory adrenocortical function after adrenalectomy in patients with breast cancer. *Lancet*, **ii**, 73.

Smith, J. A., King, R. J. B., Meggitt, B. F. & Allen, L. N. (1970) Enzyme activity, acidic nuclear proteins and prognosis in human breast cancer. *British Medical Journal*, **ii**, 698.

Sneddon, A., Steel, J. M. & Strong, J. A. (1968) Effect of thyroid function and of obesity on the discriminant function for mamary carcinoma. *Lancet*, **ii**, 792.

Stewart, J. G., Skinner, L. G. & O'Connor, P. J. (1965) Hormone therapy in metastatic breast cancer: clinical response and urinary gonadotropins. *Acta Endocrinologica (København)*, **50**, 346.

Stoll, B. A. (1959) Fluoxymesterone (Halotestin) in advanced breast carcinoma. *Medical Journal of Australia* **1**, 70.

Stoll, B. A. (1963) Corticosteroids in the therapy of advanced mammary cancer. *British Medical Journal*, **2**, 210.

Stoll, B. A. (1964a) Fact and fallacy in the hormonal control of breast cancer. *Medical Journal of Australia*, **1**, 980.

Stoll, B. A. (1964b) Hormones and breast cancer. *British Medical Journal*, **ii**, 755.

Stoll, B. A. (1965) Breast cancer and hypothyroidism. *Cancer (Philadelphia)*, **18**, 1431.

Stoll, B. A. (1967) Vaginal cytology as an aid to hormone therapy in postmenopausal breast cancer. *Cancer (Philadelphia)*, **20**, 1807.

Stoll, B. A. (1969) *Hormonal Management in Breast Cancer*. London: Pitman Medical.

Stoll, B. A. (1970) Investigation of organ culture as an aid to the hormonal management of breast cancer. *Cancer (Philadelphia)*, **25**, 1228.

Stoll, B. A. (1971) The thermoprofile as an early indicator of breast cancer response to hormonal therapy. *Cancer (Philadelphia)*, **27**, 1379.

Stoll, B. A. & Burch, W. M. (1968) Surface detection of circadian rhythm in ^{32}P content of breast cancer. *Cancer (Philadelphia)*, **21**, 193.

Strong, J. A. (1963) Hormonal control of cancer. *Proceedings of the Royal Society of Medicine*, **56**, 665.

Strong, J. A., Brown, J. B., Bruce, J., Douglas, M., Klopper, A. I. & Loraine, J. A. (1956) Sex hormone excretion after bilateral adrenalectomy and oophorectomy in patients with mammary carcinoma. *Lancet*, **ii**, 965.

Struthers, R. A. (1956) Postmenopausal oestrogen production. *British Medical Journal*, **i**, 1331.

Swyer, G. I. M., Lee, A. E. & Masterton, J. P. (1961) Oestrogen excretion of patients with breast cancer. *British Medical Journal*, **i**, 617.

Taylor, D. M., Parker, R. P., Field, E. O. & Greatorex, C. A. (1968) An interpretation of the results of measurements of the uptake of ^{32}P in human tumours. *British Journal of Radiology*, **41,** 432.

Tchao, R., Easty, G. C., Ambrose, E. J., Raven, R. W. & Bloom, H. J. G. (1968) Effects of chemotherapeutic agents and hormones on organ cultures of human tumours. *European Journal of Cancer*, **4,** 39.

Wacker, B. & Miles, C. P. (1966) Sex chromatin incidence and prognosis in breast cancer. *Cancer (Philadelphia)*, **19,** 1561.

Wade, A. P., Davis, J. C., Tweedie, M. C. K., Clarke, C. A. & Haggart, B. (1969) The discriminant factor in early carcinoma of the breast. *Lancet*, **i,** 853.

Walpole, A. L. & Paterson, E. (1949) Synthetic oestrogens in mammary cancer. *Lancet*, **ii,** 783.

Wilson, R. E., Crocker, D. W., Fairgrieve, J., Bartholomay, A. F., Emerson, K. & Moore, F. D. (1967) Adrenal structure and function in advanced carcinoma of breast. *Journal of the American Medical Association*, **199,** 474.

Wolff, B. (1957) The differential cell count in cancer of the breast and response to hormone therapy. *Guy's Hospital Reports*, **106,** 53.

Woodard, H. Q., Escher, G. C. & Farrow, J. H. (1954) Changes in the blood chemistry of patients with disseminated carcinoma of the breast during endocrine therapy. *Cancer (Philadelphia)*, **7,** 744.

Woolley-Hart, A., Twentyman, P., Corfield, J., Joslin, C., Morrison, R. & Fowler, J. F. (1968) Changes in ^{32}P counting rate in human and animal tumours. *British Journal of Radiology*, **41,** 440.

Young, S., Bulbrook, R. D. & Greenwood, F. C. (1957) The correlation between urinary estrogens and vaginal cytology. *Lancet*, **i,** 350.

Section II

Breast Cancer—Endocrine Therapy

Chapter 6

The Basis of Endocrine Therapy

BASIL A. STOLL

Malignant tumours may resemble their parent tissue in responding to changes in the level of specific circulating hormones, and breast cancer shows such 'hormonal sensitivity' in a minority of cases. Whereas in the case of thyroid, prostatic and endometrial cancer the hormone-sensitive tumours are usually those showing a very advanced degree of histological differentiation, this does not apparently apply to breast cancer. This surprising finding results from the heterogenous microscopic structure reported in the majority of breast cancers. Tumour grading based on cell of origin (Murad, 1971) may provide better correlation with clinical hormone sensitivity.

HORMONAL SENSITIVITY AND AUTONOMY

Clinical evidence of *significant* tumour response (as discussed in Chapter 5) appears in about 30 to 40 per cent of patients after being subjected to changes in the endocrine environment. The endocrine change may be spontaneous (as seen most commonly at the time of the menopause), or it may be induced by endocrine gland ablation or by additive hormone therapy. While the clinical response to additive hormone therapy usually takes the form of tumour growth inhibition, there are sometimes local or general changes which suggest growth stimulation. This is difficult to prove objectively because our clinical parameters of tumour growth are not sufficiently sensitive.

The failure of a tumour to show clinical evidence of response to endocrine change is categorised as 'tumour autonomy'. Autonomy is popularly assumed to occur in 60 to 70 per cent of breast cancers, but this is a considerable overestimate. Although every degree of response is possible, only a 50 per cent (or greater) decrease in tumour volume is generally accepted as significant. Furthermore, only a three months' (or longer) duration of response is acceptable for significant tumour remission. Yet, hormonal dependence need not necessarily involve major or prolonged shrinkage of a lesion. It should be noted that even *complete cessation* of cell division will not reduce the size of a tumour unless spontaneous cell loss is taking place at the same time, or unless death of adult cells is also caused by the endocrine change.

the case of breast cancer as it can be in the case of thyroid cancer (see Chapter 19).

HORMONAL BACKGROUND OF BREAST CANCER

Apart from genetic and viral factors (Moore et al, 1971), multiple hormonal influences affect the induction of breast cancer as is

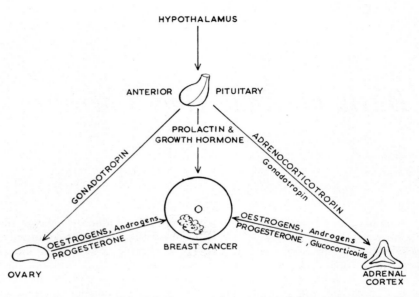

FIGURE 6.1. Diagrammatic representation of the hormonal factors which influence the growth of breast cancer in the female. (Figure reproduced from Stoll, 1969, by permission of Pitman Medical.)

When it occurs, hormonally induced inhibition of growth is temporary. The hormone-sensitive tumour regresses for a period of months or years, after which it reactivates, and its growth continues independently of further changes in the hormonal environment. It is assumed that the tumour initially contains cells of two types, sensitive and autonomous, and that the recurrent tumour is composed of autonomous cells, when the sensitive cells are eliminated by withdrawing their supporting hormone. The autonomous cells are 'de-differentiated', at least in a biological sense, although a change cannot always be demonstrated histologically in

shown diagrammatically in Figure 6.1. The development of the tumour is almost certainly influenced by oestrogens and progesterone secreted both by the ovary and the adrenal cortex. It is probably influenced by androgens secreted by the ovary and the adrenal gland, and possibly influenced by adrenal corticosteroids and by the thyroid hormones.

The pituitary also affects the growth of the tumour, indirectly through its secretion of gonadotropin and adrenocorticotropin, and directly through its secretion of the prolactin-growth hormone complex. The hormones controlling breast cancer growth are subject to homeostatic mechanisms of which a typical example is the reciprocity which exists between the gonadal and the pituitary secretions. An abnormally high oestrogen concentration in the blood, established by therapeutic administration, will lead to a decreased release of gonadotropin. Conversely, a fall in the systemic oestrogen level, due either to the natural menopause or to castration, will lead to an increased release of pituitary gonadotropin with stimulation of extraovarian sources of oestrogen (Figure 6.2).

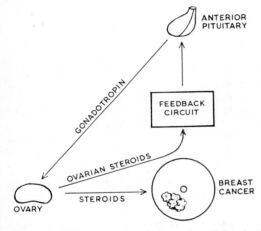

FIGURE 6.2. Diagrammatic representation of the pituitary-gonadal relationship in the female with breast cancer as a closed-cycle, feedback system. (Figure reproduced from Stoll, 1969, by permission of Pitman Medical.)

Thus, in the case of breast cancer, reactivation of tumour growth after a period of regression may be due to homeostatic mechanisms in the host, apart from the development of autonomy in the tumour cells as already mentioned. Although further episodes of tumour regression may follow subsequent endocrine ablation or additive hormone therapy, endocrine manipulation in breast cancer can be only a temporary palliative, and not a curative, procedure in our present state of knowledge.

The following paragraphs review briefly our knowledge of some relevant physiological

hormonal relationships in the female, both before and after the menopause.

The anterior lobe of the pituitary gland secretes two gonadotropins, follicle-stimulating hormone (FSH) and luteinising hormone (LH). After the menopause the systemic level of gonadotropin rises as the oestrogen level falls, and reaches its peak at about 20 years after the menopause. Persistent oestrogen secretion after the menopause can nevertheless be demonstrated biochemically (Brown, 1955) and in vaginal smear examination (Salmon and Frank, 1956). It even increases after the menopausal changes have subsided, so that significant levels may persist even in old age.

In the older postmenopausal patient, some oestrogen is presumed to arise in the adrenal cortex (Dao, 1953; Smith and Emerson, 1954) although most is derived from the food and from conversion of androgens. Oestrogen secretion from the adrenal cortex can be stimulated by ACTH as well as by FSH secretion, and can be inhibited by corticosteroid administration (Nathanson, Engel and Kelley, 1951; West, Damast and Pearson, 1958; Sandberg et al, 1958).

In the younger postmenopausal patient a portion of the systemic oestrogen may continue to be secreted by the ovarian stroma, but identification of oestrogens having an ovarian origin is difficult. Cyclical variation over the month in the oestrogen excretion level is suggestive of an ovarian origin, and this has been demonstrated in many postmenopausal patients (Brown, 1967). The failure of dexamethasone to suppress *all* oestrogen excretion is also suggestive of an extra-adrenal source of secretion (Schweppe, Jungman and Lewis, 1967). This is, however, not necessarily the ovary, as it may also lie in dietary oestrogen (Briggs, 1957), conversion of androgen to oestrogen in the body (West et al, 1956), or even in oestrogen synthesis by the tumour (Adams and Wong, 1968).

It has been claimed that the ovary may continue oestrogen secretion even in the older postmenopausal patient, because of the fall in the oestrogen excretion level which has been demonstrated after ovarian ablation up to the age of 70 (Nissen-Meyer, 1964). Other investigators do not confirm this observation (McBride, 1957; Barlow, Emerson and Saxena, 1969; Procope and Adlercreutz, 1969), and report that in women more than two years postmenopausal, the average level of oestrogen excretion is found to be no different from that of castrated women. It is therefore uncertain when the postmenopausal ovary gives up oestrogen secretion.

Major Hormonal Influences on Tumour Development

OESTROGEN

While oestrogens undoubtedly play a part in the aetiology of breast cancer, there is no direct evidence to incriminate *administered* oestrogen in the induction of human breast cancer. It has been called into question because of the occasional appearance of breast cancer during, or soon after, the therapeutic administration of oestrogens to women around the time of the menopause (Allaben and Owen, 1939; Auchinloss and Haagensen, 1940). The association is probably coincidental as one would expect a latent period of 10 to 15 years between a specific hormonal stimulus and the subsequent development of malignancy in a target organ (Bulbrook, 1966). Some authorities postulate that the hormonal status favouring the induction of breast cancer may occur as early as the first 10 years after the menarche (MacMahon and Cole, 1969). Nevertheless, it is still possible that administered oestrogen in later years may act as a co-carcinogen or 'trigger-factor' in the presence of a premalignant state of the breast.

Oestrogen administration can undoubtedly cause signs of growth *stimulation* in existing breast cancer in premenopausal women (Haddow et al, 1944; Nathanson, 1947; Taylor et al, 1948). Oestrogen therapy, even at low dosage, is therefore contraindicated in the management of menopausal symptoms in patients with a history or suspicion of breast cancer.

There is not yet enough information accumulated as to the effect that the use of oral contraceptives will have on the incidence of breast cancer in the human. However, the World Health Organisation (1966) has rightly cautioned against the use of oral contraceptives by women with a history or suspicion of breast cancer. Although the writer has reported tumour regression in some postmenopausal women following their administration (Stoll, 1967a), more information is needed as to whether their constituent hormones are more likely to *stimulate* or to *depress* the growth of existing breast cancer in premenopausal women.

It has been shown that a proportion of breast cancers can concentrate and retain oestrogen to a greater degree than normal tissue (Folca, Glascock and Irvine, 1961; Crowley et al, 1962; Ellis et al, 1969). It does not necessarily follow (although it is sometimes claimed) that there is any correlation between the oestrogen-blocking capacity of a steroid experimentally and its anti-tumour potency in the human. This remains to be proved.

It has been suggested that persistently high endogenous oestrogen levels may play a role in breast cancer induction. Hyperplasia of the ovarian cortical stroma has been noted at autopsy in 83 per cent of women with breast cancer, but in only 38 per cent of the general population (Sommers and Teloh, 1952; Sommers, Teloh and Goldman, 1953). Such pathology might be associated with an abnormally high level of oestrogen production during menstrual life. Its presence plays no special part, however, in the growth of established breast cancer, as there is no greater response rate to castration in patients with ovarian cortical hyperplasia than in other patients (Fracchia et al, 1969).

The normal range of oestrogen excretion in premenopausal women is wide, and contrary to early reports it is now accepted that there is no evidence of gross abnormality in *total* urinary oestrogen excretion in *premenopausal* women with breast cancer (Jull, Shucksmith and Bonser, 1963; Segaloff, 1967). However, it has been more recently suggested that high levels of *adrenal* oestrogen secretion may be associated with the late *postmenopausal* type of breast cancer (de Waard et al, 1964). This is difficult to prove with present methods of measurement.

It has also been suggested that the proportion of the component oestrogens may be of more importance than the total level. According to some recent reports, postmenopausal patients with breast cancer show a relatively *higher* excretion of urinary oestriol, relative to oestrone and oestradiol, than does the normal population (Marmorston, 1966; Gronroos and Aho, 1968). Another report, however, suggests a relatively *lower* oestriol excretion in such patients, and postulates that oestriol may protect against breast cancer development (Lemon, 1969). To complicate matters further, it has been shown that breast cancer tissue is itself capable of secreting oestriol (Adams and Wong, 1968). The significance in breast cancer patients of differences in the proportion of the component oestrogen levels is not clear.

ANTERIOR PITUITARY

In the control of breast cancer growth, the relative importance of anterior pituitary and ovarian hormones is still the major question. To explain the markedly different response to oestrogen therapy before and after the menopause, it has been postulated that there are two different types of breast cancer, the pituitary factor being more important in the postmenopausal type, and the oestrogen factor in the premenopausal type. It is, however, more likely that the *pituitary role is the major one in both cases*, and that oestrogens influence the growth of breast cancer mainly by an indirect effect through the pituitary gland.

Prolactin is a major stimulant of breast cancer development in experimental animals (Heuson, Walebroeck and Legros, 1970), and it has been shown that while physiological levels of oestrogen stimulate the anterior pituitary to secrete prolactin, administration of high doses of oestrogen will depress prolactin secretion (Furth and Clifton, 1958; Kim, Furth and Yannopoulos, 1963). On purely theoretical grounds, gonadotropin has also been charged with the stimulation of breast cancer development (Lazarev, 1960). Like prolactin, its secretion can either be stimulated or depressed by oestrogen administration according to the dose level (Riddle, 1963).

The hypothalamus may thus be involved in the stimulation of breast cancer because of its role in controlling pituitary function. Releasing factors for gonadotropin, growth hormone, ACTH, and TSH have been isolated in extracts of hypothalamic tissue and are normally transmitted through the hypophyseal portal system to the pituitary. An inhibiting factor for prolactin is also present in the hypothalamus, and is affected by psychotropic drugs of the phenothiazine series, as shown by the occasional appearance of galactorrhoea after their administration (Khazan et al, 1962). The writer is currently investigating agents with an effect on the hypothalamic centres in patients with breast cancer, in the hope of inducing selective 'medical hypophysectomy' (Stoll, 1971).

Spontaneous regression of advanced breast

cancer is reported in a few patients (Gurling, Scott and Baron, 1957). A possible explanation in some cases is that the pituitary fossa is the site of metastases from breast cancer, and if extensive, they may lead to a so-called 'spontaneous hypophysectomy'.

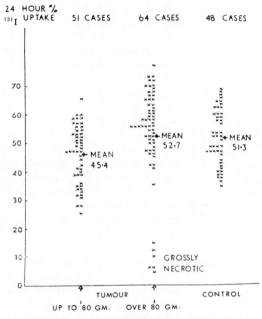

FIGURE 6.3. Percentage radioactive iodine uptake of thyroid gland at 24 hours, comparing breast cancer patients with tumours estimated up to 80 g, with those over 80 g in size. Variance ratio tests on the 'spread' of the values show a significant difference between the 'over 80 g' group and the control group ($F = 2.658$, $P < 0.01$). (Figure reproduced from Stoll, 1967, by permission of the Editor of *Cancer*, Philadelphia.)

THYROID

Many authors have commented on the findings of either a history of goitre or thyroidectomy, or signs of thyroid atrophy, in a high proportion of patients with breast cancer. This led to the suggestion that a state of hypothyroidism in the host might predispose to the development of breast cancer. Biochemical evidence of hypothyroidism has therefore been looked for in patients

with breast cancer by a number of investigators (Rawson, 1956; Edelstyn, Lyons and Welbourn, 1958; Hortling, Hiisi-Brummer and Af Bjorkesten, 1959; Marques, Bru and Espinasse, 1959; Carter, Feldman and Schwartz, 1960; Reeve et al, 1961; Dargent, Berger and Lahneche, 1962). Based mainly upon measurement of radioactive iodine uptake by the thyroid gland or of protein-bound iodine levels in the blood, their reports conflict on the existence of such an association.

One report, however, made the interesting observation that in some cases of breast cancer there was an abnormally high thyroid uptake of ^{131}I and raised protein-bound iodine level, *which returned to normal after mastectomy*, and rose again when metastasis occurred (Dargent et al, 1962). This suggested a relationship to the tumour's presence rather than to the cause of the tumour. This led me to compare the thyroid uptake of ^{131}I in 183 breast cancer patients with active tumour, to that in patients with 'cured' tumour and that in a control group (Stoll, 1965b). It was noted that not only does the presence of growing tumour modify thyroid uptake of ^{131}I, but the effect seems to vary with tumour size, and thus may be associated with iodine sequestration in the tumour (Figure 6.3). The writer therefore suggested that different proportions of patients with large tumours may account for some of the conflicting reports on the association of abnormal thyroid function tests with the presence of breast cancer.

It may be important that the thyroid function of the individual has been shown to affect the circulating level of corticosteroids, androgens and oestrogens (Goldenberg, Blodinger and Grummon, 1966). It also affects the relative proportion of the constituent oestrone, oestriol, and oestradiol fractions (Brown and Strong, 1962; Fishman et al, 1962). Thyroid function may therefore be of indirect importance in the *genesis* of breast cancer, where the role both of abnormal oestriol levels (Marmorston, 1966; Lemon,

1969) and abnormal androgen levels (Bulbrook, 1967) has recently been raised.

The prophylactic administration of thyroid hormone after mastectomy has been advised to exert a controlling effect on the growth of breast cancer (Loeser, 1954). A controlled trial has however shown that the administration of a course of tri-iodothyronine in doses of up to 120 μg daily does not influence the prognosis of breast cancer (Emery and Trotter, 1963).

ADRENAL

Metastases from breast cancer occur in the adrenal gland in a high proportion of patients (Warren and Witham, 1933; Lumb and Mackenzie, 1959), and it is possible for extensive replacement of the adrenal gland by metastases to cause unexpected regression of advanced breast cancer—the so-called 'spontaneous adrenalectomy'.

A relatively low excretion level of androgen metabolites is reported to be more common in women who subsequently develop breast cancer, and also in those patients developing early recurrence after mastectomy (Bulbrook, 1967). A low androgen excretion level is more common also in patients whose metastases do not respond to major endocrine ablation. A group of such patients was reported to show an abnormally low level of 17-desmolase secretion by the adrenal cortex (Deshpande et al, 1967), and this genetically determined enzyme abnormality may be responsible for the low excretion levels of androgen metabolites.

It has long been known that the death rate from mammary cancer in Japan is about one fifth of that in the United Kingdom. This decreased incidence was formerly ascribed to differences in breast-feeding habits, but this is now regarded as unlikely. It may also result from a genetically determined difference in the pattern of hormone secretion in Japanese women compared to women in the United Kingdom (Bulbrook, Thomas and Utsunomiya, 1964).

An early report suggested the excretion Δ^9-aetiocholenolone, an abnormal adrenocortical steroid, by patients with cancer (Dobriner et al, 1947), but later work showed that they are not specific to such patients. Similarly, the presence of adrenocortical hyperplasia has been reported in the relatively high proportion of 7·7 per cent of autopsies on patients with breast cancer (Parker and Sommers, 1956) but this may be a non-specific response to the presence of widespread cancer.

Other Influences on Tumour Development

EFFECT OF PREGNANCY AND LACTATION

Breast cancer appearing during pregnancy and lactation carries a poor prognosis, and a more rapid growth of the tumour has been suggested as the cause. A higher proportion of more anaplastic tumours has indeed been noted in patients with breast cancer associated with pregnancy or lactation (Bloom, 1955), and both this factor and the presence of vascular engorgement would worsen the prognosis.

The world literature reporting breast cancer in association with pregnancy or lactation demonstrates clearly that the poor prognosis is also associated with delay in diagnosis and treatment (White, 1954). It is noted that patients treated in the *second* half of pregnancy have the worse prognosis, and that it is in the second half of pregnancy that there is a significantly greater delay between the initial appearance of the tumour and subsequent treatment. As a result, a high proportion of patients are found to have advanced disease at the time of coming to treatment and, in addition, the risk of tumour dissemination is increased by delay at a time when maximum vascular engorgement is present in the breast.

Smaller series of breast cancer associated with pregnancy or lactation (Westberg, 1946; Holleb and Farrow, 1962; Peters, 1963) show little difference in their *overall* survival rate from that of a control group of women with breast cancer. Nevertheless, as in the larger series, they show a poor prognosis in patients treated in the second half of pregnancy, and this again is associated with a high proportion of advanced cases presumably due to delay in treatment.

The high hormonal levels occurring in pregnancy have also been suspected of increasing the activity of breast cancer. The first trimester of pregnancy is associated with a high level of circulating chorionic gonadotropin. In the second and third trimesters, placental secretion of oestrogens (especially oestriol) and progesterone increases to very high levels, and falls only when a high level of prolactin is released from the anterior pituitary following delivery. A poorer prognosis occurs in the later trimesters, but it is not due to the high oestrogen and progesterone levels, because it is found especially in those patients with delay in treatment or in those with an anaplastic tumour.

It follows that mastectomy should not be delayed in the presence of operable breast cancer in pregnancy. Further measures, such as the interruption of pregnancy followed by castration, make no difference to the prognosis in operable cases treated radically (White, 1954; Holleb and Farrow, 1962), but if the tumour is inoperable, both procedures are indicated in the hope of delaying tumour growth. It is noted in the next chapter that pregnancy does not increase the likelihood of reactivating 'cured' breast cancer.

EFFECT OF PARITY AND AGE GROUP

It has long been noted that multiparity is associated with a decreased likelihood of developing breast cancer, the risk being inversely proportional to the number of children borne (Lane-Claypon, 1926; Stocks, 1939; Peller, 1940; Clemmesen, 1951). It has subsequently been suggested that the greatest protective effect seems to be exerted if the first pregnancy occurs before the age of 20 (Stocks, 1958). Repeated high levels of oestrogen prevailing during pregnancy do not, therefore, increase predisposition to breast cancer and may in fact, protect the patient. This has been ascribed by some to the relatively high oestriol levels which occur in pregnancy (Cole and MacMahon, 1969). It is now considered doubtful whether there is any relationship between the duration of breast feeding, and the subsequent development of breast cancer (McMahon and Feinleib, 1960; Wynder, Bross and Hirayama, 1960; Lilienfeld, 1956, 1963).

There is a widespread impression that breast cancer occurring in the younger age group is more often of a higher grade of malignancy and carries a poorer prognosis. This has been reported in several series (Cade, 1950; Lewison, Trimble and Griffith, 1953; Kleinfeld, Haagensen and Cooley, 1963), although other series report a prognosis no different to that for older age groups (Richards, 1948; Scarff, 1948; Bloom, 1950). This latter opinion has been confirmed in a collected series of 549 patients under the age of 35 (Treves and Holleb, 1958), and it is also compatible that the distribution of the various histological grades of malignancy has been shown to be similar in all age groups (Lees and Park, 1949; Bloom, 1950). The effect of pregnancy and lactation is a separate influence on the prognosis of the disease in the younger age group and has been discussed above.

EFFECT OF EARLY MENOPAUSE AND CASTRATION

The proportion of women presenting with breast cancer is low between the ages of 50 and 55 (Clemmesen, 1948, 1965; Anderson et al, 1950). Since the mean age at the natural menopause is between 45 and 50, the tumour seems to be less active during the period of hormonal change following the cessation of menses. There are two alternative explanations for such an observation.

The first hypothesis is that tumour growth is slowed up in association with the failing ovarian activity occurring at the time of the menopause. There are several observations which support such a hypothesis. Spontaneous regression of breast cancer has been reported most commonly around the time of the menopause (Smithers, 1952). When the natural menopause intervenes between mastectomy and the first recurrence, the average 'free interval' is found to be longer than in other age groups (Clemmesen, 1948; Hadfield and Holt, 1956; AMA Committee on Research, 1960). The writer has noted that the highest incidence of radiologically sclerotic (slow-growing) bone metastases occurs in this group of patients, and that tumour growth is usually slow during the time that menopausal symptoms are most severe (Stoll, 1969). Finally, survival rates in breast cancer are reported to be significantly higher in the group of patients developing the disease between 41 and 50 years of age (Richards, 1948; Smithers et al, 1952; Delarue, 1955).

An alternative hypothesis to explain the low incidence of the disease around the time of the menopause is that the menopause separates two different types of breast cancer, the premenopausal and the late postmenopausal types (de Waard et al, 1964; Davis, Simons and Davis, 1964; Hems, 1967). The former type, of tumour with a peak age frequency between 40 and 50, would tend to be stimulated by oestrogen administration. The latter type, of peak frequency between 60 and 70, and pathologically characterised by a more abundant fibrous stroma, would be inhibited (Jull, 1958). This hypothesis would explain one of the major paradoxes in the hormonal therapy of breast cancer.

It would seem that early menopause may have a prophylactic value in decreasing liability to breast cancer. Several reports have shown a significantly greater proportion of previously castrated women in a control group than in a breast cancer series (Herrell, 1937; Dargent, 1949; Lilienfeld, 1956; McMahon and Feinleib, 1960). It has also been reported that breast cancer series show a higher proportion of patients with a delayed menopause compared with the normal population of the same age group (Olch, 1937; Wynder et al, 1960; AMA Committee on Research, 1960). Both these observations suggest that the longer the breast tissue is exposed to ovarian hormones, the greater the likelihood of developing breast cancer.

In summary, therefore, there is no direct evidence that the high oestrogen and progesterone levels of pregnancy increase the incidence or accelerate the growth of breast cancer in the human. There is both direct and indirect evidence however that ovarian hormones may stimulate the growth of the tumour in the premenopausal patient. The protective effect of early menopause, the predisposing effect of a late menopause, and the decreased growth rate of the tumour at the time of the menopause may be examples of such evidence. Moreover, oestrogen administration can stimulate the growth of breast cancer in premenopausal women. The commonly observed *regression* of *postmenopausal* breast cancer in response to oestrogen therapy may result from its having originated in a different hormonal environment.

Rationale of Hormonal Control in Breast Cancer

It has been a source of perplexity that two diametrically opposite methods have been used successfully for many years in the hormonal management of advanced breast cancer in women. One is the ablation of the ovaries or the adrenals, and the second is the administration of their hormonal secretion, namely oestrogens, progestins, corticosteroids and androgens. A further paradox is that cessation of oestrogen, androgen or progestin therapy may be followed by tumour regression—the so-called 'withdrawal response'—noted especially if there was tumour regression from the administration of the hormones.

'OESTROGEN DEPENDENCE' HYPOTHESIS

Castration leads to tumour regression in about one-third of premenopausal patients with advanced breast cancer. On the other hand, administration of oestrogen to premenopausal patients, or to patients whose tumour is regressing after castration, can lead to stimulation of tumour growth in some cases (Haddow et al, 1944; Nathanson, 1947; Taylor et al, 1948). These observations suggested the rationale that to create an unfavourable hormonal environment for disseminated breast cancer, one should aim at the reduction of oestrogen levels in the body, primarily by endocrine gland ablation.

To explain the temporary nature of the response to endocrine gland ablation, a temporary or incomplete withdrawal of oestrogens is postulated. Thus ovarian ablation removes a major source of oestrogen, but homeostatic mechanisms then cause increased secretion of pituitary FSH which stimulates oestrogen secretion by the adrenal cortex. Even pituitary ablation after previous oophorectomy and adrenalectomy, rarely leads to complete abolition of urinary oestrogen excretion (Greenwood and Bulbrook, 1957). A source for the oestrogens persisting in such cases is suggested to lie in accessory adrenal tissue, but this is very unlikely and the source probably lies in dietary oestrogens, in conversion of androgens to oestrogens in the body, or even in oestrogen synthesis by the tumour (Adams and Wong, 1968).

To explain failure of response to hormonal manipulation in about two-thirds of all cases, it was suggested that the growth of breast cancer in women may be either oestrogen-dependent or oestrogen-independent (Huggins and Dao, 1953; Pearson et al, 1954). If the tumour requires oestrogens for continued growth, they may be arising in the ovary or in the adrenal (Figure 6.4). Oophorectomy is the obvious step in the premenopausal patient, and if ovarian oestrogens are supporting the growth of the tumour, castration will cause objective evidence of tumour regression. This is ovary dependence. Reactivation of tumour growth at a later date is then ascribed to increasing oestrogen secretion from the adrenal cortex (Bulbrook and Greenwood, 1957).

If adrenal oestrogens are supporting the growth of tumour in the postmenopausal patient, bilateral adrenalectomy at this stage would remove the second major source of oestrogen, and again may cause tumour regression. This is adrenal dependence. When the tumour reactivates once more after temporary control by adrenalectomy, hypophyseal ablation will eliminate secretion of FSH and of ACTH. Both of these hormones are capable of stimulating ectopic adrenal sources of oestrogen which often show compensatory hyperplasia after bilateral adrenalectomy (Graham, 1953; Falls, 1955).

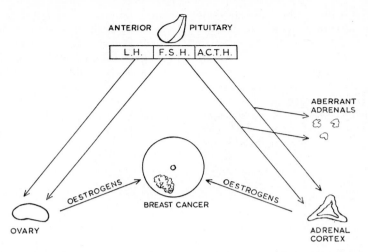

FIGURE 6.4. Diagrammatic representation of the oestrogen dependence hypothesis which has been suggested as a basis for the endocrine therapy of breast cancer in the female. (Figure reproduced from Stoll, 1969, by permission of Pitman Medical.)

INADEQUACY OF OESTROGEN DEPENDENCE HYPOTHESIS

The rationale of oestrogen reduction as a theoretical basis for endocrine control of breast cancer proved to be an over-simplification. After the introduction of biochemical methods of oestrogen assay (Brown, 1955) numerous attempts were made to correlate a favourable clinical response to castration, bilateral adrenalectomy or hypophysectomy, with a postoperative decrease in oestrogen level (Strong et al, 1956; Bulbrook et al, 1958; Gordon and Segaloff, 1958; Scowen, 1958; Hiisi-Brummer et al, 1960; McAllister et al, 1960; Irvine et al, 1961; Swyer, Lee and Masterson et al, 1961; Hortling, Hiisi-Brummer and Af Bjorkesten 1962; Palmer and Hellstrom, 1962; Jull et al, 1963).

In none of these reports could a correlation be established to a significant degree between postoperative change in oestrogen level (measured either biochemically or by cyto-hormonal evaluation of the vaginal smear) and the nature of the clinical response by the tumour. Regression of breast cancer following castration may be associated with either a higher, a lower, or an unchanged oestrogen excretion level. Tumour regression following either bilateral adrenalectomy or hypophysectomy is often associated with little change in the oestrogen excretion level. Moreover, tumour regression following hypophysectomy has not been related to the degree of adreno-cortical atrophy (Jantet et al, 1963).

Following a temporary response to ovarian or adrenal ablation, reactivation of the tumour is only rarely associated with an increase in the oestrogen excretion level. Furthermore, there is no evidence that oestrogen administration can reactivate the tumour in the presence of regression following hypophyseal ablation.

The oestrogen dependence concept is unable to explain satisfactorily the tumour regression in breast cancer commonly seen following administration of oestrogens to postmenopausal women, and first reported by Haddow (1944) and Nathanson (1946). Moreover, tumour regression is seen occasionally also in *premenopausal* women with breast cancer given very high doses of oestrogen (Nathanson, 1952; Kennedy, 1962). This applies both to the synthetic oestrogen diethylstilboestrol and to the natural conjugated equine oestrogens present in Premarin.

It is difficult to explain the observation of occasional cases of apparent tumour stimulation after major endocrine ablation (Wilson, Jessiman and Moore, 1958). Moreover, occasional patients appear to show rapid progression of tumour lesions following castration (Fracchia et al, 1969). In this connection it may be relevant that a transient rise in oestrogen excretion may immediately follow oophorectomy (Bulbrook and Greenwood, 1957), and this has been ascribed to operative 'stress' causing ACTH stimulation of adrenal oestrogen secretion.

MODIFIED OESTROGEN DEPENDENCE HYPOTHESIS

It has been noted in the previous section that administration of oestrogen may either stimulate or inhibit the growth of breast cancer in young women, according to the dose level utilised. It has therefore been suggested that there is an *optimal* dose level of oestrogen which favours tumour growth, while either higher or lower concentrations may depress tumour growth (Segaloff, 1966). This concept may explain some of the perplexities in the previous section.

The critical nature of oestrogen dosage is shown also in mouse mammary cancer induction where there is an optimum dosage of oestrogen, and doses either smaller or larger than this are not as effectual. It is possible that the control of established human breast cancer by additive hormone therapy may require individualised dose adjustment for each patient. Moreover, the optimum dose may change from time to time with changes in the patient's endogenous hormone secretion.

Such a hypothesis may explain the withdrawal response sometimes seen after oestrogen or androgen therapy. It is noted in about 30 per cent of patients whose tumour has regressed under oestrogen therapy, that when the tumour eventually reactivates, withdrawal of the steroid may be followed by a further tumour regression (Kaufman and Escher, 1961). A similar observation has been made in about 10 per cent of cases with previous evidence of remission under androgen therapy. The observation of a withdrawal response suggests that in the presence of tumour reactivation, a change in the steroidal *concentration* in the tumour environment may be more important in tumour control than changing the actual nature of the administered steroid.

Two modifications of this hypothesis have been offered:

1. There is an optimal oestrogen/androgen ratio in each individual which favours the growth of hormone-dependent breast cancer (Delarue, 1955). Change in the relative concentrations of these steroids will cause an unfavourable environment for the tumour cells, and consequent tumour regression, until its metabolism adjusts to the new environment. The importance of the androgenic environment to the growth of the tumour is suggested by the observation of a lesser likelihood of response to major endocrine ablation in the presence of abnormally low androgen secretion (Bulbrook, Greenwood and Hayward, 1960).

Administered androgens may be partly converted to oestrogens in the body (Nathanson et al, 1952; Baggett et al, 1956) and this may possibly explain the observation of exacerbation of breast cancer growth following androgen administration (Myers et al, 1955). Testosterone conversion to oestrogen has been shown even in patients who have previously been castrated and adrenalectomised (West et al, 1956). The site of conversion in such patients is uncertain but it can occur in the tumour also (Adams and Wong, 1968).

2. There is an optimal oestrogen/progesterone ratio in each individual which favours the growth of hormone-sensitive breast cancer. The tumour is either oestrogen-dependent or progesterone-dependent,

according to the environment in which the tumour develops (Jull, 1958). In older postmenopausal women the progesterone-dependent type would be more common, and tumour growth would be antagonised by increasing the oestrogen level, while in younger women the oestrogen-dependent type would be more common, and tumour growth would be antagonised by reducing the oestrogen level.

Experience with progestin therapy in breast cancer is still inadequate to lend support to this hypothesis but, as noted previously, statistical evidence also suggests that there are two types of breast cancer, a premenopausal and a postmenopausal type (Clemmesen, 1948; Anderson et al, 1950; de Waard et al, 1964; Hems, 1967).

The association of breast and endometrial cancer in the same patient occurs more frequently than would be expected from chance alone. The former is thought to arise as a result of unopposed oestrogen stimulation for considerable periods of time in a predisposed individual (see Chapter 16). Endometrial cancer responds best to progestin therapy, but if this is unsuccessful, oestrogen therapy is sometimes useful. It is interesting to note that the reverse applies to postmenopausal breast cancer (see Chapter 7).

'PITUITARY DEPENDENCE' HYPOTHESIS

A more acceptable alternative to the oestrogen dependence concept is a hypothesis based upon pituitary dependence, which postulates that breast cancer flourishes in an environment where prolactin levels are high. Reduction in the prolactin level, by whatever method it is achieved, may cause regression of tumour growth. This hypothesis has considerable support from observations on experimental mammary carcinoma and has the advantage that it applies equally to the premenopausal and the postmenopausal patient.

Since the secretion of prolactin by the anterior pituitary is normally stimulated by *physiological* levels of oestrogen in the blood (Furth and Clifton, 1958; Kim et al, 1963), ablation of oestrogen sources, whether in the ovary or in the adrenal, will decrease prolactin secretion in the premenopausal women. Administration of *high* doses of oestrogen may also decrease prolactin secretion and this may be the basis of the control of breast cancer by oestrogen therapy in the postmenopausal women (Kim et al, 1963). Hypophyseal ablation by surgery or radiation will eliminate the source of prolactin (and also incidentally the source of FSH and ACTH) in both premenopausal and postmenopausal women.

The importance of suppressing prolactin secretion in the endocrine control of breast cancer is supported by the following clinical reports:

1. The effect of oestrogens on breast cancer appears to require the presence of an intact pituitary gland. After hypophysectomy, there is no observable effect upon the tumour from oestrogen administration, even in patients with previously hormone-sensitive tumours (Pearson and Ray, 1959; Lipsett and Bergenstal, 1960; Kennedy and French, 1965).

2. Tumour regression in breast cancer after high dose oestrogen therapy is usually associated with a fall in the prolactin excretion level (Segaloff et al, 1954). A mammotropic agent, probably prolactin, has been noted in the urine of premenopausal and some postmenopausal women with breast cancer, and favourable response of the tumour to hypophysectomy was associated with abolition of this agent (Hadfield, 1957).

3. The administration of prolactin after hypophysectomy to patients with breast cancer may induce clinical evidence of exacerbation of their disease (Pearson, 1957). Biochemical evidence of exacerbation of breast cancer by injections of ovine prolactin predicts a high likelihood of tumour regression from subsequent hypophysectomy (McCalister and Welbourn, 1962).

Reports on the relationship of prolactin

excretion levels to the clinical activity of breast cancer are infrequent, because of the difficulties of separating prolactin from growth hormone. Nevertheless, the pituitary dependence hypothesis has more to commend it than the oestrogen dependence hypothesis (Pearson, 1957; Stoll, 1958). Recent discussions on the role of the pituitary hormones in the growth of human breast cancer include those of Boot (1970) and Smith and Smith (1970). The recently demonstrated superiority of hypophysectomy over adrenalectomy in a randomised trial (Hayward, 1970) suggests that prolactin may play an important part in the growth of advanced breast cancer.

Tumour Stimulation by Sex Steroids

Stimulation of the growth of breast cancer as a result of sex steroid administration is possible at any age, but is rare, and difficult to prove objectively.

SUBJECTIVE AND OBJECTIVE EVIDENCE OF AGGRAVATION

The following manifestations have been regarded as evidence of tumour stimulation, leading to the abandonment of steroid therapy:

1. Local symptomatic changes such as increased itching of soft tissue lesions, or increase in the pain of bone metastases. These are occasionally noted within a few days of instituting androgen or oestrogen administration, both in the younger and in the older patient. These symptoms, often referred to as a 'flare', may represent an immunological reaction in the tumour rather than actual increase in mitotic activity. A preliminary *increase* in tumour temperature may be noted in patients later showing clinical evidence of response to additive hormone therapy (Edelstyn, 1971).

If the patient is reassured and therapy is continued with the same agent at a reduced dosage, the symptoms often disappear and many of these patients go on to tumour regression. In a group of patients where this type of reaction after oestrogen therapy was regarded as evidence of tumour stimulation, there was no objective evidence of clinical response when castration was carried out subsequently (Lucchini, Arraztoa and Vargas, 1962).

2. A systemic reaction with fever and rigors occurs occasionally after oestrogen or androgen administration. This probably represents a pyrogenic response or idiosyncrasy to the agent used. The writer has seen repeated reactions of this type with each injection of a long-acting androgen, even although tumour regression had occurred from its administration. It is not evidence of tumour stimulation, and with continued administration, or a change to another steroid of the same group, many of these patients may achieve tumour regression at a later date.

3. True stimulation of the growth of soft tissue tumour is a rare but possible complication of sex steroid therapy. However, since such therapy is initiated only when the tumour enters a phase of active growth, the majority of cases reported to be exacerbated are probably examples of an autonomous tumour showing acute progression in spite of therapy. Rapid progression of disease when seen after surgical castration or major ablation therapy is described as 'acute failure' of therapy (Fracchia et al, 1969), and there is no reason why the same

description does not apply in the case of sex steroid therapy.

To be significant of tumour stimulation, *acceleration* of tumour growth must be objectively demonstrable, and this requires accurate serial measurements of tumour volume both before and after initiating treatment. Acceleration is proven only if the rate of growth *increases* while steroid therapy continues and then *decreases* after it is stopped. There should be no need to say that decrease in the growth rate following administration of a second steroid does not prove acceleration by the first steroid.

There does exist a very small minority of patients where true tumour stimulation occurs after *suitably chosen* sex steroid therapy. This latter phrase excludes, of course, patients with active ovarian secretion treated by oestrogen. The likelihood of tumour stimulation by oestrogens in cases other than these is less than 1 per cent (Huseby, 1958). If *true* tumour stimulation is shown, it is a sign of hormone sensitivity, and suggests that endocrine ablation should be successful in controlling tumour growth (Stoll, 1969).

Tumour stimulation by androgens may occur by conversion of androgens into oestrogens (Myers et al, 1955; West et al, 1956; Nissen-Meyer and Sanner, 1963). In postmenopausal women, a high proportion of circulating oestrogen can be derived from androgens. Stimulation of breast cancer was reported in 12 per cent of 208 patients treated with androgens by Bosboom, Meischke-DeJongh and Gerbrandy (1960), but clinical details of the manifestations are not given. In the writer's series, apart from hypercalcaemia, tumour stimulation by androgens was suspected in only 13 of 434 patients—that is 3 per cent of cases.

TUMOUR STIMULATION AND HYPERCALCAEMIA

The hypercalcaemia which occurs within one or two weeks of initiating oestrogen or androgen therapy in the presence of bone metastases is usually regarded as evidence of tumour stimulation (Moore et al, 1967). This can be true in only a proportion of cases, as hypercalcaemia occurs spontaneously in 12 to 15 per cent of patients with bone metastases from breast cancer (Kennedy et al, 1955; Jessiman et al, 1963). The cases arising *early* in steroid therapy fall into three categories which have in the past been distinguished only by hindsight. Examination of serial serum enzyme levels, including alkaline phosphatase, phosphohexose isomerase and lactic dehydrogenase, may help in their separation (see Chapter 5):

1. Initial *temporary* acceleration of tumour growth (a so-called 'flare'). Thus, hypercalcaemia was noted in 5 per cent of 269 oestrogen-treated cases and in 11 per cent of 102 androgen-treated cases (Hall, Dederick and Nevinny, 1963), but tumour regression with return of the serum calcium level to normal was noted in the majority of cases when sex hormone administration was continued. A similar observation was made by Horton and Olson (1963).

2. Stimulation of tumour growth with accelerated bone destruction. If it is proven, this observation signifies hormone sensitivity of the tumour and likelihood of a response to subsequent major endocrine ablation.

3. Spontaneous progression of disease independently of hormonal influence. If demonstrable, this type signifies that further treatment should be by cytotoxic therapy.

It is difficult to regard as tumour stimulation the appearance of hypercalcaemia in 9 per cent of 55 cortisone-treated patients (Hall et al, 1963) or its appearance shortly after hypophysectomy as noted by the writer. There is no doubt that hypercalcaemia occurs more commonly in a younger age group and 77 per cent of the writer's cases appeared within three years after the menopause. There is also no doubt that the condition occurs more commonly after androgen than after oestrogen therapy, and this may result from a specific effect of androgen metabolites on calcium metabolism in bone.

It is therefore important that repeated serum calcium estimations be carried out every third day in the first few weeks of oestrogen or androgen therapy. Hypercalcaemia is more likely in the presence of widespread bone metastases of an osteolytic type, but can occur also with osteoblastic metastases or even with occult bone metastases. There is no clear relation between the calcium level and the extent of bone metastases, and the serum phosphorus level is always found normal or raised in these patients. It has been suggested that *initial* doses of oestrogen or androgen should be small in the presence of widespread bone metastases, in order to minimise the danger of hypercalcaemia in such cases (Donovan, Bethune and Berne, 1966).

Rationale of Additive Hormone Therapy in Breast Cancer

It is a remarkable fact that the overall remission rate established in large series for the different methods of additive hormone therapy is between 20 and 30 per cent for each method. This figure may be increased if a group of patients is selected by age group, or by site of metastases, or by the length of the recurrence-free interval (see Chapter 10). However, as an overall figure, it is increased only when the steroid is used as the first endocrine method of treatment, or if the criteria of response are relaxed.

This observation does *not* imply that only 20 to 30 per cent of breast cancers are hormone sensitive, nor that the same group of patients will respond to the same degree to every method of additive hormone therapy. As mentioned previously, every degree of tumour regression is theoretically possible—from 1 to 100 per cent, but only 'clinically useful' or 'palliative' degrees are accepted as significant (see Chapter 5). Similarly, every duration of response is theoretically possible, from one day to five years or more, but here again, only 'clinically useful' durations are accepted as significant.

Short or minor degrees of remission, *if they can be proved objectively*, are just as significant of hormone sensitivity as are longer or greater degrees of remission. The problem is to find suitable parameters to measure them (see Chapter 5). If these demonstrate hormone sensitivity, even of a very minor degree, there is probably another agent at a suitable dose level, which will yield in that patient a greater or a longer remission. As seen earlier in this chapter, response to therapy by oestrogens can be modified by adjusting dose levels. Failure of response to a particular member of a group such as the progestins, does not exclude later response to other members of the group. Failure of response to one group of agents (for example, oestrogens) does not exclude the possibility of response to another group (for example, progestins).

In other words, any evidence of hormone response, *however small*, should lead to a search for an agent and a dose which will lead to significant tumour inhibition (see Chapter 10).

OESTROGEN THERAPY

About one-third of older postmenopausal women with breast cancer will show tumour regression following oestrogen therapy, either by synthetic oestrogens such as diethylstilboestrol or by natural conjugated equine oestrogens such as Premarin. Such a response is difficult to explain on the oestrogen dependence hypothesis, and some supporters of the hypothesis go so far as to regard *failure* of a tumour to regress on oestrogen therapy as a sign of oestrogen dependence (Kimel, 1957; Edelstyn, Gleadhill and Lyons, 1965).

Administration of oestrogens has a wide range of action on the endocrine system. They can affect the release of gonadotropin, prolactin and growth hormone by the anterior pituitary, and also affect the metabolism of cortisol and other hormones. Oestrogen administration can also affect calcium retention in the body, and can stimulate the reticulo-endothelial system. It is therefore not clear whether oestrogen therapy, in causing regression of breast cancer, is exerting a direct effect on the tumour or its stroma, or suppressing pituitary hormone secretion, or whether it acts by stimulation of body defence mechanisms. More than one mechanism may be involved—the first and second being the more likely—but in that case, their effects may not necessarily summate in the same direction.

DIRECT EFFECT ON TUMOUR AND ITS STROMA

The local application of oestrogen to one mammary gland in castrated rats will induce growth stimulation of only the mammary gland under treatment (MacBryde, 1939), thus suggesting a direct effect on mammary growth. It is uncertain whether the direct physiological effect of oestrogen is on the mammary epithelium or whether it tends to modify the mammary stroma, so that access of other hormones, such as prolactin, is facilitated (Mixner, Bergman and Turner, 1942). Similarly, it is uncertain whether any direct effect of therapeutic doses of oestrogen, in causing regression of breast cancer, is primarily on the epithelial elements of the tumour or on the stroma (see Chapter 7).

A direct effect on tumour growth has been noted in specimens of human breast cancer incubated in organ culture with near-pharmacological concentrations of oestrogens, androgens, or progestins (see Chapter

5). Evidence of inhibition or stimulation of growth has been demonstrated biochemically (Rienits, 1959; Altmann and Chayen, 1967) and also histologically (Kellner and Turcic, 1962; Rivera et al, 1963; Flaxel and Wellings, 1963; Mioduszewska, 1968; Tchao et al, 1968; Stoll, 1970).

Attempts to correlate the observed in vitro response with the clinical response to steroid therapy have been on small series and, so far, with little success (Hollander, Jonas and Smith, 1958; Hollander, Smith and Adamson, 1959; Kellner and Turcic, 1962; Heuson and Legros, 1963). This method measures the effect of the hormone itself, as distinct from its metabolites, and also ignores the influence of the other hormones in the body upon the tumour. Consequently, in vitro results although of scientific interest, will not necessarily predict the in vivo effects on the tumour resulting from therapeutic administration of the hormone.

INHIBITION OF PITUITARY SECRETION

It is possible to explain tumour regression in breast cancer following oestrogen therapy on the basis of pituitary inhibition. Control of prolactin secretion is probably of the greatest importance, as has been discussed earlier, but oestrogen inhibition of the pituitary involves gonadotropin secretion also.

Fall in gonadotropin excretion levels follows high dosage of natural oestrogens such as Premarin, 2·5 to 10 mg daily (Segaloff et al, 1954; Rosemberg and Engel, 1960). The level of oestrogen dosage is important as low dosage of Premarin, 0·1 to 0·25 mg daily, will cause a *rise* in gonadotropin excretion levels. Similar observations have been made with other oestrogens such as ethinyloestradiol and diethylstilboestrol.

A marked fall in the gonadotropin excretion level after high-dose oestrogen therapy in postmenopausal patients is said to be associated with a high likelihood of regression of breast cancer (Stewart, Skinner and O'Connor, 1965). There is a close correlation between prolactin and gonadotropin levels (Riddle, 1963), secretion of both hormones being stimulated by low levels and depressed by high levels of oestrogen administration.

STIMULATION OF BODY DEFENCES

The role of host defences in the control of breast cancer has recently been stressed (Crile, 1965; Bloom, Richardson and Field, 1970). It may be important that oestrogenic compounds can stimulate the reticulo-endo-thelial system (Nicol et al, 1964) and both natural and synthetic oestrogens have been shown to stimulate the activity of phagocytic cells and raise the serum gamma globulin level in animals.

The identification of abnormal antigens has been reported in some breast cancer patients (de Carvalho, 1963), and it is possible that non-specific stimulation of the reticulo-endothelial system may be *one* mechanism in the therapeutic effect of oestrogens on breast cancer (Nicol et al, 1964). However, stimulation of reticulo-endothelial activity has rarely produced regression of established tumour masses in experimental animals, possibly because the host defences appear to be overwhelmed in the presence of a large bulk of tumour. Theoretically the concomitant use of oestrogens may be useful to counteract the effect of cytotoxic therapy which can damage natural defence mechanisms, and promote acceleration or dissemination of the tumour (Magarey and Baum, 1971).

There is said to be no correlation between the stimulating effect of an oestrogen upon the reticulo-endothelial system and its oestrogenicity as measured by its effect on the reproductive tract. Moreover, steroids such as testosterone and progesterone, which have a similar effect to oestrogens in causing regression of breast cancer, are reported to have no specific effect on phagocytic activity (Nicol and Bilbey, 1957). It is interesting to note that although corticosteroids are strong depressants of the immune response, this effect can be experimentally reversed by the simultaneous administration of diethyl-stilboestrol.

ANDROGEN THERAPY

Both in postmenopausal and premenopausal women, androgen administration may lead to tumour regression in breast cancer. In addition to this, androgens may yield benefit by increasing anabolism and calcium retention, and also by stimulating erythropoiesis (see Chapter 4). Like oestrogens, androgens have a wide range of action on the female endocrine system. They can affect the release of gonadotropin and prolactin from the anterior pituitary, and of hormonal secretion from the adrenal cortex and thyroid glands.

Androgen therapy, through its metabolites, most probably acts directly on the tumour and its stroma, but in the case of some agents it may also act by suppression of specific pituitary hormones. A blocking effect on oestrogens at the target tissue is also popularly accepted as its mechanism, but is unlikely, as discussed later. If more than one mechanism is involved, the effects may not necessarily summate.

DIRECT EFFECT ON TUMOUR AND ITS STROMA

This is the most likely mechanism of androgen action on breast cancer. Observations on inhibition or stimulation by androgens of organ cultures of human breast cancer have been mentioned earlier in this chapter. The inhibitory effect of androgens upon mammary carcinoma in rats seems to involve increase in activity in the normal tissues at the expense of the malignant cells, as reflected in the activity of specific enzymes in the tissue (Rees and Huggins, 1960).

The local application of testosterone to one mammary gland of a castrated rat will induce growth stimulation of only the mammary gland under observation and not of the others (Ahren and Hamberger,

1962). As in the case of oestrogens, it is uncertain whether this direct physiological effect is on the epithelial tissues, or whether it involves the stroma. Similarly; it has not been established whether the effect of androgen in causing regression of breast cancer is primarily on the epithelial elements or on the tumour stroma.

Selective effects of androgen on different types of stroma may account for the common observation of a metastasis regressing in one tissue under androgen therapy while concomitantly progressing in another. Androgens exert control both on protein anabolism and calcium deposition in bone, and this may account for the higher proportion of remissions achieved by androgen therapy in the case of bone metastases from breast cancer. Selective efficacy of some androgenic compounds may result from the fact that the effect of androgens on the target tissue is exerted by specific metabolic end-products, which is not the case for oestrogens.

INHIBITION OF PITUITARY SECRETION

It has been suggested that the effect of androgen therapy in causing regression of breast cancer may be mediated through the anterior pituitary, by suppression of prolactin and gonadotropin. However, it has been shown that regression of breast cancer under therapy with the androgen fluoxymesterone is often associated with a *rise* in prolactin excretion levels (Segaloff et al, 1958). Again, although a fall in the gonadotropin excretion follows treatment by androgens such as testosterone propionate and methyl testosterone (Segaloff et al, 1951), this does not always apply to other androgens, such as fluoxymesterone (Segaloff et al, 1958), 2α-methyldihydrotestosterone propionate (Blackburn and Childs, 1959) or Δ^1 testololactone (Segaloff et al, 1962).

Regression of tumour following therapy with the androgen fluoxymesterone has been reported even in hypophysectomised patients (Kennedy, 1957; Beckett and Brennan, 1959; Peck and Olsen, 1963; Stoll, 1969). In the cases where ablation of pituitary tissue is assumed complete, an effect on pituitary secretion cannot be the mechanism for such androgen-induced regression of breast cancer.

OESTROGEN-BLOCKING EFFECT

Androgens may act in breast cancer by modifying the metabolism of oestradiol. They are unlikely to block the oestradiol-binding sites (Mobbs, 1970), although such blockage is common in experimental animals (Jensen, Desombre and Jungblut, 1967). No correlation has been shown between the anti-tumour efficacy of androgens in the human and their oestrogen-blocking capacity in experimental animals (Dorfman et al, 1967).

A blocking action by androgens in breast cancer is unlikely also because a combination of androgen and oestrogen therapy gives a tumour regression rate no different from that of oestrogen therapy alone (Kennedy and Brown, 1965). Furthermore, androgens given simultaneously with oestrogens to premenopausal patients with bone metastases are incapable of preventing the exacerbating influence of oestrogens (Pearson et al, 1954).

Again, if androgens block oestrogen activity in breast cancer, one might expect a higher remission rate from androgen therapy in premenopausal than in postmenopausal patients, but the opposite is the case. Finally, it is difficult to explain on this hypothesis the response of the same tumour to oestrogen and to androgen used successively, or the observation of a withdrawal response in some tumours after cessation of androgen administration (Delarue, 1955; Kaufman and Escher, 1961).

PROGESTIN THERAPY

It has been noted by the writer and others that in a proportion of patients whose tumours fail to respond to oestrogen therapy, regression resulted when progestin therapy was *added* (Stoll, 1965a; Crowley and McDonald, 1965). Decrease in pre-existing nipple pigmentation and decrease in cornification of the vaginal smear was noted in some of these cases, and suggest an ability by progestins to modify oestrogen effects at the target organ. The writer has suggested that for hormone-dependent breast cancer to respond to progestins, oestrogen priming is required, and there is therefore a higher response rate in breast cancer patients whose vaginal smear before therapy suggests the persistence of oestrogen secretion (Stoll, 1967b, c).

Many progestins of the 19-nortesterone group are metabolised to oestrogen, and this has been adduced to explain their effect on breast cancer. Such a mode of action is unlikely as the tumour response rate to progestins of the 17 α-hydroxyprogesterone group is at a similar level, although these compounds do not generally have oestrogenic metabolites. Furthermore, the writer has noted a response in 22 per cent of cases when patients with tumours previously unresponding to oestrogens were given a trial of progestin therapy (Stoll, 1967b, c).

The effect of progestin therapy on breast cancer may possibly be mediated by depression of anterior pituitary secretion, either of gonadotropin or of the prolactin/growth hormone complex. Breast cancer patients with abnormally high gonadotropin excretion levels are said to be more likely to respond to progestin therapy (Chow, Coleman and Lederis, 1966; Curwen, 1970). Response to progestin therapy is more likely to be followed by a similar response to hypophyseal ablation subsequently (Jonsson et al, 1959, Curwen, 1970). These observations favour the suggestion that the therapeutic action of progestins is exerted by depression of pituitary secretion.

The evidence on progestin depression of gonadotropin secretion is conflicting because of the cross-over in the radioimmunoassay of FSH and LH, but it is possible that a decrease in the LH level is the effect common

to the group of agents (Diczfalusy, 1965). There is evidence of progestin depression of growth hormone levels in the human, and it is accepted that there is major cross-over in the radioimmunoassay of growth hormone and prolactin in the human. The administration of progestins depresses serum prolactin levels in experimental animals (Kim, 1965).

Finally, a direct effect of progestins on the local growth of breast cancer is also possible, and the writer has demonstrated an effect of medroxyprogesterone acetate on the growth of human mammary cancer in organ culture (Stoll, 1970). A direct effect on tumour growth is suggested also by the occasional reports of tumour regression following progestin therapy even after complete hypophyseal ablation (see Chapter 8).

CORTICOSTEROID THERAPY

The administration of corticosteroids, like the operation of adrenalectomy, causes suppression of adrenal oestrogen secretion and this is widely believed to be its mode of action in controlling the growth of breast cancer. This is unlikely, however, as it has been shown that the success of corticosteroid therapy (and, for that matter, of bilateral adrenalectomy) is not correlated with subsequent decrease in oestrogen levels.

Response to corticosteroids is not correlated with either previous or subsequent response to sex hormone therapy in breast cancer and is just as likely after hypophysectomy. This has logically led to the suggestion that the effect of corticosteroids in this disease is due to a local anti-inflammatory action upon the tumour bed (Taylor, Perlia and Kofman, 1958). This would decrease vascular permeability and oedema around the tumour or its metastases, and thus relieve symptoms of pressure by the tumour. Such an action would explain rapid but transitory reduction in size (but rarely disappearance) of pulmonary metastases, metastatic skin nodules and nodes following corticosteroid therapy (see Chapter 4).

Decrease in tissue reaction around the tumour would explain the rapid but temporary improvement noted in the coma of cerebral metastases from breast cancer. Similar relief has been noted also in patients with *primary* brain tumours treated with corticosteroids, suggesting that the action is not a specific one (Kofman et al, 1957; Galicich, French and Melby, 1961).

In the case of hypercalcaemia, the effect of corticosteroids is probably by a specific action causing increased urinary calcium excretion (Gerbrandy and Hellendorn, 1957; Taylor et al, 1958). The relief of pain from bone metastases is probably mainly achieved by an action on the tumour bed because, as stated above, recalcification of bone metastases is rarely seen to follow corticosteroid therapy.

CONCLUSION

The role of ovarian hormones in the development of breast cancer in women is suggested by the protective effect of early menopause, the predisposing effect of a later menopause, and the decrease in tumour growth rate at the time of the menopause. Although there is no direct evidence that oestrogens initiate the development of breast cancer in the human, there is clinical evidence that oestrogen administration may stimulate tumour growth in the premenopausal female. To explain the inhibiting effect on breast cancer in the older postmenopausal female, it has been suggested that postmenopausal breast cancer responds differently to oestrogen administration, as a result of having developed in a different hormonal environment.

The oestrogen dependence hypothesis has been proposed to explain the regression seen in some breast cancers after castration or after bilateral adrenalectomy. This theory cannot, however, explain the regression which occurs in some tumours after what appears to be diametrically opposite therapy, that is the administration of oestrogen or progestin, or administration of corticosteroid or androgen. Furthermore, existing biochemical methods of oestrogen assay fail to show a correlation between the nature of the tumour response and a quantitative change in oestrogen excretion after endocrine ablation therapy.

A combination of a direct effect by the steroid on the tumour and an indirect effect via the pituitary is postulated in the additive hormone therapy of breast cancer. These two separate effects of a particular steroid may not be of equal importance and may not summate in their final effect on a tumour. The individual steroid members of a group may yield different metabolic end-products in the body, and this may explain the relatively greater efficacy of certain compounds in specific tissues.

References

Adams, J. B. & Wong, M. S. F. (1968) Paraendocrine behaviour of human breast carcinoma. *In vitro* transformation of steroids to physiologically active hormones. *Journal of Endocrinology*, **41**, 41.

Ahren, K. & Hamberger, L. (1962) Direct action of testosterone propionate on the rat mammary gland. *Acta Endocrinologica (København)*, **40**, 265.

Allaben, G. R. & Owen, S. E. (1939) Adenocarcinoma of the breast coincidental with strenuous endocrine therapy. *Journal of the American Medical Association*, **112**, 1933.

Altmann, F. P. & Chayen, J. (1967) A study of breast cancer by techniques of cellular biology and multiphase biochemistry. In *Cambridge Symposium on the Treatment of Carcinoma of the Breast*, p. 56, ed. Jarrett, A. S. Excerpta Medica Foundation.

AMA Committee on Research (1960) Androgens and estrogens in the treatment of disseminated mammary carcinoma. *Journal of the American Medical Association*, **172**, 1271.

Anderson, E., Reed, S. C., Huseby, R. A. & Oliver, C. P. (1950) Possible relationship between menopause and age at onset of breast cancer. *Cancer (Philadelphia)*, **3**, 410.

Auchinloss, H. & Haagensen, C. D. (1940) Cancer of the breast possibly induced by estrogenic substances. *Journal of the American Medical Association*, **114**, 1517.

Baggett, B., Engel, L. L., Savard, K. & Dorfman, R. I. (1956) The conversion of testosterone-3-C14 to C14-estradiol-17β by human ovarian tissue. *Journal of Biological Chemistry*, **221**, 931.

Barlow, J. J., Emerson, K. & Saxena, B. N. (1969) Estradiol production after ovariectomy for carcinoma of the breast. Relevance to the treatment of menopausal women. *New England Journal of Medicine*, **280**, 633.

Beckett, V. L. & Brennan, M. J. (1959) Treatment of advanced breast cancer with fluoxymesterone (Halotestin). *Surgery, Gynecology and Obstetrics*, **109**, 235.

Blackburn, C. M. & Childs, D. S. (1959) Use of 2α methyl dihydrotestosterone in the treatment of advanced carcinoma of the breast. *Proceedings of the Mayo Clinic*, **34**, 113.

Bloom, H. J. G. (1950) Further studies on prognosis of breast cancer. *British Journal of Cancer*, **4**, 347.

Bloom, H. J. G. (1955) Clinicopathological investigations; (a) Carcinoma of the breast. *British Empire Cancer Campaign. Annual Report*, **33**, 30.

Bloom, H. J. G., Richardson, W. W. & Field, J. R. (1970) Host resistance and survival in carcinoma of the breast. *British Medical Journal*, **iii**, 181.

Boot, L. M. (1970) Prolactin and mammary gland carcinogenesis. The problem of human prolactin. *International Journal of Cancer*, **5**, 167.

Bosboom, B. J. M., Meischke-De Jongh, M. L. & Gerbrandy, J. (1960) quoted by R. Nissen-Meyer (1964) *Acta Endocrinologica (København)*, **44**, 334.

Briggs, G. M. (1957) Estrogen residues in meat – public health aspects. *Journal of the American Medical Association*, **164**, 1473.

Brown, J. B. (1955) A chemical method for the determination of oestriol, oestrone and oestradiol in human urine. *Biochemical Journal*, **60**, 185.

Brown, J. B. (1967) Personal communication.

Brown, J. B. & Strong, J. A. (1962) The metabolism of oestrogens in relation to thyroid function. *Acta Endocrinologica (København) Supplement*, **67**, 90.

Bulbrook, R. D. (1966) Hormonal factors in the etiology and treatment of breast cancer. *Canadian Cancer Conference*, **6**, 36.

Bulbrook, R. D. (1967) Studies on the endocrinology of breast cancer. In *Cambridge Symposium on the Treatment of Carcinoma of the Breast*, p. 40, ed. Jarrett, A. S. Excerpta Medica Foundation.

Bulbrook, R. D. & Greenwood, F. C. (1957) Persistence of urinary oestrogen excretion after oophorectomy and adrenalectomy. *British Medical Journal*, **i**, 662.

Bulbrook, R. D., Greenwood, F. C., Hadfield, G. J. & Scowen, E. F. (1958) Oophorectomy in breast cancer. An attempt to correlate clinical results with oestrogen production. *British Medical Journal*, **ii**, 7.

Bulbrook, R. D., Greenwood, F. C. & Hayward, J. L. (1960) Selection of breast cancer patients for adrenalectomy or hypophysectomy by determination of urinary 17 hydroxycorticosteroids and aetiocholanolone. *Lancet*, **i**, 1154.

Bulbrook, R. D., Thomas, B. S. & Utsunomiya, J. (1964) Urinary 11-deoxy-17 oxosteroids in British and Japanese women with reference to the incidence of breast cancer. *Nature (London)*, **201**, 4915.

Cade, S. (1950) *Malignant Disease and its Treatment by Radium*, Vol. 3, p. 74. Bristol: Wright.

Carter, A. C., Feldman, E. B. & Schwartz, H. L. (1960) Levels of serum PBI in patients with metastatic carcinoma of the breast. *Journal of Clinical Endocrinology*, **20**, 477.

Chow, Y. F., Coleman, J. R. & Lederis, K. (1966) quoted by Briggs, M. H., Caldwell, A. D. S. & Pitchford, A. E. (1967) *Hospital Medicine*, **2**, 63.

Clemmesen, J. (1948) Carcinoma of breast. Results from statistical research. *British Journal of Radiology*, **21**, 583.

Clemmesen, J. (1951) On the etiology of some human cancers. *Journal of the National Cancer Institute*, **12**, 1.

Clemmesen, J. (1965) Statistical studies in the aetiology of malignant neoplasms: I Review and results. *Acta pathologica et microbiologica Scandinavia Supplement* 174, **1**, 254.

Cole, P. & MacMahon, B. (1969) Oestrogen fractions during early reproductive life in the aetiology of breast cancer. *Lancet*, **i**, 604.

Crile, G. Jr (1965) Rationals of simple mastectomy without radiation for clinical stage 1 carcinoma of the breast. *Surgery, Gynecology and Obstetrics*, **120**, 975.

Crowley, L. G., Demetriou, J. A., McDonald, I., Kotin, P., Kushinsky, S. & Donovan, A. J. (1962) Levels of exogenous estrogens in tissues in human mammary carcinoma. *Surgical Forum*, **13**, 103.

Crowley, L. G. & McDonald, I. (1965) Delalutin and estrogens for the treatment of advanced mammary carcinoma in the postmenopausal woman. *Cancer (Philadelphia)*, **18**, 346.

Curwen, S. (1970) The treatment of advanced carcinoma of the breast with SH 420. *Clinical Radiology*, **21**, 219.

Dao, T. L. Y. (1953) Estrogen excretion in women with mammary cancer before and after adrenalectomy. *Science*, **118**, 21.

Dargent, M. (1949) Carcinoma of the breast in castrated women. *British Medical Journal*, **ii**, 54.

Dargent, M., Berger, M. & Lahneche, B. (1962) Thyroid function in breast cancer patients. *Acta Unio internationalis contra cancrum*, **18**, 915.

Davis, H. H., Simons, M. & Davis, J. B. (1964) Cystic disease of the breast relationship to carcinoma. *Cancer (Philadelphia)*, **17**, 957.

De Carvalho, S. (1963) Preliminary experimentation with specific immuno-therapy of neoplastic disease in man. *Cancer (Philadelphia)*, **16**, 306.

Delarue, N. C. (1955) Fundamental concepts determining a philosophy of treatment in mammary carcinoma. *Canadian Medical Association Journal*, **73**, 597.

Deshpande, N., Jensen, V., Bulbrook, R. D. & Doouss, T. W. (1967) *In vivo* steroidogenesis by the human adrenal gland. *Steroids*, **9**, 393.

De Waard, F., Baanders-van Halewijn, E. A. & Huizinga, J. (1964) The bimodal age distribution of patients with mammary carcinoma. *Cancer (Philadelphia)*, **17**, 141.

Diczfalusy, E. (1965) Probable mode of action of oral contraceptives. *British Medical Journal*, **ii**, 1394.

Dobriner, K., Lieberman, S., Hariton, L., Sarett, L. H. & Rhoads, C. P. (1947) The isolation of delta-9-etiocholenolone from human urine. *Journal of Biological Chemistry*, **169**, 221.

Donovan, A. J., Bethune, J. E. & Berne, T. V. (1966) Hypercalcemia in patients with advanced mammary cancer and osseous metastases. *American Surgeon*, **32**, 673.

Dorfman, R. I., Baba, S., Abe, O., Harada, T. & Rooks, W. H. (1967) The influence of drostalone on a transplantable rat mammary fibroadenoma and carcinogen induced adenocarcinoma. In *Cambridge Symposium on the Treatment of Carcinoma of the Breast*, p. 15, ed. Jarrett, A. S. Excerpta Medica Foundation.

Edelstyn, G. (1971) Personal communication.

Edelstyn, G., Gleadhill, C. & Lyons, A. (1965) A rational approach to hypophysectomy. *British Journal of Surgery*, **52**, 953.

Edelstyn, G. A., Lyons, A. R. & Welbourn, R. B. (1958) Thyroid function in patients with mammary cancer. *Lancet*, **i**, 670.

Ellis, F. G., Berne, T. U., Deshpande, R., Belzer, F. O. & Bulbrook, R. D. (1969) The uptake of tritiated steroids by human breast carcinoma. *Surgery, Gynecology and Obstetrics*, **128**, 975.

Emery, E. S. & Trotter, W. R. (1963) Tri-iodo-thyronine in advanced breast cancer. *Lancet*, **i**, 358.

Falls, J. L. (1955) Accessory adrenal cortex in the broad ligament: incidence and functional significance. *Cancer (Philadelphia)*, **8**, 143.

Fishman, J., Hellman, L., Zumoff, B. & Gallagher, T. F. (1962) Influence of thyroid hormone on estrogen metabolism in man. *Journal of Clinical Endocrinology*, **22**, 389.

Flaxel, J. & Wellings, S. R. (1963) Toxic effects of testosterone on organ cultures of mammary carcinoma cells of C3H/CRGL mice. *Federation Proceedings*, **22**, 331.

Folca, P. J., Glascock, R. F. & Irvine, W. T. (1961) Studies with tritium labelled hexoestrol in advanced breast cancer. *Lancet*, **ii**, 796.

Fracchia, A. A., Farrow, J. D., de Palo, A. G., Connelly, D. P. & Huvos, R. G. (1969) Castration for primary inoperable recurrent breast carcinoma. *Surgery, Gynecology and Obstetrics*, **128**, 1226.

Furth, J. & Clifton, K. H. (1958) Experimental observations on mammotropes and the mammary gland. In *Endocrine Aspects of Breast Cancer*, p. 276, ed. Currie, A. R. and Illingsworth, C. F. W. Edinburgh: Livingstone.

Galicich, J. H., French, L. A. & Melby, J. C. (1961) Use of dexamethasone in the treatment of cerebral oedema resulting from brain tumours and brain surgery. *Journal Lancet*, **81**, 46.

Gerbrandy, J. & Hellendorn, H. B. A. (1957) The diagnostic value of calciuria during hormonal treatment of metastasised mammary carcinoma. *Acta Endocrinologica (København)* Supplement 31, 275.

Goldenberg, I. S., Blodinger, P. H. & Grummon, R. A. (1966) Some observations on thyroid and adrenocortical interrelationships. *Surgery*, **59**, 522.

Gordon, D. L. & Segaloff, A. (1958) Castration as a palliative therapy for advanced breast cancer. In *Breast Cancer*, p. 187, ed. Segaloff, A. St Louis: C. V. Mosby.

Graham, L. S. (1953) Celiac accessory adrenal glands. *Cancer (Philadelphia)*, **6**, 149.

Greenwood, F. C. & Bulbrook, R. D. (1957) Effect of hypophysectomy on urinary oestrogen in breast cancer. *British Medical Journal*, **i**, 666.

Gronroos, M. & Aho, A. J. (1968) Estrogen metabolism in postmenopausal women with primary and recurrent breast cancer. *European Journal of Cancer*, **4**, 523.

Gurling, K. H., Scott, G. B. D. & Baron, D. N. (1957) Metastases in pituitary tissue removed at hypophysectomy in women with mammary carcinoma. *British Journal of Cancer*, **11**, 519.

Haddow, A., Watkinson, J. M., Paterson, E. & Koller, P. (1944) Influence of synthetic oestrogens upon advanced malignant disease. *British Medical Journal*, **ii**, 393.

Hadfield, G. (1957) The nature and origin of the mammotropic agent present in human female urine. *Lancet*, **i**, 1058.

Hadfield, G. J. & Holt, J. A. G. (1956) The physiological castration syndrome on breast cancer. *British Medical Journal*, **ii**, 972.

Hall, T. C., Dederick, M. M. & Nevinny, H. B. (1963) Prognostic value of hormonally induced hypercalcaemia in breast cancer. *Cancer Chemotherapy Reports*, **30**, 21.

Hayward, J. L. (1970) Clinical trials comparing transfrontal hypophysectomy with adrenalectomy and with transethmoidal hypophysectomy. In *Second Tenovus Workshop*, ed. Joslin, C. A. F. and Gleave, E. N. Cardiff: Tenovus Workshop.

Hems, G. (1967) Two types of breast cancer. *British Medical Journal*, **iii**, 496.

Herrell, W. E. (1937) The relative incidence of oophorectomy in women with and without carcinoma of the breast. *American Journal of Cancer*, **29**, 659.

Heuson, J. C. & Legros, N. (1963) *In vitro* effect of testosterone and 17β-Estradiol on L-leucine 14C incorporation into human breast cancer. *Cancer (Philadelphia)*, **16**, 404.

Heuson, J. C., Walebroeck, V. G. C. & Legros, N. (1970) Growth inhibition of rat mammary carcinoma and endocrine changes produced by ergocryptine, a suppressor of lactation and nidation. *European Journal of Cancer*, **6**, 353.

Hiisi-Brummer, L., Hortling, H., Malmio, K. & Af Bjorkesten, G. (1960) The effect of hypophysectomy on the oestrogen effect in the body as measured by the vaginal smear technique in metastasising mammary cancer. *Acta Endocrinologica (København)*, 81.

Hollander, V. P., Jonas, H. & Smith, D. E. (1958) Estradiol-sensitive isocitric dehydrogenase in non-cancerous and cancerous human breast tissue. *Cancer (Philadelphia)*, **11**, 803.

Hollander, V. P., Smith, D. E. & Adamson, T. E. (1959) Studies on estrogen-sensitive transhydrogenase: the effect of estradiol 17β in ketoglutarate production in non-cancerous and cancerous human breast tissue. *Cancer (Philadelphia)*, **12**, 135.

Holleb, A. I. & Farrow, J. H. (1962) The relation of carcinoma of the breast and pregnancy in 283 cases. *Surgery, Gynecology and Obstetrics*, **115**, 64.

Horton, J. & Olson, K. B. (1963) Hypercalcaemia associated with cancer of the breast and other organs, quoted in *Current Concepts in Cancer*, ed. Segaloff, A., Meyer, K. K. and Debakey, S. Baltimore: Williams & Wilkins.

Hortling, H., Hiisi-Brummer, L. & Af Bjorkesten, G. A. (1959) Thyroid function in cases of mammary cancer. *Annales medicinae internae Fenniae (Helsinki)*, **48**, Supplement 28, 50.

Hortling, H., Hiisi-Brummer, L. & Af Bjorkesten, G. A. (1962) Endocrine therapy of metastasising breast cancer. *Acta medica Scandinavica*, **172**, Supplement 385.

Huggins, C. & Dao, T. L. Y. (1953) Adrenalectomy and oophorectomy in treatment of advanced carcinoma of the breast. *Journal of the American Medical Association*, **151**, 1388.

Huseby, R. A. (1958) The use of estrogen in the treatment of advanced human breast cancer. In *Breast Cancer*, p. 206, ed. Segaloff, A. St. Louis: C. V. Mosby.

Irvine, W. T., Aitken, E. H., Rendleman, D. L. & Folca, P. J. (1961) Urinary oestrogen measurement after oophorectomy and adrenalectomy for advanced breast cancer. *Lancet*, **ii**, 791.

Jantet, G., Crocker, D. W., Masanori, S. & Morre, F. D. (1963) Adrenal suppression in disseminated carcinoma of the breast (1) The effect on adrenal morphology of hypophysectomy and corticosteroid treatment. *New England Journal of Medicine*, **269**, 1.

Jensen, E. V., Desombre, E. R. & Jungblut, P. W. (1967) Estrogen receptors in hormone responsive tissues and tumour. In *Endogenous Factors Influencing Host-tumor Balance*, ed. Wissler, R. W., Dao, T. and Wood, S. Jr. Chicago: University of Chicago Press.

Jessiman, A. G., Emerson, K., Shah, R. C. & Moore, F. D. (1963) Hypercalcemia in carcinoma of the breast, *Annals of Surgery*, **157**, 377.

Jonsson, U., Colsky, J., Lessner, H. E., Roath, O. S., Alper, R. G. & Jones, R. Jr (1959) Clinical and pharmacological observations on the effects of 9α-bromo-11β ketoprogesterone on patients with carcinoma of the breast. *Cancer (Philadelphia)*, **12**, 509.

Jull, J. W. (1958) Hormonal mechanisms in mammary carcinogenesis. In *Endocrine Aspects of Breast Cancer*, p. 305, ed. Currie, A. R. and Illingsworth, C. F. W. Edinburgh: Livingstone.

Jull, J. W., Shucksmith, H. S. & Bonser, G. M. (1963) A study of urinary estrogen excretion in relation to breast cancer. *Journal of Clinical Endocrinology*, **23**, 433.

Kaufman, R. J. & Escher, G. C. (1961) Rebound regression in advanced mammary carcinoma. *Surgery, Gynecology and Obstetrics*, **113**, 635.

Kellner, G. & Turcic, G. (1962) The importance of tissue culture for hormonal therapy of mammary carcinoma. *Klinische Medizin (Wien)*, **17**, 83.

Kennedy, B. J. (1957) Present status of hormone therapy in advanced breast cancer. *Radiology*, **69**, 330.

Kennedy, B. J. (1962) Massive estrogen administration in premenopausal women with metastatic breast cancer. *Cancer (Philadelphia)*, **15**, 641.

Kennedy, B. J. & Brown, J. H. (1965) Combined estrogenic and androgenic hormone therapy in advanced breast cancer. *Cancer (Philadelphia)*, **18**, 431.

Kennedy, B. J. & French, L. (1965) Hypophysectomy in advanced breast cancer. *American Journal of Surgery*, **110**, 411.

Kennedy, B. J., Nathanson, I. T., Tibbetts, D. M. & Aub. J. C. (1955) Biochemical alterations during steroid hormone therapy of advanced breast cancer *American Journal of Medicine*, **19**, 337.

Khazan, N., Primo, C. H., Danon, A., Assael, M., Sulman, F. G. & Winnik, H. Z. (1962) The mammotropic effect of tranquillising drugs. *Archives internationales de pharmacodynamie et de thérapie*, **141**, 29.

Kim, U. (1965) Pituitary function and hormonal therapy of experimental breast cancer. *Cancer Research*, **13**, 445.

Kim, U., Furth, J. & Yannopoulos, K. (1963) Observations on hormonal control of mammary cancer: I Estrogen and mammotropes. *Journal of the National Cancer Institute*, **31**, 233.

Kimel, V. M. (1957) Clinical cytological correlations of mammary carcinoma based upon sex chromatin counts. *Cancer (Philadelphia)*, **10**, 922.

Kleinfeld, G., Haagensen, C. D. & Cooley, E. (1963) Age and menstrual status as prognostic factors in carcinoma of the breast. *Annals of Surgery*, **156**, 600.

Kofman, S., Garvin, J. S., Nagamani, D. & Taylor, S. G. III (1957) Treatment of cerebral metastases from breast carcinoma with prednisolone. *Journal of the American Medical Association*, **163**, 1473.

Lane-Claypon, J. E. (1926) A further report on cancer of the breast with special reference to its associated antecedent conditions. In *Ministry of Health Report on Public Health and Medical Subjects*, No. 32. London: H.M.S.O.

Lazarev, N. J. (1960) New developments in the hormone therapy of malignant tumours. In *Cancer Progress (1960)*, p. 204, ed. Raven, R. W. London: Butterworths.

Lees, J. C. & Park, W. W. (1949) The malignancy of cancer at different ages: a histological study. *British Journal of Cancer*, **3**, 186.

Lemon, H. M. (1969) Endocrine influences on human mammary cancer formation. *Cancer (Philadelphia)*, **23**, 781.

Lewison, E. F., Trimble, F. H. & Griffith, P. C. (1953) Results of surgical treatment of breast cancer at Johns Hopkins Hospital. *Journal of the American Medical Association*, **153**, 905.

Lilienfeld, A. M. (1956) The relationship of cancer of the female to artificial menopause and marital status. *Cancer (Philadelphia)*, **9**, 927.

Lilienfeld, A. M. (1963) The epidemiology of breast cancer. *Cancer Research*, **23**, 1503.

Lipsett, M. B. & Bergenstal, D. M. (1960) Lack of effect of human growth hormone and ovine prolactin in cancer in man. *Cancer Research*, **20**, 1172.

Loeser, A. A. (1954) A new therapy for prevention of post-operative recurrences in genital and breast cancer. *British Medical Journal*, **ii**, 1380.

Lucchini, A., Arraztoa, J. & Vargas, L. (1962) Metalysis syndrome and effectiveness of subcutaneous implantation of hexestrol in the treatment of breast cancer metastases. *Cancer (Philadelphia)*, **15**, 181.

Lumb, G. & Mackenzie, D. H. (1959) The incidence of metastases in adrenal glands and ovaries removed for carcinoma of the breast. *Cancer (Philadelphia)*, **12**, 521.

McAllister, R. A., Sim, A. W., Hobkirk, R., Stewart, H., Blair, D. W. & Forrest, A. P. M. (1960) Urinary oestrogens after endocrine ablation. *Lancet*, **i**, 1102.

McBride, J. M. (1957) Estrogen excretion levels in the normal postmenopausal woman. *Journal of Clinical Endocrinology*, **17**, 1440.

MacBryde, C. M. (1939) The production of breast growth in the human female. *Journal of the American Medical Association*, **112**, 1045.

McCalister, A. & Welbourn, R. B. (1962) Stimulation of mammary cancer by prolactin and the clinical response to hypophysectomy. *British Medical Journal*, **i**, 1669.

MacMahon, B. & Cole, P. (1969) Endocrinology and epidemiology of breast cancer. *Cancer (Philadelphia)*, **24**, 1146.

McMahon, B. & Feinleib, M. (1960) Breast cancer in relation to nursing and menopausal history. *Journal of the National Cancer Institute*, **24**, 733.

Magarey, C. J. & Baum, M. (1971) Oestrogen as a reticuloendothelial stimulant in patients with cancer. *British Medical Journal*, **ii**, 367.

Marmorston, J. (1966) Urinary hormone metabolic levels in patients with cancer of the breast, prostate and lung. *Annals of the New York Academy of Science*, **125**, 959.

Marques, P., Bru, A. & Espinasse, A. (1959) Role du fonctionnement thyroidien dans le pronostic du cancer du sein. *Bulletin de l'Association français pour l'etude du cancer*, **46**, 645.

Mioduszewska, O. (1968) In *Prognostic Factors in Breast Cancer*, p. 347, ed. Forrest, A. P. M. and Kunkler, P. B. Edinburgh: Livingstone.

Mixner, J. P., Bergman, A. J. & Turner, C. W. (1942) Relation of mammogenic lobule-alveolar growth factor of the anterior pituitary to other anterior pituitary hormones. *Endocrinology*, **31**, 461.

Mobbs, B. G. (1970) The effect of testosterone treatment on the uptake of oestradiol 17β by DMBA induced rat mammary tumours. *Journal of Endocrinology*, **48**, 293.

Moore, D. H., Charney, J., Kramarsky, B., Lasforgues, E. Y., Sarkar, N. H., Brennan, M. J., Burrows, J. H., Sirsat, S. M., Paymaster, J. C. & Vaudja, A. B. (1971) Search for a human breast cancer virus. *Nature (London)*, **229**, 611.

Moore, F. D., Woodrow, S. I., Aliopoulios, M. R. & Wilson, R. E. (1967) Carcinoma of the breast. A decade of new results with old concepts. *New England Journal of Medicine*, **277**, 460.

Murad, T. M. (1971) A proposed histochemical and electron microscopic classification of human breast cancer according to cell of origin. *Cancer (Philadelphia)*, **27**, 288.

Myers, W. P. L., West, C. D., Pearson, O. H. & Karnofsky, D. A. (1955) Androgen induced exacerbation of human breast cancer as measured by calcium excretion. *Proceedings of the American Association for Cancer Research*, **2**, 36.

Nathanson, I. T. (1946) The effect of stilboestrol on advanced cancer of the breast. *Cancer Research*, **6**, 484.

Nathanson, I. T. (1947) Hormonal alteration of advanced cancer of the breast. *Surgical Clinics of North America*, **27**, 1144.

Nathanson, I. T. (1952) Clinical investigative experience with steroid hormones in breast cancer. *Cancer (Philadelphia)*, **5**, 754.

Nathanson, I. T., Engel, L. L. & Kelley, R. M. (1951) The effect of ACTH on the urinary excretion of steroids in neoplastic disease. In *Proceedings of the Second Clinical ACTH Conference*, p. 54. New York: Blakiston.

Nathanson, I. T., Engel, L. L., Kelley, R. M., Ekman, G., Spaulding, K. H. & Elliott, J. (1952) The effect of androgens on the urinary excretion of keto-steroids, non ketonic alcohols and estrogens. *Journal of Clinical Endocrinology*, **12**, 1172.

Nicol, T. & Bilbey, D. L. J. (1957) Reversal by diethylstilboestrol of the depressant effect of cortisone on the phagocytic activity of the reticulo-endothelial system. *Nature (London)*, **179**, 1137.

Nicol, T., Bilbey, D. L. J., Charles, L. M., Cordingley, J. L. & Vernon Roberts, B. (1964) Oestrogen, the natural stimulant of body defence. *Journal of Endocrinology*, **30**, 277.

Nissen-Meyer, R. (1964) Prophylactic endocrine treatment in carcinoma of the breast. *Clinical Radiology*, **15**, 152.

Nissen-Meyer, R. & Sanner, T. (1963) The excretion of oestrone, pregnanediol and pregnanetriol in breast cancer patients. *Acta Endocrinologica (København)*, **44**, 334.

Olch, I. Y. (1937) The menopausal age in women with cancer of the breast. *American Journal of Cancer*, **30**, 563.

Palmer, J. D. & Hellstrom, J. (1962) The use of urinary estrogen estimations as a means of predicting response to oophorectomy and adrenalectomy in breast cancer. *Canadian Journal of Surgery*, **5**, 180.

Parker, T. G. & Sommers, S. C. (1956) Adrenal cortical hyperplasia accompanying cancer. *Archives of Surgery*, **72**, 495.

Pearson, O. H. (1957) Observations on the role of androgens and estrogens in body balance. *Archives of Internal Medicine*, **100**, 724.

Pearson, O. H. & Ray, B. S. (1959) Results of hypophysectomy in the treatment of metastatic mammary cancer. *Cancer (Philadelphia)*, **12**, 85.

Pearson, O. H., West, C. D., Hollander, V. P. & Treves, N. E. (1954) Evaluation of endocrine therapy of advanced breast cancer. *Journal of the American Medical Association*, **154**, 234.

Peck, F. C. & Olson, K. B. (1963) The treatment of advanced breast cancer by hypophysectomy. *New York State Journal of Medicine*, **63**, 2191.

Peller, S. (1940) Cancer and its relations to pregnancy, to delivery and to marital and social status. *Surgery, Gynecology and Obstetrics*, **71**, 1.

Peters, M. V. (1963) Carcinoma of the breast associated with pregnancy and lactation. *Proceedings of the Tenth Clinical Conference*, p. 161, Canada: Ontario Research Foundation.

Procope, B. J. & Adlercreutz, H. (1969) Studies on the influence of age on oestrogen in postmenopausal women with atrophic endometrium and normal liver function. *Acta Endocrinologica (København)*, **62**, 461.

Rawson, R. W. (1956) Today's thyroidologists and their beckoning frontiers—presidential address. *Journal of Clinical Endocrinology*, **16**, 1405.

Rees, E. D. & Huggins, C. (1960) Steroid influences on respiration, glycolysis, and levels of pyridine nucleotide linked dehydrogenases of experimental mammary cancers. *Cancer Research*, **20**, 963.

Reeve, T. S., Rundle, F. F., Hales, I. B., Myhill, J. & Croydon, M. (1961) Thyroid function in the presence of breast cancer. *Lancet*, **i**, 632.

Richards, G. E. (1948) Mammary cancer, the place of surgery and of radiotherapy in its management. *British Journal of Radiology*, **21**, 109.

Riddle, O. (1963) Prolactin in vertebrate function and organisation. *Journal of the National Cancer Institute*, **31**, 1039.

Rienits, K. G. (1959) The effects of estrone and testosterone on respiration of human mammary cancer *in vitro*. *Cancer (Philadelphia)*, **21**, 958.

Rivera, E. M., Elias, J. J., Bern, H. A., Napalkov, N. P. & Pitelka, D. R. (1963) Toxic effects of steroid hormones on organ cultures of mouse mammary tumours. *Journal of the National Cancer Institute*, **31**, 671.

Rosemberg, E. & Engel, I. (1960) The influence of steroids on urinary gonadotropin excretion in a postmenopausal woman. *Journal of Clinical Endocrinology*, **20**, 1576.

Salmon, U. J. & Frank, R. T. (1956) Hormonal factors affecting vaginal smears in castrates and after the menopause. *Proceedings of the Society for Experimental Biology and Medicine*, **33**, 612.

Sandberg, H., Paulsen, C. A., Leach, R. B. & Maddock, W. O. (1958) Estrogen excretion in ovariectomised women receiving adrenocorticotropin. *Journal of Clinical Endocrinology*, **18**, 1268.

Scarff, R. W. (1948) Prognosis in carcinoma of the breast. *British Journal of Radiology*, **21**, 594.

Schweppe, J. S., Jungman, R. A. & Lewis, I. (1967) Urine steroid excretion in postmenopausal cancer of the breast. *Cancer (Philadelphia)*, **20**, 155.

Scowen, E. F. (1958) Oestrogen excretion after hypophysectomy in breast cancer. In *Endocrine Aspects of Breast Cancer*, p. 208, ed. Currie, A. R. and Illingsworth, C. F. Edinburgh: Livingstone.

Segaloff, A. (1966) Hormones and breast cancer. *Recent Progress in Hormone Research*, **22**, 351.

Segaloff, A. (1967) Pituitary hormones influencing breast cancer. In *Current Concepts in Breast Cancer*, p. 94, ed. Segaloff, A. Meyer, K. K. and Debakey, S. Baltimore: Williams & Wilkins.

Segaloff, A., Bowers, C. Y., Rongone, E. L., Murison, P. J. & Schlosser, J. (1958) Hormonal therapy in cancer of the breast: XIII The effect of fluoxymesterone therapy on clinical course and hormonal excretion. *Cancer (Philadelphia)*, **11**, 1187.

Segaloff, A., Gordon, D., Carabasi, R. A., Horwitt, B. N., Schlosser, J. V. & Murison, P. J. (1954) Hormonal therapy in cancer of the breast: VII Effect of conjugated estrogens (equine) on clinical course and hormonal excretion. *Cancer (Philadelphia)*, **7**, 758.

Segaloff, A., Gordon, D., Horwitt, B. N., Schlosser, J. V. & Murison, P. J. (1951) Hormonal therapy in cancer of the breast: I The effect of testosterone propionate on clinical course and hormonal excretion. *Cancer (Philadelphia)*, **4**, 319.

Segaloff, A., Weeth, J. B., Meyer, K. K., Rongone, E. L. & Cunningham, M. E. G. (1962) Hormonal therapy in cancer of the breast: Effect of oral administration of delta-testololactone on clinical course and hormonal excretion. *Cancer (Philadelphia)*, **15**, 633.

Smith, O. W. & Emerson, K. Jr (1954) Urinary estrogens and related compounds in postmenopausal women with mammary cancer: effect of cortisone treatment. *Proceedings of the Society for Experimental Biology and Medicine*, **85**, 264.

Smith, O. W. & Smith, G. V. (1970) Urinary oestrogen profiles and the aetiology of breast cancer. *Lancet*, **i**, 1152.

Smithers, D. W. (1952) Cancer of the breast and the menopause. *Journal of the Faculty of Radiologists*, **4**, 89.

Smithers, D. W., Rigby-Jones, P., Galton, D. A. G. & Payne, P. N. (1952) Cancer of the breast—a review. *British Journal of Radiology Supplement* 4, 1.

Sommers, S. C. & Teloh, H. A. (1952) Ovarian stromal hyperplasia in breast cancer. *Archives of Pathology*, **53**, 160.

Sommers, S. C., Teloh, H. A. & Goldman, G. (1953) Ovarian influence upon survival in breast cancer. *Archives of Surgery*, **67**, 916.

Stewart, J., Skinner, L. G. & O'Connor, P. J. (1965) Hormone therapy in metastatic breast cancer: clinical response and urinary gonadotropins. *Acta Endocrinologica (København)*, **50**, 345.

Stocks, P., (1939) Distribution in England and Wales of cancer of various organs. *British Empire Cancer Campaign. Annual Report*, 308.

Stocks, P. (1958) Statistical investigations concerning the causation of various forms of human cancer. In *Cancer*, vol. 3, ed. Raven, R. W. London: Butterworth.

Stoll, B. A. (1958) Endocrine factors in the aetiology and treatment of cancer of the breast and prostate. In *Modern Trends in Endocrinology*, p. 212, vol. 1, ed. Gardiner Hill, H. London: Butterworth.

Stoll, B. A. (1965a) Progestogens and oestrogens in the treatment of breast cancer. In *Recent Advances in Ovarian and Synthetic Steroids*, ed. Shearman, R. Sydney: Globe.

Stoll, B. A. (1965b) Breast cancer and hypothyroidism. *Cancer (Philadelphia)*, **18**, 1431.

Stoll, B. A. (1967a) Effect of Lyndiol, an oral contraceptive, on breast cancer. *British Medical Journal*, **i**, 150.

Stoll, B. A. (1967b) Vaginal cytology as an aid to hormone therapy in postmenopausal breast cancer. *Cancer (Philadelphia)*, **20**, 1807.

Stoll, B. A. (1967c) Progestin therapy of breast cancer—comparison of agents. *British Medical Journal*, **ii**, 338.

Stoll, B. A. (1969) *Hormonal Management in Breast Cancer*. London: Pitman Medical and Philadelphia: J. B. Lippincott Co.

Stoll, B. A. (1970) Investigation of organ culture as an aid to the hormonal management of breast cancer. *Cancer (Philadelphia)*, **25**, 1228.

Stoll, B. A. (1971) Unpublished.

Strong, J. A., Brown, J. B., Bruce, J., Douglas, M., Klopper, A. I. & Loraine, J. A. (1956) Sex hormone excretion after bilateral adrenalectomy and oophorectomy in patients with mammary carcinoma. *Lancet*, **ii**, 955.

Swyer, G. I. M., Lee, A. E. & Masterson, J. P. (1961) Oestrogen excretion of patients with breast cancer. *British Medical Journal*, **i**, 617.

Taylor, S. G., Perlia, C. P. & Kofman, S. (1958) Cortical steroids in the treatment of disseminated breast cancer. In *Breast Cancer*, p. 217, ed. Segaloff, A. St Louis: C. V. Mosby.

Taylor, S. G., Slaughter, D. P., Smejkal, W., Fowler, E. F. & Preston, F. W. (1948) The effect of sex hormones on advanced carcinoma of the breast. *Cancer (Philadelphia)*, **1**, 604.

Tchao, R., Easty, G., Ambrose, E. J., Raven, R. W. & Bloom, H. J. G. (1968) Effects of chemotherapeutic agents and hormones on organ cultures of human tumours. *European Journal of Cancer*, **4**, 39.

Treves, N. & Holleb, A. I. (1958) A report of 549 cases of breast cancer in women 35 years of age or younger. *Surgery, Gynecology and Obstetrics*, **107**, 271.

Warren, S. & Witham, E. M. (1933) Studies on tumour metastasis: distribution of metastases on cancer of the breast. *Surgery, Gynecology and Obstetrics*, **57**, 81.

West, C. D., Damast, B. & Pearson, O. H. (1958) Adrenal estrogens in patients with metastatic breast cancer. *Journal of Clinical Investigation*, **37**, 341.

West, C. D., Damast, B. L., Sarro, S. D. & Pearson, O. H. (1956) Conversion of testosterone to oestrogens in castrated adrenalectomised human females. *Journal of Biological Chemistry*, **218**, 409.

Westberg, S. V. (1946) Prognosis of breast cancer for pregnant and nursing women. *Acta obstetrica et gynecologica Scandinavica*, 25, Supplement No. 4, 239.

White, T. T. (1954) Carcinoma of the breast and pregnancy. Analysis of 920 cases collected from the literature and new cases. *Annals of Surgery*, **139**, 9.

World Health Organisation Report (1966) *Clinical Aspects of Oral Gestagens* (Technical Report, No. 326), p. 19. Geneva: W.H.O.

Wilson, R. E., Jessiman, A. G. & Moore, F. D. (1958) Severe exacerbation of cancer of the breast after oophorectomy and adrenalectomy. Report of four cases. *New England Journal of Medicine*, **258**, 312.

Wynder, E. L., Bross, I. J. & Hirayama, T. (1960) A study on the epidemiology of cancer of the breast. *Cancer (Philadelphia)*, **13**, 559.

Chapter 7

Castration and Oestrogen Therapy

BASIL A. STOLL

For purely empirical reasons, the choice of initial endocrine therapy in the woman with recurrent, metastatic or inoperable breast cancer depends primarily on the presence or absence of measurable oestrogen excretion.

SELECTION OF PRIMARY THERAPY

For all *premenopausal* patients, castration is recommended as the initial method of endocrine therapy. If the patient is well enough, an attempt at surgical castration is worth while even in the presence of metastases in the liver, pleura, lung or brain, and tumour regression has been reported even in 22 per cent of cases with liver metastases (Dao, 1967). Most would agree that the presence of very extensive visceral metastases contraindicates operation, however, because of the poor response rate and high postoperative mortality (Fracchia et al, 1969).

Androgen therapy is not recommended as an alternative since it has the disadvantage of virilisation, and does not provide as high a proportion of remissions or as prolonged remissions as does castration (Pearson et al, 1955; AMA Committee on Research, 1960; Taylor, 1962; Stoll, 1969). There is no evidence given to support the authoritative affirmation that 'in the advanced disease therapeutic castration or androgen therapy seem equally effective' (Hayward, 1970). Androgens should be advised in premenopausal cases only if the patient is too ill for surgical castration, and even under these circumstances, it is best combined with radiation castration.

For *postmenopausal patients within five years of the menopause*, the writer recommends that serial weekly estimations of urinary oestrogen excretion, or cytohormonal evaluation of serial vaginal smears, should be carried out. If the oestrogen excretion levels are above 10 μg in 24 hours, or if they show cyclical fluctuation in level, ovarian activity is likely (Brown, 1967), and castration is advised as the initial endocrine therapy just as in the premenopausal patient. Examination of the vaginal smear pattern provides a simpler method of selecting such patients for castration (Munguia et al, 1960; Hortling, Hiisi-Brummer and Af Bjorkesten, 1962; Donegan, 1967; Stoll, 1967) because adrenal oestrogens are said to have little effect upon the vaginal smear of recently postmenopausal women (Struthers, 1956; Adlercreutz, 1969).

Most authorities believe that oestrogen secretion by the ovaries is unlikely to persist more than *two* years after the menopause (McBride, 1957; Barlow, Emerson and Saxena, 1969; Procope and Adlercreutz, 1969), and that castration is valueless after that time. Although Nissen-Meyer (1964) has reported that the ovarian stroma may continue oestrogen secretion for many years after the menopause, his work is unconfirmed.

The writer has reported the value of cytohormonal evaluation of serial vaginal smears also in deciding whether castration is necessary for the younger patient with breast cancer who has had a hysterectomy in the preceding five years, and in whom it is uncertain whether ovarian activity persists (Stoll, 1967). The ovaries usually atrophy within a year or two of hysterectomy due to interference with their blood supply, but persistently high oestrogenic activity has been demonstrated for several years after hysterectomy in the vaginal smear of some of these patients.

If an unselected group of patients past the menopause is subjected to castration, the overall tumour remission rate in breast cancer is less than 10 per cent (Treves and Finkbeiner, 1958; Fracchia et al, 1969; Barlow et al, 1969). However, by selecting for castration only those postmenopausal patients with a high oestrogen excretion level, a higher proportion will show regression of breast cancer and the others will be saved an unnecessary operation (Block et al, 1960). The vaginal smear pattern can be used to select patients in this way (Munguia et al, 1960; Stoll, 1967).

For postmenopausal patients within five years of the menopause, oestrogen administration is recommended as the initial therapy only if the vaginal smear shows *no evidence of oestrogen excretion* (Stoll, 1969). Oestrogen administration is contraindicated in patients with a high or cyclical oestrogen excretion, because of the danger of tumour stimulation. Nor is it advised in recently postmenopausal patients where oestrogen excretion persists, even if not at a high level nor with a cyclical rhythm. Androgen therapy is preferred by the writer in such cases, and this applies to most patients between two and five years postmenopausal (see Chapter 8).

Good results from oestrogen therapy in advanced breast cancer are obtained in patients *more than five years postmenopausal*, and the highest remission rates and the longest duration of response are seen in patients more than 10 years postmenopausal. It has therefore been suggested that oestrogen therapy be given a trial even before palliative radiotherapy in older patients with advanced breast cancer, because of the poorer response to oestrogen in irradiated tissue (Huseby, 1958; Kennedy, 1969). The writer prefers, however, to follow a 'sequential' plan of therapy even in old women (Stoll, 1958), keeping oestrogen therapy in reserve until after surgical or radiation treatment have failed to control the disease. This is partly because oestrogen therapy may not be tolerated, and also because tumour response occurs only in the minority of patients treated by oestrogens.

It has been stated that therapeutic doses of oestrogen carry a danger of stimulating the growth of breast cancer in up to 50 per cent of premenopausal women (Pearson, 1957). Surprisingly, it has also been shown that *very high* doses of oestrogen (either synthetic or natural—diethylstilboestrol 400 to 1000 mg daily or Premarin 100 to 800 mg daily) may cause *regression* of breast cancer in some premenopausal women (Nathanson, 1952; Kennedy, 1962).

Therapeutic Castration

TECHNIQUE OF CASTRATION IN RELATION TO RESPONSE

The simplest effective endocrine method of achieving tumour regression in the premenopausal patient with advanced breast cancer is by therapeutic castration. Objective evidence of tumour regression after *surgical*

methods has been compared in a randomised controlled trial, with no significant difference in the recurrence or survival rates up to five years between the two methods (Nissen-Meyer, 1965). Moreover, there is no difference reported in the residual oestrogen levels following castration, whether carried out by surgery or by radiation, nor any change

TABLE 7.1. *Major reports of response to castration in patients with breast cancer, in relation to the method used*

Author	Total cases	Percentage with regressing tumour	
Treves and Finkbeiner, 1958	176	*37*	
Taylor, 1962	398	*29·7*	Surgical
Hall et al, 1963b	282	*24·5*	castration
Dao, 1967	202	*34*	
Fracchia et al, 1969	466	*34·5*	
Adair et al, 1945	304	*15*	
Thayssen, 1948	99	*32*	Radiation
Douglas, 1952	175	*20*	castration
Stoll, 1964	162	*14·8*	

castration has been noted in between 24·5 per cent and 37 per cent of patients in the larger series reported (Table 7.1). Those groups utilising the more rigid criteria of response report the lower remission rates— 29·7 and 24·5 per cent respectively (Taylor, 1962; Hall et al, 1963b). Objective evidence of tumour regression after *radiation* castration is noted in between 14·8 per cent and 32 per cent of patients in the larger series reported (Table 7.1).

The effect on the tumour is, *in the long term*, probably similar from either method of castration. Prophylactic castration by both

in the residual oestrogen level if oophorectomy is carried out after *adequate* radiation of the ovaries (Struthers, 1956; Gordon and Segaloff, 1958; Block, Vial and Pullen, 1958; Diczfalusy et al, 1959; Nissen-Meyer and Sanner, 1963).

However, whereas oestrogen levels fall sharply within two to three days of surgical castration, it may take as long as three to five months for them to reach comparable levels even after the relatively high dose of 1200 to 1600 R in four days to the ovaries (Nathanson, Rice and Meigs, 1940; Block et al, 1958). It has been suggested in one report that, although more delayed, the effect on hormone secretion is more prolonged from radiation castration (Lalanne et al, 1967).

Failure to allow for this delay in response to radiation probably explains the relatively lower tumour remission rate reported from radiation castration in some series of breast cancer. Whereas relief of pain of bone metastases is usually noted within a week of oophorectomy, and objective evidence of tumour regression within two months, it usually takes from one to three months for menses to cease following radiation castration, and tumour remission is correspondingly delayed for three to four months.

In occasional cases, the writer has seen the onset of tumour regression even before the menses ceased following radiation castration, and this suggests that *complete* ablation of ovarian function may not be necessary for tumour control to occur. This observation is analogous to that seen in the case of hypophyseal ablation, where it is reported in most series that complete ablation of hormonal secretion is not necessary to achieve tumour regression.

It is likely that irradiation of the ovaries, as sometimes performed in past years, was inadequate for permanent castration. In patients under the age of 40 given 450 R to the ovaries as a single dose, 33 per cent later showed recurrence of menstrual bleeding (Paterson and Russell, 1959). In the writer's experience, a fractionated dose of 1200 R in 10 to 14 days is adequate to ensure permanent cessation of menses in practically every woman over 40 years of age. However, the interstitial secreting cells of the ovary are probably more resistant to radiation than is the follicle, and, in addition, the ovaries of younger women are probably more resistant to radiation than are those of women over 40 years of age (Nathanson and Kelley, 1952). A relatively higher dose is therefore advisable in women under the age of 40, such as 1500 to 2000 R in 14 to 21 days. The writer has shown that fractionation of

treatment over 10 days or longer is associated with a higher response rate in breast cancer than a shorter overall period (Stoll, 1969).

SELECTION OF METHOD

Surgical castration is preferred in cases of clinical urgency because of the delayed response to radiation. This urgent category would include the presence of painful bone deposits or metastases in the lung, pleura, brain or liver. Surgical castration is also advised in all cases where there is associated gynaecological disease requiring surgery, or where dissemination was early and the tumour growth rapid. A short 'free' interval between mastectomy and recurrence also requires surgical castration, although the likelihood of response is low in such cases (see later).

Radiation castration may be preferred, on the other hand, when there are multiple peritoneal metastases, or when bone metastases are limited to the pelvic bones. Castration and palliative irradiation can then be carried out by the same fields. In cases of clinical urgency, but where surgical castration is not possible, androgen or corticosteroid therapy are added to radiation castration, depending on whether the metastases are osseous or visceral, respectively.

A theoretical disadvantage of castration is that any procedure causing 'acute stress' leads to an outpouring of ACTH, which may possibly stimulate increased oestrogen secretion from the adrenal cortex (Nathanson, Engel and Kelley, 1951). Thus, an immediate *increase* in oestrogen secretion has been noted to follow oophorectomy in some patients (Bulbrook and Greenwood, 1957), presumably due to the operative stress. This may possibly account for the occasional appearance of hypercalcaemia after oophorectomy (Wilson, Jessiman and Moore, 1958). The suggestion that a short course of corticosteroids may be useful after castration, for the purpose of counteracting increased ACTH secretion (Nissen-Meyer and Vogt, 1959) might apply also to radiation castration with higher dosage or in the case of a very ill patient (see later).

PALLIATION FROM CASTRATION

In the majority of therapeutic castration series, the mean duration of tumour regression is between 10 and 14 months (Lewison, 1965). It may, however, be as long as 25 months (Hortling et al, 1962) and such an average period of tumour regression is as long as that reported from major endocrine

patients with a short recurrence-free interval following mastectomy (Table 7.2).

Tumour regression following castration in breast cancer is shown by shrinkage of the primary breast tumour, metastatic nodes or nodules (Plate 7.1, facing p. 208). It may also be manifested by regression of visceral metastases in liver, brain or lungs, or by delay in reaccumulation of serous effusions or recalcification in lytic bone metastases (Figure 7.1). It is commonly noted that metastatic lesions in different systems may

TABLE 7.2. *The average length of free interval between mastectomy and first recurrence, in patients responding to castration as against those not responding* (Stoll, 1969)

Author	Total cases	Average recurrence-free interval if:	
		Regression of tumour	No regression of tumour
Treves and Finkbeiner, 1958	191	24 months	14 months
Taylor, 1962	398	32 months	20·9 months
Stoll, 1964	162	20·3 months	20·9 months

Reproduced by permission of Pitman Medical.

ablation, although the quality of remission from castration is considered by some to be inferior (Hayward, 1970).

An average *survival* of 31·2 months following castration is noted in responding cases of breast cancer compared to only 8·8 months in nonresponding cases—a considerable extension of survival (Taylor, 1962). It has been suggested that prolonged survival in responding cases may not be the result of castration, but may reflect the natural history of a slower growing tumour, and that this is the type most likely to respond to castration. This is not confirmed in the writer's series where patients with a long recurrence-free interval show no significant difference in response rate to castration, from those

not be controlled equally. Thus, a malignant pleural effusion may appear while bone lesions are healing, or preexisting lytic lesions in bone may develop a sclerotic appearance while new lytic lesions are appearing.

Many patients obtain relief of pain within two to seven days of surgical castration but subsequently show no radiographic evidence of healing in bone metastases. Gain in weight or return to near normal activity are often associated with the pain relief, even in the absence of objective evidence of bone healing. Improvement of this type, and even changes in haemoglobin or serum calcium levels, are not acceptable as objective evidence of tumour remission in patients with bone metastases, although they provide valuable palliation to the patient (see Chapter 5).

FACTORS INFLUENCING RESPONSE

There are several clinical factors which affect the likelihood of tumour remission after castration. It is important to note that the change in oestrogen excretion levels in breast cancer patients following castration, cannot be related to the likelihood of tumour

breast and soft-tissue tumour in 22·6 per cent and visceral metastases in 18·6 per cent of cases following oophorectomy (Taylor, 1962). The same report showed tumour regression in 16·3 per cent of patients under 35, following oophorectomy, but in 31·6 per cent of patients over 35 years of age. A lower remission rate, was, however, not found in premenopausal patients under the age of 40 in the writer's series of 162 patients, treated by x-ray castration (Table 7.3).

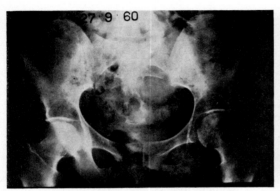 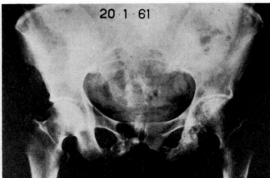

FIGURE 7.1. Radiographs to show recalcification of metastases from breast cancer in the ischium and acetabulum, within four months of surgical castration. (Figure reproduced from Stoll, 1969, by permission of Pitman Medical.)

regression. Associated with regression of tumour growth following castration, oestrogen excretion may either decrease, increase or remain unchanged in level.

Response to castration by patients with recurrent breast cancer is said to be more likely in association with a longer recurrence-free interval since mastectomy (McDonald, 1962) although not confirmed in the writer's series (Table 7.2). This characteristic has not been linked with any specific histological type in the case of breast cancer, although in the case of endometrial, prostatic and thyroid cancer, it is only well-differentiated tumours which are likely to respond.

The likelihood of favourable response to castration is also governed by the tumour site and age group of the patient. Bone metastases respond in 38·7 per cent of cases,

A higher remission rate from oophorectomy has been shown in patients with regular menses than in those with irregular menses (Fracchia et al, 1969) and a higher remission rate has been shown also in those patients found to have metastases in the ovary at castration (Osborne and Pitts, 1961). The significance of these observations is not clear.

Patients whose tumour growth has responded favourably to castration have a considerably higher likelihood of a similar response later both to additive hormonal and endocrine ablative therapy. A review of three collected series totalling 282 patients concludes that of patients who have responded favourably to castration, 23 per cent will respond similarly to subsequent additive hormonal therapy of different types, while of the castration non-responders, only 7 per cent will respond to such therapy (Hall et al, 1963b).

Response to major endocrine ablation is much more likely in those patients with a short remission from castration (up to 15 months) than in those with a longer remission. 'If the oophorectomy remission is prolonged then all available remission time would seem to have been, as it were, used up' (Stewart, 1970). A similar observation does not apply to additive hormonal therapy given after castration, or even to one type of additive therapy after another, for example androgen therapy after oestrogen therapy (Stoll, 1969).

TABLE 7.3. *Response to radiation castration in patients with breast cancer, in relation to age group and in relation to whether androgen was added concurrently* (Stoll, 1969)

		Cases with regressing tumour	Percentage with regressing tumour	
Age group	Up to 39	11 of 59	*18·7*	} Difference not significant
	Over 40	13 of 103	*12·6*	
Method used	Castration alone	15 of 95	*15·8*	} Difference not significant
	Castration with added androgens	9 of 67	*13·4*	

Reproduced by permission of Pitman Medical.

Castration Combined with Additive Hormone Therapy

Objective evidence of tumour growth remission has been claimed in 51 per cent of breast cancer patients for an average duration of 18 months, following the combination of x-ray castration with cortisone 50 mg daily (Nissen-Meyer and Vogt, 1959). Another report has noted similarly that the administration of prednisolone, 20 mg daily, after oophorectomy improves the palliative results (Brinkley and Kingsley-Pillers, 1960). It is interesting to note, however, that there is no correlation between the likelihood of clinical benefit in such cases and the degree of adrenal suppression as shown by ketosteroid or oestrogen excretion levels (Eley and Riddell, 1960). Therefore, the benefit from corticosteroid therapy after oophorectomy is more likely to be from a local effect on the tumour, and not from adrenal oestrogen suppression as was suggested by Nissen-Meyer and Vogt (1959).

Corticosteroid treatment as a routine procedure after castration is not recommended by the writer because of the unwanted side-effects following prolonged corticosteroid dosage. Nevertheless, a *short* course of prednisolone after castration, at a dosage of at least 30 mg daily, may be beneficial in the

6

presence of lung, liver or brain metastases, or in a very ill patient. Corticosteroid therapy should also always be added to castration in the presence of hypercalcaemia, because the results of castration alone are poor in this condition (Fracchia et al, 1969).

It has been suggested that the results of castration in breast cancer may be improved by the concomitant administration of androgens (Poppe and Gregl, 1961; Hortling et al, 1962). In the writer's series (Table 7.3) and in that of Donegan (1967), there was no significant improvement in the *overall* tumour remission rates after castration from the addition of androgens. Nevertheless, it was noted by the writer that in patients with bone metastases, the proportion showing recalcification was higher when androgens were added, and androgens are especially useful in the presence of severe myelophthisic anaemia. It may also be useful to add androgen therapy to castration in patients under 35 years of age, because of the poorer results from castration alone reported in this age group (Taylor, 1962).

The virilising side-effects of androgens need to be justified, so that apart from these two categories of patients, it is better to reserve androgens until the tumour reactivates after castration. Objective evidence of tumour regression from androgen therapy will then occur in up to 30 per cent of those patients previously responding favourably to castration (Escher, 1958). Moreover, even in those patients not having previously responded to castration, androgen therapy commonly leads to prolonged relief of pain from bone metastases.

The administration of thyroid hormone was long ago suggested as an adjuvant to the effect of castration in breast cancer (Beatson, 1896). So far, there is no evidence to justify its use, but a randomised trial is being carried out to assess its possible benefit (Lewison, 1962). There are still some who believe that thyroid hormone administration has a prophylactic effect against recurrence, although the value of prophylactic tri-iodothyronine administration in breast cancer was not proved in a clinical trial (Emery and Trotter, 1963).

'Prophylactic' Castration

Because therapeutic castration can sometimes lead to temporary regression of tumour growth in breast cancer, it was logical to expect castration carried out at the time of mastectomy to delay the onset of recurrence in a proportion of patients. Such castration has been variously described as 'prophylactic', 'early' or 'postoperative'. Several retrospective surveys have suggested an increase in the mean recurrence-free interval, or an increased survival in prophylactically castrated patients (Siegert, 1952; Smith and Smith, 1953; Horsely, 1957; Treves, 1957; Kennedy et al, 1964).

THE PLACE OF PROPHYLACTIC CASTRATION

It requires prospective randomised trials to assess scientifically the value of prophylactic castration, and the results of such trials have not been available until recently. For *surgical* prophylactic castration, two recent trials of this type (Nevinny et al, 1969; Ravdin et al,

1970) have shown no significant overall increase in the mean recurrence-free interval or total survival time in large series of patients who were castrated. This applies both to patients with and without axillary node involvement at operation.

However, if women with four or more involved axillary nodes are assessed separately, there appears to be a 29 per cent reduction of recurrences in the castration group at 18 months, although this advantage is lost at 36 months. This same advantage is noted from thiotepa therapy at mastectomy in premenopausal patients (Ravdin et al, 1970). The total survival time is not significantly improved by either procedure. It seems therefore that temporary retardation of tumour growth resulting from prophylactic castration is demonstrable only in patients who are likely to have widespread subclinical metastases. In the early operable case, there is no advantage or justification for its use.

A prospective randomised trial of prophylactic *x-ray* castration (Cole, 1964) could not demonstrate an acceptably significant decrease in recurrence rate, or increase in the 5 or 10-year survival rate, in the castrated series although the recurrence-free interval was significantly improved (Cole, 1970). The castration dosage was only 450 R, and patients up to two years postmenopausal were included in the trial. These factors would militate against significant evidence of benefit.

Another randomised trial of prophylactic x-ray castration in breast cancer demonstrated an improvement in the survival and recurrence rates not only in premenopausal women, but surprisingly also in *post*menopausal women up to 70 years of age (Nissen-Meyer, 1967). Ovarian secretion of oestrogens appeared to continue long after the menopause in some of these cases, as in each five-year group up to the age of 70 the urinary output of oestrogen was said to be lower in the castrated than in the control group.

Ovarian secretion of oestrogens in older postmenopausal women has, however, not been confirmed by others (Barlow et al, 1969; Procope and Aldercreutz, 1969). Furthermore, an earlier study had noted no improvement in five-year survival rates in breast cancer, when postmenopausal patients up to 69 years of age received an x-ray castration dose to the ovaries prophylactically at the time of mastectomy (McWhirter, 1957). The results are awaited of a further clinical trial which aims to correlate the results of prophylactic x-ray castration in breast cancer patients aged between 35 and 59, with hormone assays before castration (Meakin et al, 1968).

To sum up, therefore, it is likely that the effect of prophylactic castration, like that of all endocrine therapy in breast cancer, is merely a temporary retarding influence upon the growth of disseminated tumour. Although, on a theoretical basis, the hormonal changes following prophylactic castration may decrease the viability of cells liberated at mastectomy, there is no evidence of an increased cure rate from the use of prophylactic castration. Against its possible beneficial effect must also be placed the possibility of increased susceptibility to cardiovascular disease (Oliver and Boyd, 1959; Parrish et al, 1967), although this is not confirmed by others (Novak and Williams, 1960). Other sequelae of castration in females are predisposition to early osteoporosis, thinning of the scalp hair, dryness of the skin and loss of libido (Ansfield, 1967).

Prophylactic castration must therefore be justified in each individual by a high likelihood of benefit. Having already been subjected to a mutilating breast resection and a tiring course of irradiation, prophylactic castration is an additional psychological and physical burden to the patient. In patients found to have extensive axillary node metastases, the likelihood of disseminated but subclinical metastases is very high. Prophylactic castration is therefore advised in such cases as it may be effective in postponing clinical evidence of recurrence, thus giving the patient *a longer period free from anxiety,* even if not providing a longer survival. It also avoids the disadvantage of castration postponed until recurrence occurs, when it may find the patient too ill from pulmonary, hepatic, or cerebral metastases to benefit.

Prophylactic castration may be advised also in less advanced disease, in the presence of an anaplastic tumour, which would predict a poor prognosis, or in patients for whom regular follow-up examination is likely to be difficult. Fundamentally, the choice of timing for castration should be based upon whether or not residual tumour is assumed to persist after operation, and, in that sense, postoperative castration is 'therapeutic' and not 'prophylactic'.

Whether prophylactic castration should be surgical or radiotherapeutic depends on the urgency of the condition as reflected in the tumour's rate of growth, histology and extent of spread. It must also be taken into account that while radiotherapeutic castration can be carried out simultaneously with postoperative irradiation of the operation area, surgical castration requires an additional operation.

PROPHYLACTIC CASTRATION IN RELATION TO PREGNANCY AND OVARIAN PATHOLOGY

The avoidance of further pregnancy has been quoted as an additional reason in favour of prophylactic castration in breast cancer. There is, however, no valid evidence that pregnancy worsens the prognosis in patients with breast cancer which has been treated radically. It is usual nevertheless to advise postponement of child-bearing for several years after mastectomy if the prognosis appears poor in order to avoid the possible orphaning of an infant.

A review of the literature on pregnancy in breast cancer patients reported a five-year survival rate of 49 per cent in patients per-mitted to undergo pregnancy following radical surgical treatment for breast cancer, a figure similar to the survival rate in a series in which pregnancy did not occur (White, 1954). Similar conclusions were reached in subsequent series also (Holleb and Farrow, 1962; Peters, 1963; Cooper and Butterfield, 1970). Since pregnancy is usually postponed for a few years after radical treatment of breast cancer, this would eliminate patients with more actively malignant tumours, and the point, therefore, is not conclusively proven.

Unsuspected ovarian metastases have been found at laparotomy or autopsy in a high proportion of women with advanced breast cancer (Warren and Witham, 1933; Abrams, Spiro and Goldstein, 1950; Lumb and Mac-kenzie, 1959). This has been quoted as a reason for carrying out prophylactic castra-tion at the time of mastectomy in all pre-menopausal cases (Sicard, 1948). However, the presence of ovarian metastases is usually indicative of widespread disease, and their removal could hardly affect the prognosis.

Hyperplasia of the ovarian cortical stroma (which is said to be associated with a high level of oestrogen secretion), is found in 83 per cent of autopsies in patients with breast cancer (Sommers and Teloh, 1952; Sommers, Teloh and Goldman, 1953), and this incidence is said to be considerably higher than in the normal population. It has been suggested as a reason favouring surgical rather than radia-tion castration, because the ovarian stroma is relatively radioresistant compared to the follicle. Nevertheless, numerous authors have reported that there is no correlation between the likelihood of tumour response to castra-tion, and the change in oestrogen excretion levels after such treatment (see Chapter 6). An advantage is therefore not obvious for surgical over radiation castration on this basis.

Oestrogen Therapy

Oestrogen therapy is the simplest effective method of endocrine therapy for the post-menopausal patient with advanced breast cancer, in whom oestrogen secretion has ceased. Its use in relationship to major endocrine ablation therapy is discussed in Chapter 9.

reviewing his personal series of 407 patients treated with oestrogens and using more rigid criteria, reported objective evidence of tumour regression in 31 per cent of cases (Stoll, 1964). A randomised trial of hormone therapy by Kennedy (1965) in 114 post-menopausal women showed remission in

TABLE 7.4. *Favourable clinical response to oestrogen therapy compared to that from androgen therapy in breast cancer, in relation to menopausal age group* (Stoll, 1969, and A.M.A. Committee on Research, 1960)

Years since menopause	Percentage with regressing tumour after:			
	Androgens		Oestrogens	
	Stoll, 1969	A.M.A. 1960	Stoll, 1969	A.M.A. 1960
0–5	*10*	*17*	*9*	*13**
6–9	*28**	*13**	*28**	*38**
10 or more	*22*	*27*	*36*	*38*
Overall percentage regression	*15*	*21*	*31*	*37*
Cases	434	580	407	364

* Represents small series of cases.

Reproduced by permission of Pitman Medical.

THE PLACE OF OESTROGEN THERAPY

The AMA Committee on Research (1960) assembled 364 cases of postmenopausal women with breast cancer treated by oestrogens, of whom 37 per cent showed objective evidence of tumour regression. The writer in

29·1 per cent of patients treated by diethylstilboestrol.

There is no doubt that in patients more than five years postmenopausal, the *overall* results of oestrogen therapy are superior to those of androgen therapy (Table 7.4) although, as noted later, this does not apply to bone metastases. Furthermore, the average duration of tumour regression from oestrogen therapy is 16·5 months, which is longer than that resulting from androgens (10·9 months). These figures in the writer's series are comparable because uniform criteria of regression have been used in both series (see Chapter 5).

Prolongation of life appears to follow oestrogen therapy in patients with hormone-sensitive breast cancer. The mean survival time after treatment was 27·3 months for patients responding favourably to oestrogen, compared to 10·4 months for non-responders (AMA Committee on Research, 1960). In the presence of lung or pleural metastases, the writer has shown 31 per cent of oestrogen-treated patients to survive over 12 months, compared to 7·5 per cent of untreated patients (Stoll and Ellis, 1953).

It has been suggested that the prolonged survival observed in patients with breast cancer responding to hormone therapy may occur because these tumours belong to a slowly growing group. The evidence of prolonged survival in patients receiving high doses of oestrogens is important, however, because long-term high dosage oestrogen therapy has been accused of an unfavourable effect on the cardiovascular system (Sellwood, 1970).

The tumour remission rate from oestrogen therapy in breast cancer has long been noted to be higher with increasing number of years past the menopause (Stoll, 1950). Up to five years after the menopause, the remission rate is 9 per cent from oestrogen therapy, between six and nine years postmenopausal it is 28 per cent, and after 10 years postmenopausal it is 36 per cent in the writer's series (Table 7.4). Regression occurred in 49 per cent of patients over 70 when at least two months' therapy was given (Stoll and Ackland, 1970).

Remission rates from oestrogen therapy are higher than those for androgen therapy in the case of soft-tissue and visceral lesions (Stoll, 1950). For these sites, the remission rates are 36 and 28 per cent respectively for oestrogen therapy, as against 16 and 11 per cent for androgen therapy in the writer's series (Table 8.1). In the case of bone metastases, however, there is a higher remission rate from androgen therapy than from oestrogen therapy—19 per cent as against 7 per cent. Thus, when both types of metastasis coexist in the patient, it is not unusual to see soft tissue tumour regressing, while bone metastases are uncontrolled by oestrogen therapy. The reverse experience is more common with androgen therapy.

It has long been noted that slow growing cancers clinically described as 'atrophic scirrhous' tumours in older patients tend to have a higher likelihood of remission from oestrogen therapy (Stoll, 1950). A third factor influencing the remission rate (apart from the age of the patient and site of metastases) is the length of 'free' interval between mastectomy and recurrence. Tumour regression from additive hormone therapy was noted in 16 per cent of patients with a recurrence-free interval of less than two years, compared to 22 per cent of those with a free interval of over two years (Escher and Kaufman, 1963). This has not been correlated with tumour histology, and while an early report suggested that highly cellular breast cancer is more likely to respond to oestrogen therapy (Haddow et al, 1944), later reports noted the opposite finding (Emerson, Kennedy and Nathanson, 1949; Wolff, 1957). Most series show no correlation between tumour histology and the likelihood of response to additive hormonal therapy (AMA Committee, 1960).

PALLIATION FROM OESTROGEN ADMINISTRATION

It should be emphasised that a trial of oestrogens should not be abandoned under three months, except in the presence of proven exacerbation of the disease (see later), or of gross intolerance to the agent. The first evidence of tumour regression in breast cancer usually appears about six weeks after commencing oestrogen therapy, but is often delayed for a further two to six weeks, especially in the presence of slowly growing disease. The writer therefore strongly disagrees with the advice that if favourable response to oestrogen therapy does not occur within one month, further administration is unlikely to be of value (Forrest, 1965). Recalcification of osteolytic bone metastases usually takes between three and six months to appear.

In the writer's series the average duration of objective response from oestrogen therapy in breast cancer is 16·5 months, but for soft tissue lesions the duration of tumour remission tends to be longer than that for bone or visceral lesions. Remissions for as long as five years are occasionally seen, especially in the older patient, but this may reflect the more common clinically 'atrophic scirrhous' type of cancer in these patients.

Large ulcerated primary breast cancer may heal completely after oestrogen therapy, especially in the elderly patient (Plate 7.2, facing p. 208). A dusky wrinkled appearance of the skin at the ulcer periphery is the first sign of regression, and this is followed by flattening of the everted tumour edges, and the appearance of bleeding granulation tissue in the ulcer base. Scarring and shrinkage of the breast result when healing finally occurs in a primary breast cancer. Regression of tumour tends to be more delayed and less complete in areas previously subjected to radiation therapy, presumably because of the impaired vascular supply. For this reason, some authorities prefer trial of oestrogen therapy to be carried out *before* radiation therapy (Kennedy, 1969).

Oestrogen therapy will also cause regression of metastatic skin nodules or enlarged metastatic nodes, but often this is not uniform in all the lesions (Plate 7.3, following p. 208). Sometimes the primary tumour heals, while the metastatic nodes show no evidence of regression, and sometimes nodules regress in one area but spread in another. There is no relationship between the size of a lesion and the likelihood of its regression on oestrogen therapy. Larger nodules may regress before smaller ones, unlike the response to corticosteroid therapy where, in general, only the smallest nodules regress. The remission rate for recurrent nodules is 22 per cent in irradiated tissue, compared to 46 per cent for unirradiated tissue (Kennedy, 1969).

In a series of 61 patients reported by the writer (Stoll and Ellis, 1953), regression of lung or pleural metastases followed oestrogen therapy in 26 per cent of cases, and was associated with a longer survival than in untreated cases (Figure 7.2). Radiographic evidence of regression of lung metastases appeared within two to three months of initiating oestrogen therapy, and was noted for all types of metastasis: large rounded opacities, generalised mottling, or lymphatic permeation. Nevertheless, the disappearance of lymphatic permeation of the lungs (lymphangitis carcinomatosa) is usually very temporary. While measurable decrease in size of a cytologically proven peritoneal or pleural effusion is generally accepted as a sign of tumour remission, delay for months in the reaccumulation of an effusion previously requiring frequent paracentesis, is not acceptable as tumour regression to some authorities.

Relief of pain from bone metastases may be noted after two to four weeks of oestrogen therapy, but in the writer's experience it is usually of shorter duration than the pain relief achieved from the use of androgen therapy. Recalcification of osteolytic bone metastases may eventually appear radiographically in a small proportion of the patients achieving pain relief from oestrogen therapy, but it takes at least three months for the first signs to appear (Figure 7.3). The presence of hypercalcaemia requires corticosteroid or sodium phosphate therapy. Large metastases in the liver or brain rarely respond to oestrogen therapy, and corticosteroid therapy is preferred also in such cases.

Subjective benefit in the form of a general feeling of well-being and increase in energy,

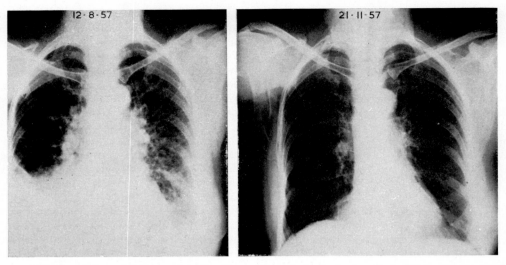

FIGURE 7.2. Radiographs to show regression of malignant pleural effusion in a patient with breast cancer, within three months of therapy with ethinyloestradiol 0·5 mg tds. The patient survived for nine years on intermittent hormonal therapy before final recurrence and death from the disease. (Figure reproduced from Stoll, 1969, by permission of Pitman Medical.)

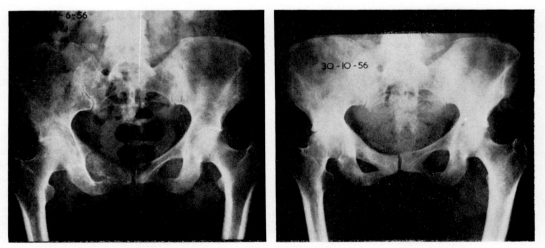

FIGURE 7.3. Radiographs to show recalcification of metastases from breast cancer in ischium and pubis, within four months of instituting ethinyloestradiol therapy 0·5 mg tds. (Figure reproduced from Stoll, 1969, by permission of Pitman Medical.)

such as is seen from androgen administration, rarely results from high dose oestrogen therapy in postmenopausal women. Such an effect has been widely claimed however from low doses of oestrogen popularly recommended as 'replacement' therapy at the menopause.

WITHDRAWAL RESPONSE

After oestrogen therapy has lost its control, cessation of the agent may lead to a further period of remission called a 'withdrawal response'. New therapy should therefore be delayed two months for this reason (Segaloff et al, 1954; Delarue, 1955). Such delay is not reasonable in the presence of rapidly advancing disease, and in these circumstances, either immediate corticosteroid therapy or major endocrine ablation are necessary. Objective evidence of a withdrawal response is claimed in as many as 31 per cent of patients who have previously responded favourably to oestrogen therapy, and surprisingly, also in 3·6 per cent of those who have *not* responded (Kaufman and Escher, 1961). Its cause is uncertain, but it is more likely to reflect a response by a hormone-sensitive tumour to change in the hormonal environment (see Chapter 6) rather than to the withdrawal of a stimulating influence, as has been suggested by some.

The average duration of a withdrawal response of this type is 10 months, and is, in the writer's experience, shorter than that of the primary response in the individual. A third period of response may occasionally be achieved if further oestrogen therapy is given after the withdrawal response has been lost (Stoll, 1969). Since both the extent and duration of a withdrawal response in an individual are usually related to the extent and duration of the previous tumour regression in that patient (Huseby, 1958), withdrawal response is barely to be expected in patients who have not obtained a primary response.

SECONDARY OESTROGEN THERAPY

In spite of statements to the contrary (Dao, 1970), secondary response to oestrogen therapy *does* occur after response by breast cancer to androgens, although the remission rate is considerably lower than the 31 per cent expected from oestrogen therapy given as the first choice. Remission rates in some series are as low as 4 per cent from secondary oestrogen therapy (Witt et al, 1963), but was 20 per cent in the writer's series, when applied to patients with a previous favourable response to androgen therapy (Stoll, 1969).

Oestrogen therapy given alone after failure of hypophysectomy yields no observable clinical benefit (Pearson and Ray, 1959; Lipsett and Bergenstal, 1960; Kennedy and French, 1965), and this would suggest the necessity for pituitary hormones to mediate oestrogen effects upon breast cancer. Nevertheless, objective evidence of tumour regression has been reported in several patients from treatment with a combination of progesterone and oestradiol after hypophyseal ablation (Landau, Ehrlich and Huggins, 1962).

OESTROGEN COMBINATION THERAPY

It has been suggested that breast cancer which has ceased to respond to oestrogen therapy may respond again if tri-iodothyronine in high dosage is added (Bacigalupo, 1959; Luehrs, 1961). In an attempt to confirm this, the writer prescribed maximum tolerated doses of either tri-iodothyronine or thyroid hormone with oestrogen therapy, in patients whose tumour had failed to regress previously on oestrogen therapy alone. There was no evidence that thyroid hormone sensitised breast cancer to the effect of diethylstilboestrol therapy (Stoll, 1962).

It has also been suggested that oestrogen therapy must always be accompanied by brief courses of cortisone therapy in order to depress secretion of progesterone by the adrenal cortex (Larionov, 1965). It is postulated on a theoretical basis that progesterone tends to counteract the beneficial effect of oestrogen therapy on cancer of the breast, although this is contrary to the clinical experience of Landau et al (1962). This theoretical rationale for cortisone therapy is doubtful, but a short course of prednisone therapy may be usefully associated with the initiation of oestrogen therapy in very ill patients. The general condition is often dramatically improved, and the danger of hypercalcaemia may be lessened in the presence of bone metastases.

A combination of oestrogen with progestin therapy has been found to cause remission in 28 per cent of patients with breast cancer, not previously responding to oestrogen therapy (Stoll, 1969). A similar observation has been reported by Berndt (1970). It has been suggested in Chapter 6 that progestins can modify oestrogen effects at the target organ.

The administration of oestrogen in combination with cyclophosphamide therapy does not sensitise the tumour to the effect of cyclophosphamide, as is said to occur from the use of androgen (Meakin, 1969).

OESTROGEN EFFECTS AT MOLECULAR AND HISTOLOGICAL LEVELS

The selective uptake of oestrogen by breast cancer in vivo and in vitro has been discussed in Chapter 5. These investigations have, so far, little application to the clinical management of breast cancer.

Characteristic of oestrogen is its marked affinity for target tissues such as the breast, uterus, vagina and anterior pituitary gland. Oestrogen receptors there show an affinity for oestradiol, but not for oestrone. Cells which are stimulated by oestradiol contain a receptor protein to which the circulating oestrogen becomes bound. There is a specific receptor in the cytoplasm, and from here the oestrogen is transferred to another receptor protein in the nucleus. Interference with growth in the target tissue is thought to result from the attachment of the protein-oestrogen complex to the DNA of the nucleus.

The concentration of oestrogen required for physiological activity at the target organ is from 500 to 1000 times less than that for progesterone or androgen (Jensen, 1964). Furthermore, while the nature of the latter steroids change as they move from the cytoplasmic to the nuclear receptor, oestrogens are not metabolised at the target organ. A remarkable feature too is that physiological and biochemical responses to oestrogen may appear within one to two hours of its administration (Jensen, 1964).

Oestrogen initiates or stimulates growth in responsive tissues, and its physiological effects at a molecular level in the target organ may occur as a result of one, or more, of the following mechanisms:

(a) Effect on the permeability of the cell membrane or subcellular membranes.
(b) Altering the availability of enzymes, or itself acting as coenzyme in transhydrogenation or in protein synthesis.
(c) Increasing RNA synthesis in the cell.

The biological action of oestrogen on breast cancer may however be quite different from its physiological effect. It has been shown that stimulation of the normal mammary epithelium may be seen in breast cancer patients on oestrogen therapy, at the same time as the tumour tissue is showing depression of activity (Huseby and Thomas, 1954). This has led to the suggestion that oestrogen therapy may increase the mitotic activity of the normal tissue cells at the expense of the malignant cells. A similar observation in animals is that oestrogen administration will inhibit the activity of certain dehydrogenase systems in rat mammary carcinoma, while the level of their activity is raised in the adjacent normal mammary tissues (Rees and Huggins, 1960).

The initial histological change in breast cancer accompanying regression under oestrogen therapy is a vacuolisation of the cytoplasm in the tumour cells, associated with a loosening of the connective tissue fibrils around the cells (Koller, 1944; Emerson et al, 1953; Emerson, Kennedy and Taft, 1960). The latter is accompanied by biochemical evidence of increase in the turnover of chon-droitin sulphate and hyaluronic acid (Sino-hara and Sky-Peck, 1964). There follows infiltration of the stroma with lymphocytes and plasma cells, while the malignant cells now show pyknosis and fragmentation of the nuclei. Finally, the round-cell infiltration subsides, leaving a mass of hyaline connective tissue which in some cases encloses a few clumps of surviving cancer cells in the inter-stices.

It is therefore uncertain whether the effect of oestrogens on breast cancer is primarily on the epithelial elements of the tumour or on the stroma, since necrosis of the malignant cells, and loosening and round-cell infiltra-tion of the connective tissue, seem to proceed simultaneously. In experimental trans-planted tumours, the lymphocyte and the plasma cell are the principal cells involved in the host reaction against cancer.

TUMOUR STIMULATION BY OESTROGENS

Having noted the appearance of hyper-calcaemia in 20 per cent of 84 oestrogen-treated patients, Moore et al (1967) consider this form of therapy to be contraindicated under the age of 65, because of the risk of tumour stimulation. This is an extreme view-point. While oestrogen at the usual thera-peutic dosage may stimulate the growth of breast cancer in premenopausal women (Pearson, 1957), and possibly also in *recently* postmenopausal women with persistent oestro-gen excretion, McDonald (1963) has not found a single case of true tumour stimulation in patients more than one year postmenopausal.

Tumour stimulation by endocrine therapy is very difficult to prove objectively (see Chapter 6), but it is generally agreed that the likelihood of stimulation of breast cancer by oestrogens is extremely low in patients more than 5 years postmenopausal. Further-more, if postmenopausal women of any age group are properly selected for oestrogen therapy by vaginal smear examination as described previously, exacerbation of tumour is likely in less than 1 per cent of cases (Huseby, 1958).

Subjective symptoms such as increase in itching of skin lesions or increase in pain of bone deposits are occasionally seen after oestrogen administration. However, an ac-celeration of tumour growth must be *objec-tively* demonstrated in order to be significant of stimulation under therapy, and accurate serial measurements of tumour volume before and after treatment are necessary to confirm it. Rapid progression of disease is described as 'acute failure' of therapy when seen after surgical castration (Fracchia et al, 1969), and there is no reason why this term should not apply equally after additive hormone therapy. If proven, however, oestrogen-induced tumour acceleration is a sign of hormone sensitivity and suggests that sub-sequent major endocrine ablation should be successful in controlling tumour growth.

General malaise, rigors and pyrexia occur occasionally after oestrogen administration and probably represent idiosyncrasy to the agent used. There is no proof that such symptoms represent evidence of tumour stimulation, as with persistence of oestrogen therapy many of these patients go on to tumour healing. Moreover, few of them benefit objectively if oestrogen therapy is discontinued and the patient subjected to castration (Lucchini, Arraztoa and Vargas, 1962).

The hypercalcaemia which sometimes follows within a week or two of the institution of oestrogen therapy in the presence of bone metastases is said to be evidence of tumour stimulation (Moore et al, 1967). However, this can be true in only a proportion of cases. In a series of 269 oestrogen-treated patients, hypercalcaemia was noted in only 5 per cent (Hall, Dederick and Nevinny, 1963a) and, in the majority of these cases, clinical evidence of tumour growth remission occurred when oestrogen therapy was persisted with in spite of the hypercalcaemia. It should also be remembered that hypercalcaemia is reported to occur *spontaneously* in 12 to 15 per cent of patients with bone metastases from breast cancer (Kennedy et al, 1955; Jessiman et al, 1963). Nevertheless, frequent checks of the serum calcium level are advisable in the first two weeks of oestrogen therapy in the presence of bone metastases, and initial small doses of oestrogens may minimise the danger of hypercalcaemia (Donovan, Bethune and Berne, 1966).

Hypercalcaemia occurring *late* in a course of oestrogen therapy suggests a loss of tumour control by the hormone, rather than stimulation of activity. Whether occurring early or late, the raised serum calcium will return to normal in the majority of cases when oestrogen therapy is stopped, hydration maintained, and treatment instituted with corticosteroids and sodium phosphate. Later treatment is by cytotoxic agents or by major endocrine ablation (Beckett, 1969), in the hope of long-term control of the tumour. The latter method is preferred if the patient is over five years postmenopausal and showed a long recurrence-free interval between mastectomy and metastasis.

CHOICE OF OESTROGEN AND DOSAGE

Administration of oestrogens may be either continuous or intermittent. In continuous therapy, oestrogens are maintained for as long as control of tumour growth persists. When oestrogen therapy is stopped on reactivation of the disease, a withdrawal response may occur in a minority of cases. Alternatively, treatment may be intermittent, with discontinuation of oestrogens as soon as complete regression of visible tumour has occurred. In such cases, tumour regression is often maintained for many months after stopping therapy and, when the disease reactivates, further regression may occur when the oestrogen is reinstituted.

Intermittent administration is preferred by the writer, since it may postpone the development of autonomy in the tumour as a result of alternating its hormonal environment. The intermittent method also decreases the hazards of oestrogen administration (see later) and is safer in patients with evidence of mild cardiac failure, because fluid retention is not maintained. The continuous method may be more convenient if serious side-effects are absent, but its use may necessitate increase of the dose at intervals as noted later. It is important to note that when tumour control is lost to either method of administration, there is no evidence that a change of oestrogenic agent will regain control of tumour growth.

Diethylstilboestrol is a synthetic non-steroidal oestrogen of high potency and low cost. It has the added advantage of oral administration, so that if complications arise, treatment can be quickly discontinued.

Dienoestrol has approximately one fifth of the oestrogenic potency of stilboestrol, and has no obvious advantage over the latter.

Diethylstilboestrol is usually prescribed at a dose of 5 mg tds. This dosage has been compared by the writer with that of 0·5 mg tds in a randomised trial on breast cancer, and both the remission rates and gastric tolerance were found to be similar (Stoll, 1950). The higher dose is recommended for at least the first months of therapy, until response can be established. Very high oestrogen dosage (600 mg oestradiol undecylate weekly), has been found to yield a similar remission rate to that of 5 mg tds of stilboestrol noted above (Kennedy, 1967), and there is no advantage in exceeding this latter dose of stilboestrol. An early trial of dienoestrol in breast cancer suggested that 20 mg dienoestrol daily was significantly more effective than was 1 to 2 mg (Walpole and Paterson, 1949). The lower dose is equivalent in oestrogenic activity to only 0·25 mg diethylstilboestrol daily, and this dose may be below the minimum required for the control of breast cancer.

It appears therefore, that within a wide therapeutic range, there is no increase in remission rate resulting from increase in oestrogen dosage. However, there is some evidence that increasing the dose of diethyl-stilboestrol beyond 15 mg daily may re-establish tumour control *when the latter dose becomes ineffective.* The vaginal smear is a biological indicator of the patient's oestrogen

dose of 0·1 to 0·5 mg tds. It is sometimes tolerated by patients who cannot tolerate diethylstilboestrol.

Hexoestrol has been given orally at the massive dosage of 1 g daily (Mrazek et al, 1968). There is no obvious advantage from its use.

Oestradiol monobenzoate may be administered

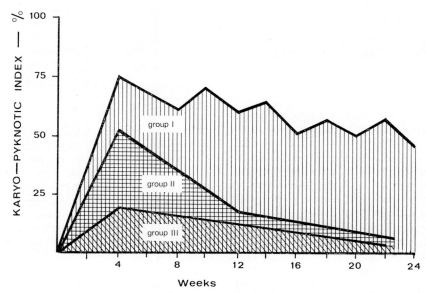

FIGURE 7.4. Diagrammatic representation of the vaginal smear response to oestrogen therapy, followed up in serial manner. Categorised into three group patterns:

Group 1: a rise in karyopyknotic index above 60 per cent, followed by a gradual fall over a period of six months or longer.

Group 2: a rise in the KPI to 50 per cent (approx.), followed by a rapid fall after 8 weeks.

Group 3: no rise in the KPI above 25 per cent throughout treatment. (Figure reproduced from Stoll, 1967, by permission of the Editor of *Cancer*, Philadelphia.)

utilisation in the body, and, if it is found that inadequate vaginal keratinisation is associated with a lessening tumour response, it is advisable to increase the oestrogen dose, or even change from oral to parenteral prescription (Figure 7.4). The writer has confirmed a correlation between the degree of vaginal keratinisation and the likelihood of breast cancer regression from oestrogen therapy (Liu, 1957; Stoll, 1967).

Ethinyloestradiol is also given orally, but at a

parenterally if there is any difficulty in the patient's cooperation in oral dosage.

Premarin is a mixture of conjugated oestrogens derived from the urine of pregnant mares, and can be given either orally or intravenously. It is relatively expensive, but taken at a dosage of 2·5 to 5 mg daily it is, in the writer's experience, almost free of side-effects such as nausea or vomiting.

Depot injections of oestrogens such as the undecylate or valerate esters can be used for maintenance therapy, but have the disadvantage that in the presence of urgent complications such as hypercalcaemia or heart failure, their action cannot be swiftly terminated.

Implants of oestrogens, such as α-oestradiol 25 mg or hexoestrol 500 mg, are used for maintenance therapy and are usually replaced at two-monthly intervals. The same objection applies as for depot injections.

UNWANTED AND TOXIC EFFECTS OF OESTROGENS

GASTRIC INTOLERANCE

The ability of the liver to inactivate oestrogens may be impaired in patients with liver damage (Pincus et al, 1951), and this may account for the variation in tolerance to different oestrogens from patient to patient. It is interesting to note that even massive doses of oestradiol undecylate 600 mg by weekly intramuscular injection (Kennedy, 1967), or hexoestrol 1 g orally daily (Mrazek et al, 1968), can be well tolerated.

Approximately 20 per cent of women complain of vomiting when taking diethylstilboestrol 5 mg three times daily, and anorexia or nausea are even more common. The writer has found that the symptoms may be controlled by taking pyridoxine hydrochloride 30 mg daily concurrently, until the patient develops tolerance to oestrogen therapy. It may be relevant that high doses of oestrogen result in an increased excretion of abnormal tryptophane metabolites in the urine unless adequate pyridoxal phosphate is present in the body (Rose, 1966). Premarin is much less likely to cause vomiting than diethylstilboestrol and can be used to start oestrogen therapy (Stoll, 1969). It is usually found that the patient will then tolerate diethylstilboestrol after a few weeks' therapy.

SODIUM RETENTION

Swelling of the ankles is seen in almost every patient taking oestrogens at the dose levels recommended, and is due to sodium retention by the kidney. In patients with a mild degree of heart failure, symptoms are usually increased after taking oestrogens at the dosage recommended. Lower dosage may be tried, or a trial of diuretics and a restricted sodium diet may be useful in such cases. In patients with severe heart failure, oestrogens are better avoided completely, although short intermittent courses of administration have achieved regression of breast cancer in patients with lesser degrees of heart failure (Stoll, 1969).

UTERINE BLEEDING

'Withdrawal' bleeding occurs in the majority of postmenopausal females when oestrogen therapy is interrupted, and the patient should be forewarned of this to avoid anxiety. Mucous cervical discharge is not uncommon in patients while on oestrogen therapy for breast cancer but 'breakthrough' uterine bleeding occurs only in a minority of patients. Bleeding can usually be stopped in such cases by *increasing* the dose of stilboestrol to 20 or even 30 mg daily, whereas stopping oestrogen administration will usually intensify and prolong the bleeding.

It has been suggested that there may be an increased risk of developing uterine cancer in breast cancer patients after long-term administration of large doses of oestrogens. If a patient on oestrogen therapy complains of excessive or prolonged bleeding, diagnostic curettage of the uterus is indicated. Endometrial hyperplasia is commonly found but the incidence of uterine cancer in such cases is said to be negligible (Koller, 1966). The addition of progestins will counteract the tendency of oestrogens to cause endometrial hyperplasia.

METABOLIC AND VASCULAR EFFECTS

Thrombophlebitis is not uncommon in patients with advanced cancer, and recent reports suggest that oestrogen administration may possibly increase the risk by an effect on both fibrinolytic and coagulation processes (Poller and Thomson, 1966).

The oestrogen component of oral contraceptives has been implicated in causing hypertension, impairment of glucose tolerance, venous thromboembolic disease and impairment of liver function. By reason of their age, postmenopausal women are already predisposed to these metabolic and vascular changes, which may be intensified by oestrogen administration. On the other hand, adequate oestrogen replacement is said to prevent osteoporosis and coronary artery disease in this age group.

It seems important that a nationwide study should be set up to determine for breast cancer (as has been done for prostatic cancer in the USA) whether the dangers of oestrogen therapy should cause hesitation in their prescription to the older postmenopausal women with advanced breast cancer.

MINOR SIDE-EFFECTS

In the older patient especially, dribbling of urine associated with cough or straining is often troublesome during oestrogen therapy. It is particularly marked in patients suffering from cystocoel, and the prescription of tolazoline 100 mg daily has been found useful by the writer in such cases.

Almost all patients on diethylstilboestrol therapy note pigmentation of the nipples and areola. Occasionally, pigmentation is noted also in recent scars. Fullness and tenderness of the breasts is common when beginning therapy. Dizziness, excessive tiredness or pelvic cramps, are also occasional complaints in patients receiving oestrogen therapy at therapeutic dosage for breast cancer.

Idiosyncrasy to oestrogen therapy is manifested by fever and rigors after administration. It occurs rarely, but its importance is that it is likely to be misinterpreted as exacerbation of tumour activity.

CONCLUSION

Therapeutic castration, either by surgery or by radiation, is advised as the initial step in the endocrine therapy of premenopausal patients with recurrent or advanced breast cancer, and will induce objective evidence of tumour response in about 30 per cent of cases for an average of one to two years. Life is prolonged by an average of 22 months in responding cases, but in a further proportion there results subjective improvement which is unassociated with objective signs of tumour regression. Castration is advised also in the early postmenopausal patient if there is evidence of persistent oestrogen secretion by the ovary.

Although response is much more likely in the case of bone and soft tissue lesions, castration is well worth a trial also in patients with visceral metastases such as those in the lungs, liver or brain. Concomitant corticosteroid therapy is usual in such cases. Prophylactic castration at the time of mastectomy is advisable only in the presence of extensively invaded axillary nodes. Total life expectation is probably not increased, but clinical evidence of recurrence is postponed in such cases.

Oestrogen therapy is advised as the initial step in endocrine therapy for postmenopausal patients in whom there is no evidence of oestrogen secretion. It will induce tumour regression in about 30 per cent of cases for an average of 16 months and life is prolonged by an average of 17 months in responding cases. Objective evidence of tumour regression is most common in the presence of soft tissue metastases in older patients, but lung and pleural metastases not uncommonly respond also. A remarkable feature is that a second growth remission is not uncommon on withdrawal of oestrogen therapy.

Dosage of diethylstilboestrol recommended is between 1·5 and 15 mg daily, but the adequacy of oestrogen intake is best assured by serial examination of the vaginal smear. Continuous and intermittent methods of oestrogen administration each have a place in management. In spite of opinions to the contrary, stimulation of tumour growth by oestrogens is extremely rare. In patients more than 10 years postmenopausal, the dangers of fluid retention are a more serious problem than that of tumour exacerbation.

References

Abrams, H. L., Spiro, R. & Goldstein, N. (1950) Metastases in carcinoma: analysis of 1000 autopsied cases. *Cancer (Philadelphia)*, **3**, 74.

Adair, F. E. Treves, N., Farrow, J. H. & Scharnagel, I. M. (1945) Clinical effects of surgical and X-ray castration in mammary cancer. *Journal of the American Medical Association*, **128**, 161.

Adlercreutz, H. (1969) Personal Communication.

AMA Committee on Research (1960) Androgens and estrogens in the treatment of disseminated mammary carcinoma. *Journal of the American Medical Association*, **172**, 1271.

Ansfield, D. (1967) In Symposium on cancer of the breast. *Cancer (Philadelphia)*, **201**, 1065.

Bacigalupo, C. (1959) Certain aspects and results of hormone therapy in oncology. *Problems of Oncology (New York)*, **5** (8), 51.

Barlow, J. J., Emerson, K. & Saxena, B. N. (1969) Estradiol production after ovariectomy for carcinoma of the breast. Relevance to the treatment of menopausal women. *New England Journal of Medicine*, **280**, 633.

Berndt, G. (1970) Management of metastasising mammary carcinoma with oestrogen gestagen combination therapy by SH834. *Deutsche medizinische Wocenschrift*, **95**, 2399.

Beatson, G. T. (1896) On the treatment of inoperable cases of carcinoma of the mamma. Suggestion for a new method of treatment with illustrative cases. *Lancet*, **ii**, 104, 162.

Beckett, U. L. (1969) Hypercalcemia associated with estrogen administration in patients with breast carcinoma. *Cancer (Philadelphia)*, **23**, 109.

Block, G. E., Lampe, I., Vial, A. B. & Collier, F. A. (1960) Therapeutic castration for advanced mammary cancer. *Surgery*, **67**, 877.

Block, G. E., Vial, A. B. & Pullen, F. W. (1958) Estrogen excretion following operative and irradiation castration in cases of mammary cancer. *Surgery*, **43**, 415.

Brinkley, D. M. & Kingsley-Pillers, E. (1960) Treatment of advanced carcinoma of the breast by bilateral oophorectomy and prednisone. *Lancet*, **i**, 123.

Brown, J. B. (1967) Personal communication.

Bulbrook, R. D. & Greenwood, F. C. (1957) Persistence of urinary oestrogen excretion after oophorectomy and adrenalectomy. *British Medical Journal*, **i**, 662.

Cole, M. P. (1964) The place of radiotherapy in the management of early breast cancer. A report of two clinical trials. *British Journal of Surgery*, **51**, 216.

Cole, M. (1970) Prophylactic compared with therapeutic X-ray artificial menopause. In *Second Tenovus Workshop on Breast Cancer*, ed. Joslin, C. A. F. and Gleave, E. N. Cardiff: Tenovus Workshop.

Cooper, D. R. & Butterfield, J. (1970) Pregnancy subsequent to mastectomy for cancer of the breast. *Annals of Surgery*, **171**, 429.

Dao, T. L. (1967) Current concepts in the management of advanced breast malignancies. *Cancer Chemotherapy Abstracts*, **8**, 568.

Dao, T. L. D. (1970) Discussion, p. 47. In *Second Tenovus Workshop, on Breast Cancer*, ed. Joslin, C. A. F. and Gleave, E. N. Cardiff: Tenovus Workshop.

Delarue, N. C. (1955) Fundamental concepts determining a philosophy of treatment in mammary carcinoma. *Canadian Medical Association Journal*, **73**, 597.

Diczfalusy, E., Notter, G., Edsmyr, F. & Westman, A. (1959) Estrogen excretion in breast cancer patients before and after ovarian irradiation and oophorectomy. *Journal of Clinical Endocrinology*, **19**, 1230.

Donegan, W. L. (1967) Endocrine ablation, hormone therapy, and chemotherapy. In *Cancer of the Breast*, ed. Spratt, J. S. and Donegan, W. L. Philadelphia: Saunders.

Donovan, A. J., Bethune, J. E. & Berne, T. V. (1966) Hypercalcemia in patients with advanced mammary cancer and osseous metastases. *American Surgeon*, **32**, 673.

Douglas, M. (1952) The treatment of advanced breast cancer by hormone therapy. *British Journal of Cancer*, **6**, 32.

Eley, A. & Riddell, V. (1960) Treatment of advanced carcinoma of the breast by oophorectomy and prednisone. *Lancet*, **i**, 278.

Emerson, W. J., Kennedy, B. J., Graham, J. N. & Nathanson, I. T. (1953) Pathology of primary and recurrent carcinoma of the human breast after administration of steroid hormones. *Cancer (Philadelphia)*, **6**, 641.

Emerson, W., Kennedy, B. J. & Nathanson, L. T. (1949) Histological alterations in cancer of the breast in patients treated with steroid hormones. *Cancer Research*, **9**, 551.

Emerson, W. J., Kennedy, B. J. & Taft, E. B. (1960) Correlation of histological alterations in breast cancer with response to hormone therapy. *Cancer (Philadelphia)*, **13**, 1047.

Emery, E. S. & Trotter, W. R. (1963) Tri-iodothyronine in advanced breast cancer. *Lancet*, **i**, 358.

Escher, G. (1958) Panel discussion. In *Breast Cancer*, p. 225, ed. Segaloff, A. St Louis: C. V. Mosby.

Escher, G. C. & Kaufman, R. J. (1963) Advanced breast carcinoma—factors influencing survival. *Acta Unio internationalis contra cancrum*, **19**, 1039.

Forrest, A. P. M. (1965) Endocrine treatment of breast cancer. *Israel Journal of Medical Science*, **1**, 259.

Fracchia, A. A., Farrow, J. H., de Palo, A. J., Connelly, D. P. & Huvos, R. G. (1969) Castration for primary inoperable or recurrent breast carcinoma. *Surgery, Gynecology and Obstetrics*, **128**, 1226.

Gordon, D. L. & Segaloff, A. (1958) Castration as a palliative therapy for advanced breast cancer. In *Breast Cancer*, p. 187, ed. Segaloff, A. St Louis: C. V. Mosby.

Gow, S. & MacGillivray, J. (1971) Metabolic, hormonal and vascular changes after synthetic oestrogen therapy in oophorectomised women. *British Medical Journal*, **ii**, 73.

Haddow, W., Watkinson, J. M., Paterson, E. & Koller, P. (1944) Influence of synthetic oestrogens upon advanced malignant disease. *British Medical Journal*, **ii**, 393.

Hall, T. C., Dederick, M. M. & Nevinny, H. B. (1963a) Prognostic value of hormonally induced hypercalcemia in breast cancer, *Cancer Chemotherapy Reports*, **30**, 21.

Hall, T. C., Dederick, M. M., Nevinny, H. B. & Muench, H. (1963b) Prognostic value of response of patients with breast cancer to therapeutic castration. *Cancer Chemotherapy Reports*, **31**, 47.

Hayward, J. (1970) Treatment of the advanced disease. *British Medical Journal*, **ii**, 469.

Holleb, A. I. & Farrow, J. H. (1962) The relation of carcinoma of the breast and pregnancy in 283 cases. *Surgery, Gynecology and Obstetrics*, **115**, 65.

Horsely, G. W. (1957) Prophylactic oophorectomy in treatment of cancer of the breast. *American Surgeon*, **23**, 396.

Hortling, H., Hiisi-Brummer, L. & Af Bjorkesten, G. A. (1962) Endocrine therapy of metastatising breast cancer. *Acta Medica Scandinavica*, **172**, Supplement, 385.

Huseby, R. A. (1958) The use of estrogen in the treatment of advanced human breast cancer. In *Breast Cancer*, p. 206, ed. Segaloff, A. St Louis: C. V. Mosby.

Huseby, R. A. & Thomas, L. B. (1954) Histological and histochemical alterations in the normal breast tissues of patients with advanced breast cancer being treated with estrogenic hormones. *Cancer (Philadelphia)*, **7**, 54.

Jensen, E. V. (1964) Metabolic fate of sex hormones in target tissues with regard to tissue specificity. *Proceedings of the 2nd International Congress on Endocrinology.*

Jessiman, A. G., Emerson, K., Shah, R. C. & Moore, F. D. (1963) Hypercalcemia in carcinoma of the breast. *Annals of Surgery*, **157**, 377.

Kaufman, R. F. & Escher, G. C. (1961) Rebound regression in advanced mammary carcinoma. *Surgery, Gynecology and Obstetrics*, **113**, 635.

Kennedy, B. J. (1962) Massive estrogen administration in premenopausal women with metastatic breast cancer. *Cancer (Philadelphia)*, **15**, 641.

Kennedy, B. J. (1965) Hormonal control of breast cancer. *Annals of Internal Medicine*, **63**, 329.

Kennedy, B. J. (1967) Effect of massive doses of estradiol undecylate in advanced breast cancer. *Cancer Chemotherapy Report*, **51**, 491.

Kennedy, B. J. (1969) Hormone therapy in inoperable breast cancer. *Cancer (Philadelphia)*, **24**, 1345.

Kennedy, B. J. & French, L. (1965) Hypophysectomy in advanced breast cancer. *American Journal of Surgery*, **110**, 411.

Kennedy, B. J., Mielke, P. W. & Fortuny, I. E. (1964) Therapeutic castration versus prophylactic castration in breast cancer. *Surgery, Gynecology and Obstetrics*, **118**, 524.

Kennedy, B. J., Nathanson, I. T., Tibbetts, D. M. & Aub, J. C. (1955) Biochemical alternations during steroid hormone therapy of advanced breast cancer. *American Journal of Medicine*, **19**, 337.

Koller, P. C. (1944) Addendum—cytology of serial biopsies from a case of carcinoma of the breast treated with stilboestrol. *British Medical Journal*, **ii**, 398.

Koller, O. (1966) The risk of development of uterine cancer in patients with breast cancer after long term treatment with oestrogen in massive doses. *Acta obstetrica et gynecologca Scandinavica*, **45**, 111.

Lalanne, C. M., Juret, P., Hourtoule, F. & Sarazin, D. (1967) Castration in breast cancer—surgery or radiation. *Acta Radiologica*, **6**, 323.

Landau, R. L., Ehrlich, E. N. & Huggins, C. (1962) Estradiol benzoate and progesterone in advanced human breast cancer. *Journal of the American Medical Association*, **182**, 632.

Larionov, L. F. (1965) *Cancer Chemotherapy*, p. 459. Oxford: Pergamon Press.

Lewison, E. F. (1962) Prophylactic versus therapeutic castration in the total treatment of breast cancer. *Obstetrics and Gynecology, Scandinavica*, **17**, 769.

Lewison, E. F. (1965) Castration in the treatment of advanced breast cancer. *Cancer (Philadelphia)*, **18**, 1558.

Lipsett, M. B. & Bergenstal, D. M. (1960) Lack of effect of human growth hormone and ovine prolactin on cancer in man. *Cancer Research*, **20**, 1172.

Liu, W. (1957) Vaginal cytology in breast cancer patients. *Surgery, Gynecology and Obstetrics*, **105**, 421.

Lucchini, A., Arraztoa, J. & Vargas, L. (1962) Metastalysis syndrome and effectiveness of subcutaneous implantation of hexestrol in the treatment of breast cancer metastases. *Cancer (Philadelphia)*, **15**, 189.

Luehrs, W. (1961) Conference on biochemistry of human cancer. *British Medical Journal*, **i**, 1752.

Lumb, G. & Mackenzie, D. H. (1959) The incidence of metastases in adrenal glands and ovaries removed for carcinoma of the breast. *Cancer (Philadelphia)*, **12**, 521.

McBride, J. M. (1957) Estrogen excretion levels in the normal postmenopausal woman. *Journal of Clinical Endocrinology*, **17**, 1440.

McDonald, I. (1962) Endocrine ablation in disseminated mammary carcinoma. *Surgery, Gynecology and Obstetrics*, **115**, 215.

McDonald, I. (1963) Letter, Disseminated mammary carcinoma. *Journal of the American Medical Association*, **186**, 273.

McWhirter, R. (1957) Some factors influencing prognosis in breast cancer. *Journal of the Faculty of Radiologists*, **8**, 220.

Meakin, J. W., Allt, W. E. C., Beale, F. A., Brown, T. C., Bulbrook, R. D., Clark, K. M., Fitzpatrick, P. F., Hawkins, N. V., Hayward, J. L. & Jenkin, R. D. T. (1968) A preliminary report of two studies of adjuvant treatment of primary breast cancer. In *Prognostic Factors in Breast Cancer*, ed. Forrest, A. P. M. and Kunkler, P. B. Edinburgh: Livingstone.

Meakin, J. W. (1969) Effect of chemotherapeutic agents on hormone dependent neoplasms and tissues. *Annual Report of the Ontario Cancer Research Foundation*, p. 151.

Moore, F. D., Woodrow, S. I., Aliapoulios, M. A. & Wilson, R. E. (1967) Carcinoma of the breast. A decade of new results with old concepts. *New England Journal of Medicine*, **277**, 460.

Mrazek, W., Andrews, N. C., Bisel, H. F., Wilson, W. L., Hummel, R. P. (1968) Clinical study of hexestrol. *Cancer Chemotherapy Report*, **52**, 751.

Munguia, M. H., Pina, A., Franco, P. E., Rivadeneyra, G. J., Velasco Arce, H. J. M. & Montano, G. (1960) Vaginal cytology in advanced mammary cancer. I Selection of patients for oophorectomy. English abstract in *Cancer Chemotherapy Abstracts*, **2**, 83.

Nathanson, I. T. (1947) Hormonal alteration of advanced cancer of the breast. *Surgical Clinics of North America*, **27**, 1144.

Nathanson, I. T. (1952) Clinical investigative experience with steroid hormones in breast cancer. *Cancer (Philadelphia)*, **5**, 754.

Nathanson, I. T., Engel, L. L. & Kelley, R. M. (1951) The effect of ACTH on the urinary excretion of steroids in neoplastic disease. In *Proceedings of the Second Clinical ACTH Conference*, p. 54. New York: Blakiston.

Nathanson, I. T. & Kelley, R. M. (1952) Hormonal treatment of cancer. *New England Journal of Medicine*, **246**, 135.

Nathanson, I. T., Rice, C. & Meigs, J. V. (1940) Hormonal studies on artificial menopause produced by roentgen rays. *American Journal of Obstetrics and Gynecology*, **40**, 936.

Nevinny, H. B., Nevinny, D., Rosoff, C. B., Hall, T. C. & Muench, H. (1969) Prophylactic oophorectomy in breast cancer therapy—preliminary report. *American Journal of Surgery*, **117**, 531.

Nissen-Meyer, R. (1964) Prophylactic endocrine treatment in carcinoma of the breast. *Clinical Radiology*, **15**, 152.

Nissen-Meyer, R. (1965) Castration as part of the primary treatment for operable female breast cancer. *Acta Radiologica* (Stockholm). Supplement, p. 249.

Nissen-Meyer, R. (1967) The role of prophylactic castration in the therapy of human mammary cancer. *European Journal of Cancer*, **3**, 395.

Nissen-Meyer, R. & Sanner, T. (1963) The excretion of oestrone, pregnanediol, and pregnanetriol in breast cancer patients. *Acta endocrinologica (København)*, **44**, 334.

Nissen-Meyer, R. & Vogt, J. H. (1959) Cortisone treatment of metastatic breast cancer. *Acta Unio internationalis contra cancrum*, **15**, 1140.

Novak, E. R. & Williams, T. J. (1960) Autopsy comparisons of cardiovascular changes in the castrated and normal woman. *American Journal of Obstetrics and Gynecology*, **80**, 863.

Oliver, M. F. & Boyd, G. S. (1959) Effect of bilateral oophorectomy on coronary artery disease and serum lipid levels. *Lancet*, **ii**, 691.

Osborne, M. P. & Pitts, R. M. (1961) Therapeutic oophorectomy for advanced breast cancer. *Cancer (Philadelphia)*, **14**, 126.

Parrish, H. M., Carr, C. A., Hall, D. G. & King, T. M. (1967) Coronary disease in castrated women. *American Journal of Obstetrics and Gynecology*, **99**, 105.

Paterson, R. & Russeil, M. H. (1959) Breast cancer: value of irradiation of the ovaries. *Journal of the Faculty of Radiologists*, **10**, 130.

Pearson, O. H. (1957) Observations on the role of androgens and estrogens in body balance. *Archives of Internal Medicine*, **100**, 724.

Pearson, O. H. & Ray, B. S. (1959) Results of hypophysectomy in the treatment of metastatic mammary carcinoma. *Cancer (Philadelphia)*, **12**, 85.

Pearson, O. H., West, C. D., Li, M. C., McLean, J. P. & Treves, N. (1955) Endocrine therapy of metastatic breast cancer. *Archives of Internal Medicine*, **95**, 357.

Peters, M. V. (1963) Carcinoma of the breast associated with pregnancy and lactation. *Proceedings of the Tenth Clinical Conference*, p. 161. Canada: Ontario Research Foundation.

Pincus, I. J., Rakoff, A. E., Cohn, E. M. & Tumen, H. J. (1951) Hormonal studies in patients with chronic liver disease. *Gastroenterology*, **19**, 735.

Poller, L. & Thomson, J. M. (1966) Clotting factors during oral contraception—further report. *British Medical Journal*, **ii**, 23.

Poppe, H. & Gregl, A. (1961) Quoted in Hortling *et al.* (1962).

Procope, B. J. & Adlercreutz, H. (1969) Studies on the influence of age on oestrogen in postmenopausal women with atrophic endometrium and normal liver function. *Acta endocrinologica (København)*, **62**, 461.

Ravdin, R. G., Lewison, E. F., Slack, N. H., Gardner, B., State, D. & Fisher, B. (1970) Results of a clinical trial concerning the worth of prophylactic oophorectomy for breast cancer. *Surgery, Gynecology and Obstetrics*, **131**, 1055.

Rees, E. D. & Huggins, C. (1960) Steroid influences on respiration, glycolysis, and levels of pyridine nucleotide linked dehydrogenases of experimental mammary cancers. *Cancer Research*, **20**, 963.

Rose, D. P. (1966) Excretion of xanthurenic acid in the urine of women taking progestogen–oestrogen preparations. *Nature (London)*, **210**, 196.

Segaloff, A., Gordon, D., Carabasi, R. A., Horwitt, B. N., Schlosser, J. V. & Murison, P. J. (1954) Hormonal therapy in cancer of the breast: VII Effect of conjugated estrogens (equine) on clinical course and hormonal excretion. *Cancer (Philadelphia)*, **7**, 758.

Sellwood, R. (1970) Discussion, p. 86. In *Second Tenovus Workshop on Breast Cancer*, ed. Joslin, C. A. and Gleave, E. N. Cardiff: Tenovus Workshop.

Sicard, A. (1948) La frequence de metastases ovariennes des cancers du sein. *Presse médicale*, **56**, 606.

Siegert, A. (1952) Castration and mammary carcinoma. *Strahlentherapie*, **87**, 62.

Sinohara, H. and Sky-Peck, H. H. (1964) The effects of estradiol on acid mucopolysaccharide metabolism in oophorectomised rats. *Archives of Biochemistry and Biophysics*, **106**, 138.

Smith, G. V. & Smith, O. W. (1953) Carcinoma of the breast. Results and evaluation of X-radiation and relation of age and surgical castration to length of survival. *Surgery, Gynecology and Obstetrics*, **97**, 508.

Sommers, S. C. & Teloh, H. A. (1952) Ovarian stromal hyperplasia in breast cancer. *Archives of Pathology*, **53**, 160.

Sommers, S. C., Teloh, H. A. & Goldman, G. (1953) Ovarian influence upon survival in breast cancer. *Archives of Surgery*, **67**, 916.

Stewart, H. (1970) Oophorectomy response as an index to further endocrine ablation. In *Second Tenovus Workshop on Breast Cancer*, ed. Joslin, C. A. F. and Gleave, E. N. Cardiff: Tenovus Workshop.

Stoll, B. A. (1950) Hormone therapy in relation to radiotherapy in the treatment of advanced carcinoma of the breast. *Proceedings of the Royal Society of Medicine*, **43**, 875.

Stoll, B. A. (1958) Endocrine factors in the aetiology and treatment of cancer of the breast and prostate. In *Modern Trends in Endocrinology*, p. 212, vol. 1, ed. Gardiner Hill, H. London: Butterworth.

Stoll, B. A. (1962) A clinical trial of tri-iodothyronine as a hormone potentiator in advanced breast cancer. *British Journal of Cancer*, **16**, 436.

Stoll, B. A. (1964) Fact and fallacy in the hormonal control of breast cancer. *Medical Journal of Australia*, **1**, 980.

Stoll, B. A. (1967) Vaginal cytology as an aid to hormone therapy in postmenopausal breast cancer. *Cancer (Philadelphia)*, **20**, 1807.

Stoll, B. A. (1969) *Hormonal Management in Breast Cancer*. London: Pitman Medical and Philadelphia: Lippincott.

Stoll, B. A. & Ackland, T. H. (1970) Management of breast cancer in old age. *British Medical Journal*, **iv**, 201.

Stoll, B. A. & Ellis, F. (1953) Treatment by oestrogens of pulmonary metastases from breast cancer. *British Medical Journal*, **ii**, 796.

Struthers, R. A. (1956) Postmenopausal oestrogen production. *British Medical Journal*, **i**, 1331.

Taylor, S. G. (1962) Endocrine ablation in disseminated mammary carcinoma. *Surgery, Gynecology and Obstetrics*, **115**, 443.

Thayssen, V. E. (1948) The influence of castration by roentgen on carcinoma of the breast. *Acta Radiologica*, **29**, 189.

Treves, N. (1957) An evaluation of prophylactic castration in the treatment of mammary carcinoma. *Cancer (Philadelphia)*, **10**, 393.

Treves, N. & Finkbeiner, J. A. (1958) An evaluation of therapeutic surgical castration in the treatment of metastatic, recurrent and primary inoperable mammary carcinoma in women. *Cancer (Philadelphia)*, **11**, 421.

Walpole, A. L. & Paterson, E. (1949) Synthetic oestrogens in mammary cancer. *Lancet*, **ii**, 783.

Warren, S. & Witham, E. M. (1933) Studies on tumour metastasis; distribution of metastases in cancer of the breast. *Surgery, Gynecology and Obstetrics*, **57**, 81.

White, T. T. (1954) Carcinoma of the breast and pregnancy. Analysis of 920 cases collected from the literature and new cases. *Annals of Surgery*, **139**, 9.

Wilson, R. E., Jessiman, A. G. & Moore, F. D. (1958) Severe exacerbation of cancer of the breast after oophorectomy and adrenalectomy. Report of four cases. *New England Journal of Medicine*, **258**, 312.

Witt, J. A., Gardner, B., Gordan, G. S., Graham, W. P. & Thomas, A. N. (1963) Secondary hormonal therapy of disseminated breast cancer. Comparison of hypophysectomy, replacement therapy, estrogens, and androgens. *Archives of Internal Medicine*, **111**, 557.

Wolff, B. (1957) The differential cell count in cancer of the breast and response to hormone therapy. *Guy's Hospital Report*, **106**, 53.

Chapter 8

Androgen, Corticosteroid and Progestin Therapy

BASIL A. STOLL

Steroid therapy is commonly utilised as an alternative to major endocrine ablation, when primary therapy by castration or by oestrogens has either failed or ceased to control tumour growth in advanced cancer. The decision to postpone major endocrine ablation and to institute steroid therapy by androgens, corticosteroids, or progestins is difficult, and the selection of the correct steroid for the individual case is summarised in Chapter 10.

Androgen Therapy

The use of androgen therapy in the management of advanced breast cancer is still debated emotionally (see Chapter 22). In the past, the androgen most widely reported was testosterone propionate (Adair, 1947; Stoll, 1950), and the prolonged therapy necessary for the control of breast cancer was associated, in the case of this agent, with a considerable degree of virilisation. In the last 10 years, equally effective, but less virilising, androgens have been introduced. In spite of this, opposition to the use of androgen therapy in breast cancer is still maintained by some authorities (Juret, 1966; Pearson,

1967), on the basis that the overall remission rate does not justify the possibility of virilisation from their use.

INDICATIONS FOR PRIMARY THERAPY

Androgen therapy is practised in some centres as an alternative to castration, as the primary endocrine therapy in premenopausal breast cancer patients. It should be emphasised that although high doses of androgen can cause temporary amenorrhoea, the results of androgen therapy are undoubtedly inferior to those of castration in the treatment of premenopausal patients with breast cancer. The writer found not a single case of significant tumour regression among 22 such cases treated by androgens (Stoll, 1969). Another series reported tumour regression in only 13 per cent of premenopausal patients treated by androgen therapy, compared to 44 per cent for those treated by surgical castration (Pearson et al, 1955). Furthermore, the mean duration of remission reported for androgen therapy in premenopausal patients is between 8 and 12 months, compared to between 10 and 25 months for castration (Hortling, Hiisi-Brummer and Af Bjorkesten, 1962; CCNSC Breast Cancer Group, 1964).

Therefore, both because of the more frequent and more prolonged remissions following castration (AMA Committee on Research, 1960; Taylor, 1962), and because of the avoidance of virilisation, practically all authorities prefer castration as the primary endocrine treatment in premenopausal women with advanced breast cancer. Androgen therapy is prescribed as an *alternative* to castration, only if the patient is too ill for surgical castration, and under these circumstances irradiation of the ovaries or corticosteroid therapy are usually added. Androgen therapy may be prescribed in *addition* to castration in patients under the age of 35, or in the presence of bone metastases at any age, in order to increase the likelihood of remission (Stoll, 1969).

In the case of *postmenopausal* breast cancer patients also, the overall results of androgens as primary endocrine treatment are inferior to those of oestrogen therapy (Table 8.1). Thus, objective evidence of tumour regression was reported by the AMA Committee on Research (1960) in 21 per cent of 420 postmenopausal women, and by the CCNSC Breast Cancer Group (1964a) in 21·5 per cent of such patients with advanced breast cancer treated by androgens. The writer, reviewing his personal series of 434 androgen-treated patients, and using rigid criteria of response, noted regression in only 15 per cent of cases (Stoll, 1964). Though *overall* remission figures are inferior to those from oestrogen therapy (Table 8.1), in the case of bone metastases the remission rates from androgen therapy are considerably higher than those of oestrogen therapy, in the writer's experience.

There is another indication for primary androgen therapy in postmenopausal patients: cases where oestrogen therapy are contraindicated. It has been mentioned in Chapter 7 that if oestrogen excretion (as reflected in the vaginal smear or urinary assay) is at a high level or with a cyclical rhythm in the first five years after the menopause, it is presumed to originate in the ovaries, and castration is advised. Even in the presence of *significant but not cyclical* oestrogen excretion, there is still a possibility that oestrogen administration may cause stimulation of breast cancer growth. In these circumstances, androgens are given as primary endocrine therapy in the presence of bone metastases, while progestin therapy is preferred for soft tissue metastases.

The first five years after the menopause are a 'difficult' age group for endocrine therapy, and tumour response both to sex steroids and to major endocrine ablation is poor. Nevertheless, the longer the free period between mastectomy and tumour recurrence, the greater the likelihood of remission from androgen therapy (Escher and Kaufman, 1961). If the menopause has intervened between mastectomy and the first evidence of recurrence, a long recurrence-free interval is, in the writer's experience, usually associated with the presence of mixed sclerotic and lytic bone metastases, and indicates a high likelihood of response to androgen therapy.

There is considerable extension of survival in patients responding to androgen therapy compared to non-responding cases. According to the AMA Committee on Research (1960), the mean survival is 19·1 and 9·7

Unfortunately, response rates to androgen therapy are also poor in this difficult age group. Thus, the CCNSC Breast Cancer Group (1964a) reports a regression rate of only 8·7 per cent from androgen therapy in women castrated less than one year, and it was only 10 per cent overall in the writer's series of women treated within five years of the menopause.

It is important to note, however, that bone metastases respond to androgen therapy almost as well in these younger women as

TABLE 8.1. *Response to androgen therapy in breast cancer, compared to that from oestrogen therapy, in relation to the dominant site of metastasis* (Stoll, 1969 and A.M.A. Committee on Research, 1960)

	Total cases	Percentage regression according to site of metastasis:			Overall percentage regression
		Local	Bone	Visceral	
ANDROGENS					
Stoll, 1969	434	*16*	*19*	*11*	*15*
A.M.A., 1960	266	*23*	*24*	*29**	*21*
OESTROGENS					
Stoll, 1969	407	*36*	*7*	*28*	*31*
A.M.A., 1960	166	*38*	*27**	*40**	*37*

* Represents small series of which significance is doubtful.

months in the respective groups, and according to the CCNSC Breast Cancer Group (1964), 23 and 9 months respectively. However, as mentioned previously under oestrogen therapy, it has been suggested that hormone-responsive tumours belong to a slowly growing group, and that this may account for the prolonged survival in such patients.

SECONDARY THERAPY BY ANDROGENS

A trial of steroid therapy is usually advised as secondary treatment after failure of response to therapeutic castration, because of the poor response rate from major endocrine ablation in the first five years after the menopause.

they do in the older (Figure 8.1). Thus, even within five years of the menopause, the regression rate for bone metastases approaches 20 per cent and the relief of pain without tumour healing is noted in a further proportion of patients with bone metastases treated by androgens. However, in the case of soft tissue metastases appearing within five years after castration, androgen therapy needs to be combined with cytotoxic agents, because of the poor response to androgens alone. Progestin therapy is an alternative form of treatment in such cases.

Postmenopausal women who have lost tumour control from oestrogen therapy may also undergo trial of androgens, as long as symptoms are not urgent. The overall remission rate from androgen therapy increases considerably with age (Table 8.2). In the writer's series, there was a 22 per cent response rate to androgens after previous response to oestrogens (Stoll, 1969). Others have noted response in 30 per cent of such cases (Escher and Kaufman, 1961), and even in 15 per cent of cases where previous hormone therapy had been ineffective (Witt

(Table 8.1). The opposite opinion quoted by the AMA Committee on Research (1960) was based on response, in a small series, of 9 out of 33 oestrogen treated cases. Furthermore, as noted earlier, response in bone metastases to androgens is less dependent on age group than response in other types of metastasis (Figure 8.1). This may possibly reflect a non-specific role of androgens in the

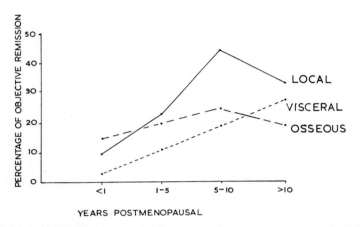

FIGURE 8.1. Clinical response of breast cancer to testosterone propionate therapy in relation to the number of years postmenopausal, and according to the predominant site of metastasis. (Modified from C.C.N.S.C. Breast Cancer Group, 1962. Figure reproduced from Stoll, 1969, by permission of Pitman Medical.)

et al, 1963). It is interesting to note that while there are no reports of benefit from the administration of oestrogens after failure of hypophysectomy, the androgen fluoxymesterone has been reported to cause tumour regression even in patients regarded as completely hypophysectomised (Kennedy, 1958; Beckett and Brennan, 1959; Peck and Olsen, 1963; Stoll, 1969).

USE OF ANDROGEN THERAPY FOR BONE METASTASES

The response rate in bone metastases is, in the writer's experience, markedly higher from androgen therapy, whether primary or secondary, than it is from oestrogen therapy

calcium metabolism of bone, apart from a specific effect upon tumour growth.

In patients with bone metastases, therefore, a trial of androgen therapy is recommended in all age groups and whatever the response to primary therapy, before bilateral adrenalectomy or hypophyseal ablation are considered. Relief of pain by fluoxymesterone therapy was achieved in 82 per cent of cases treated by the writer (Stoll, 1959). It should be noted, however, that in the presence of hypercalcaemia, it is necessary urgently to institute phosphate or corticosteroid therapy in order to reduce the serum calcium level. This is usually followed by major endocrine ablation or cytotoxic therapy in an attempt to achieve tumour control.

PROPHYLACTIC THERAPY BY ANDROGENS

To decrease the likelihood of recurrence after mastectomy, the prophylactic administration of androgens was suggested many years ago (Prudente, 1945; Loeser, 1954), and Loeser

oenanthate injected intramuscularly at intervals, or the instillation of 1 g of androgen ester into the wound-bed at mastectomy. More recent methods include the prescription of less virilising androgens, such as fluoxymesterone, given orally at a dose of 5 to 15 mg daily for prolonged periods.

TABLE 8.2. *Response to androgen therapy in breast cancer according to menopausal age group.* (Stoll, 1969 series and C.C.N.S.C. Breast Cancer Group, 1964a)

Age group (Years after menopause)	Total cases	Percentage regression
STOLL, 1969		
0–5	212	10
>5	222	24
C.C.N.S.C., 1964		
<1	92	8·7
1–5	100	17
5–10	82	25·6
>10	247	26·7

Reproduced by permission of Pitman Medical.

advised a combination of androgen with thyroid hormone for this purpose. The practice fell into disuse, however, because of the virilising effects of long-continued testosterone administration at the dosage level recommended.

There has been renewal of interest in androgen prophylaxis, because of a recent suggestion that patients with a low level of androgen excretion may have a poorer prognosis following mastectomy for breast cancer (Bulbrook, 1966), and because of the recent development of androgens with lesser tendencies to virilisation. A clinical trial of androgen prophylaxis after mastectomy is under way (Meakin et al, 1968) but no reports are so far available of the results.

Methods of prophylactic androgen administration which have been suggested include 250 mg crystalline testosterone by subcutaneous implant, 250 mg testosterone

PALLIATION FROM ANDROGEN THERAPY

It usually requires six weeks of androgen therapy before the earliest signs of shrinkage appear in the primary breast tumour, skin nodules or metastatic nodes. By eight weeks, about half of all potential regressions are present but, in the remainder, the writer has found that regression of soft tissue deposits may be delayed as long as 16 weeks in the case of slowly growing tumours. A trial of therapy should therefore not be abandoned before three months unless there are urgent manifestations of advancing disease, or urgent side-effects necessitating termination of treatment.

Regression in large ulcerated tumours is less commonly seen after androgen therapy than after oestrogen therapy. Again, while the primary tumour may regress, metastatic nodes often remain unchanged in size. Smaller nodules of breast cancer tend to disappear completely (Plates 8.1 and 8.2, following p. 208) while there is a tendency for larger nodules to become umbilicated and covered with a dark greasy scab (Stoll, 1950). Regression of recurrent nodules is always less marked if they lie within a previously irradiated area, presumably because of the decreased vascularity.

was it followed by objective evidence of tumour regression in osseous metastases (Figures 8.2 and 8.3). Pain relief usually appears within one or two weeks of beginning treatment, and commonly results in improved appetite and consequent gain in weight.

Furthermore, the haemoglobin level often rises after androgen therapy in patients with bone metastases, due as much to a stimulating effect on erythropoiesis, as to reduction in the

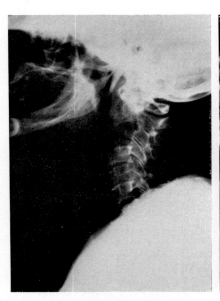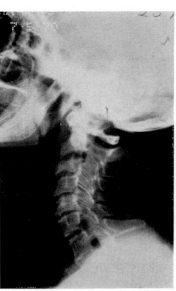

FIGURE 8.2. Radiographs to show recalcification of metastases from breast cancer in cervical vertebrae, within nine months of instituting therapy by fluoxymesterone 10 mg tds. The only other treatment was immobilisation by a collar.

The average duration of regression of soft tissue lesions from androgen therapy is only 6·9 months in the writer's series, similar to that from corticosteroid or progestin therapy. The duration of regression can, however, be increased by combining androgen with cytotoxic therapy (see later).

It was emphasised above that relief of pain from bone metastases is very common from androgen therapy, relief being noted in 82 per cent of patients receiving fluoxymesterone therapy in the writer's series (Stoll, 1958b). However, in only a minority of these cases

marrow replacement by tumour (Gardner and Pringle, 1961). Radiological evidence of recalcification in bone metastases cannot be expected before at least three months of androgen therapy but, when it occurs, may occasionally be followed by reconstitution of bony trabeculae. The average duration of control of bone metastases without new metastases appearing, is 13·2 months in the writer's series, yet it is not uncommon for androgens to maintain control of the pain of bone metastases for several years.

Subjective benefit in the form of gain in

weight, and increase in appetite and energy, is often associated with the anabolic effect of androgen therapy, except in the presence of widespread disease. Regression of lung and pleural metastases is not uncommon following androgen therapy (Stoll, 1950), although regression of other visceral metastases is rarely seen.

ANDROGEN WITHDRAWAL RESPONSE

Following cessation of steroid therapy in breast cancer, there is a possibility of a

although in the experience of Kaufman and Escher (1961) a withdrawal response is encountered also in 2·2 per cent of patients *not* responding to androgen therapy. The rarity of its occurrence in such cases does not justify a waiting period before further therapy.

In occasional cases, a third tumour regression may be achieved from androgen administration after the withdrawal response has been lost (Stoll, 1969). This paradoxical series of responses suggests that changes in the steroid *concentration* of the environment of the tumour may be more important in

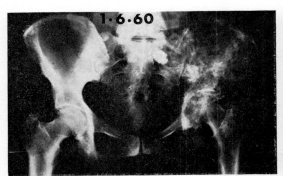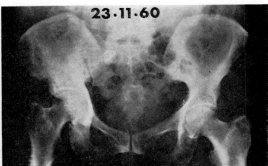

FIGURE 8.3. Radiographs to show recalcification of metastases from breast cancer in the ilium, ischium and pubis within five months of instituting fluoxymesterone 10 mg tds. (Figure reproduced from Stoll, 1969, by permission of Pitman Medical.)

'withdrawal response' (Segaloff et al, 1954b; Delarue, 1955). Tumour regression follows withdrawal of androgen therapy in about 10 per cent of those patients who have shown temporary response to therapy. Its average duration is said to be 10 months but, in the writer's experience, its duration is always shorter than that of the original response.

Because of the possibility of a withdrawal response, two months' delay should be allowed after stopping androgen therapy before initiating new endocrine therapy. This does not apply in the presence of rapidly advancing disease, when immediate corticosteroid therapy or major endocrine ablation is usually indicated. Neither does it apply in the absence of a response to androgen therapy,

tumour control, than the actual *nature* of the steroid being administered.

HYPERCALCAEMIA IN ANDROGEN THERAPY

Hypercalcaemia occurring within two weeks of initiating androgen therapy is discussed in Chapter 6. Hypercalcaemia occurring *late* in the course of androgen therapy indicates a loss of tumour control by the hormone rather than stimulation of tumour activity. Cessation of hormone administration is indicated, but rarely leads to fall in the serum calcium level. A low calcium diet and a high fluid intake are instituted in all cases, associated with therapy by oral or intravenous sodium or potassium phosphate (Goldsmith and Ingbar, 1966; Thalassinos and Joplin, 1968).

Prednisolone or prednisone up to a dosage of 100 mg daily is prescribed if the serum calcium level has not fallen after these measures (Figure 8.4). This will increase urinary calcium excretion and reduce serum calcium levels in nearly all patients, but dosage must

(Nevinny, Dederick and Hall, 1960; Hall, Dederick and Nevinny, 1963).

ANDROGENS IN COMBINATION THERAPY

WITH OESTROGEN

A combination of androgen and oestrogen given concurrently has been suggested in the

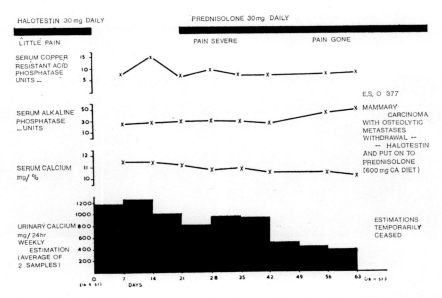

FIGURE 8.4. The effect of prednisolone 10 mg tds on the urinary calcium excretion and on the serum calcium and enzyme levels, in a patient with bone metastases from breast cancer. (Figure reproduced from Stoll, 1959, by permission of the Editor, Medical Journal of Australia.)

be high and usually requires systemic administration because of coma or vomiting. Chelating agents such as sodium edetate (EDTA) can also temporarily increase urinary calcium excretion, but may lead to kidney damage.

Major endocrine ablation is considered after the hypercalcaemic crisis has been controlled and, in fact, may be necessary to obtain control in very severe or resistant cases (Thalassinos and Joplin, 1968; Moon, 1968). The use of cytotoxic agents, particularly methotrexate 2·5 mg daily, is also claimed to be useful in resistant cases

therapy of advanced breast cancer, but a clinical trial has led to no better results than those obtained by oestrogen therapy alone (Kennedy and Brown, 1965). It is better to use the agents separately and consecutively. Life may be prolonged by achieving two distinct remissions, and this is more likely to occur in the older postmenopausal patient.

WITH RADIOACTIVE PHOSPHORUS

Androgen administration is said to increase the uptake of radioactive phosphorus in breast cancer metastases (Hertz, 1950). On this basis, a combination of androgen and ^{32}P has been suggested in the treatment of patients with osseous metastases from breast cancer, especially those which have not previously responded to androgen therapy alone.

The technique involves the preliminary administration of testosterone propionate 50 mg or nandrolone phenylpropionate 50 mg, intramuscularly daily for four days. Half dosage is then continued for a further

propionate will protect the bone marrow, but not the tumour, against the cytotoxic effect of massive doses of the alkylating agent thiotepa (Watson and Turner, 1959; Cree, 1960). This assumption has not been confirmed by the writer, and several reports (Rider, 1960; Stoll, 1962, 1963a; Lyons and Edelstyn, 1962) have noted deaths from toxicity in between 11 per cent and 63 per cent of patients treated by the technique recommended (Table 8.3). Furthermore, temporary objective evidence of tumour remission was

TABLE 8.3. *Reported incidence of tumour regression and deaths from toxicity following combined thiotepa and testosterone propionate therapy in breast cancer* (Stoll, 1963)

Author	Toxicity deaths in:	Tumour regression in:
Watson and Turner, 1959	0 of 23	22 of 23*
Cree, 1960	0 of 11	10 of 11*
Rider, 1960	7 of 11	3 of 11
Lyons and Edelstyn, 1963	5 of 46	17 of 46
Stoll and Matar, 1961	2 of 9	7 of 9†

* Added oophorectomy in premenopausal patients
† Half the recommended thiotepa dosage
Reproduced by permission of the Editor, *British Medical Journal.*

eight days, while 1·5 mCi of ^{32}P is injected intravenously daily. Treatment is usually complicated by the subsequent appearance of leucopenia and severe thrombocytopenia, but repair of bone destruction is claimed to follow in 50 per cent of patients, and relief of pain for up to 18 months in 87 per cent of patients (Mandel and Chiat, 1962; Riordan and Browne, 1966). In a small personal series, the writer has noted up to six months' pain relief in a minority of patients treated by this technique, after failure of other hormonal methods.

WITH ALKYLATING AGENTS

It has been suggested that in the treatment of breast cancer, the use of testosterone

noted in only 37 per cent of the surviving cases (Edelstyn, Gleadhill and Lyons, 1968) and the technique therefore has no obvious curative value to justify its risks.

Nevertheless, there are indications for a combination of androgen and alkylating agents in clinical therapy, because androgen premedication has been shown to increase the susceptibility of experimental mammary cancer to alkylating agents (Meakin, 1969). A combination of thiotepa and the androgen nandrolone decanoate has been reported to yield good clinical palliation in 68 per cent of patients with advanced breast cancer, compared to 35 per cent from the androgen alone (Bond and Arthur, 1966).

The writer has found that the addition of either thiotepa or 5-fluorouracil to androgen therapy will increase the duration of control of soft-tissue metastases, and increase the remission rate in the 'difficult' years for endocrine therapy, that is the five years following the menopause. However, in the presence of extensive bone metastases, the writer prefers the addition to androgen therapy of the alkylating agent cyclophosphamide, at the relatively low oral maintenance dosage of 100 to 150 mg daily. This is better tolerated over a long period by a damaged bone marrow (Stoll, 1970b).

CHOICE OF AGENT AND DOSAGE

The androgens which were first found useful in the control of breast cancer tended to have marked virilising properties. With the development of newer agents, however, it is no longer true that control of breast cancer by androgens must *necessarily* involve virilisation of a significant degree (see Plate 8.1, following p. 208).

There are two dosage regimes possible. In the continuous method of androgen therapy, steroid administration is maintained for as long as tumour regression persists. A withdrawal response may be observed in the tumour when therapy is stopped, and, although rare, a third regression may be obtained by restarting androgens after withdrawal response has been lost. In the intermittent method, on the other hand, steroid administration is stopped when tumour regression is complete in observable lesions, and started again only when reactivation of tumour is observed. Tumour regression is usually maintained for some months following cessation of therapy and, when reactivation occurs, further regression of the tumour often follows a further course of androgen therapy.

It is important to note that when response is finally lost to either method, there is no evidence that a change of androgenic agent, or increase in dose, will regain control of tumour growth. The intermittent method of androgen administration is preferred by the writer, as it appears to postpone the development of autonomy in the tumour, and is associated with a lesser degree of virilisation in the patient.

Testosterone propionate, 100 mg three times weekly intramuscularly, has been widely used until about 10 years ago. Apart from occasional nausea, it is well tolerated, but virilisation is usually severe.

Methyltestosterone is inactivated by the gastric juices but absorbed by the buccal mucosa. Given at a dosage of 150 to 200 mg orally daily, the response rate in breast cancer is similar to that from testosterone propionate given intramuscularly, and is associated with approximately the same degree of virilisation.

Fluoxymesterone has been widely tested for over 10 years since it was first reported in breast cancer by the writer and others (Stoll, 1958a, 1959; Kennedy, 1958; Segaloff et al, 1958). The tumour remission rate, subdivided both by site of metastasis and also by age group, has been shown in controlled trials to be no different from 20 mg fluoxymesterone daily than it is from testosterone propionate 100 mg three times weekly. Fluoxymesterone administration is, however, associated with much reduced signs of virilisation, and this has been confirmed in large controlled trials (CCNSC Breast Cancer Group, 1964b).

Doses of 25 to 40 mg fluoxymesterone daily lead to even higher regression rates in the writer's experience (Table 8.4) but, if persisted with, will lead to an increase in the proportion of patients virilised. This higher *loading dose* is recommended for at least the first 8 to 12 weeks of treatment, but is subsequently decreased when control of tumour growth has been established. Fluoxymesterone dosage of 15 mg daily, reported in some trials (Sellwood, 1970) is, in the writer's experience, inadequate except as maintenance dosage for breast cancer of low activity.

7α,17α-Dimethyltestosterone, given orally at a dose of 150 to 200 mg daily, has yielded objective evidence of tumour response in 40 per cent of a small series of postmenopausal patients with advanced breast cancer (Cantino, Eisenberg and Gordan, 1966; Gordan, Halden and Walter, 1970). Its anabolic properties are associated with improvement in appetite and pain relief. Virilisation is moderate from its use, but there may be evidence of minor hepatotoxicity. It merits further investigation.

2α-Methyldihydrotestosterone propionate has been claimed to be as effective as testosterone propionate in the treatment of breast cancer but less virilising (Blackburn and Childs, 1959; Goldenberg and Hayes, 1961; Thomas et al, 1962). The writer's experience does not confirm this claim. This agent is reported to block the oestrogen uptake of breast cancer in tissue culture, but there is no correlation between clinical anti-tumour potency

TABLE 8.4. *Fluoxymesterone dosage in relation to response by breast cancer and the incidence of virilisation in the patient* (Stoll, 1959)

Fluoxymesterone daily dose	Percentage with regression	Percentage with virilisation
15–20 mg	*40*	*15*
25–40 mg	*58*	*35*

Nandrolone decanoate (50 mg monthly intramuscularly) and *nandrolone phenylpropionate* (25 mg weekly intramuscularly) have their protagonists (Hortling, Malmio and Hiisi-Brummer, 1961; Ford, 1959). These are long-acting androgens with no less an incidence of virilisation and hypercalcaemia than fluoxymesterone. While their efficacy in the presence of bone metastases is at a comparable level, the writer has found their effect on soft tissue and visceral lesions to be markedly inferior to that of fluoxymesterone. Depot compounds are also dangerous if the patient develops hypercalcaemia, because their absorption cannot be swiftly terminated.

Δ^1-*Testololactone* has been claimed to yield remission in breast cancer without evidence of pituitary depression or obvious signs of virilisation (Segaloff et al, 1962). A recent controlled trial with this agent, at a dosage of 150 mg daily, notes regression of soft tissue tumour in 18 per cent of patients (Goldenberg, 1969), but in a much smaller proportion in other types of metastasis. The major interest of this compound is, that being hormonally inert, its effect upon breast cancer may be a direct one upon the tumour tissue.

and experimental anti-oestrogenicity among androgenic compounds.

'*Anabolic*' androgens have occasionally been claimed to show a controlling effect on advanced breast cancer. Norethandrolone has gonadotropin-inhibiting properties and, following its administration, occasional examples of tumour regression have been claimed in breast cancer (Pommatau et al, 1961).

UNWANTED AND TOXIC EFFECTS OF ANDROGENS

Some pharmacological effects of androgen administration are of advantage to the cancer patient, and increase in appetite and energy commonly result, especially in postmenopausal patients.

MASCULINISATION

Increase of hair growth on the upper lip, chin, trunk and limbs is noted in the majority of women given testosterone propionate or methyltestosterone at the dosage suggested, for longer than three months. Thinning and fall of the scalp hair is often preceded by a temporary phase of greasiness and thickened growth. Acne of the shoulders and seborrhoea of the facial skin are often associated with the increased hirsutism, and all these signs of masculinisation take several months to clear after stopping therapy.

Hirsutism of a significant degree is noted by the patient in about one-third of breast cancer patients taking the relatively large dose of 25 to 40 mg fluoxymesterone daily for longer than three months (Table 8.4), while a therapeutic *trial* of this hormone for three months is usually free of this complication. If tumour regression or pain relief result, the patient is usually willing to continue medication, and accept the risk of unwanted side-effects, but if there is no response to the trial, the hormone is stopped and no side-effects ensue.

Deepening of the voice also occurs with androgen therapy, and is due to decreased tension in the laryngeal muscles associated with thickening of the submucosa of the larynx. Younger patients are more sensitive to androgens in this respect and, once established, restoration of normal voice is rare when androgens are discontinued. Increase of libido and irritability are sometimes complained of, but hypertrophy of the clitoris usually passes unnoticed by the patient. Androgen has a beneficial effect in the early postmenopausal patient in controlling hot flushes and other climacteric symptoms.

FLUID RETENTION AND GASTROINTESTINAL INTOLERANCE

Cardiac embarrassment due to fluid retention occurs less commonly than from oestrogen therapy, and rarely necessitates interruption of androgen therapy. Oedema of the ankles and generalised increase in weight are seen especially in younger patients. Vomiting and abdominal cramps also occur, but much less frequently than with oestrogen therapy.

HEPATOTOXIC EFFECTS

All androgens which are substituted in the 17α position—those that are effective when given by mouth—may have hepatotoxic effects, and methyltestosterone may, in occasional cases, cause evidence of liver damage. Although the appearance of jaundice and biliary stasis has been reported also in one patient following treatment by fluoxymesterone (Beckett and Brennan, 1959), the rarity of its occurrence does not prejudice the choice of this agent for therapy.

Corticosteroid Therapy

Cortisone administration is followed by diminished oestrogen secretion from the adrenal glands (Wilkins et al, 1952), and long-continued cortisone administration can cause atrophy of the adrenal cortex. This is the basis of the so-called 'medical adrenalectomy' practised in late breast cancer, and tumour remission has been claimed in 51 per cent of patients, from a combination of castration and corticosteroid therapy (Nissen-Meyer and Vogt, 1959; Brinkley and Kingsley-Pillers, 1960). The addition of castration is not essential and numerous reports have shown that corticosteroid therapy given alone can also lead to tumour remission (Segaloff et al, 1954a; West et al, 1954; Read, 1957; Kofman et al, 1957; Taylor, Perlia and Kofman, 1958; Kolodziejska, 1959; Lemon,

1959; Gilse, 1962; Gardner, Thomas and Gordan, 1962; Stoll, 1960a, 1963b; Ker and Stewart, 1966; Foley et al, 1966).

INDICATIONS AND PALLIATIVE RESULTS

The multiplicity of reports on the corticosteroid therapy of advanced breast cancer is unfortunately not associated with agreement as to the stage of the disease most suitable for such therapy. Nor do the reports agree on the proportion of patients likely to show evidence of tumour regression, or on the most effective agents and their optimal dose levels.

All observers are in accord on one point however—that in seriously ill patients with advanced breast cancer, subjective benefit from corticosteroid therapy is often dramatic. Pain arising from metastases in bone, pleura, liver or soft tissues may be rapidly reduced. Dyspnoea from lung metastases is often relieved, and both appetite and well-being are improved, sometimes to the extent of euphoria. Corticosteroids, too, are the only steroidal group used in the therapy of breast cancer which can be administered without fear of stimulating the activity of the disease.

Significant regression in the size of tumour masses occurs, in the writer's experience, in only about 15 per cent of cases (Stoll, 1963b). Nevertheless, corticosteroid therapy is particularly valuable for rapid reduction of the intolerable itching and pain of rapidly growing skin infiltration, and of the painful lymphoedema of an arm due to apical axillary infiltration by tumour. In spite of dramatic symptomatic relief, the writer has remarked that the degree of tumour regression after corticosteroid therapy is rarely complete, even in small lesions, and it rarely lasts longer than nine months, except in the case of tumours of low activity.

Although relief of pain from bone metastases is common, sclerosis of lytic bone metastases is rarely seen in the radiographs after corticosteroid therapy alone. Similarly, although relief of coma from brain metastases,

of dyspnoea from lung metastases and of pain from liver metastases, are all common, they are short lived and rarely associated with objective evidence of tumour regression. The latter is, however, much more likely if corticosteroid therapy is combined with cytotoxic agents, and in such circumstances remission may last a year or longer (see later). Regression of metastatic pleural and pericardial effusions may occur rapidly following corticosteroid therapy (Figure 8.5).

In view of the foregoing, it is surprising that visceral metastases have been reported more widespread at autopsy in corticosteroid-treated patients, than in those treated by major endocrine ablation (Sherlock and Hartmann, 1962). A possible explanation is that patients with very widespread visceral metastases are more likely to be selected for corticosteroid therapy.

Hypercalcaemia can usually be controlled by corticosteroid therapy, even when other therapy has failed. As soon as the serum calcium level is brought down to normal, either major endocrine ablation or cytotoxic therapy should be considered in the hope of long-term control of the tumour. Surprisingly, the appearance of hypercalcaemia was reported in 5 out of 45 patients, while they were receiving corticosteroids for the treatment of bone metastases in breast cancer (Hall et al, 1963).

FACTORS INFLUENCING RESPONSE, AND MODE OF ACTION

Response to corticosteroid therapy is said to be greater in primary than in recurrent breast cancer (Ker and Stewart, 1966), and in some cases this may reflect a lesser response in damaged tissues. In the writer's experience, response is considerably more marked in smaller nodules than in larger soft tissue lesions.

It has been suggested by one authority that surgical castration must precede corticosteroid therapy in breast cancer, because such therapy does not inhibit ovarian, but

7

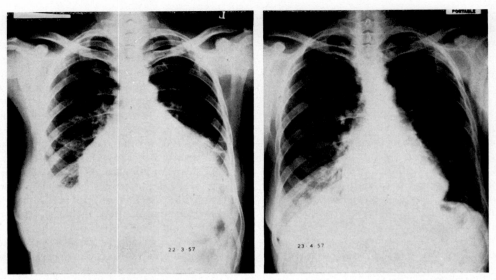

FIGURE 8.5. Radiographs to show regression of malignant pericardial effusion secondary to breast cancer, after four weeks of prednisolone 10 mg tds. (Figure reproduced from Stoll, 1969, by permission of Pitman Medical.)

only adrenal, secretion (Lemon, 1959). Nevertheless, the writer and others have shown that objective evidence of tumour regression can follow corticosteroid therapy also in premenopausal patients (Gardner et al, 1962; Stoll, 1963b). In the writer's experience also, the likelihood of tumour regression from corticosteroid therapy is not related either to the patient's age group or to the previous response to sex hormone therapy (Table 8.5). All these observations have led to the suggestion that corticosteroid effects in breast cancer are due mainly to an effect on the *host* tissues (see Chapter 4).

Cortisone suppression of urinary calcium excretion has been suggested as a means of predicting sex hormone sensitivity in breast cancer (Emerson and Jessiman, 1956). This

TABLE 8.5. *Response of breast cancer to corticosteroid therapy in relation to menopausal age group and previous response to sex hormones* (Stoll, 1963b)

Age group	Cases with regression	Percentage regression
Within 5 years of menopause	21 of 79	27 ⎫
Over 5 years postmenopausal	16 of 75	21 ⎬ Difference not significant
Previous response to sex hormones	9 of 24	37 ⎫
Previous failure of sex hormones	13 of 59	22 ⎬ Difference not significant

appears unlikely in view of the observation that corticosteroid administration can also control the hypercalciuria associated with types of cancer not generally regarded as sex hormone dependent (see Chapter 5).

CORTICOSTEROID THERAPY AND MAJOR ENDOCRINE ABLATION

Several authors have suggested that the palliation resulting from corticosteroid therapy is as good as that from hypophysectomy or bilateral adrenalectomy, in the treatment of advanced breast cancer (Nissen-Meyer and Vogt, 1959; Lemon, 1961; Bethune, 1964). Nevertheless, controlled studies have shown that *objective* evidence of tumour regression following corticosteroid administration is neither as prolonged nor as complete as that following adrenalectomy (Dao, Tan and Brooks, 1961; Forrest et al, 1968). The average length of remission from corticosteroid therapy is 6·5 to 8·5 months (Lemon, 1959; Stoll, 1963b), while that for adrenalectomy is 18 to 24 months. Over-estimation of the degree of benefit from corticosteroid therapy is probably influenced by subjective criteria of response.

Although it has been suggested that response by breast cancer to corticosteroid therapy may be used to predict the likelihood of a similar response to adrenalectomy (Fracchia et al, 1959), the writer has shown that this is not so (Stoll, 1963b). Response to adrenalectomy or to hypophyseal ablation has been shown in 14 per cent of patients in whom previous corticosteroid therapy has been unsuccessful (Ker and Stewart, 1966). Nevertheless, a preliminary course of corticosteroids, will cause marked subjective benefit in seriously ill patients, and may improve their condition sufficiently to face later major ablative surgery (Hellstrom and Franksson, 1958). The preoperative corticosteroid therapy does not appear to prejudice the subsequent postoperative management of the patient.

CORTICOSTEROIDS IN COMBINATION THERAPY

WITH THYROID HORMONE

Objective evidence of tumour regression was claimed in 48 per cent of patients with breast cancer treated by prednisolone combined with tri-iodothyronine (Lemon, 1959). A synergic effect from this combination has been confirmed in controlled trials (Segaloff, 1971) and is also claimed from the addition of liothyronine to prednisolone (Gardner et al, 1962).

WITH CYTOTOXIC AGENTS

In an assessment by the writer of prednisolone combined with an alkylating agent in the treatment of advanced cancer of all types, it was only in the case of breast cancer that an additive effect was apparent (Stoll, 1960b). The benefit from the addition of the alkylating agent was most marked in the case of intrathoracic metastases from breast cancer where 55 per cent of patients responded (Stoll, 1963b) (Table 8.6). This synergic effect is remarkable as alkylating agents given alone are said rarely to yield any evidence of benefit in such cases (Hurley et al, 1961) (Figures 8.6 and 8.7).

It is therefore advised that, in the presence of severe symptoms arising from lung metastases in breast cancer, immediate treatment should be initiated with prednisolone and an alkylating agent in combination (Stoll, 1963b). Sex hormone therapy by oestrogen or androgen (according to the patient's age), is *added later* when symptoms have improved. After a few weeks of such triple therapy, an attempt is made to taper off the therapy with prednisolone and alkylating agent. This combination yields rapid but transient subjective improvement in the *majority* of patients, while the sex hormone therapy may induce a delayed but more prolonged objective remission in the hormone-sensitive tumours.

TABLE 8.6. *Response of intrathoracic metastases of breast cancer to prednisolone,*
with or without added nitromin (Stoll, 1963b)

Therapy	Cases with regression	Percentage regression	
Prednisolone	2 of 33	6	Difference significant
Prednisolone with nitromin	17 of 31	55	$P < 0.05$

Reproduced by permission of the Editor, *British Medical Journal.*

In the presence also of metastatic peritoneal or pleural effusions, a combination of prednisolone and an alkylating agent is often very useful. In such a case, a loading dose of thiotepa (see Chapter 9) is injected into the serous cavity after paracentesis, and followed by a maintenance course of this agent by intracavitary or systemic administration. This is combined with orally administered prednisolone and reaccumulation of the effusion may be delayed for a year or longer in such cases.

Combination therapy may also be used in the presence of widespread bone metastases

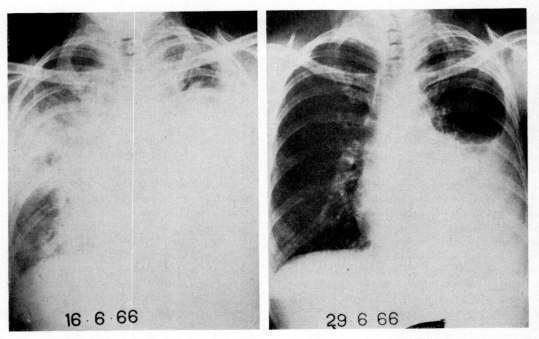

FIGURE 8.6. Radiographs to show regression of pulmonary metastases from breast cancer within two weeks of initiating therapy with prednisolone combined with thiotepa. (Figure reproduced from Stoll, 1969, by permission of Pitman Medical.)

after loss of control by castration or androgen therapy, and, by this means, adrenalectomy or hypophyseal ablation may be postponed for a considerable time. A continuous low dosage regime of cyclophosphamide, combined with prednisolone, has been found by the writer to be especially valuable in the presence of leucoerythroblastic anaemia, as this alkylating agent is usually well tolerated over a long period, even by a damaged bone marrow (Stoll, 1970b).

50 to 100 mg prednisolone or prednisone daily. It has been suggested that these larger doses of corticosteroids are followed by better control of symptoms in breast cancer (Taylor et al, 1958). This may be true but, in the writer's experience, there appears to be little advantage, yet a considerable increase in unwanted side-effects, in using in *all* cases of breast cancer, a dosage of prednisolone or prednisone higher than 30 mg daily.

Dosage levels of 25 to 30 mg daily are

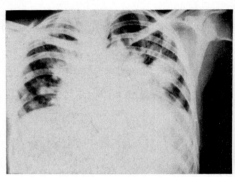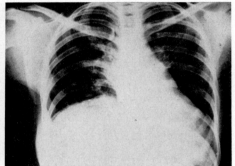

FIGURE 8.7. Radiographs to show regression of pulmonary metastases from breast cancer within three weeks of instituting therapy with prednisolone combined with nitrogen mustard oxide. (Figure reproduced from Stoll, 1960, by permission of the Editor, *Acta Unio Internationalis Contra Cancrum*.)

Corticosteroid therapy in combination with other alkylating agents has been reported by several authors in the treatment of advanced breast cancer (McCarthy, 1955; Curreri and McIver, 1956; Freckman et al, 1964). The last authors claim tumour regression in 34 per cent of a series treated by a combination of prednisolone and chlorambucil. A combination of prednisolone with weekly injections of the antimetabolite 5-fluorouracil has recently been recommended for patients who are unfit for, or unlikely to benefit from, bilateral adrenalectomy (Moore et al, 1967).

CORTICOSTEROID DOSAGE AND SIDE-EFFECTS

The earlier reports in the literature on corticosteroid therapy in breast cancer advised a dosage of 200 to 400 mg cortisone daily or

recommended in the majority of cases. The unwanted side-effects resulting from six to nine months' administration of prednisolone even at this dosage usually involve a gross gain in weight, rounding of the face and slight increase of hirsutism, but occasionally there may appear also dyspepsia, glycosuria or hypertension. Elderly patients with cardiac disease may not tolerate even 20 mg prednisolone daily. It has been suggested recently that the administration of a morning dose of 25 mg every 24 or 48 hours leads to similar benefit in breast cancer to that of 10 mg tds, but with lessened unwanted side-effects. By its timing, it leads also to a lesser depression of the pituitary-adrenal axis, but it is often not well tolerated.

Increase in dosage up to 100 mg prednisolone daily may be necessary for patients not responding to lower dosage, and, in the presence of severe symptoms, the possibility of palliation is weighed against the dangers of severe side-effects from the steroid. *Initial* high doses of up to 100 mg daily, and systemic administration, are always necessary in emergencies such as hypercalcaemia (Connor et al, 1956), acute dyspnoea due to pulmonary or mediastinal metastases, or coma due to cerebral metastases from breast cancer.

In such cases, dosage should be reduced to 60 mg prednisolone daily as soon as control of symptoms is achieved, and to 25 to 30 mg daily as soon as the patient is ambulatory. Attempts are often made to reduce the dose still further, but these are rarely successful, and, as the disease progresses, it is more often found necessary to *increase* the dose of corticosteroid in order to maintain control over the symptoms.

Dosage of less than 15 mg prednisolone (or 50 mg cortisone) daily has not been demonstrated to cause objective evidence of tumour regression in breast cancer (Dao et al, 1961; Stoll, 1963b). The commonly prescribed dose of prednisolone 5 mg tds is, in the writer's experience, marginal in its palliative effect on breast cancer. It is usually found that tumours claimed to be under long-term control by 15 mg prednisolone daily are examples of very slowly progressing disease. Corticosteroids are better tapered off completely in such cases, and larger doses used in intermittent courses when necessary.

Reports have shown prednisone and prednisolone to be of equal effectiveness in the treatment of breast cancer, and less likely to cause serum electrolyte disturbance than cortisone. Betamethasone or paramethasone in pharmacologically equivalent dosage to prednisone are no more successful in the writer's experience. Dexamethasone 2 mg tds can be used as an alternative to prednisone 10 mg tds (Stoll, 1960a) and is claimed to cause even less danger of electrolyte disturbance.

Progestin Therapy

THE PLACE OF PROGESTIN THERAPY

The place of progestins in advanced breast cancer is still uncertain, because relatively small series of patients with advanced breast cancer have been reported, with widely varying results. Also, because of the proliferation of new synthetic progestins in recent years, a wide variety of agents has been used in these trials, and there is still considerable uncertainty as to the most efficacious group of progestins in the treatment of breast cancer. To make assessment even more difficult, some series reported are of treatment by a progestin alone (Jonsson et al, 1959;

Lewin, Spencer and Herrmann, 1959; Douglas, Loraine and Strong, 1960; Jolles, 1962; Bucalossi, Dipietro and Gennari, 1963; Stoll, 1965; Sonkin and Coudeyras, 1966; Notter and Wicklund, 1967; Wolff and Juret, 1967; Curwen, 1963, 1970; Clavel, 1970), while others are by a progestin in combination with oestrogen (Landau, Ehrlich and Huggins, 1962; Crowley and McDonald, 1965; Kennedy, 1965; Notter, 1966; Stoll, 1967a; Berndt, 1970).

Opinion is divided as to the most suitable stage to intoduce progestins into the sequential endocrine management of breast cancer. Because of its lower response rate, progestin therapy undoubtedly takes second place to castration and oestrogen therapy in the management of premenopausal and post-menopausal cases respectively. However, because of its relative freedom from side-effects, there is an increasing tendency to carry out a trial of progestin therapy before major endocrine surgery, or instead of a trial of androgens or corticosteroids.

PALLIATIVE RESULTS

A review of the literature suggests that tumour response to progestin therapy occurs overall in about 25 per cent of all cases treated (Briggs, Caldwell and Pitchford, 1967). The response rate noted by the writer in 137 patients with soft tissue metastases was 19 per cent (Stoll, 1969), similar to that from androgen therapy. It is generally agreed that favourable response to progestin therapy in advanced breast cancer is most likely in the case of soft tissue lesions (Jolles, 1962; Curwen, 1963; Stoll, 1966; Juret, 1966; Jones et al, 1971) and that regression rates are higher when progestin therapy is used as the first method of hormonal treatment (Edelstyn, 1970). It is also agreed that regression is usually less complete in the case of larger tumours, and in tumours growing in previously irradiated tissue, presumably because of the decreased vascularity in both cases.

The earliest signs of tumour regression in the soft tissue lesions of breast cancer are usually apparent about six to eight weeks after starting progestin therapy, but may be delayed for up to four months in the case of slowly growing tumours. The subsequent duration of tumour regression is, in the writer's experience, only six to nine months, although after loss of control, a further withdrawal response has been obtained in occasional cases (Plate 8.3, following p. 208). Other reports claim response occasionally lasting for more than two years (Curwen, 1970; Edelstyn, 1970).

Whereas most series note regression of soft tissue lesions to be usually associated with *progression* of metastases in other systems, some small series claim tumour regression in up to 50 per cent of cases with bone metastases and in up to 70 per cent of those with lung metastases (Clavel, 1970; Notter, 1970; Pommatau, 1970). This is not the usual experience, however, and it has even been suggested that, in the presence of bone metastases, the likelihood of hypercalcaemia is increased by medroxyprogesterone therapy (Kaufman et al, 1964). If this is regarded as evidence of tumour stimulation, it is remarkable for a progestin which is said to have no oestrogenic or androgenic metabolites (see Chapter 6).

Subjective benefit is fortunately common from the administration of progestins. Gain in weight and increase in appetite are noted with most of these agents, and euphoria similar to that seen from corticosteroid therapy was also noted by the writer, particularly from administration of the agent dimethisterone (Stoll, 1967c).

INDICATIONS FOR THERAPY

In the writer's opinion, progestins are indicated as primary endocrine therapy as an alternative to androgens in the presence of soft-tissue metastases, in early post-menopausal patients with significant, but not cyclical, oestrogen excretion. As secondary endocrine therapy, progestins are indicated as an alternative to androgens, after doubtful response to castration or oestrogen therapy, again in the presence of soft-tissue metastases. Response to progestins was noted by the writer in 18 per cent of patients with soft tissue metastases who had failed to respond to oestrogens, and response to a progestin/oestrogen combination in 28 per cent of such cases (Stoll, 1967a, c). Other reports confirm that the combination may be more effective than progestins alone (Berndt, 1970).

Major endocrine ablation may thus be postponed in the absence of urgent symptoms. Adrenalectomy or hypophyseal ablation are still possible after an attempt at progestin therapy, and, conversely, progestin therapy is reported to be occasionally effective also after failure or loss of response to hypophyseal ablation (Curwen, 1963; Pommatau, 1970). In the writer's opinion, the predominance of bone metastases makes a trial of androgen therapy preferable to progestin therapy, and the predominance of widespread visceral metastases makes a trial of corticosteroid therapy preferable.

FACTORS INFLUENCING RESPONSE

The writer has found no significant variation in the response rate to progestin therapy with the age of the patient and, in this respect, response to progestins differs from that to oestrogens or androgens (Stoll, 1967c; Clavel, 1970). Tumour response is just as likely in the first five years after the menopause (the 'difficult' age group for endocrine therapy) as in older patients (Table 8.7). Although some series report progestin therapy to be more effective in the older age groups (Curwen, 1963; Juret, 1966; Pommatau, 1970; Edelstyn, 1970), the writer has not found it as effective as oestrogens in the older patient. It is interesting to note that progestin therapy has been reported to cause regression of breast cancer in premenopausal patients also (Bucalossi et al, 1963; Ennuyer and Chemama, 1970), although the writer would prefer the use of castration in such cases.

A greater likelihood of response to progestin therapy has been suggested in those patients with a history of a previous response to sex hormone therapy (Curwen, 1963), but this has not been confirmed (Table 8.7). As noted above, the writer has observed response to progestins in the *absence* of previous response to oestrogens, and this suggests that the mechanism of action is different for the two types of agent (Stoll, 1967c). Nevertheless, as in the case of oestrogen therapy, response is more likely to progestins if there is a longer recurrence-free interval following mastectomy

(Edelstyn, 1970), and in the presence of soft-tissue metastases.

Bonte, Decoster and Ide (1970) have suggested that patients with evidence *before* progestin therapy, of oestrogenic stimulation in the vaginal smear which is neutralised by such therapy, are much more likely to show regression in endometrial cancer. This does not apply to breast cancer in the writer's experience (Stoll, 1967c). However, it is noted that the presence of oestrogenic stimulation in the vaginal smear *before* progestin therapy is associated with a 29 per cent likelihood of response by breast cancer to progestins, while an atrophic pattern is associated with only a 6 per cent likelihood of such response (Stoll, 1967b). Like Bonte's observation, this may reflect the ability by progestins to modify oestrogen effects at the target organ (see Chapter 6). The cytohormonal pattern of the vaginal smear has a similar predictive value in the case of treatment by the oral contraceptive Lyndiol, a combination of lynoestrenol and mestranol (Stoll, 1967a).

AGENTS, DOSAGE AND SIDE-EFFECTS

The active progestins available have marked qualitative differences in their oestrogenicity, androgenicity, pituitary-inhibiting properties, and metabolic activity. The relative importance of each of these properties in the control of breast cancer by progestins is unknown (see Chapter 6), but the androgenic and oestrogenic metabolites of each compound are certainly of importance in deciding the unwanted side-effects.

Progestins can be divided into three main chemical groups: derivatives of 19-nortestosterone, of 17α-hydroxyprogesterone, and of testosterone respectively (Table 8.8). The 19-nortestosterone derivatives probably yield oestrogenic metabolites and the group tends also to be androgenic in experimental animals. The 17α-hydroxyprogesterone and the testosterone derivatives, on the other hand, are unlikely to possess inherent oestrogenicity,

TABLE 8.7. *Response of breast cancer to progestin therapy in relation to menopausal age group and previous response to sex hormones* (Stoll, 1967a, c)

Age group	Cases with regression	Percentage regression	
Within 5 years of menopause	7 of 30	*23*	
Over 5 years postmenopausal	14 of 77	*18*	Difference not significant
Previous response to sex hormones	2 of 13	*16*	
Previous failure of sex hormones	10 of 49	*20*	Difference not significant

and in fact, some tend to have a pronounced anti-oestrogenic effect. For this reason, these latter groups are probably safer in the treatment of the *younger* postmenopausal patient.

Agents belonging to the three groups of progestins have been compared by the writer in the management of soft-tissue lesions from breast cancer (Stoll, 1966, 1967c). Tumour regression was noted in 18 per cent of the series overall, and there was no significant difference in the tumour remission rate between the three groups (Table 8.8)

although differences in the nature and incidence of side-effects was noted (see later). It was also shown that patients failing to show favourable tumour response to a progestin of one group may yet respond to trial of a member of another group.

The writer has reported the use of Lyndiol, a commercially available oral contraceptive in the treatment of breast cancer (Stoll, 1967a). It contains lynoestrenol (a progestin of the 19-nortestosterone group) combined with an oestrogen, mestranol. Regression of soft tissue tumour was noted in 22 per cent of

TABLE 8.8. *Response to progestin therapy in breast cancer, according to agent used* (Stoll, 1967c)

Progestin daily dose		Cases with regression	Percentage regression
19-Nortestosterone derivatives		3 of 19	*16*
Norethisterone acetate	60 mg		
Lynoestrenol	30 mg		
17α-Hydroxyprogesterone derivatives		5 of 28	*18*
Medroxyprogesterone	200–400 mg		
Melengestrol, Megestrol	30–120 mg		
Testosterone derivatives		4 of 18	*22*
Dimethisterone	300 mg		

Reproduced by permission of the Editor, *British Medical Journal*.

65 postmenopausal patients, the tumour remission rate being similar from the contraceptive does as from a dose six times as high.

It is important to note that 28 per cent of patients who had previously failed to respond to oestrogen therapy, subsequently responded to therapy with Lyndiol. All the treated patients were *postmenopausal*, and it is not possible to deduce from this observation the likely effect of progestin/oestrogen combinations on the development of breast cancer in *premenopausal* women taking them for contraceptive purposes.

In previously hypophysectomised patients, tumour regression was observed in two of seven cases following treatment by a combination of oestradiol and progesterone (Landau et al, 1962), and in two of four cases following treatment by a combination of stilboestrol and 17α-hydroxyprogesterone caproate (Kennedy, 1965). It is very interesting to note that oestrogen therapy alone has never been shown to yield a response in breast cancer after hypophysectomy.

It is claimed that the use of 17α-hydroxyprogesterone caproate for therapy is associated with almost complete absence of unwanted side-effects (Jolles, 1962; Juret, 1966). However, progestin therapy with other agents at the dosage used for the treatment of breast cancer is, in the writer's experience, occasionally associated with backache, headache, breast tension, and leg or abdominal cramps (Stoll, 1967c). Nausea or vomiting may occasionally be severe enough to stop treatment, especially with members of the 19-nortestosterone group. Mental depression or minor degrees of irritability have been noted in some patients, but euphoria in others, while gain in weight and increase in appetite have already been referred to.

Both biochemical and histological evidence of liver damage have been reported by the writer and others in some patients following the administration of progestational agents of the 19-nortestosterone group (Eisalo, Jarvinen and Luukkainen, 1964; Stoll et al,

1965; Stoll, Andrews and Motteram, 1966). The incidence of unwanted side-effects tends to be proportionate to the progestin dosage used. Since there is no evidence that the high dosage of these agents generally used yields a greater tumour response rate than lower dosage (Stoll, 1967a), it is advised by the writer that the initial loading dose should be high, and after 8 to 12 weeks when control of the tumour growth has been established, dosage is gradually reduced to maintenance levels.

CONCLUSION

Androgens should be used as primary endocrine therapy in postmenopausal patients with evidence of persistent, but not cyclical, oestrogen secretion. They are used as secondary therapy after failure of primary treatment by castration or oestrogens, especially in the presence of bone metastases. Objective evidence of tumour regression occurs overall in about 15 per cent of cases, but may be as high as 30 per cent in selected groups of patients. The average period of tumour control is only from 9 to 12 months, but may be prolonged by combination with cytotoxic agents.

The anabolic effects of androgens are valuable in most patients, and the pain of bone metastases is often relieved without radiographic evidence of bone healing. Virilisation is the major disadvantage of androgen therapy, but is not inevitable with the newer agents.

Corticosteroid therapy is indicated especially for patients who are too ill for major endocrine ablation and for those who are not likely to respond to such therapy. It is also indicated as emergency treatment in the presence of hypercalcaemia, lung or brain metastases. Corticosteroids are most valuable for their ability to relieve pain due to tumour infiltration, and induce euphoria within a few days. There is no correlation between the likelihood of benefit from corticosteroid therapy and that from previous or subsequent endocrine manipulation. Benefit is also independent of age and whether the patient is pre- or post-menopausal and it is likely that response is mainly through an anti-inflammatory reaction around the tumour. Except in the case of very slowly growing tumour, the usual duration of response is between six and nine months.

Progestational agents are indicated as an alternative to androgens in patients with soft-tissue metastases, and may cause tumour regression in cases which have failed to respond to primary therapy by oestrogens. Response is noted in about 20 per cent of treated cases for an average of six to nine months. These agents have the advantage that they are relatively free from unwanted side-effects and are occasionally effective in the 'difficult' groups for endocrine therapy—the first five years after the menopause, and the post-hypophysectomy group.

References

Adair, F. E. (1947) The use of the male sex hormone in women with breast cancer. *Surgery, Gynecology and Obstetrics*, **84**, 719.

AMA Committee on Research (1960) Androgens and estrogens in the treatment of disseminated mammary carcinoma. *Journal of the American Medical Association*, **172**, 1271.

Beckett, V. L. & Brennan, M. J. (1959) Treatment of advanced breast cancer with fluoxymesterone (Halotestin). *Surgery, Gynecology and Obstetrics*, **109**, 235.

Berndt, G. (1970) Management of metastasising mammary carcinoma with oestrogen gestagen combination therapy by SH 834. *Deutsche Medizinische Wochenschrift*, **95**, 2399.

Bethune, G. W. (1964) Cortisone in the palliative treatment of breast cancer. *Canadian Journal of Surgery*, **7**, 289.

Blackburn, C. M. & Childs, D. S. (1959) Use of 2α methyl dihydrotestosterone in the treatment of advanced cancer of the breast. *Proceedings of the Mayo Clinic*, **34**, 113.

Bond, W. H. & Arthur, K. (1966) Some observations on the use of cytotoxic drugs and anabolic steroids in the treatment of breast carcinomatosis. In *The Value of Cytotoxic Agents and Anabolic Steroids in the Treatment of Advanced Malignant Disease*, p. 57, ed. Abrahamson, M. London: Parcener Press.

Bonte, J., Decoster, J. M. & Ide, P. (1970) Radiosensitivation of endometrial adenocarcinoma by means of medroxyprogesterone. *Cancer (Philadelphia)*, **25**, 907.

Briggs, M. H., Caldwell, A. D. S. & Pitchford, A. G. (1967) The treatment of cancer by progestogens. *Hospital Medicine*, **2**, 63.

Brinkley, D. M. & Kingsley-Pillers, E. (1960) Treatment of advanced carcinoma of the breast by bilateral oophorectomy and prednisone. *Lancet*, **i**, 123.

Bucalossi, P., Dipietro, S. & Gennari, L. (1963) Hormonal treatment of metastatic breast carcinoma with a synthetic progestin—methyl acetoxy progesterone. *Practitioner*, **191**, 702. English abstract.

Bulbrook, R. D. (1966) Hormonal factors in the etiology and treatment of breast cancer. *Canadian Cancer Conference*, **6**, 36.

Cantino, J. J., Eisenberg, E. & Gordan, G. S. (1966) Antitumor efficacy of 7α, 17αDimethyl testosterone in disseminated breast cancer. *Cancer (Philadelphia)*, **19**, 817.

C.C.N.S.C. Breast Cancer Group (1964) Testosterone propionate therapy in breast cancer. *Journal of the American Medical Association*, **188**, 1069.

C.C.N.S.C. Breast Cancer Group (1964b) Trials of fluoxymesterone. *Cancer Chemotherapy Reports*, 41, Supplement 1.

Clavel, B. (1970) Personal communication.

Connor, T. B., Hopkins, T. R., Thomas, W. C. Jr, Carey, R. H. & Howard, J. E. (1956) The use of cortisone and ACTH in hypercalcemic states. *Journal of Clinical Endocrinology*, **16**, 945.

Cree, I. C. (1960) Toxic marrow failure after treatment of carcinoma with cytotoxic drugs. *British Medical Journal*, **ii**, 1499.

Crowley, R. G. & McDonald, I. (1965) Delalutin and estrogens for the treatment of advanced mammary carcinoma in the postmenopausal women. *Cancer (Philadelphia)*, **18**, 346.

Curreri, A. R. & McIver, F. A. (1956) OPSPA with and without corticosteroids in the treatment of human cancer. *Proceedings of the American Association for Cancer Research*, **2**, 101.

Curwen, S. (1963) The value of norethisterone acetate in the treatment of advanced carcinoma of the breast. *Clinical Radiology*, **14**, 445.

Curwen, S. (1970) The treatment of advanced carcinoma of the breast with SH 420. *Clinical Radiology*, **21**, 219.

Dao, T. L. Y., Tan, E. & Brooks, V. (1961) A comparative evaluation of adrenalectomy and cortisone in the treatment of advanced mammary carcinoma. *Cancer (Philadelphia)*, **14**, 1259.

Delarue, N. C. (1955) Fundamental concepts determining a philosophy of treatment in mammary carcinoma. *Canadian Medical Association Journal*, **73**, 597.

Douglas, M., Loraine, J. A. & Strong, J. A. (1960) Studies with 19 norethisterone oenanthate in mammary carcinoma. *Proceedings of the Royal Society of Medicine*, **53**, 427.

Edelstyn, G. (1970) Personal communication.

Edelstyn, G., Gleadhill, C. & Lyons, A. (1968) Total hypophysectomy for advanced breast cancer. *Clinical Radiology*, **19**, 426.

Eisalo, A., Jarvinen, P. A. & Luukkainen, T. (1964) Hepatic impairment during the intake of contraceptive pills: clinical trials with postmenopausal women. *British Medical Journal*, **ii**, 426.

Emerson, K. & Jessiman, A. G. (1956) Hormonal influences on the growth and progression of cancer: Tests for hormone dependency in mammary and prostate cancer. *New England Journal of Medicine*, **254**, 252.

Ennuyer, A. & Chemama, M. (1970) Personal communication.

Escher, G. C. & Kaufman, R. J. (1961) Current views on the management of metastatic mammary carcinoma. *Medical Clinics of North America*, **45**, 613.

Foley, J. F., Lemon, H. M., Meyer, L. R. & Miller, D. M. (1966) Glucocorticoids in the treatment of breast cancer. *Proceedings of the American Association for Cancer Research*, **7**, 21.

Ford, H. T. (1959) Durabolin and Deca-Durabolin in the treatment of advanced mammary cancer. *British Empire Cancer Campaign. Annual Report*, **37**, 267.

Forrest, A. P. M., Benson, E. A., Ker, H., Jones, V., Kunkler, P. B. & Campbell, H. (1968) Controlled studies in advanced breast cancer. In *Prognostic Factors in Breast Cancer*, ed. Forrest, A. P. M. and Kunkler, P. B. Edinburgh: Livingstone.

Fracchia, A. A., Holleb, A. I., Farrow, J. H., Treves, N. E., Randall, H. T., Finkbeiner, J. A. & Whitmore, Jr, W. F. (1959) Results of bilateral adrenalectomy in the management of incurable breast cancer. *Cancer (Philadelphia)*, **12**, 58.

Freckman, H. A., Fry, H. L., Mendex, F. L. & Maurer, E. R. (1964) Chlorambucil, Prednisone therapy for disseminated breast cancer. *Journal of the American Medical Association*, **189**, 23.

Gardner, F. H. & Pringle, J. C. Jr (1961) Androgens and erythropeiesis: I Preliminary clinical observations. *Archives of Internal Medicine*, **107**, 846.

Gardner, B., Thomas, A. N. & Gordan, G. S. (1962) Anti-tumor efficacy of prednisone and sodium liothyronine in advanced breast cancer. *Cancer (Philadelphia)*, **15**, 334.

Gilse, H. A. Van (1962) Long-term treatment with corticosteroids of patients with metastatic breast cancer. *Cancer Chemotherapy Reports*, **16**, 293.

Goldenberg, J. S. (1969) Clinical trial of $\triangle^1$-testololactone, medroxyprogesterone and oxyolone acetate in advanced female breast cancer. *Cancer (Philadelphia)*, **23**, 109.

Goldenberg, J. S. & Hayes, M. A. (1961) Hormonal therapy of metastatic female breast carcinoma. 2α methyl dihydrotestosterone propionate. *Cancer (Philadelphia)*, **14**, 705.

Goldsmith, R. S. & Ingbar, S. H. (1966) Inorganic phosphate treatment of hypercalcemia of diverse etiologies. *New England Journal of Medicine*, **274**, 1.

Gordan, G. S., Halden, A. & Walter, R. M. (1970) Antitumor efficacy of 7α,17α-Dimethyl testosterone in advanced female breast cancer. *California Medicine*, **113**, 1.

Hall, T. C., Dederick, M. M. & Nevinny, H. B. (1963) Prognostic value of hormonally induced hypercalcemia in breast cancer. *Cancer Chemotherapy Reports*, **30**, 21.

Hellstrom, J. & Franksson, C. (1958) Adrenalectomy in cancer of the breast. In *Endocrine aspects of Breast Cancer*, p. 5, ed. Currie, A. R. and Illingsworth, C. F. W. Edinburgh: Livingstone.

Hertz, S. (1950) The modifying effect of steroid therapy on human neoplastic tissue as judged by 32P studies. *Journal of Clinical Investigation*, **29**, 821.

Hortling, H., Hiisi-Brummer, L. & Af Bjorkesten, G. A. (1962) Endocrine therapy of metastatising breast cancer. *Acta Medica Scandinavica*, **172**, Suppl. 385.

Hortling, H., Malmio, K. & Hiisi-Brummer, L. (1961) Norandrostenolone in the treatment of metastasising mammary cancer. *Acta Endocrinologica (København) Suppl.*, **63**, 132.

Hurley, J. D., Trump, D. S., Flatley, T. J. & Riesch, J. D. (1961) A method of selecting patients for cancer chemotherapy. *Archives of Surgery*, **83**, 611.

Jolles, B. (1962) Progesterone in the treatment of advanced malignant tumours of the breast, ovary and uterus. *British Journal of Cancer*, **16**, 209.

Jones, V. (1970) A prospective trial of oestrogens, androgens and progestagens for the treatment of advanced cancer of the breast. In *Second Tenovus Workshop on Breast Cancer*, ed. Joslin, C. A. F. and Gleave, E. N. Cardiff.

Jones, V., Roberts, M. M., Joslin, C. A. F., Gleave, E. N., Jones, R. E., Campbell, H., Davies, D. K. L. & Forrest, A. P. M. (1971) Progestogens and advanced breast cancer. *Lancet*, **i**, 1049.

Jonsson, U., Colsky, J., Lessner, H. E., Roath, A. S., Alper, R. G. & Jones, R. Jr (1959) Clinical and pharmacological observations of the effects of 9α bromo-11 ketoprogesterone on patients with carcinoma of the breast. *Cancer (Philadelphia)*, **12**, 509.

Juret, P. (1966) *Endocrine Surgery in Human Cancers*. Springfield: Charles C. Thomas.

Kaufman, R. J. & Escher, G. C. (1961) Rebound regression in advanced mammary carcinoma. *Surgery, Gynecology and Obstetrics*, **113**, 635.

Kaufman, R. J., Rothschild, E. O., Escher, G. C. & Myers, W. P. L. (1964) Hypercalcemia in mammary carcinoma following the administration of a progestational agent. *Journal of Clinical Endocrinology*, **24**, 1235.

Kennedy, B. J. (1958) Fluoxymesterone therapy in advanced breast cancer. *New England Journal of Medicine*, **259**, 673.

Kennedy, B. J. (1965) Hormone therapy for advanced breast cancer. *Cancer (Philadelphia)*, **18**, 1551.

Kennedy, B. J. & Brown, J. H. (1965) Combined estrogenic and androgenic hormone therapy in advanced breast cancer. *Cancer (Philadelphia)*, **18**, 431.

Ker, H. R. & Stewart, H. J. (1966) Clinical trial of steroid therapy in advanced breast cancer. *British Journal of Surgery*, **53**, 151.

Kofman, S., Garvin, J. S., Nagamani, D. & Taylor, S. G. III (1957) Treatment of cerebral metastases from breast carcinoma with prednisolone. *Journal of the American Medical Association*, **163**, 1473.

Kolodziejska, H. (1959) Hormone treatment of patients with well advanced forms of cancer of the breast. *Problems in Oncology (New York)*, **5** (11), 45.

Landau, R. L., Ehrlich, E. N. & Huggins, C. (1962) Estradiol benzoate and progesterone in advanced human breast cancer. *Journal of the American Medical Association*, **182**, 632.

Lemon, H. M. (1959) Prednisone therapy of advanced mammary cancer. *Cancer (Philadelphia)*, **12**, 93.

Lemon, H. M. (1961) Discussion of hormonal therapy of breast cancer. In *Biological Activities of Steroids in Relation to Cancer*, p. 375, ed. Pincus, G. and Vollmer, E. P. New York: Academic Press.

Lewin, I., Spencer, H. & Herrmann, J. (1959) Clinical and metabolic effects of 17α ethinyl-19 nortestosterone in mammary cancer. *Proceedings of the American Association for Cancer Research*, **3**, 37.

Loeser, A. A. (1954) A new therapy for prevention of post-operative recurrences in genital and breast cancer. *British Medical Journal*, **ii**, 1380.

Lyons, A. & Edelstyn, G. (1962) ThioTEPA in treatment of advanced breast cancer. *British Medical Journal*, **ii**, 1280.

McCarthy, W. D. (1955) The palliation and remission of cancer with combined corticosteroid and nitrogen mustard therapy; report of 100 cases. *New England Journal of Medicine*, **252**, 467.

Mandel, P. R. & Chiat, H. (1962) Radioactive phosphorus for carcinoma of the breast with diffuse metastatic bone disease. *New York Journal of Medicine*, **62**, 1970.

Meakin, J. W., Allt, W. E. C., Beale, F. A., Brown, T. C., Bulbrook, R. D., Clark, K. M., Fitzpatrick, P. F., Hawkins, N. V., Hayward, J. L. & Jenkin, R. D. T. (1968) A preliminary report of two studies of adjuvant treatment of primary breast cancer. In *Prognostic Factors in Breast Cancer*, ed. Forrest, A. P. M. and Kunkler, P. B. Edinburgh: Livingstone.

Meakin, J. W. (1969) Effect of chemotherapeutic agents on hormone dependent neoplasms and tissues. *Annual Report of the Canadian Research Foundation*, p. 151.

Moon, W. J. (1968) Personal communication.

Moore, F. D., Woodrow, S. I., Aliapoulois, M. A. & Wilson, R. E. (1967) Carcinoma of the breast. A decade of new results with old concepts. *New England Journal of Medicine*, **277**, 460.

Nevinny, H. B., Dederick, M. M. & Hall, T. C. (1960) Effect of methotrexate on hormone induced hypercalcemia. *Clinical Research*, **8**, 251.

Nissen-Meyer, R. and Vogt, J. H. (1959) Cortisone treatment of metastatic breast cancer. *Acta Unio internationalis contra cancrum*, **15**, 1140.

Notter, C. (1966) Toxic effects of progestogens and estrogens in breast cancer. *Cancer Chemotherapy Abstracts*, **7**, 408.

Notter, G. (1970) Personal communication.

Notter, G. & Wicklund, H. (1967) Treatment of inoperable and metastasising cancer of the breast with progestational hormones. *Cancer Chemotherapy Abstracts*, **8**, 455.

Pearson, O. H. (1967) Hormone dependence of tumours in man. In *Modern Trends in Endocrinology*, vol. 3, p. 242, ed. Gardiner, H. Hill. London: Butterworth.

Pearson, O. H., West, C. D., Li, M. C., McLean, J. P. & Treves, N. (1955) Endocrine therapy of metastatic breast cancer. *Archives of Internal Medicine*, **95**, 357.

Peck, F. C. & Olson, K. B. (1963) The treatment of advanced breast cancer by hypophysectomy. *New York State Journal of Medicine*, **63**, 2191.

Prudente, A. (1945) Postoperative prophylaxis of recurrent mammary cancer with testosterone propionate. *Surgery, Gynecology and Obstetrics*, **80**, 575.

Pommatau, E. (1970) Personal communication.

Pommatau, E., Poulain, S., Maurel, C., Vauterin, C. & Olivier, L. (1961) Initial results of the treatment of advanced breast cancer with Nilevar (norethandrolone). *Cancer Chemotherapy Abstracts*, **2**, 747 (English abstract).

Read, L. J. (1957) Metastatic breast cancer: hormonal manipulation in the palliative treatment. *Virginia Medical Monthly*, **84**, 57.

Rider, W. D. (1960) Bradford approach to breast cancer. *British Medical Journal*, **i**, 1501.

Riordan, D. J. & Browne, P. A. (1966) The treatment of secondary deposits in bone from carcinoma of the breast with radiophosphorus and Durabolin. *Journal of the Irish Medical Association*, **49**, 40.

Segaloff, A., Bowers, C. Y., Rongone, E. L., Murison, P. J. & Schlosser, J. (1958) Hormonal therapy in cancer of the breast: XIII The effect of fluoxymesterone therapy on clinical course and hormonal excretion. *Cancer (Philadelphia)*, **11**, 1187.

Segaloff, A. (1971) Personal communications.

Segaloff, A., Carabasi, R. A., Horwitt, B. N., Schlosser, J. V. & Murison, P. J. (1954a) Hormonal therapy in cancer of the breast: VI Effect of ACTH and cortisone on clinical course and hormonal excretion. *Cancer (Philadelphia)*, **7**, 331.

Segaloff, A., Gordon, D., Carabasi, R. A., Horwitt, B. N., Schlosser, J. V. & Murison, P. J. (1954b) Hormonal therapy in cancer of the breast: VII Effect of conjugated estrogens (equine) on clinical course and hormonal excretion. *Cancer (Philadelphia)*, **7**, 758.

Segaloff, A., Weeth, J. B., Meyer, K. K., Rongone, E. L. & Cunningham, M. E. G. (1962) Hormonal therapy in cancer of the breast. Effect of oral administration of delta-testololactaone on clinical course and hormonal excretion. *Cancer (Philadelphia)*, **15**, 633.

Sellwood, R. (1970) Early or late Yttrium 90 implant compared with other forms of treatment. In *Second Tenovus Workshop on Breast Cancer*, ed. Joslin, C. A. F. and Gleave, E. N. Cardiff:

Sherlock, P. & Hartmann, W. H. (1962) Adrenal steroids and the pattern of metastases of breast cancer. *Journal of the American Medical Association*, **18**, 313.

Sonkin, R. & Coudeyras, M. (1966) Summary of results obtained with high doses of Norethindrone in the treatment of advanced genital cancer. *Cancer Chemotherapy Abstracts*, **7**, 685.

Stoll, B. A. (1950) Hormone therapy in relation to radiotherapy in the treatment of advanced carcinoma of the breast. *Proceedings of the Royal Society of Medicine*, **43**, 875.

Stoll, B. A. (1958a) Fluoxymesterone in advanced breast cancer. *Proceedings of the 7th International Cancer Congress*, 382.

Stoll, B. A. (1958b) Endocrine factors in the aetiology and treatment of cancer of the breast and prostate. In *Modern Trends in Endocrinology*, p. 212, vol. 1, ed. Gardiner Hill, H. London: Butterworth.

Stoll, B. A. (1959) Fluoxymesterone (Halotestin) in advanced breast carcinoma. *Medical Journal of Australia*, **1**, 70.

Stoll, B. A. (1960a) Dexamethasone in advanced breast cancer. *Cancer (Philadelphia)*, **13**, 1704.

Stoll, B. A. (1960b) Nitromin and corticosteroids in the treatment of advanced cancer. *Acta Unio internationalis contra cancrum*, **16**, 919.

Stoll, B. A. (1962) Cyclophosphamide in disseminated malignant disease. *British Medical Journal*, **i**, 475.

Stoll, B. A. (1963a) ThioTEPA and breast cancer. *British Medical Journal*, **1**, 54.

Stoll, B. A. (1963b) Corticosteroids in the therapy of advanced mammary cancer. *British Medical Journal*, **ii**, 210.

Stoll, B. A. (1964) Fact and fallacy in the hormonal control of breast cancer. *Medical Journal of Australia*, **1**, 980.

Stoll, B. A. (1965) Progestogens and oestrogens in the treatment of breast cancer. In *Recent Advances in Ovarian and Synthetic Steroids*, ed. Shearman, R. Sydney: Globe.

Stoll, B. A. (1966) Therapy by progestational agents in advanced breast cancer. *Medical Journal of Australia*, **1**, 331.

Stoll, B. A. (1967a) Effect of Lyndiol, an oral contraceptive, on breast cancer. *British Medical Journal*, **i**, 150.

Stoll, B. A. (1967b) Vaginal cytology as an aid to hormone therapy in postmenopausal breast cancer. *Cancer (Philadelphia)*, **20**, 1807.

Stoll, B. A. (1967c) Progestin therapy of breast cancer—comparison of agents. *British Medical Journal*, **2**, 338.

Stoll, B. A. (1969) *Hormonal Management in Breast Cancer*. London: Pitman Medical. Philadelphia: Lippincott.

Stoll, B. A. (1970a) Investigation of organ culture as an aid to the hormonal management of breast cancer. *Cancer (Philadelphia)*, **25**, 1228.

Stoll, B. A. (1970b) Evaluation of cyclophosphamide dosage schedules in breast cancer. *British Journal of Cancer*, **24**, 475.

Stoll, B. A., Andrews, J. T., Motteram, R. & Upfill, J. (1965) Oral contraceptives and liver damage. *British Medical Journal*, **1**, 723.

Stoll, B. A., Andrews, J. T. & Motteram, R. (1966) Liver damage from oral contraceptives. *British Medical Journal*, **1**, 960.

Stoll, B. A. & Matar, J. (1961) Cyclophosphamide in advanced breast cancer—a clinical and haematological appraisal. *British Medical Journal*, **ii**, 283.

Taylor, S. G. (1962) Endocrine ablation in disseminated mammary carcinoma. *Surgery, Gynecology and Obstetrics*, **115**, 443.

Taylor, S. G., Perlia, C. P. & Kofman, S. (1958) Cortical steroids in the treatment of disseminated breast cancer. In *Breast Cancer*, p. 217, ed. Segaloff, A. St. Louis: C. V. Mosby.

Thalassinos, N. & Joplin, G. F. (1968) Phosphate treatment of hypercalcemia due to carcinoma. *British Medical Journal*, **iv**, 14.

Thomas, A. N., Gordan, G. S., Goldman, L. & Lowe, R. (1962) Anti-tumour efficacy of 2x methyl dihydrotestosterone propionate in advanced breast cancer. *Cancer (Philadelphia)*, **15,** 176.

Watson, G. W. & Turner, R. L. (1959) Breast cancer, A new approach to therapy. *British Medical Journal.* **i,** 1315.

West, C. D., Li, M. C., Maclean, J. P., Escher, G. C. & Pearson, O. H. (1954) Cortisone induced remissions in women with metastatic mammary cancer. *Proceedings of the American Association for Cancer Research*, **1,** No. 2, 51.

Wilkins, L., Gardner, L. I., Crigler, J. F., Silverman, S. H. & Migeon, C. J. (1952) Comparison of oral and intramuscular administration of cortisone with a note on the suppressive action of compounds F and B on the adrenal. *Journal of Clinical Endocrinology*, **12,** 257.

Witt, J. A., Gardner, B., Gordan, G. S., Graham, W. P. & Thomas, A. N. (1963) Secondary hormonal therapy of disseminated breast cancer. Comparison of hypophysectomy, replacement therapy, estrogens and androgens. *Archives of Internal Medicine*, **111,** 557.

Wolff, J. P. & Juret, P. (1967) Use of progesterone in the treatment of uterine body carcinoma and of breast carcinoma. *Cancer Chemotherapy Abstracts*, **8,** 569.

Chapter 9

Major Endocrine Ablation and Cytotoxic Therapy

BASIL A. STOLL

Major endocrine ablation may be considered in advanced breast cancer when relapse occurs after primary therapy by castration or oestrogen, in the premenopausal and postmenopausal patient respectively. This applies especially in the presence of urgent symptoms and a history of a favourable response to castration. Cytotoxic therapy is usually reserved until after loss of control by major endocrine ablation, but may have a place earlier, especially in the first five years after the menopause when it is used in combination with steroid therapy (see Chapter 8).

Major Endocrine Ablation Therapy

For a discussion of the technical aspects of adrenalectomy or of the different methods of hypophyseal ablation, Chapter 22 and the review by Juret (1966) can be consulted. This section will be confined to the timing of ablation, the selection of patients for major endocrine ablation, and the selection of the most suitable method of ablation for the individual patient.

THE TIMING OF MAJOR ENDOCRINE ABLATION

If the oestrogen dependence hypothesis is correct, the benefit to breast cancer patients from major ablation—either from bilateral adrenalectomy and oophorectomy, or from hypophysectomy—should exceed that of lesser procedures, such as castration or additive hormone therapy. It has therefore been repeatedly advised that major endocrine ablation should be the first step in endocrine therapy for recurrence or metastasis (Jessiman, Matson and Moore, 1959; McCalister et al, 1961; Irvine et al, 1961; Nelson and

possible *after* a favourable response to castration or oestrogen therapy, the reverse does not apply.

There is no reason to advise bilateral adrenalectomy as the initial therapy in the *pre*menopausal patient. The remission rate and the mean duration of survival following adrenalectomy (or hypophysectomy) in the premenopausal patient are not significantly different from those following castration

TABLE 9.1. *Comparison of castration and major endocrine ablation in premenopausal patients with breast cancer* (after Taylor, 1962)

	Total cases	Percentage with regression	Mean survival of responders (months)
Oophorectomy	387	*29·7*	31·2
Bilateral adrenalectomy after oophorectomy	232	*33·2*	27·7
Hypophysectomy after oophorectomy	74	*31·1*	35·8

Dragstedt, 1961; Dao and Nemoto, 1965; Cade, 1966; Hunt and Nemoto, 1970; Ferguson, 1970). This suggestion might at first sight appear to be supported by the high tumour remission rates claimed in the literature—up to 51 per cent for bilateral adrenalectomy, and up to 57 per cent for hypophyseal ablation.

Nevertheless, from a critical assessment of pooled series of cases, it has been estimated that either hypophysectomy or bilateral adrenalectomy yields an average 31 to 32 per cent tumour remission rate, a postoperative mortality of 13 to 15 per cent, and a mean survival following operation of 21 to 22 months (Joint Committee on Endocrine Ablative Procedures in Disseminated Mammary Carcinoma, 1961). Against these more modest remission rates must be offset the not inconsiderable mortality and morbidity of the operations. Furthermore, whereas a second response from major ablation is still

alone (Table 9.1). Moreover, following a favourable response to castration, there is still a 40 per cent likelihood of a similar response to subsequent bilateral adrenalectomy (McDonald, 1962). If, on the other hand, there has been no response to castration, adrenalectomy is not usually advised, and major surgery can thus be avoided in the majority of premenopausal patients if castration is practised as the initial method of endocrine therapy.

There is equally no reason to advise bilateral adrenalectomy as the initial therapy in the *post*menopausal patient in preference to additive hormone therapy. It is, however, essential to select the correct additive hormone therapy for the patient.

In a randomised comparison of early adrenalectomy as against adrenalectomy postponed until after a trial of *oestrogen* therapy, there was no difference in the overall response between the two series (Dao, 1970).

In a previous trial, early adrenalectomy was found markedly superior to *androgen* therapy in such cases (Dao and Nemoto, 1965). Nevertheless, overall figures do not indicate the choice of additive hormone in the *individual* patient. Thus, whereas oestrogen therapy is better for the postmenopausal patient with soft tissue lesions, androgens are more useful for bone metastases (see Chapter 10).

The argument has been advanced that ablation. This applies both to premenopausal and postmenopausal patients.

In the first series (Atkins et al, 1966; Hayward et al, 1970), one group of patients was treated either by oestrogen or androgen therapy (apart from localised radiotherapy) and referred for major endocrine ablation only if, and when, 'conservative' therapy failed. The second group of patients was submitted to major ablation at the first

TABLE 9.2. *Response to primary steroid therapy followed in some cases by major endocrine ablation, compared to that from immediate endocrine ablation in breast cancer* (after Hayward et al, 1970)

	Operation group	'Conservative' group
Remission from hormones	—	16%⎫ 28%
Remission from operation	30%	12%⎭
Mean survival	14·94 months	15·46 months
Mean period of remission	8·98 months	7·65 months

during attempts at additive hormone therapy in late breast cancer, the patient may die or become so ill that the possibility of subsequent ablative therapy is lost, as occurred in 43 per cent of the series treated by androgens (Dao and Nemoto, 1965). It has also been noted that the response rate to major ablation is lower in patients who have received previous additive therapy (Dao and Nemoto, 1965; Atkins et al, 1966). Thus some of the patients who fail to respond to additive therapy lose a chance of possible response to major ablation. It is unfortunate that we have no means of identifying such patients beforehand, but on the other hand, over half of those who respond to additive therapy are saved an operation.

Three prospective randomised clinical trials have demonstrated that breast cancer patients *as a group* are not deprived of any life expectation by an attempt at conservative therapy before proceeding to major endocrine

sign of recurrence or metastasis after mastectomy. It is noted in Table 9.2 that the remission rate of 30 per cent, and mean survival time of 15 months for the operation group, are almost identical with those for the conservative therapy group.

There was therefore no clinical advantage gained from early major endocrine ablation, and by starting treatment with conservative therapy, the unresponsive cases, forming 70 per cent of the total, were spared a major operation. Equivalent survival periods have been demonstrated also in two other randomised trials of 'early' as against 'late' pituitary ablation by radioactive yttrium, in both premenopausal and postmenopausal cases (Sellwood et al, 1968; Stewart et al, 1969).

An evaluation of 'prophylactic' bilateral adrenalectomy (ablation carried out at the time of mastectomy) demonstrated no improvement in prognosis from its practice (Patey, 1960; Patey and Nabarro, 1970).

There is therefore no evidence either from the results of 'prophylactic' adrenalectomy or from those of 'prophylactic' castration (see Chapter 7) to support the opinion that in breast cancer it is 'reasonable to suppose that the longer the disease is left untreated, the more likely it is to become independent of hormonal control' (McCalister et al, 1961).

SELECTION OF PATIENTS FOR MAJOR ENDOCRINE ABLATION

Most authorities agree that the nature of the response to castration is of the greatest assistance in the prediction of response to subsequent major endocrine ablation therapy. Of a group of patients with breast cancer showing tumour remission from castration, 52 per cent subsequently responded to hypophysectomy and 40 per cent to bilateral adrenalectomy (McDonald, 1962). Of those *not* responding to castration, only 14 per cent and 10 per cent respectively showed a tumour remission from subsequent major ablation therapy. Response to major endocrine ablation is, according to one report, much more likely in those patients with a short remission from castration (up to 15 months) than in those with a longer remission (Stewart, 1970).

The more rigid the criteria of response to castration, the greater its predictive value as to the likelihood of subsequent response to major endocrine ablation. Thus, rigidly selected castration responders are said *always* to respond to subsequent hypophysectomy (Pearson and Ray, 1960), while similarly selected castration non-responders are said *never* to respond favourably to subsequent adrenalectomy (Escher, 1958). This method of selecting patients for major endocrine ablation is therefore of the greatest value (Delarue et al, 1967; Welbourn, 1967), but unfortunately can be applied in only a very small proportion of patients. It should be noted that when the second response does occur in such cases, it is not necessarily

associated with a further reduction in the oestrogen excretion level.

There is some doubt as to whether the nature of the response to additive hormone therapy can help in the selection of patients for subsequent major endocrine ablation. Several authorities claim a correlation between favourable response to oestrogen or androgen therapy and subsequent response to hypophysectomy (Jessiman et al, 1959; Pearson and Ray, 1960; Kennedy and French, 1965), but this is not confirmed by all (Atkins et al, 1966). It has even been suggested that *failure* to respond to oestrogen therapy favours the likelihood of a good response to hypophyseal ablation (Edelstyn, Gleadhill and Lyons, 1968). Again, a correlation is claimed by some between favourable response to oestrogen or androgen therapy and subsequent response to bilateral adrenalectomy (Douglas, 1957; Hellstrom and Franksson, 1958), but this is not confirmed by all (Byron et al, 1962; Dao and Nemoto, 1965; Fracchia, Randall and Farrow, 1967).

It is important to note that the likelihood of a favourable response to hypophyseal ablation by radioactive yttrium is not clearly related to the nature of previous response either to castration or to additive hormone therapy (Ahlquist, Jackson and Stewart, 1968).

The longer the recurrence-free interval between mastectomy and the first evidence of recurrence, the more likely is tumour remission following bilateral adrenalectomy or hypophysectomy (Hellstrom and Franksson, 1958; Luft et al, 1958; Pearson and Ray, 1960; Boesen, Radley, Smith and Baron, 1961; Cade, 1966). Whereas 33 per cent of patients with a recurrence-free interval of less than one year show tumour regression after hypophysectomy, the proportion is 66 per cent if the interval is over four years (Pearson and Ray, 1960). The response curve rises sharply after two years' recurrence-free interval (Atkins et al, 1968).

The effect of the size and site of metastasis, and the age group of the patient, on the likelihood of response to major endocrine ablation is discussed later under each technique. The use of the 'discriminant function', or other biochemical criteria for selecting patients more likely to respond to major ablation therapy, is discussed in Chapter 5, but it can be stated here that the discriminant function appears to be more useful in predicting the response to hypophysectomy than to bilateral adrenalectomy (Atkins et al, 1968).

28 and 51 per cent of operated cases. Objective tumour remission rates for hypophysectomy and for pituitary ablation by radio-active yttrium are listed similarly in Table 9.4 and they show variations between 18 and 57 per cent of operated cases.

The results of bilateral adrenalectomy and transfrontal hypophysectomy were compared in a retrospective analysis of 673 collected patients (Joint Committee, 1961).

TABLE 9.3. *Major reports of palliation from bilateral adrenalectomy in patients with breast cancer*

Author	Total cases	Percentage regression
Dao and Huggins, 1955	95	*41*
Cade, 1958	137	*49*
Hellstrom and Franksson, 1958	150	*51*
Daicoff et al, 1962	455	*28*
Byron et al, 1962	248	*38*
Fracchia et al, 1967	500	*35*

As in the case of other methods of endocrine therapy in breast cancer, most authorities have been unable to establish a correlation between histological grading of the tumour and the likelihood of response to major endocrine ablation (Smith and Emerson, 1954; Peters, 1956; Lipsett et al, 1957; Cade, 1958; Pyrah, 1958; Block et al, 1959; Swyer, Lee and Masterson, 1961; Delarue et al, 1967). A few authors have suggested that the more differentiated tumours are likely to respond favourably (Dao and Huggins, 1953; Galante, Fournier and Wood, 1957; Boesen, 1967), but histological grading of breast cancer is difficult because of the heterogeneous microscopic structure.

SELECTION OF METHOD FOR MAJOR ENDOCRINE ABLATION

Table 9.3 lists the percentage of patients showing objective evidence of tumour regression in breast cancer in the larger adrenalectomy series, and shows variations between

As mentioned previously, overall tumour remission rates of between 31 and 32 per cent were found to be similar for both methods (Table 9.5) and the postoperative mortality rates for the two procedures were also similar—13 and 14 per cent. The average survival of patients responding favourably to the operations was between 20 and 22 months.

Similar results for the two methods were originally reported in the Guy's Hospital randomised trial (Atkins et al, 1960), but reanalysis 10 years later, shows a response rate of 36 per cent for transfrontal hypophysectomy, compared to only 23 per cent for bilateral adrenalectomy (Hayward et al, 1970). Mean remission periods and mean survival of responders are also about 10 months longer for hypophysectomy than for adrenalectomy (Table 9.5).

Thus a considerable advantage has been demonstrated for the results of transfrontal hypophysectomy in the randomised trial, although adrenalectomy may still be the

TABLE 9.4. *Major reports of palliation from hypophyseal ablation in patients with breast cancer*

Author	Total cases	Percentage with regression	Method of ablation
Pearson and Ray, 1960	333	42 ⎫	Transfrontal
Boesen et al, 1961	111	42 ⎬	
Reed and Pizey, 1967	95	18	Transsphenoidal
Juret et al, 1962	150	37 ⎫	⁹⁰Y implant
Forrest, 1965	138	28 ⎬	
Edelstyn et al, 1968	102	57	⁹⁰Y after surgery

operation of choice when skilled neuro-surgery is not available (Hayward, 1970). Complete ablation of all pituitary tissue is difficult and has caused various modifications in technique to be proposed. The original transfrontal approach, with curettage of the fossa, is the popular method and has been used in the majority of reported series. Postoperative packing of the fossa with radioactive yttrium in wax (Edelstyn et al, 1968) has been suggested for completeness of ablation.

Access to the pituitary fossa is not as good by the transsphenoidal approach and complete removal of the gland is difficult. Nevertheless, the technique has no higher a complication rate than the transfrontal approach in the hands of experienced surgeons (Hayward, 1970), and its reported results in the palliation of breast cancer are encouraging. Section of the pituitary stalk, and interposition of an inert disc between the two cut ends, is also reported to have yielded remission of tumour growth in some cases of advanced breast cancer.

Radioactive sources—radon, radioactive gold, or radioactive yttrium—have been used for interstitial irradiation of the pituitary. Table 9.4 shows the results only of the radioactive yttrium method, as the other methods have been abandoned because of the danger of damage to the optic tracts and

TABLE 9.5. *Remission from bilateral adrenalectomy compared to that from hypophysectomy in advanced breast cancer*

Author		Bilateral adrenalectomy	Hypophysectomy
Joint Committee, 1961	Total cases	404	467
	Response rate	31·7%	31·3%
	Mean survival	22 months	20·6 months
	Postoperative mortality	13%	14%
Hayward et al, 1970	Total cases	77	70
	Response rate	23%	36%
	Mean remission	26·3 months	37·1 months
	Mean survival of responders	31·6 months	40·8 months

to the motor nerves of the eyes. Other methods used for hypophyseal ablation in breast cancer include the use of ultrasonic radiation (Arslan, 1966), heavy particle irradiation by a cyclotron (Lawrence, 1967), and cryogenic therapy (Bleasel and Lazarus, 1965; Wilson et al, 1966; Norrell et al, 1970). The palliative results of these newer techniques have not yet been sufficiently evaluated.

The salvage and morbidity to be expected from bilateral adrenalectomy or hypophyseal ablation in advanced breast cancer *depends, in the main, on the experience of available specialists*. Postoperative serum electrolyte problems are less common following hypophyseal ablation (due to aldosterone secretion being relatively unaffected), but hypothyroidism and diabetes insipidus require replacement therapy. Radioactive yttrium implantation or transsphenoidal hypophysectomy are preferred in the very ill patient, in whom more drastic ablative procedures are contraindicated.

RESPONSE TO BILATERAL ADRENALECTOMY

Pain relief occurs in the majority of patients with bone metastases following bilateral adrenalectomy, but it bears no relationship in the individual patient to the likelihood of tumour regression. Relief of pain from bone metastases often occurs within two to three days of adrenalectomy, its cause is uncertain and it is often very transient (see Chapter 22).

Objective evidence of remission following adrenalectomy is less frequent, but in the ease of local soft tissue and bone metastases it is claimed in 40 to 50 per cent of cases (Hellstrom and Franksson, 1958; Fracchia et al, 1959). One report claims regression of lung and pleural metastasis in a similar proportion of cases (Dao, 1970). Regression of brain, liver, and peritoneal metastases, on the other hand, occurs in only 10 to 20 per cent of cases, and it is generally agreed that in the presence of *large* brain, liver or peritoneal metastases, adrenalectomy is

contraindicated (van Prohaska, Houttuin and Kocandrle, 1966). Most reports agree that regression of lesions in one system is often associated with progression of lesions in another system, a common observation in all types of endocrine therapy in breast cancer.

Tumour regression from bilateral adrenalectomy has a mean duration of 26·3 months (Hayward et al, 1970). Prolongation of survival as a result of operation was shown in 455 adrenalectomised patients, among whom 12·5 per cent survived five years compared to 3·7 per cent in non-operated cases (Daicoff, Harmon and van Prohaska, 1962).

The likelihood of response to adrenalectomy has been related earlier in the chapter to previous response to castration or additive hormone therapy and to the length of the recurrence-free interval. The age of the patient in relation to the menopause probably also influences the likelihood of response to adrenalectomy. A higher response rate has been noted over the age of 50 in a large series of patients (Fracchia et al, 1959), although other authors show no correlation between tumour remission rate and age group (Dao and Huggins, 1955; Galante et al, 1957; Hellstrom and Franksson, 1958; Cade, 1966). According to Atkins et al (1968) the poorest palliative results from bilateral adrenalectomy are within the first six years following the menopause, the 'difficult' age group for endocrine therapy of all types.

ADRENALECTOMY, CORTICOSTEROID THERAPY AND CASTRATION

Survival after bilateral adrenalectomy without cortisone maintenance therapy has been reported in occasional cases, and such survival has been ascribed to cortisone secretion by accessory adrenal tissue (Lipsett et al, 1957). Nevertheless, the usual hormonal maintenance therapy after major endocrine ablation involves fractionated dosage to a total of 37·5 mg cortisone daily. When daily dosage of cortisone replacement reaches 75 mg daily, or of prednisone 15 mg daily, there is a possibility that relief of pain ascribed to the operation, may be due, at least in part, to corticosteroid effects.

Bilateral adrenalectomy is rarely carried out by itself but oophorectomy is usually performed at the same time, even in patients long postmenopausal. Postmenopausal secretion of steroids by the ovary is presumed to affect the growth of breast cancer because comparative remission rates reported for bilateral adrenalectomy alone, and from its combination with oophorectomy, are 40 and 52 per cent respectively (Hellstrom and Franksson, 1958) or 36 and 44·5 per cent respectively (Fracchia et al, 1967). The addition of castration not only increases the proportion responding, but is said also to increase the duration of tumour growth remission. Since it is generally accepted that oestrogen secretion by the ovaries is unlikely to persist more than two years after the menopause, the benefit must be ascribed to removal of androgens or other steroid secreted by the ovaries.

Comparison of cortisone therapy and bilateral adrenalectomy in the palliation of breast cancer has been made in the previous chapter.

RESPONSE TO HYPOPHYSECTOMY

Objective evidence of tumour regression from hypophysectomy is said to be most common in the case of local soft tissue, bone, lung or pleural metastases, being claimed in 40 to 50 per cent of such patients (Pearson and Ray, 1960). Tumour regression is claimed even in 35 per cent of those with liver or brain metastases. Nevertheless, most authorities agree that hypophysectomy is advisable only if liver or brain metastases are *small* in size (McCalister et al, 1961).

The likelihood of remission from hypophysectomy is also influenced by the age of the patient. The highest response rates are in the premenopausal age group, and in patients over the age of 60 (Pearson and Ray, 1960), and the poorest results are within the first six years following the menopause (Atkins et al, 1968). The likelihood of response to hypophysectomy has been related earlier in the chapter to previous response to castration or additive hormone therapy and to the length of the recurrence-free interval.

The mean duration of tumour remission following hypophysectomy is 37·1 months (Hayward et al, 1970) and prolongation of survival occurs in responding cases. It is also possible that responding cases belong to a group of slowly growing tumours, and that is the reason for the prolonged survival (Taylor and Perlia, 1960).

Response may be achieved from hypophyseal ablation for an average duration of 12 to 18 months in up to 20 per cent of those patients who have failed to respond either to previous castration, or bilateral adrenalectomy (Pearson and Ray, 1960). Because of the lower likelihood of response in such patients, hypophyseal ablation by the transsphenoidal route or by radioactive yttrium implant is preferred, although the operations are not as complete anatomically as transfrontal hypophysectomy.

Relief of pain from bone metastases occurs within two or three days of hypophyseal ablation in the majority of cases treated, but is often transient and unassociated with objective evidence of tumour regression or the healing of bone metastases. It has been suggested that in the case of hypophyseal implantation by radioactive yttrium, the analgesic effect cannot always be ascribed to an endocrine response in the tumour, as this procedure is able to relieve the pain of bone metastases secondary to cancers of the rectum and cervix also (Juret, Hayem and Thomas, 1962). The analgesic effect of such implants into the pituitary may be due to trauma to the diencephalon, or to the adjacent sympathetic plexus, and a similar mechanism may explain the relief of pain which follows pituitary stalk section.

PARAMETERS OF HYPOPHYSEAL ABLATION

The likelihood of breast cancer regression following hypophyseal ablation is not related to changes in the oestrogen or androgen excretion levels after operation (Beck et al, 1966). The source of persistent oestrogen excretion noted in the majority of patients after hypophysectomy is uncertain (see Chapter 6).

The *anatomical* completeness of pituitary ablation does appear to be correlated with tumour response rate. Thus transfrontal hypophysectomy, with its better exposure of the gland, yields higher remission rates in breast cancer than either transsphenoidal hypophysectomy or radioactive yttrium ablation of the pituitary. Transfrontal hypophysectomy followed by packing of the fossa with radioactive yttrium in wax should provide even more complete ablation. It is claimed to have yielded a 57 per cent remission rate in one series, compared to 20 per cent from resection alone, although the incidence of ocular damage is 11 per cent and 4 per cent respectively in the two series (Edelstyn et al, 1968). Cryogenic hypophysectomy is claimed to show at autopsy a more complete destruction of the pituitary than either transfrontal or transsphenoidal hypophysectomy (Norrell et al, 1970), but reported series are so far inadequate to demonstrate superior remission rates in breast cancer.

In spite of these observations that techniques of pituitary ablation which are anatomically more complete yield higher remission rates, no correlation has been shown between completeness of ablation measured by *endocrine* parameters and the remission rate in breast cancer (Hortling, Af Bjorkesten and Hiisi-Brummer, 1957;

Pearson and Ray, 1960; Beck et al, 1966; Norrell et al, 1970).

Commonly used endocrine parameters include changes in the radioactive iodine uptake by the thyroid, the serum protein-bound iodine, and the urinary ketosteroid excretion levels measured before and after the operation. Special measurements include response to metyrapone or insulin as a measure of integrity of the hypothalamo-pituitary-adrenal axis. The disappearance of urinary gonadotropin excretion is also said to be a sensitive indicator of complete ablation (McCullagh et al, 1965), while the disappearance of growth hormone is the indicator most favoured by Norrell et al (1970).

The failure to correlate remissions in breast cancer with disappearance of hormonal parameters such as TSH, ACTH, gonadotropin and growth hormone mentioned above may be because these hormones have little influence on the growth of breast cancer. The pituitary hormone more likely to be involved is prolactin, and its assay in the human has only just been reported.

Another possible clue to this dilemma is the claim that the development of diabetes insipidus after transsphenoidal hypophysectomy is said to be associated with a greater likelihood of remission in breast cancer (Bateman, 1962; Reed and Pizey, 1967). Damage to the pituitary stalk may be associated with an effect on the hypothalamic centres controlling pituitary secretion, and damage to the centres may be more important than the extent of destruction of the hypophysis.

A complicating factor is that persistence of hormonal secretion after apparently complete anatomical ablation of the pituitary may be due to compensatory hyperplasia of pituitary tissue cells in the wall of the pharynx (Muller, 1958).

Cytotoxic Chemotherapy

It is essential for the clinician who attempts hormonal palliation of late breast cancer to know the benefits, limitations and toxicity to be expected from the administration of available cytotoxic agents.

COMBINATION WITH STEROID THERAPY

There are several situations in the course of late breast cancer when cytotoxic therapy is used additively with endocrine methods, and the combination of cytotoxic agents either with corticosteroids or with androgen therapy has been referred to in Chapter 8.

The writer has noted objective evidence of response in 55 per cent of patients, when the alkylating agent nitrogen mustard oxide is associated with prednisolone in the treatment of lung or pleural metastases from breast cancer (Stoll, 1960c). A combination of an alkylating agent with a corticosteroid may provide dramatic relief of symptoms in a very ill patient with rapidly advancing pleural effusion, ascites, pulmonary or liver metastases. The combination also tends to prolong the duration of objective remissions beyond the usual maximum of nine months, noted either from cytotoxic therapy alone or from corticosteroids alone, in the treatment of breast cancer.

Mention has been made in Chapter 8 of therapy by a combination of androgens with alkylating agents, particularly in the presence of bone metastases. The androgen is thought to counteract marrow depression, but it is recently reported that preliminary androgen administration increases the sensitivity of experimental mammary carcinoma to cyclophosphamide (Meakin, 1970). Whatever its mechanism, the combination of androgen with alkylating agents may yield

prolonged objective remissions in patients with breast cancer, apart from subjective benefit and relief of pain from metastases (Figure 9.1).

PROPHYLACTIC CHEMOTHERAPY

Prophylactic systemic chemotherapy has been suggested at the time of radical cancer surgery, because of the sharp rise which has been observed in the number of malignant cells in the circulation during surgery (Cole et al, 1958). Various agents were tried, and from a nation-wide controlled trial in the USA it has recently been concluded that prophylactic thiotepa administration can lead to a significant decrease in the tumour recurrence rate in the case of breast cancer (Fisher et al, 1968). This improvement was confined to premenopausal patients with four or more involved axillary nodes and, in such cases, a 21 to 38 per cent decrease was found in the recurrence rate at 18 months after mastectomy. A similar trial of 5-fluorouracil for prophylactic purposes found it unsatisfactory.

Decrease in the tumour recurrence rate could result from a cytotoxic effect upon malignant cells liberated at operation. In the case of breast cancer, it could also result from an indirect endocrine effect, because significant decrease in the recurrence rate was noted only in *premenopausal* women. Amenorrhoea has been noted even before systemic toxicity in premenopausal women following thiotepa administration (Sears, Eckles and Kirschbaum, 1960) and ovarian atrophy may follow high dosage thiotepa therapy (Bateman and Carlton, 1960).

An effect upon ovarian secretion was postulated by the writer as a major cause for the tumour control occasionally observed from thiotepa administration in young women with breast cancer (Stoll, 1963). A recent clinical trial has compared the effect of prophylactic oophorectomy with that of prophylactic thiotepa administration upon the recurrence rate in premenopausal patients with early breast cancer (Lewison, 1969). Both methods cause a similar decrease in

has been suggested as an alternative in this group, especially in the presence of soft tissue and visceral metastases (Segaloff, 1967; Ahman, Bisel and Hahn, 1967).

It is interesting to note in Table 9.6 that all available cytotoxic agents effective in the palliation of breast cancer achieve regression of tumour in about 20 to 30 per cent of

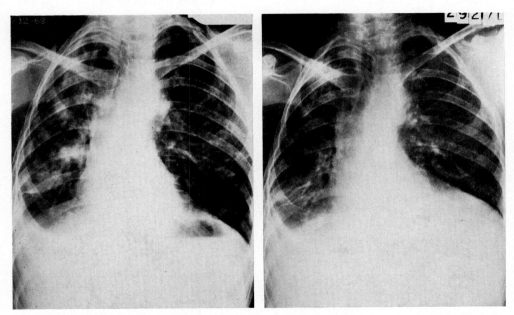

FIGURE 9.1. Radiographs to show regression of pulmonary metastases from breast cancer within seven weeks of instituting therapy with fluoxymesterone 10 mg tds and cyclophosphamide 50 mg bd. This patient had previously undergone transfrontal hypophysectomy which controlled the disease for seven years.

the recurrence rate in patients with four or more involved axillary nodes (Ravdin et al, 1970).

PALLIATIVE CHEMOTHERAPY

Cytotoxic chemotherapy is generally advised in breast cancer when palliation by other methods is unlikely. Thus, since the response rate to endocrine therapy is poor in patients who are less than two years postmenopausal and with a short recurrence—free interval, the administration of 5-fluorouracil

patients, when dosage of the agents is taken to moderate levels of haemopoietic or gastrointestinal toxicity. The writer has shown that there is no advantage to be gained by increasing the dose of the cytotoxic agents to induce extrmee toxicity in such cases as it will not increase the remission rate in breast cancer (Stoll, 1962, 1970; Bross et al, 1966; Fracchia et al, 1970a).

Cytotoxic agents carry no danger of exacerbating the growth of breast cancer, and this advantage coupled with their 20 to 30 per cent remission rate should make them potential rivals to endocrine therapy in the initial management of inoperable breast cancer. However, when used by themselves, they are less effective *qualitatively* than hormonal agents: regression of soft tissue tumour masses is rarely complete, recalcification of osteolytic metastases is rarely seen, and the periods of tumour remission achieved are usually only between three and six months (Table 9.6).

in breast cancer as are stressed for hormonal therapy (Chapter 5). Objective evidence of tumour regression must be differentiated from subjective benefit, and decrease in the size of all visible lesions should be *significant* and maintained for a reasonable time period. A recent assessment of response to cytotoxic chemotherapy in 253 patients reports a 7 per cent remission rate if a 50 per cent decrease in lesion size was demanded, or a

TABLE 9.6. *Major reports of palliation from cytotoxic agent therapy in patients with breast cancer*

Author		Total cases	Percentage with regression	Average duration of tumour regression (months)
Conference, 1958	Alkylating agents	724	*26*	4
Brennan et al, 1964	5-Fluorouracil	296	*21*	6
CCNSC Cooperative Breast Cancer Group, 1967	Methotrexate	96	*17*	5
Goldenberg, 1963 } Frei, 1965 }	Vinblastine Vincristine	79 135	*17*} *29*}	3 to 4

In addition, unlike steroidal agents, the use of cytotoxic agents is rarely associated with a subjective feeling of well-being. Toxic side-effects are almost inevitable and often a danger to life, while bone-marrow depression, alopecia, ulceration of the mouth, vomiting, and diarrhoea are frequently seen. It is important to avoid burdening an ill patient with additional side-effects of this nature and degree, unless the palliation which can be expected is worthwhile. For this reason there is an increasing tendency to use lower, less toxic dosage of these agents, particularly in combination with steroid therapy.

FACTORS INFLUENCING RESPONSE

The same criteria of response must be used in assessing the results of cytotoxic chemotherapy

48 per cent remission rate if a 10 per cent decrease was accepted (Rimm, Ahlstrom and Bross, 1966). In assessing response it should be remembered that regression of a lesion may be considerably delayed following cytotoxic therapy, as even complete cessation of cell division will not reduce the tumour size, unless spontaneous cell loss is taking place at the same time.

The histology, vascularity, and metabolic activity of the same type of tumour varies widely from patient to patient, and this may explain why the response of breast cancer to cytotoxic chemotherapy is unpredictable. Nevertheless, attempts have been made, as in the hormonal therapy of breast cancer, to elucidate biological determinants of response in the patient.

It is uncertain whether response of breast

cancer to cytotoxic agents is more likely if there has been a previous response to endocrine therapy. Whereas one reported series shows such a correlation (Hurley et al, 1961), another was unable to confirm it for either cyclophosphamide or 5-fluorouracil therapy (Ravdin and Eisman, 1967). Furthermore, response to cyclophosphamide is just as likely after, as before, hypophysectomy (Joslin, 1970) and there is no relationship between the likelihood of response and the age of the patient relative to the menopause (Cole, 1970).

It is generally agreed that, if used earlier in the disease, the remissions achieved by cytotoxic therapy tend to occur more frequently and to be of longer duration, probably because the volume of the tumour is smaller. Previous x-ray irradiation of the part decreases the likelihood of a tumour response to cytotoxic therapy, presumably because of interference with the tumour vascularity. The history of recent cytotoxic chemotherapy of any type will reduce the likelihood of tumour response to a second course and this may result from decreased tolerance of the bone marrow to further therapy. It is generally agreed also that cytotoxic therapy used in the presence of large masses of tumour is less likely to be effective, and tumour ablation by surgery has therefore been suggested before cytotoxic therapy, in order to increase the concentration in the remaining tumour volume.

Although the *rapidity* of response is generally greater for anaplastic tumours, the histological grade of a breast cancer has not been clearly correlated with the likelihood of its response to cytotoxic chemotherapy. Whereas it has been noted that the likelihood of response to cyclophosphamide is greater for slowly growing tumours (Edelstyn et al, 1968), it is reported that 5-fluorouracil therapy is more likely to yield response in rapidly growing tumours (Ravdin and Eisman, 1967).

Metastases in bone show tumour regression much less frequently than do soft-tissue metastases and, in the case of extensive bone metastases, the writer prefers a combination of cytotoxic therapy with androgen therapy (Stoll, 1970). Whereas nodular lung metastases and early liver metastases occasionally respond to cytotoxic chemotherapy, lymphogenous permeation of the lungs and large liver metastases rarely do so (Fracchia et al, 1970a). In the case of extensive lung, liver, pleural or peritoneal metastases, the writer prefers to combine cytotoxic chemotherapy with corticosteroid therapy, and dramatic response is sometimes seen from this combination (Stoll, 1960, 1969).

Response to cytotoxic agents in the treatment of breast cancer is usually very temporary, the average duration being from three to six months. Tumour resistance may develop either as a result of proliferation of surviving resistant cells in the tumour, or alternatively, as a result of the tumour metabolism by-passing the blocked enzymatic pathways in nucleoprotein synthesis. It is claimed that response may occur in a tumour to a second cytotoxic agent after the development of resistance to the first agent, but this is rare in the writer's experience.

METHODS OF ADMINISTRATION

INTRACAVITARY THERAPY

In the control of recurrent effusions due to tumour deposits on a serous surface, cytotoxic agents either alone or in combination with corticosteroid therapy have been found particularly useful. The rate of reaccumulation of fluid is decreased in the majority of treated cases although it often takes four to six weeks to manifest. Failure to respond in such a case is usually associated with a transudate of low specific gravity.

The writer has found intracavitary nitrogen mustard therapy to be as effective as colloidal radioactive gold instillation in controlling metastatic pleural effusions (Bonte, Storaasli and Weisberger, 1956; Weisberger, 1958), and it involves a much less complicated procedure. Dosage is 0·4 mg/kg in 20 ml saline, split in the case of bilateral effusions. Although the local irritant effect of nitrogen mustard may be an advantage in causing pleurodesis in pleural effusions, this effect does not recommend its use for intraperitoneal instillation. Pleurodesis by talc insufflation, or alternatively by intracavitary quinacrine, may be preferred in the presence of a damaged bone marrow.

Whereas nitrogen mustard almost invariably causes severe nausea and vomiting, thiotepa can be given repeatedly with only occasional nausea, and has the added advantage that it can be given intraperitoneally also. Injected intracavitarily, the local concentration of the agent remains high, and because of slower absorption from the serous cavities, approximately twice the dose can be tolerated as would be when given systemically. Dosage is 0·5 to 1 mg/kg in 20 to 40 ml saline repeated at one to four weeks' interval.

Reaccumulation of fluid in the serous cavity is delayed two months or longer in 27·5 per cent of breast cancer patients following nitrogen mustard or thiotepa instillation (Fracchia et al, 1970b), and survival for one to five years is claimed from thiotepa therapy in 17 per cent of such cases (Bateman, 1967).

SYSTEMIC THERAPY

In the presence of extensive tumour recurrence or of distant metastases, cytotoxic agents are administered systemically, in the hope of achieving a higher uptake within the more rapidly dividing tumour cells than in the more slowly dividing cells of the host.

In order to do this in practice, the ideal aim is to increase both the *concentration* of the agent in the tumour bed and the *time* for which the tumour cells are exposed to it. Closed-circuit high dose perfusion with a cytotoxic agent would provide the highest local concentration, but this can be applied only to an isolated part and for a limited period. Systemic therapy for a prolonged

period would be the most suitable method of finding the nuclei of all the tumour cells in their most sensitive phase before division, but if dosage is high this would entail considerable marrow toxicity. Intermittent high single doses will kill only a small percentage of the tumour cells because of the short effective concentration in the blood and the high percentage of resistant cells.

In the case of breast cancer, the choice in practice therefore lies between *intermittent courses* of high dosage of the agent and *continuous maintenance* therapy with lower dosage. The route of administration is usually intravenous for the former and oral for the latter. There is, however, a recent report of regional intra-arterial infusion for breast cancer for 5 to 15 days which claims objective response in 42 per cent of cases for an average of 14·7 months (Freckman, 1970). Agents used included 5-fluorouracil, vinblastine, cyclophosphamide, or methotrexate associated with oral administration of prednisolone 30 mg daily. The latter undoubtedly contributed to the good remission rate.

CHOICE OF CYTOTOXIC AGENTS

ALKYLATING AGENTS

Alkylating agents interfere with nucleoprotein synthesis and with the duplication of chromosomes. *Nitrogen mustard* was the first of the group to be introduced into clinical practice, but is now used in breast cancer only in the management of pleural effusions. The most commonly administered systemic agents in breast cancer are the related agents *thiotepa* and *cyclophosphamide* (Endoxana, Cytoxan), but the use of *phenylalanine nitrogen mustard* (melphalan), *chlorambucil* (Leukeran) and *nitrogen mustard oxide* (nitromin) has also been reported.

Signs of toxicity by the group affect mainly the bone marrow, causing leucopenia and thrombocytopenia and, if severe, a tendency to haemorrhages. In addition, nausea, vomiting, or alopecia may follow the use of individual agents. The first sign of regression in advanced breast cancer usually takes about six weeks to manifest, and the final degree of tumour shrinkage is usually incomplete (Plates 9.1 and 9.2, facing p. 209). The average duration of response is about four months, and a second tumour response is rarely obtained from the use of a different member of the group later.

A report on 724 collected cases of breast

thrombocyte-sparing effect, but unfortunately it tends to cause alopecia which is most marked when intermittent high dosage schedules are used (Stoll and Matar, 1961). The writer now prefers a loading dose of 20 to 30 mg/kg divided into two or three intravenous doses, followed by oral maintenance dosage of 2 to 3 mg/kg daily. This continuous low-dosage technique gives a similar degree of palliation in breast cancer, but with less

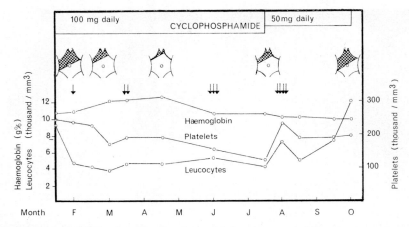

FIGURE 9.2. Clinical record and blood count of patient with breast cancer with temporary regression of grossly enlarged liver following a prolonged course of cyclophosphamide therapy at low dosage. (Arrows represent adjustment of dose levels.)

cancer treated by alkylating agents, noted objective evidence of tumour regression in 26 per cent of the total (Conference, 1958). In spite of the wide variation in tumour remission rates reported for different alkylating agents in breast cancer, it is the writer's experience that using uniform criteria of response, the choice between the various agents is merely one of convenience and consideration of side-effects.

The use of thiotepa rarely causes nausea or vomiting of any extent. A loading dose of 0·5 to 1 mg/kg is given intramuscularly (intravenous therapy is not essential), followed by half this dose at one to two-week intervals. Cyclophosphamide can be given either orally or parenterally and has a

toxicity than the intermittent high-dosage technique (Stoll, 1970) (Figures 9.2 and 9.3).

Phenylalanine mustard can be given orally or parenterally. Although not widely used in the treatment of breast cancer, tumour regression has been reported in 11 per cent of one series (Silva, Smart and Rochlin, 1965) and in 30 per cent of another (CCNSC Breast Cancer Group, 1966). Nitrogen mustard oxide can also be given orally with minimal side-effects apart from moderate marrow depression (Stoll, 1956, 1960c).

ANTIMETABOLITES

Pyrimidines such as uracil may be chemically changed so that when metabolised by the cell in the synthesis of nucleoprotein they prevent proper coding of RNA.

Remission rates reported from the use of *5-fluorouracil* in breast cancer vary from 16 to 42 per cent (Ansfield and Curreri, 1963; Hurley et al, 1961). Judged by the rigid criteria of the CCNSC Breast Cancer Group, the response rate was reported to be 21 per cent in 296 patients (Brennan, Talley and San Diego, 1964). In various series,

The average duration of tumour control from the fluorinated pyrimidines is about six months. This is somewhat longer than from the alkylating agents, but the toxicity from the fluorinated pyrimidines is much greater. The treatment mortality rate is about 5 per cent from intensive treatment, and signs of toxicity include severe diarrhoea, stomatitis, nausea and vomiting, apart from marrow depression.

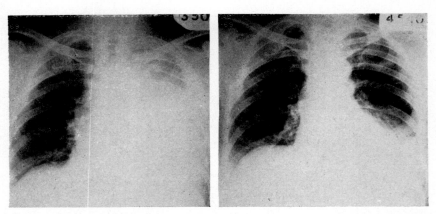

FIGURE 9.3. Radiographs to show regression of malignant pleural effusion after nine weeks of cyclophosphamide therapy at a dose of 50 mg bd. This patient had previously failed to respond to oestrogen therapy.

5-fluorodeoxyuridine has been reported to induce regression of breast cancer in between 12 and 48 per cent of patients (Ansfield and Curreri, 1963; Dao and Grinberg, 1963; Nevinny, 1964).

The two agents probably induce similar remission rates in breast cancer, when allowance is made for different criteria of response. In this respect Ansfield and Curreri (1963) accept the maintenance of a 25 per cent reduction in size for two months as evidence of favourable response in a tumour, whereas others demand a higher degree of remission and for a longer period.

The standard course of 5-fluorouracil recommended originally (Ansfield and Curreri, 1963) is 15 mg/kg intravenously daily for three to five days followed by 7·5 mg/kg every two or three days until toxicity appears.

The modest remission rate reported from this intensive technique, and its short duration, do not justify the high risk of severe toxicity and the occasional drug deaths. For this reason, there has been an increasing tendency to use a dose of 10 to 15 mg/kg at weekly intervals by rapid intravenous injection, especially for the treatment of ambulatory patients. This results in similar palliation of breast cancer (Jacobs, Luce and Wood, 1968) but with a decreased toxicity and mortality.

Methotrexate (Amethopterin) is a antimetabolite which prevents the conversion of folic acid into cirtrovorum factor, and toxic symptoms can thus be reversed by the administration of citrovorum factor, if given within four hours of methotrexate administration. A 41 per cent tumour remission rate

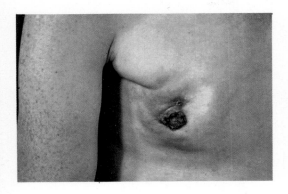
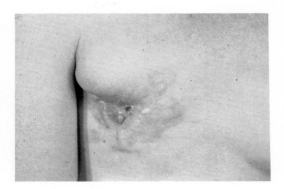

PLATE 7.1. Photographs to show healing of malignant ulceration of the breast within 6 months of surgical castration (Stoll, 1969). (Reproduced by permission of Pitman Medical)

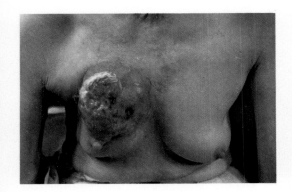
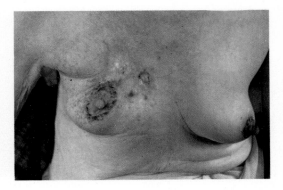

PLATE 7.2. Photographs to show regression of malignant ulceration of the breast within 9 months of stilboestrol therapy 5 mg tds (Stoll, 1969). (Reproduced by permission of Pitman Medical)

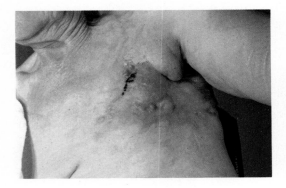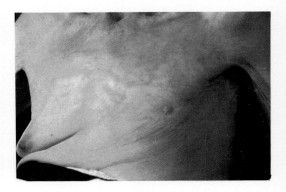

PLATE 7.3. Photographs to show regression of malignant ulceration of the breast within 4 months of ethinyl oestradiol therapy 0·5 mg tds (Stoll, 1969). (Reproduced by permission of Pitman Medical)

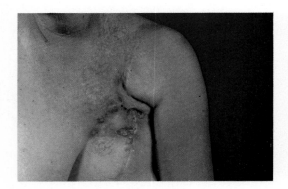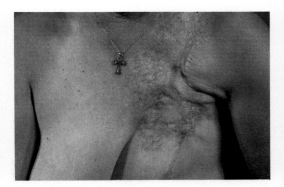

PLATE 8.1. Photographs to show healing of malignant ulceration of the chest wall within 3 months of fluoxymesterone therapy 10 mg tds (Stoll, 1959). (Reproduced by permission of the Editor, *Medical Journal of Australia*.)

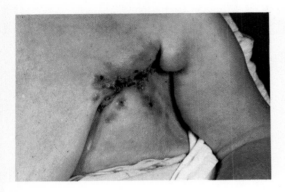
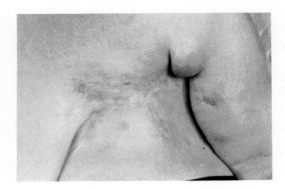

PLATE 8.2. Photographs to show healing of malignant ulceration of the chest wall within 4 months of Lyndiol therapy 1 mg tds (Stoll, 1966). (Reproduced by permission of the Editor, *Medical Journal of Australia*.)

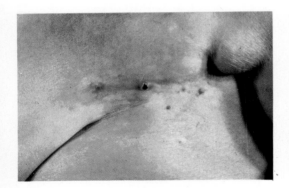
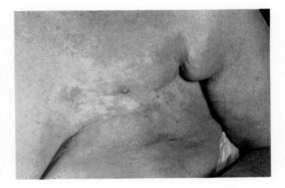

PLATE 8.3. Same patient as in Plate 8.2. Photographs to show recurrence of tumour after 15 months Lyndiol therapy, and its disappearance 6 months after stopping therapy (Stoll, 1967). (Reproduced by permission of the Editor, *British Medical Journal*.)

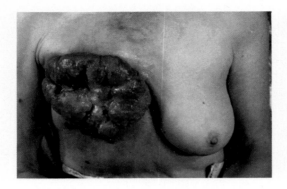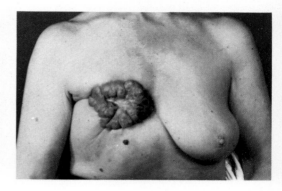

PLATE 9.1. Photographs to show partial regression of massive breast cancer following a course of 345 mg Thiotepa in 17 weeks (Stoll, 1969). (Reproduced by permission of Pitman Medical)

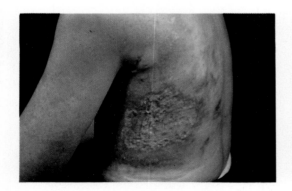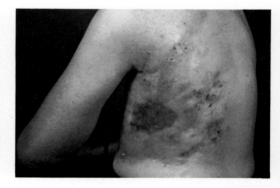

PLATE 9.2. Photographs to show partial regression of malignant ulceration of the chest wall following a course of 285 mg Thiotepa in 22 weeks (Stoll, 1969). (Reproduced by permission of Pitman Medical)

has been reported from the use of methotrexate in advanced breast cancer (Vogler, Furtado and Huguley, 1968) but a randomised comparison of cytotoxic agents (CCNSC Breast Cancer Group, 1967) reported regression in only 17 per cent of those treated by methotrexate compared to 25 per cent of those treated by the fluorinated pyrimidines. However, it was reported that in the methotrexate series the response was more prolonged although slower in its onset, and the proportion of survivors at one year was considerably higher. In a retrospective survey, methotrexate was claimed to yield the highest response rate of seven cytotoxic agents in breast cancer (Fracchia et al, 1970a).

Oral dosage of methotrexate is generally 5 mg daily in two divided doses, but doses of 20 to 25 mg daily can be tolerated by rapid intravenous administration because of rapid excretion by the kidney. Treatment courses are generally for four to five days and are repeated at three to four-week intervals, but dosage is ceased at the first appearance of mouth ulceration or diarrhoea. Other signs of toxicity are mainly haemopoietic and gastrointestinal.

The use of *combination chemotherapy* in breast cancer has long been practised as a means of prolonging response by blocking several pathways of tumour metabolism, and thus delaying the onset of drug resistance (Stoll, 1955, 1959). A 60 per cent response rate in soft tissue, brain or lung metastases has been reported in breast cancer patients treated by a combination of thiotepa and methotrexate (Greenspan, 1964, 1965). A 50 per cent response rate is reported in a series treated by a combination of cyclophosphamide and methotrexate (Haab et al, 1967; Brunner, 1969). Several groups are at present investigating the results of 'triple' and 'quadruple' therapy by various combinations of cyclophosphamide, methotrexate, 5-fluorouracil and vincristine.

Vinblastine is a plant alkaloid extracted from the periwinkle flower. It acts as a spindle poison, but is included here among the antimetabolites because its cytotoxic effects can be reversed experimentally by administration of coenzyme A and various amino acids. Vinblastine therapy is claimed in one breast cancer series to have induced objective evidence of tumour regression in 23 per cent of patients for an average period of three to four months (Frei, 1965), but another series reported no responders from its administration in breast cancer patients (Goldenberg, 1963). Toxicity affects mainly the bone marrow, but recovery occurs fairly rapidly.

Favourable response to *vincristine*, which is related to vinblastine, is said to occur within three to four weeks of starting treatment, and sometimes in the absence of response to previous cytotoxic therapy (Goldenberg, 1964). It has been reported to yield remission of tumour growth in 29 per cent of 135 collected breast cancer patients (Gailani, 1963; Mittelman, Grinberg and Dao, 1963; Frei, 1965). Toxicity from this agent is, however, frequently severe, and includes neurological symptoms in addition to alopecia, leucopenia and gastrointestinal symptoms.

ANTIBIOTICS

The use of *Mitomycin C* has been sporadically reported in the treatment of advanced breast cancer for the last 10 years. Remission of tumour growth was reported in 45 per cent of 20 patients by the writer and others (Colsky et al, 1960; Stoll, 1960b), and a review of Japanese reports showed remission in 42 per cent of 26 breast cancer cases (Frank and Osterburg, 1960). Reports of toxic effects of the agent upon the marrow have tended to limit the clinical use of Mitomycin C outside Japan. However, recent trial reports remission in 36 per cent of 42 patients with breast cancer, and suggests that wider use should be made of this agent (Moore et al, 1968).

Carzinophilin has been reported by Kurokawa and Saito (1959) to have a palliative effect upon advanced breast cancer. The toxic side-effects upon the bone marrow are

8

minimal, and its use is still being reported from Japan. The writer reported no benefit from its administration to a small series of breast cancer patients (Stoll, 1960a).

CONCLUSION

Both bilateral adrenalectomy and hypophyseal ablation yield objective evidence of tumour regression in about 30 per cent of patients with advanced breast cancer for an average duration of 24 to 36 months. These regression rates are little different from those resulting from primary castration or oestrogen therapy, and their longer average duration must be set against the not inconsiderable postoperative mortality associated with such major surgery.

For this reason major endocrine ablation is indicated only after loss of response to these primary methods of endocrine therapy, and may achieve a second response in such cases. Hypophysectomy yields superior results, but the choice of method for major ablation therapy depends mainly upon the available specialists. Radioactive yttrium or transnasal methods of pituitary ablation are preferred in patients who are too ill for the major procedures or those who have not responded to primary methods of endocrine therapy. Pain relief in bone metastases is very common within a few days of major endocrine ablation but is often not related to radiographic evidence of recalcification in metastases.

Intracavitary injection of cytotoxic agents may control metastatic serous effusions for periods of one to two years. Systemic chemotherapy may lead to objective evidence of tumour regression in 20 to 30 per cent of cases, but such regression is generally incomplete, and lasts for a period of only three to six months on average. The possibility of such a remission must be weighed against the toxic side-effects commonly associated with the use of these agents.

Cytotoxic agents are used most commonly in the control of soft-tissue tumour in patients who have either not responded or are unlikely to respond to endocrine therapy. In combination with corticosteroid therapy they may lead to dramatic relief of symptoms associated with rapidly growing visceral metastases, although such effect is generally short lived. In combination with androgens they may result in objective evidence of regression in bone metastases for a prolonged period.

References

Ahlquist, K. A., Jackson, A. W. & Stewart, J. C. (1968) Urinary steroid values as a guide to prognosis in cancer. *British Medical Journal*, **i**, 217.

Ahmann, D. L., Bisel, H. F. & Hahn, R. G. (1967) An evaluation of 5 fluorouracil in the treatment of advanced breast cancer. *Cancer Chemotherapy Abstracts*, **8**, 51.

Ansfield, F. J. & Curreri, A. R. (1963) Further clinical comparison between 5 fluorouracil and 5 fluorodeoxyuridine. *Cancer Chemotherapy Reports*, **32**, 101.

Arslan, M. (1966) Ultrasonic hypophysectomy. *Journal of Laryngology and Otology*, **80**, 73.

Atkins, H. J. B., Falconer, M. A., Hayward, J. L., Maclean, K. S., Schurr, P. H. & Armitage, P. (1960) Adrenalectomy and hypophysectomy for advanced cancer of the breast. *Lancet*, **i**, 1148.

Atkins, H., Falconer, M. A., Hayward, J. L., Maclean, K. S. & Schurr, P. H. (1966) The timing of adrenalectomy and of hypophysectomy in the treatment of advanced breast cancer. *Lancet*, **i**, 827.

Atkins, H., Bulbrook, R. D., Falconer, M. A., Hayward, J. L., MacLean, K. S. & Schurr, P. H. (1968) Ten years experience of steroid assays in the management of breast cancer. *Lancet*, **ii**, 1256.

Bateman, G. H. (1962) Transsphenoidal hypophysectomy. *Journal of Laryngology and Otology*, **76**, 442.

Bateman, J. (1967) Maintenance chemotherapy in advanced cancer. *Cancer Chemotherapy Reports*, **8**, 471.

Bateman, J. C. & Carlton, H. (1960) The role of chemotherapy in the treatment of breast cancer. *Surgery*, **47**, 895.

Beck, J. C., Blair, A. J., Griffiths, M. M., Rosenfeld, M. W. & McGarry, E. E. (1966) In search of hormonal factors as an aid in predicting the outcome of breast carcinoma. *Canadian Cancer Conference*, **6**, 3.

Bleasel, K. & Lazarus, L. (1965) Cryogenic hypophysectomy. *Medical Journal of Australia*, **2**, 148.

Block, G. E., Vial, A. B., McCarthy, J. D., Porter, C. W. & Coller, F. A. (1959) Adrenalectomy in advanced mammary cancer. *Surgery, Gynecology and Obstetrics*, **108**, 651.

Boesen, E., Radley-Smith, E. J. & Baron, D. N. (1961) Further experience with hypophysectomy in advanced breast cancer. *British Medical Journal*, **ii**, 790.

Boesen, E. (1967) Hormonal therapy in disseminated cancer. *Hospital Medicine*, **1**, 886.

Bonte, F. J., Storaasli, J. P. & Weisberger, A. S. (1956) Comparative evaluation of radioactive colloidal gold and nitrogen mustard in the treatment of serous effusions of neoplastic origin. *Radiology*, **67**, 63.

Brennan, M. J., Talley, R. W. & San Diego, E. L. (1964) quoted by Jacobs et al. (1968).

Bross, I. D. J., Rimm, A. A., Sack, N. H., Ausman, R. K. & Jones, R. (1966) Is toxicity really necessary? *Cancer (Philadelphia)*, **19**, 780.

Brunner, K. W. (1969) Polychemotherapy in hormone resistant breast cancer. *Schweizerische Medizinische Wochenschrift*, **99**, 1298.

Byron, R., Yonemoto, R. H., Bashore, R., Bierman, H. R., Cronemiller, P. & Masters, H. (1962) Bilateral adrenalectomy in advanced breast cancer. *Surgery*, **52**, 725.

Cade, S. (1958) Adrenalectomy in cancer of the breast. In *Endocrine Aspects of Breast Cancer*, p. 2, ed. Currie, A. R. and Illingsworth, C. F. W. Edinburgh: Livingstone.

Cade, S. (1966) Adrenalectomy for disseminated breast cancer. *British Medical Journal*, **ii**, 613.

C.C.N.S.C. Breast Cancer Group (1966) Melphalan in advanced breast cancer. *Cancer Chemotherapy Reports*, **50**, 271.

C.C.N.S.C. Breast Cancer Group (1967) Comparison of antimetabolites in the treatment of breast and colon cancer. *Journal of the American Medical Association*, **200**, 770.

Cole, M. P. (1970) Decadurabolin compared with cyclophosphamide. In *Second Tenovus Workshop on Breast Cancer*, ed. Joslin, C. A. F. and Gleave, E. N. Cardiff: Tenovus Workshop.

Cole, W. H., Robert, S., Watne, A., McDonald, G. & McGrew, E. (1958) The dissemination of cancer cells. *Bulletin of the New York Academy of Science*, **34**, 163.

Colsky, J., Escher, G. C., Evans, A., Mitus, A., Li, M. C., Roath, S., Sullivan, R. D., Sykes, M. P. & Tan, C. T. T. (1960) Preliminary clinical pharmacology of Mitomycin C. Personal communication.

Conference (1958) Comparative clinical and biological effects of alkylating agents. *Annals of the New York Academy of Science*, **68**, 657.

Daicoff, G. R., Harmon, R. & Van Prohaska, J. (1962) Effect of adrenalectomy on mammary carcinoma. *Archives of Surgery*, **85**, 800.

Dao, T. L. (1970) Early compared with late adrenalectomy. In *Second Tenovus Workshop on Breast Cancer*, ed. Joslin, C. A. F. and Gleave, E. N. Cardiff: Tenovus Workshop.

Dao, T. L. Y. & Grinberg, R. (1963) Fluorinated pyrimidines in the treatment of breast cancer patients with liver metastases. *Cancer Chemotherapy Reports*, **27**, 71.

Dao, T. L. Y. & Huggins, C. (1955) Bilateral adrenalectomy in the treatment of cancer of the breast. *Archives of Surgery*, **71**, 645.

Dao, T. L. Y. & Nemoto, T. (1965) An evaluation of adrenalectomy and androgen in disseminated mammary carcinoma. *Surgery, Gynecology and Obstetrics*, **121**, 1257.

Delarue, N. C., Peters, U., Anderson, W. S. & Starr, J. (1967) A re-evaluation of the place of major extirpation in the management of patients with metastatic mammary carcinoma. *Canadian Medical Association Journal*, **96**, 637.

Douglas, M., (1957) Indications for adrenalectomy and hypophysectomy in advanced breast cancer. *Acta endocrinologica (København) Suppl.*, **31**, 307.

Edelstyn, G., Gleadhill, C. & Lyons, A. (1968) Total hypophysectomy for advanced breast cancer. *Clinical Radiology*, **19**, 426.

Escher, G. (1958) Panel discussion. In *Breast Cancer*, p. 225, ed. Segaloff, A. St. Louis: C. V. Mosby.

Ferguson, D. J. (1970) Planning appropriate operations for cancer of the breast. *Surgical Clinics of North America*, **50**, 213.

Fisher, B., Radvin, R. G., Ausman, R. K., Slack, N. H., Moore, G. E. & Noer, R. J. (1968) Surgical adjuvant chemotherapy in cancer of the breast. *Annals of Surgery*, **168**, 337.

Forrest, A. P. M. (1965) Endocrine treatment of breast cancer. *Israel Journal of Medical Science*, **1**, 259.

Fracchia, A. A., Holleb, A. I., Farrow, J. H., Treves, N. E., Randall, H. T., Finkbeiner, J. A. & Whitmore, Jr, W. F. (1959) Results of bilateral adrenalectomy in the management of incurable breast cancer. *Cancer (Philadelphia)*, **12**, 58.

Fracchia, A. A., Randall, H. T. & Farrow, J. H. (1967) The results of adrenalectomy in advanced breast cancer in 500 consecutive patients. *Surgery, Gynecology and Obstetrics*, **125**, 747.

Fracchia, A. A., Farrow, J. H., Adam, Y. G., Monroy, J. & Knapper, W. H. (1970a) Systemic chemotherapy for advanced breast cancer. *Cancer (Philadelphia)*, **26**, 424.

Fracchia, A. A., Knapper, W. H., Carey, J. T. & Farrow, J. H. (1970b) Intrapleural chemotherapy for effusion from metastatic breast carcinoma. *Cancer (Philadelphia)*, **26**, 626.

Frank, W. & Osterberg, A. E. (1960) Mitomycin C—an evaluation of the Japanese reports. *Cancer Chemotherapy Reports*, **9**, 114.

Freckman, H. A. (1970) Chemotherapy of breast cancer by regional intra-arterial transfusion. *Cancer (Philadelphia)*, **26**, 560.

Frei, E. (1965) Chemotherapy of breast cancer. *Annals of Internal Medicine*, **63**, 334.

Gailani, S. (1963) Phase II studies on Vincristine in human cancer. *Proceedings of the American Association for Cancer Research*, **4**, 21.

Galante, M., Fournier, D. J. & Wood, D. A. (1957) Adrenalectomy for metastatic breast carcinoma. *Journal of the American Medical Association*, **163**, 1011.

Goldenberg, I. S. (1963) Vinblastine sulphate therapy of women with advanced breast cancer. *Cancer Chemotherapy Reports*, **29**, 111.

Goldenberg, I. S. (1964) Vincristine therapy of women with advanced breast cancer. *Cancer Chemotherapy Reports*, **41**, 7.

Greenspan, E. M. (1964) Combinations of methotrexate, thiotepa and 5-fluorouracil in advanced breast carcinoma. *Proceedings of the American Association for Cancer Research*, **5**, 23.

Greenspan, E. M. (1965) Results of four drug sequential combination chemotherapy of breast carcinoma in relation to predominant organ metastases. *Proceedings of the American Association for Cancer Research*, **6**, 24.

Haab, O. P., Martz, G., Brunner, H. E., Brunner, K. W., Sonntag, R., Ryssel, H. J., Maurice, P. & Alberto, O. (1967) Combined chemotherapy for metastasising mammary carcinoma. *Cancer Chemotherapy Abstract*, **8**, 456.

Hayward, J. L., Atkins, H. J. B., Falconer, M. A., MacLean, K. S., Salmon, L. F. W., Schurr, P. H. and Shahcen, C. H. (1970) Clinical trials comparing transfrontal hypophysectomy with adrenalectomy and with transethmoidal hypophysectomy. In *Second Tenovus Workshop on Breast Cancer*, ed. Joslin, C. A. F. and Gleave, E. N. Cardiff: Tenovus Workshop.

Hayward, J. L. (1970) A comparison of early hypophysectomy or adrenalectomy with late hypophysectomy. In *Second Tenovus Workshop on Breast Cancer*, Joslin, C. A. F. and Gleave, E. N. Cardiff: Tenovus Workshop.

Hellstrom, J. & Franksson, C. (1958) Adrenalectomy in cancer of the breast. In *Endocrine Aspects of Breast Cancer*, p. 5, ed. Currie, A. R. and Illingsworth, C. F. W. Edinburgh: Livingstone.

Hortling, H., Af Bjorkesten, G. & Hiisi-Brummer, L. (1957) Experience with hypophysectomy in mammary cancer patients. *Acta endocrinologica (København)*, **31**, 289.

Hurley, J. D., Trump, D. S., Flatley, T. J. & Riesch, J. D. (1961) A method of selecting patients for cancer chemotherapy. *Archives of Surgery*, **83**, 611.

Hunt, P. S. & Nemoto, T. (1970) The management of advanced breast cancer. *Medical Journal of Australia*, **2**, 591.

Irvine, W. T., Aitken, E. H., Rendleman, D. L. & Folca, P. J. (1961) Urinary oestrogen measurements after oophorectomy and adrenalectomy for advanced breast cancer. *Lancet*, **ii**, 791.

Jacobs, E. M., Luce, J. K. & Wood, D. A. (1968) Treatment of cancer with weekly intravenous 5 fluorouracil. *Cancer (Philadelphia)*, **22**, 1233.

Jessiman, A. G. (1958) In *Endocrine Aspects of Breast Cancer*, p. 26, ed. Currie, A. P. and Illingsworth, C. F. W. Edinburgh: Livingstone.

Jessiman, A. G., Matson, D. D. & Moore, F. D. (1959) Hypophysectomy in the treatment of breast cancer. *New England Journal of Medicine*, **261**, 1199.

Joint Committee on Endocrine Ablative Procedures in Disseminated Mammary Carcinoma (1961). *Journal of the American Medical Association*, **175**, 137, 787.

Joslin, C. A. (1970) Cyclophosphamide and its relation to endocrine ablation. In *Second Tenovus Workshop on Breast Cancer*, ed. Joslin, C. A. F. and Gleave, E. N. Cardiff: Tenovus Workshop.

Juret, P. (1966) *Endocrine Surgery in Human Cancers*, Springfield: Charles C. Thomas.

Juret, P., Hayem, M. & Thomas, M. (1962) quoted In *Endocrine Surgery in Human Cancers*, p. 237, by Juret, P. Springfield: Charles C. Thomas, 1966.

Kennedy, B. J. & French, L. (1965) Hypophysectomy in advanced breast cancer. *American Journal of Surgery*, **110**, 411.

Kurokawa, T. & Saito, T. (1959) Chemotherapy of malignant tumours, *Acta Unio internationalis contra cancrum*, **15** (suppl.), 159.

Lawrence, J. H. (1967) quoted by Hayward, J. In *Hormones and Human Breast Cancer*. London: Heinemann.

Lewison, E. F. (1969) Castration in the treatment of operable breast cancer. *Cancer (Philadelphia)*, **24**, 1297.

Lipsett, M. B., Whitmore, W. F., Treves, N., West, C. D., Randall, H. T. & Pearson, O. H. (1957) Bilateral adrenalectomy in the palliation of metastatic breast cancer. *Cancer (Philadelphia)*, **10**, 111.

Luft, R., Olivecrona, H., Ikkos, D., Nilsson, L. B. & Mossberg, H. (1958) Hypophysectomy in the management of metastatic carcinoma of the breast. In *Endocrine Aspects of Breast Cancer*, p. 27, ed. Currie, A. R. and Illingsworth, C. F. W. Edinburgh: Livingstone.

McCalister, A., Welbourn, R. B., Edelstyn, G. J. A., Lyons, A. R., Taylor, A. R., Gleadhill, C. A., Gordon, D. S. & Cole, J. O. Y. (1961) Factors influencing response to hypophysectomy for advanced cancer of the breast. *British Medical Journal*, **i**, 613.

McCullagh, E. P., Feldstein, M. A., Tweed, D. C. & Dohn, D. F. (1965) A study of pituitary function after intrasellar implantation of ^{90}Yt. *Journal of Clinical Endocrinology*, **25**, 832.

McDonald, I. (1962) Endocrine ablation in disseminated mammary carcinoma. *Surgery, Gynecology and Obstetrics*, **115**, 215.

Meakin, J. W. (1970) Effect of chemotherapeutic agents on hormone dependent neoplasms and tissues. *Annual Report of the Ontario Cancer Research Foundation*, p. 151.

Mittelman, A., Grinberg, R. & Dao, T. L. (1963) Clinical experiences with Vincristine in women with breast cancer. *Proceedings of the American Association for Cancer Research*, **4**, 44.

Moore, G. E., Bross, J. D. T., Ausman, R., Nadler, S., Jones, R. Jr, Slack, N. & Rimm, A. A. (1968) Effect of Mitomycin C in 346 patients with advanced cancer. *Cancer Chemotherapy Reports*, **52**, 675.

Muller, W. (1958) On the pharyngeal hypophysis. In *Endocrine Aspects of Breast Cancer*, p. 106, ed. Currie, A. R. and Illingsworth, C. F. W. Edinburgh: Livingstone.

Nelson, T. S. & Dragstedt, L. R. (1961) Adrenalectomy and oophorectomy for breast cancer. *Journal of the American Medical Association*, **175**, 379.

Nevinny, H. B. (1964) Comparative study of 5 fluorouracil, 5 fluorodeoxyuridine and methotrexate in patients with advanced cancer. *Proceedings of the American Association for Cancer Research*, **5**, 47.

Norrell, H., Alves, A. M., Winternitz, N. W. & Maddy, J. (1970) A clinico-pathological analysis of cryohypophysectomy in patients with advanced cancer. *Cancer (Philadelphia)*, **25**, 1050.

Patey, D. H. (1960) Early (prophylactic) oophorectomy and adrenalectomy in carcinoma of the breast—an interim report. *British Journal of Cancer*, **14**, 457.

Patey, D. H. & Nabarro, J. D. N. (1970) Early (prophylactic) oophorectomy and adrenalectomy in carcinoma of the breast. A ten year follow-up. *British Journal of Cancer*, **24**, 16.

Pearson, O. H. & Ray, B. S. (1960) Hypophysectomy in the treatment of metastatic mammary cancer. *American Journal of Surgery*, **99**, 544.

Peters, M. V. (1956) The influence of hormone therapy on metastatic mammary carcinoma. *Surgery, Gynecology and Obstetrics*, **102**, 545.

Pyrah, L. N. (1958) The results of adrenalectomy with gonadectomy in breast cancer. In *Endocrine Aspects of Breast Cancer*, p. 22, ed. Currie, A. R. and Illingsworth, C. F. W. Edinburgh: Livingstone.

Ravdin, R. G. & Eisman, S. H. (1967) Disseminated breast cancer; relationship of response to endocrine manipulation, Cytoxan and fluorouracil. In *Current Concepts in Breast Cancer*, p. 200, ed. Segaloff, A., Meyer, K. K. and Debakey, S. Baltimore: Williams and Wilkins.

Ravdin, R. G., Lewison, E. F., Slack, N. H., Gardner, B., State, D. & Fisher, B. (1970) Results of a clinical trial concerning the worth of prophylactic oophorectomy for breast cancer. *Surgery, Gynecology and Obstetrics*, **131**, 1055.

Reed, P. I. & Pizey, N. C. D. (1967) Trans-sphenoidal hypophysectomy in the treatment of advanced breast cancer. *British Journal of Surgery*, **54**, 369.

Rimm, A. A., Ahlstrom, J. K. & Bross, I. D. J. (1966) What is objective response? *Proceedings of the American Association for Cancer Research*, **7**, 59.

Sears, M. E., Eckles, N. & Kirschbaum, A. (1960) Thiotepa induced amenorrhoea associated with prolonged regression of human breast cancer. *Proceedings of the American Association for Cancer Research*, **3**, 150.

Segaloff, A. (1967) Progress in the treatment of cancer. In *Cambridge Symposium on the Treatment of Carcinoma of the Breast*, p. 8, ed. Jarrett, A. S. Excerpta Medica Foundation.

Sellwood, R. A., Davey, J., Galaska, C. S. B., Li, J. & Burr, J. L. (1968) A clinical trial to compare early and late pituitary ablation in advanced cancer of the breast. *British Journal of Surgery*, **55**, 870.

Silva, A. R. M., Smart, C. R. & Rochlin, D. B. (1965) Chemotherapy of breast cancer. *Surgery, Gynecology and Obstetrics*, **121**, 494.

Smith, O. W. & Emerson, K. Jr (1954) Urinary estrogens and related compounds in postmenopausal women with mammary cancer—effect of cortisone treatment. *Proceedings of the Society for Experimental Biology and Medicine*, **85**, 264.

Stewart, H. (1970) Oophorectomy response as an index to further endocrine ablation. In *Second Tenovus Workshop on Breast Cancer*, ed. Joslin, C. A. F. and Gleave, E. N. Cardiff: Tenovus Workshop.

Stewart, H. J., Forrest, A. P. M., Roberts, M. M., Jones, R. E. A., Jones, V. & Campbell, H. (1969) Early pituitary implantation with Yttrium 90 for advanced breast cancer. *Lancet*, **ii**, 817.

Stoll, B. A. (1955) Chemotherapy in cancer. *Medical Journal of Australia*, **2**, 322.

Stoll, B. A. (1956) Advanced cancer treated with Nitromin. *Medical Journal of Australia*, **2**, 882.

Stoll, B. A. (1959) Recent advances in the chemotherapy of cancer. *Medical Journal of Australia*, **2**, 240.

Stoll, B. A. (1960a) Carzinophilin in advanced breast cancer. *Cancer (Philadelphia)*, **13**, 439.

Stoll, B. A. (1960b) Mitomycin C in advanced breast carcinoma—preliminary report. *Asian Medical Journal*, **3**, 1.

Stoll, B. A. (1960c) Nitromin and corticosteroids in the treatment of advanced cancer. *Acta Unio internationalis contra cancrum*, **16**, 919.

Stoll, B. A. (1962) Cyclophosphamide in disseminated malignant disease. *British Medical Journal*, **i**, 475.

Stoll, B. A. (1963) Thiotepa and breast cancer. *British Medical Journal*, **i**, 54.

Stoll, B. A. (1969) *Hormonal Management in Breast Cancer*. London: Pitman Medical.

Stoll, B. A. (1970) Evaluation of cyclophosphamide dosage schedules in breast cancer. *British Journal of Cancer*, in press.

Stoll, B. A. & Matar, J. (1961). Cyclophosphamide in advanced breast cancer—a clinical and haematological appraisal. *British Medical Journal*, **ii,** 283.

Swyer, G. I. M., Lee, A. E. & Masterson, J. P. (1961) Oestrogen excretion of patients with breast cancer. *British Medical Journal*, **i,** 617.

Taylor, S. G. (1962) Endocrine ablation in disseminated mammary carcinoma. *Surgery, Gynecology and Obstetrics*, **115,** 443.

Taylor, S. G. & Perlia, C. P. (1960) Evaluation of endocrine ablative surgery in the treatment of mammary carcinoma: a preliminary study on survival. In *Biological Activities of Steroids in Relation to Cancer*, p. 343, ed. Pincus, G. and Vollmer, E. P. New York: Academic Press.

Van Prohaska, J., Houttuin, E. & Kocandrle, U. (1966) Mammary carcinoma metastases response to bilateral adrenalectomy and oophorectomy. *Archives of Surgery*, **92,** 530.

Vogler, W. R., Furtado, V. P. & Huguley, C. M. (1968) Methotrexate for advanced cancer of the breast. *Cancer (Philadelphia)*, **21,** 26.

Weisberger, A. S. (1958) Direct instillation of nitrogen mustard in the management of malignant effusions. *Annals of the New York Academy of Science*, **68,** 1091.

Welbourn, R. B. (1967) Endocrine aspects of advanced mammary cancer. *Annals of the Royal College of Surgeons (Supplement)*, **41,** 131.

Wilson, C. B., Winternitz, W. W., Bertain, V. & Sizemore, G. (1966) Stereotaxic cryosurgery of the pituitary gland in carcinoma of the breast and other disorders. *Journal of the American Medical Association*, **19,** 8587.

Chapter 10

Synopsis of Endocrine Management in the Female and in the Male

BASIL A. STOLL

The relative merits and limitations of the established methods of endocrine therapy have been considered in the previous chapters. The very multiplicity of methods and agents available for endocrine palliation in late breast cancer has led to considerable confusion in the choice of treatment. The following survey attempts to place these therapeutic methods in perspective and in a rational order, and summarises their application to the individual patient. The case of the female patient with breast cancer will be considered first.

INDIVIDUALISATION OF THERAPY

It must be emphasised that only one patient in three with advanced breast cancer will show significant clinical response to hormonal manipulation of any kind. Because of this, and because of the very limited life expectation at this stage of the disease, every effort must be made to recognise not only those patients likely to benefit from endocrine therapy, but also the method of endocrine therapy most likely to yield benefit in that patient *at that particular stage of the disease.* If several alternative methods seem to offer a more or less equivalent prospect of palliation, humane considerations should dictate that the least noxious form of treatment is utilised first of all.

The writer's recommended sequence of treatment is outlined in the flow chart (Table 10.1), and is amplified later in the chapter. It will be noted that it is subdivided into nine subgroups by taking into account the age of the patient relative to the menopause, and also the predominant site of metastases. These are the major factors in a group which the writer terms 'biological determinants of hormonal response'. These are the factors which, to our present knowledge, influence the likelihood of hormonal

TABLE 10.1. *Scheme of sequential management in the hormonal therapy of female breast cancer*

		Soft tissue metastases	Bone metastases	Visceral metastases
Premenopausal (or if oestrogen excretion cyclical)	1.	Castration (Surgical or RT)	Oophorectomy (± Androgens)	Oophorectomy (± Corticoids)
	2.	Progestins *or* Androgens *or* *Adrenalectomy	Androgens plus Cytotoxics *or* *Adrenalectomy	Corticoids plus Cytotoxics *or* Adrenalectomy
	3.	†Hypophysectomy	†Hypophysectomy	†Hypophysectomy
Within 5 years of menopause (or if oestrogen excretion, but not cyclical)	1.	Progestins *or* Androgens	Androgens	Androgens *or* Progestins
	2.	Androgens plus Cytotoxics	Androgens plus Cytotoxics	Corticoids plus Cytotoxics
	3.	†Hypophysectomy	†Hypophysectomy	†Hypophysectomy
Over 5 years postmenopausal (or if oestrogen excretion, absent)	1.	Oestrogens	Androgens *or* Oestrogens	Oestrogens
	2.	Progestins *or* Androgens *or* *Adrenalectomy	Androgens plus Cytotoxics *or* *Adrenalectomy	Corticoids plus Cytotoxics *or* Adrenalectomy
	3.	†Hypophysectomy	†Hypophysectomy	†Hypophysectomy

* If good response to primary endocrine method, then adrenalectomy may be preferred to steroid therapy if the disease is advancing rapidly. If no objective response to primary endocrine method, there may still be a response by soft tissue metastases to progestins, by bone metastases to an androgen/cytotoxic combination, or by visceral metastases to a corticosteroid/cytotoxic combination. Further treatment in such cases is by radioactive yttrium ablation of the hypophysis.

† Following hypophysectomy, progestins may yield a response in the case of soft tissue metastases, or androgens in the case of bone metastases. Otherwise palliation is by radiotherapy or by cytotoxic agents.

response, by taking into account the host defence as well as the tumour potential (Stoll, 1969). Other biological determinants of hormonal response which may lead to a modification in the sequence of treatment *within* each subgroup are:

Extent of major metastases.
Duration of free-interval before the first recurrence.
Histology of tumour and hormonal profile of the patient.
Response to previous endocrine therapy.

For the last factor to be meaningful, it is essential that the nature of the response should have been established by *objective* measurements, and also, if possible, with the assistance

of biochemical and other indices of tumour activity (see Chapter 5).

The sequence of treatment within each subgroup may also need to be modified if the patient is very ill, or if symptoms are urgent and the disease is progressing rapidly. To take into account all these modifying factors, the physician presented with a woman suffering from advanced breast cancer can be helped to select the appropriate endocrine therapy by the answers to the following questions.

HOW ILL IS THE PATIENT?

The possible benefit to the patient from any form of endocrine therapy must be weighed against its possible deleterious effects. The patient who is very ill with widespread bone, liver, lung or brain metastases should obviously not be burdened with toxic or heroic forms of therapy. In such cases, corticosteroid therapy acts rapidly, and the undesirable side-effects of even large doses are of little consequence in a short course of treatment. It will cause euphoria and increase in appetite, and will often relieve the pain of bone, soft tissue, and liver metastases, correct hypercalcaemia, and decrease pressure symptoms in the brain or thoracic cavity.

If, and when, the general condition of the patient improves, it is then worth adding a *well-tolerated* cytotoxic agent in fractionated dosage. If further improvement then occurs, consideration can be given to hypophyseal ablation (either by transnasal hypophysectomy or by radioactive yttrium implant) in the older patient, or surgical castration in the premenopausal patient.

HOW URGENT ARE THE SYMPTOMS?

In the presence of rapidly advancing disease, it is obviously inadvisable to rely on slowly acting forms of endocrine therapy by themselves. This would apply to x-ray castration, oestrogen, androgen or progestin therapy. The presence of pain from bone metastases or from rapidly growing soft tissue tumour, requires urgent administration of radiation therapy if the disease is localised. If the tumour is so widespread that radiation is not possible, the choice lies between corticosteroid therapy and an attempt at surgical castration or major endocrine ablation.

The presence of extensive liver, lung or brain metastases suggests a limited expectation of life, and the first attempt at palliation should be by the administration of corticosteroid therapy combined with a cytotoxic agent, as mentioned in the section above. If the symptoms improve, then a trial of either oestrogen, androgen or progestin therapy may be added later according to the patient's

age group and the predominant site of metastasis. The effect of sex hormones is likely to be more prolonged (although more uncertain and more delayed) than that of the corticosteroid/cytotoxic combination.

On the other hand, in the presence of asymptomatic, slowly growing nodules or nodes, or even metastases in bone, liver or lung, endocrine treatment may be withheld completely. The patient may be better left in ignorance of these metastases for as long as possible, because endocrine control of tumour growth has only a limited duration, and is better kept in reserve for as long as symptoms are absent.

WHAT IS THE PATIENT'S AGE IN RELATION TO THE MENOPAUSE?

In premenopausal women, castration is the primary endocrine therapy of choice, and under the age of 35 or in the presence of bone metastases, the further addition of androgen therapy may increase the likelihood of palliation. It should be taken into account that major endocrine ablation is more effective in younger women and in women over the age of 60, than in the intermediate age group. The poorest results are in the five-year period following the menopause, the 'difficult' period for *every* form of endocrine therapy in breast cancer. The only patients in this group to show a hormonal response are usually those with a long recurrence-free interval, that is those in whom tumour growth has possibly been slowed up already by the intervening menopause.

Oestrogen therapy is not advised in the presence of persistent significant levels of oestrogen excretion by the postmenopausal patient (see Chapter 7). The older the patient, the more likely is a response to either oestrogen or androgen therapy. Corticosteroid therapy has the advantage that its benefits are independent of age group, and this applies also to progestin therapy in the writer's experience. Benefit from androgen therapy also appears to be less age dependent in the presence of bone metastases.

WHAT IS THE SITE AND EXTENT OF THE MAJOR METASTASES?

It is in the case of bone metastases that castration, bilateral adrenalectomy, hypophyseal ablation and androgen therapy lead to their best results, and of the four methods, hypophyseal ablation gives the highest remission rate. The palliation of soft tissue metastases by these four methods is not as successful, and in the case of visceral metastases they are least effective.

In the case of oestrogen and progestin therapy, on the other hand, the results are best in the treatment of soft tissue metastases, less satisfactory for visceral metastases such as those in the lung, pleura, or peritoneum, and least satisfactory for bone metastases. Corticosteroid therapy, unlike all the other methods mentioned, shows its most dramatic palliation in the case of brain, lung and liver metastases. It is interesting to note that bilateral adrenalectomy is *least* useful for metastases at these sites, suggesting that the term 'medical adrenalectomy' is an unsuitable description for corticone therapy in breast cancer.

Smaller lesions respond, in general, better than do larger lesions to endocrine therapy, but there are exceptions according to the site of metastasis. In the case of large visceral lesions in the liver or brain, major endocrine ablation yields very poor results, whereas corticosteroid therapy sometimes yields dramatic, although short lived, palliation in such cases. In the case of bone metastases, radiographic evidence of recalcification following castration, androgen therapy or major endocrine ablation, is as common in larger lesions as in smaller lesions, presumably because of the good vascularity of bone metastases. Soft tissue lesions in irradiated tissues usually respond poorly to any form of endocrine therapy, because of the poor vascularity of the stromal tissue.

WHAT WAS THE RECURRENCE-FREE INTERVAL?

A long recurrence-free interval might be expected to be associated with a slowly growing highly differentiated adenocarcinoma, but many of the cases do not demonstrate any such correlation. The heterogeneous microscopic structure of the majority of breast cancers often defies histological grading or typing, but this may not be the only reason for the absence of a correlation. Tumours may vary their growth rate during their life history in the body (Smithers, 1968), and a long free interval between mastectomy and the first recurrence may also signify slowing of tumour growth associated with immune mechanisms or with sensitivity to endogenous hormonal change. Whatever its cause, the longer the recurrence-free interval, the greater is the likelihood of favourable response to every form of endocrine therapy except corticosteroid therapy.

If the menopause has intervened between mastectomy and the first evidence of recurrence, a short recurrence-free interval indicates a low likelihood of hormone sensitivity, and usually a tumour rapidly progressing to death. A long recurrence-free interval in such cases (especially if associated with the presence of mixed sclerotic and lytic bone metastases) indicates, in the writer's experience, a high likelihood of sensitivity to hormonal manipulation. In neither case is there likely to be a response by the recurrence to castration. The choice between oestrogen and androgen therapy at this stage depends on the site of metastases and the result of serial examination of the cytohormonal pattern of the vaginal smear, or of the urinary oestrogen excretion (see Table 10.1).

WHAT WAS THE PATIENT'S RESPONSE TO PREVIOUS ENDOCRINE THERAPY?

In patients with a history of *objective* response to castration, there is a likelihood of subsequent favourable response to hypophysectomy in approximately 50 per cent of cases, to bilateral adrenalectomy in 40 per cent of cases, to androgen therapy in 30 per cent of cases and to oestrogen therapy in 20 per cent of cases. These figures compare with a 10 to 15 per cent likelihood or response to adrenalectomy or hypophysectomy in patients who have *failed* to respond to castration previously. Response to major endocrine ablation appears to be more likely in those patients with a short remission following castration (up to 15 months) than in those with a longer remission (Stewart, 1970).

It is uncertain whether a history of objective response to oestrogen or androgen therapy favours the likelihood of subsequent response to major endocrine ablation. A previous response to androgen therapy does, however, predict the likelihood of secondary response to oestrogens in 20 per cent of the cases in the writer's experience.

It is important to note that there are certain methods of endocrine therapy, such as hypophyseal ablation by radioactive yttrium, progestin and corticosteroid therapy, response to which is *not* clearly related to previous response to castration or sex steroid therapy. These methods of endocrine therapy may therefore be worth a trial in patients who show no response to primary or to secondary endocrine therapy.

WHAT IS THE TUMOUR HISTOLOGY AND THE PATIENT'S HORMONAL PROFILE?

The significance of these two factors in the determination of hormonal response is more uncertain than those previously mentioned. Most authorities have been unable to establish a correlation between histological grading in breast cancer, and the likelihood of response to major endocrine ablation or to oestrogen therapy. A few authors have suggested that as in the case of thyroid, prostatic and endometrial cancer, the more differentiated tumours are more likely to show a response. The general failure to confirm this in the case of breast cancer, may result from the difficulties in its grading and typing. A recent report suggests that tumour grading based on cell of origin (Murad, 1971), may provide better correlation with clinical hormone sensitivity.

The pretreatment hormonal profile of patients with breast cancer has been investigated by estimating the urinary excretion of steroids such as oestrogens, androgens, corticoids and their metabolites, or of peptides such as gonadotropin or prolactin. One or more of these assays have been suggested for use as indices in predicting tumour response to endocrine therapy (see Chapter 5). The one given the widest trials is Bulbrook's 'discriminant function' which now claims to distinguish patients with either a 35 per cent or a 16 per cent likelihood of response to major endocrine ablation.

It has been suggested that breast cancer in abnormally hirsute women is more likely to respond to oestrogens, while androgens should be used for those with a 'female configuration'. Such contrasexual hormone therapy may well have a scientific basis but the choice of steroid therapy based upon the physical appearance of the patient (Cornil, 1949; Green, 1966) has not been confirmed by hormonal excretion studies. The significance of the tumour sex chromatin in determining hormonal sensitivity is also uncertain (see Chapter 5).

Sequential Therapy

In view of the controlling influence exerted by the anterior pituitary over the other endocrine glands, the remission of tumour growth achieved by early hypophyseal ablation might be expected to equal that achieved by preliminary trial of lesser procedures.

This has been confirmed in clinical trials (see Chapter 9) but, because of the existence of hormone sensitivity in only a *minority* of patients' tumours, and because of the morbidity and mortality of hypophyseal ablation, the writer has for many years strongly advocated a sequential endocrine attack on the tumour. The aim is to derive the longest possible time in remission from more simple procedures, before proceeding to a trial of hypophyseal ablation in *selected* patients.

Endocrine therapy is merely a temporary palliative procedure in women with advanced breast cancer. The average duration of tumour growth control, and of consequent increase in survival, is only 12 to 24 months from the minor methods of therapy, but *several methods can be used sequentially with additive results*. By selecting for the individual patient suitable methods of endocrine therapy in combination with radiotherapy, cytotoxic agents and general medical care, the extra months of life achieved can be useful and pain-free. There is no justification for burdening the patient with severe mental or physical suffering, or the risk of a high operative mortality, unless justified by a *substantial likelihood* of achieving useful and pain-free survival. The physician treating late breast cancer requires considerable experience and compassion in order to make the correct choice of treatment.

Sequential endocrine management of advanced breast cancer is conveniently divided into three stages:

1. Primary therapy by castration or oestrogens (see Chapter 7).
2. Additive hormone therapy by androgens, progestins or corticosteroids (see Chapter 8).
3. Major endocrine ablation therapy (see Chapter 9).

In the presence of symptoms from localised manifestations of the tumour, surgery and radiotherapy may also have a place at any stage in the treatment.

PRELIMINARY SURGERY OR RADIOTHERAPY

It is important to stress that surgery and radiotherapy should be used to the limit of their ability in the management of recurrent or inoperable breast cancer *before* endocrine therapy is considered. Even if hormone sensitivity is present, endocrine control of tumour growth will have only a limited duration in the patient, and is therefore better kept in reserve for as long as possible.

Palliative simple mastectomy may be practised for the removal of a mobile ulcerated breast tumour even in the presence of metastases, *as long as malignant tissue is not transected by the operation.* Wide excision of a solitary skin nodule, or dissection of a mobile axillary node which has appeared many years after mastectomy, may be followed by freedom from further recurrence for a prolonged period.

Radiotherapy is practised for the palliation of localised soft tissue or bone lesions if they are causing symptoms. The growth of the primary tumour, multiple skin nodules, parasternal recurrence, axillary or supra-clavicular nodes, can be controlled in this way for periods usually ranging from 6 to 24 months. Energetic radiotherapy to a solitary slowly growing metastasis may be followed by a considerable interval before the appearance of other metastases.

The relief of pain from bone metastases which follows within two weeks of radiation is almost diagnostic, and subsequent recalcification of bone metastases is not uncommon. Bone metastases liable to pathological fracture should be irradiated urgently and, if weight bearing, should be submitted to internal fixation if the patient's general condition justifies it. Pressure symptoms due to cerebral or mediastinal metastases can also be relieved by radiation, although usually only for a short period. Laminectomy is indicated as an emergency on the appearance of symptoms suggesting pressure from metastases upon the spinal cord, radiation therapy being postponed until *after* the operation.

'PROPHYLACTIC' CASTRATION

Castration may have been carried out at the time of mastectomy. It has recently been shown that it significantly delays recurrence of tumour only in the presence of widespread axillary node metastases at operation. Whether prophylactic castration should be surgical or radiotherapeutic in such cases depends on the tumour rate of growth, the histology and the degree of spread, as radiotherapeutic castration takes three to six months to establish its effect (see Chapter 7).

PRIMARY ENDOCRINE THERAPY

The presence or absence of measurable oestrogen secretion in the body will decide the primary form of endocrine therapy in advanced breast cancer—castration or oestrogen therapy. Ovarian oestrogen secretion is, of course, assumed in premenopausal women, but in women within five years following the menopause, the vaginal smear pattern or the urinary oestrogen excretion should be assayed weekly for a month. Oestrogen levels above 10 μg in 24 hours, or cyclical fluctuation in oestrogen secretion, are not uncommon and are suggestive of persistent ovarian secretion.

Evidence of active tumour growth and assessment of regression should be based both on clinical measurement and on serial estimation of biochemical indices of tumour activity, such as the phosphohexose isomerase and lactic dehydrogenase levels in the serum (see Chapter 5). If bone metastases are present, serial estimations of serum calcium and serum alkaline phosphatase are required in addition. After these initial investigations, management of the patient is as follows.

PATIENTS WITH PERSISTENT OVARIAN SECRETION

Therapeutic castration is advised as the primary method of endocrine treatment for all premenopausal patients with recurrent, metastatic or inoperable primary breast cancer. It is indicated also for postmenopausal patients if serial estimation of the vaginal smear pattern or urinary oestrogen excretion suggests persistent ovarian secretion.

Castration by surgery is preferred in cases of clinical urgency, including the presence of 'inflammatory' carcinoma, hypercalcaemia and painful bone metastases, and in the presence of lung, pleural, brain or liver metastases. Radiation castration is equally effective in ablating oestrogen secretion, but is suitable only for slowly growing soft tissue tumours, as it requires three to six months to show an effect.

Following castration, periodic assays of the vaginal smear pattern or of the urinary oestrogen excretion are useful to assist in the decision on further treatment when tumour control is lost. In addition to clinical measurements of the lesions, the writer recommends periodic measurements of the relevant indices of tumour activity in order to confirm a clinical estimate of tumour control. (It should be remembered that in the presence of bone metastases, the serum alkaline phosphatase level may show an initial 'flare' before demonstrating a slow fall towards normal.)

A short course of corticosteroid therapy may useful precede surgical castration in the patient with hypercalcaemia, or in the ill patient with visceral metastases. Added androgen therapy, started immediately after castration, is advised in the presence of bone metastases, or in the case of patients under 35 years of age.

Castration is the simplest effective endocrine method of achieving tumour regression in the premenopausal patient. In the larger published series of surgical or radiation castration, the reported tumour remission rate varies between 15 and 37 per cent. The average duration of control in responding cases is between 10 and 25 months, and life is prolonged on an average from 18 to 22 months in responding cases, compared to untreated cases.

There is a difference in the response rate according to the site of metastases. Bone metastases are the most likely to respond, with relief of pain within one or two weeks, and the earliest signs of recalcification of lytic lesions within about three months. Objective evidence of regression of breast tumour, metastatic nodules or nodes is less likely and usually takes at least eight weeks to manifest. Although regression of visceral metastases in the liver, brain, lungs or serous cavities is the least likely, an attempt at castration is worthwhile in such cases, possibly in combination with corticosteroid therapy.

The patient's age may influence the remission rate, in that tumour regression from castration is said to be less likely in women under 35 years of age. On the other hand, the history of a recurrence-free period after mastectomy of over two years increases the likelihood of response to castration.

'Medical castration' by androgens as primary therapy carries with it the unwanted side-effect of masculinisation, and yields a much lower percentage, and shorter duration, of objectively demonstrable tumour remission. For these reasons androgens are better used as secondary therapy, and in patients responding favourably to surgical or radiation castration there is a 30 per cent likelihood of a second tumour remission from androgen therapy later.

POSTMENOPAUSAL PATIENTS WITH CESSATION OF OVARIAN SECRETION

In some patients within five years following the menopause, serial urinary estimations or vaginal smear examination may show persistence of oestrogen secretion but below 10 μg in 24 hours and with no evidence of cyclical fluctuation. For these patients, progestins or androgens are preferred as the primary method of endocrine treatment, because oestrogen therapy in such patients involves a danger of tumour exacerbation. This is the 'difficult' group of patients for every type of endocrine therapy in breast cancer.

The addition of cytotoxic agents to androgen therapy will increase the likelihood of remission in this age group, and also prolong its duration. For this purpose 5-fluorouracil or methotrexate are suggested by the writer in the presence of soft tissue metastases, while alkylating agents, such as cyclophosphamide in continuous low dosage, are safer in the presence of bone or visceral metastases. Alternatively, progestin therapy can be used for soft tissue metastases in this age group. In the presence of hypercalcaemia, or in the very ill patient with liver, peritoneal or brain metastases, corticosteroid therapy is preferred to either progestin or androgen therapy. Its administration also may be combined with cytotoxic therapy, particularly the use of alkylating agents.

Oestrogen therapy is advised as the primary method of endocrine treatment only in the *absence* of significant oestrogen excretion. The presence of an atrophic pattern in the vaginal smear suggests such treatment to be safe. The risk of tumour aggravation is, in any case, very low in patients more than five years postmenopausal, and oestrogens yield a higher proportion of tumour remissions in older postmenopausal women than does any other method of endocrine therapy.

In the patients for whom oestrogen therapy is prescribed, monthly assays of the vaginal smear pattern are useful. By this means can be determined the lowest possible dosage of oestrogen for the patient, compatible with achieving a karyopyknotic (cornification) index in the vaginal smear of 50 per cent or more. There is no need to increase the dose of oestrogen as long as the disease appears clinically to be under control and biochemical parameters of tumour activity remain low.

If, however, serial observations show a rising trend in the level of these indices, and the cornification index of the vaginal smear falls below 50 per cent, then the dose of oestrogen should be increased (taking into account the patient's cardiovascular condition). If this fails to raise the index, parenteral forms of oestrogen therapy such as oestradiol monobenzoate or stilboestrol diphosphate may be tried as an alternative, in case oestrogen absorption in the bowel is at fault.

In the larger published series, the tumour remission rate for oestrogen therapy in advanced breast cancer has been reported as being between 29 and 37 per cent, the remission rate increasing with increasing number of years past the menopause. The writer has noted tumour regression in 49 per cent of patients over 70 when oestrogen administration was adequate. The average duration of tumour control is 16 months, and life is prolonged on an average by 17 months in favourably responding cases compared with untreated cases. Tumour response to oestrogen therapy is more likely in patients with a history of a recurrence-free period after mastectomy of over two years.

The earliest signs of tumour regression appears within six to eight weeks of initiating therapy, and a trial of oestrogen cannot be declared a failure unless maintained for at least three months. The healing of a large ulcerated primary tumour, or the regression of metastatic nodules or nodes, is common in elderly patients after oestrogen therapy. However, relief of pain from bone metastases and recalcification of lytic metastases are seen less commonly from oestrogen therapy. Thus, in the presence of widespread, painful bone metastases the writer prefers to initiate treatment with androgens. Regression of visceral metastases, especially of lung and pleural infiltration, is not uncommon from oestrogen therapy in the older patient, and in responding cases there is sometimes prolongation of survival for several years.

Oestrogen therapy is given continuously by most physicians, being maintained for as long as tumour control persists. The writer prefers intermittent therapy, administration being stopped when tumour regression is maximal and when the tumour reactivates in such a case, further oestrogen therapy may cause a second regression. The intermittent method decreases the hazards of oestrogen therapy (see Chapter 7) and is particularly useful in older patients if the drug administration is associated with serious side-effects, such as fluid retention or cardiac embarrassment.

SECONDARY ENDOCRINE THERAPY

Clinical evidence of relapse appears on the average after one to two years, response to oestrogen therapy, whether continuous or intermittent methods are used. When the tumour no longer responds to oestrogen therapy, the mere stopping of oestrogen administration will yield a withdrawal response in approximately 30 per cent of cases. Advantage should be taken of such a possibility and, except in cases with urgent symptoms, the writer suggests at least two months free from therapy after loss of tumour control from oestrogens, before proceeding to another form of endocrine therapy.

In the majority of patients, clinical evidence of relapse appears within 18 months of castration. If, when tumour reactivation occurs after castration, it is found that the cornification index of the vaginal smear or the oestrogen excretion level are rising, then tumour autonomy may not necessarily be the cause of the relapse.

Further endocrine management, after failure of response or loss of response to castration or to oestrogen therapy, depends on the urgency of the symptoms. If *urgent*, and if there was a good response to the primary endocrine method, a trial of bilateral adrenalectomy is advised, and remission is likely in 40 per cent of these patients. If the patient's symptoms are urgent, but there was no objective response to the primary endocrine method, then a corticosteroid/cytotoxic combination is advised for visceral metastases, or an androgen/cytotoxic combination for bone metastases.

If the patient's symptoms are *not urgent*, major endocrine ablation may be postponed, and a trial of steroid therapy by androgens, progestins or corticosteroids is indicated. The steroid is selected after consideration of the 'biological determinants of hormonal response' in the patient, as described at the beginning of this chapter. In addition, if it is possible, the hormonal sensitivity of the tumour to sex steroids may be looked for by the isomerase inhibition test (see Chapter 5).

ANDROGEN THERAPY

When tumour reactivation occurs after previous response to castration, objective response to androgens is likely in about 30 per cent of cases. In patients not previously responding to castration, response to androgen therapy is seen *overall* in fewer than 10 per cent of cases, but, in the writer's experience, the proportion is likely to be much higher in the case of bone metastases. After loss of response to previous oestrogen therapy, a secondary response to androgen therapy is likely overall in about 20 to 30 per cent of cases, but again in a higher proportion in the presence of bone metastases.

In the larger published series the overall tumour remission rate from androgen therapy has been reported as being between 15 and 22 per cent. The average duration of tumour control is from 8 to 11 months, and life is prolonged on an average by 9 to 14 months in responding cases compared with untreated cases. As in the case of oestrogens, tumour response to androgen therapy is more likely with a history of a long recurrence-free interval after mastectomy, and the tumour remission rate tends to increase with increasing number of years past the menopause. Objective evidence of response to androgens is rare in the first five years after the menopause, except in the presence of osteoblastic bone metastases, or a recurrence-free interval straddling the menopause, or the history of response to previous castration.

The earliest signs of tumour regression may appear within six to eight weeks of initiating androgen therapy but is often delayed, so that a trial cannot be declared a failure unless continued for at least three months. Although response by bone metastases is more likely, regression of the primary breast tumour, local soft tissue and visceral metastases is less likely, from androgen than from oestrogen therapy. Commonly there is subjective benefit in the form of gain in weight and increase in appetite as a result of the anabolic effect of androgen therapy, and improvement in anaemia due to a stimulating effect on erythropoiesis.

Androgen therapy is given continuously by most physicians, being maintained for as long as tumour regression lasts. On stopping hormone administration, a 'withdrawal' response may be seen in 10 per cent of the cases. As an alternative, androgen therapy may be given intermittently, administration being stopped when tumour regression is maximal. This method is preferred by the writer because of the lesser tendency to masculinisation which is associated with its use. When the tumour reactivates in such cases, a further course of therapy may yield a second regression.

When there has been no response to castration or to oestrogen therapy previously, a combination of cytotoxic therapy and androgen gives a greater likelihood and more prolonged remission than either method alone. It is especially useful in the first five years after the menopause, when the response rate to major endocrine ablation is very low. The addition of an alkylating type of cytotoxic agent is recommended in the presence of bone metastases, but in the presence of soft tissue metastases the addition of 5-fluorouracil or methotrexate is preferred.

A trial of androgen therapy is therefore indicated especially if there has been a good response to primary endocrine therapy, but in all cases with widespread bone metastases. In such cases, it is usually more effective than primary oestrogen therapy. Androgens should always be considered before pituitary ablation, in the treatment of bone metastases, except in the presence of hypercalcaemia, when corticosteroid or phosphate therapy are indicated instead.

PROGESTIN THERAPY

Progestins are often useful as primary therapy in the management of soft tissue metastases in the recently postmenopausal patient with significant, but not cyclical, oestrogen excretion levels. Progestins are also useful as secondary therapy in the presence of soft tissue or visceral metastases in patients who have shown a doubtful response to primary castration or oestrogen therapy. Such patients rarely respond to secondary androgen therapy except in the presence of bone metastases. Beneficial response to secondary progestin therapy is not clearly related to previous hormonal response, in the writer's experience.

Progestin therapy leads to its best results in the treatment of soft tissue tumour involving the breast, metastatic nodules or nodes, while regression of bone or visceral metastases is rare from its use. The earliest signs of tumour regression usually appear within six to eight weeks of initiating therapy, and although the average duration of tumour control is nine months, long remissions are claimed in some reports. 'Withdrawal' response similar to that seen after oestrogen or androgen therapy, has been noted by the writer also with progestin therapy. Subjective benefit is fortunately common with these agents, associated with a gain in weight and improvement in appetite, and unwanted side-effects are usually mild at the recommended dosage.

Because of the relative absence of side-effects, progestins are often used as an alternative to androgens, especially in the presence of soft tissue metastases. A trial of progestin therapy is indicated before pituitary ablation is considered, in patients with slowly growing soft tissue or visceral metastases which have failed to respond to primary therapy by oestrogens or castration. It is interesting to note that in combination with small doses of oestrogen, progestin therapy may cause tumour regression in breast cancer even *after* hypophysectomy, whereas oestrogen therapy alone has never been shown to cause a response at this stage.

SECONDARY OESTROGEN THERAPY

Secondary oestrogen therapy may be effective in patients treated primarily by androgens, but is safe only if serial vaginal smears show absence of significant oestrogen secretion. There is an *overall* likelihood of tumour remission in 20 per cent of cases from secondary oestrogen therapy following previous favourable response to androgen therapy. The likelihood of response to secondary oestrogen therapy is, however, higher in the presence of soft tissue metastases, and increases with increasing postmenopausal age.

CORTICOSTEROID THERAPY

Corticosteroid therapy is useful even in the absence of objective response to primary therapy, and is particularly indicated if insensitivity to sex hormones is suggested by the isomerase inhibition test. In addition, corticosteroids are always preferred to other forms of steroid therapy in the case of a very ill patient with extensive visceral metastases involving the liver, lung, pleura, brain or peritoneal cavity. They are useful also in the relief of pain from widely disseminated bone metastases and, together with phosphates, corticosteroids are life-saving agents in the reduction of the serum calcium level in hypercalcaemia.

The likelihood of benefit from corticosteroid therapy is independent of previous response to sex hormone manipulation, and is also independent of the patient's age group relative to the menopause. For these reasons, it has been suggested that the effect of corticosteroids in breast cancer is not that of a 'medical adrenalectomy' but is mainly exerted through an anti-inflammatory mechanism which decreases vascular permeability around the tumour and its metastases.

Corticosteroid therapy, especially in combination with alkylating agents, usually causes rapid but temporary improvement in the pain of liver metastases, in the coma of cerebral metastases, or in the dyspnoea from pulmonary metastases. Metastatic pleural and peritoneal effusions often decrease in size under such therapy. The regression of soft tissue metastases and the recalcification of lytic bone metastases following corticosteroids alone are rarely complete and rarely last longer than nine months. However, a combination of corticosteroids with alkylating agents may lead to remissions lasting a year or longer even in the presence of extensive bone, soft tissue, pleural or peritoneal metastases.

The great advantage of corticosteroid therapy is the feeling of well-being and the relief of pain it induces within a few days in the majority of patients treated. The steroid, usually in combination with a well-tolerated alkylating agent, is especially useful in the treatment of patients who are too ill for any form of endocrine ablative surgery, and in those who have shown no objective response to the primary method of endocrine therapy.

MAJOR ENDOCRINE ABLATION THERAPY

When relapse occurs after successful primary therapy by castration or oestrogen, major endocrine ablation may be indicated in the presence of urgent symptoms. When relapse occurs after secondary steroid therapy, there is no endocrine alternative to major ablation therapy. It yields approximately 40 per cent likelihood of remission if the patient is more than five years postmenopausal, if there has been a long recurrence-free interval, or if there was a favourable response to castration. The likelihood of remission is said to be about 35 per cent if the urinary 'discriminant function' is positive. In all other cases the likelihood of remission is less than 5 per cent.

The choice between bilateral adrenalectomy and transfrontal hypophysectomy has been widely debated. The latter has shown superior results in controlled trials but requires the services of a skilled neurosurgeon. The relatively minor morbidity of the radioactive yttrium or transnasal methods of pituitary ablation may be justified in patients who appear to be too ill for more major endocrine ablation therapy, or in those who have not responded either to primary therapy by castration or oestrogens, or to secondary additive hormone therapy.

BILATERAL ADRENALECTOMY

The likelihood of response to adrenalectomy varies according to the site of metastasis. Tumour regression is more likely in the case of metastases in bone, soft tissue, lung or pleura, and is less likely for those in the brain, liver or peritoneum. In the presence of *large* liver, brain or peritoneal metastases the operation is contraindicated (although corticosteroid therapy is often beneficial in such cases). Relief of the pain of bone metastases is sometimes dramatic after adrenalectomy but is often transitory, and only in a minority of patients is it followed by recalcification of lytic bone metastases. The mechanism of this transitory pain relief is uncertain (see Chapter 22).

Bilateral adrenalectomy may be advised instead of steroid therapy by progestins or androgens, if the disease is advancing rapidly, and there was a good response to the primary method of endocrine therapy. There is little doubt that added ovariectomy increases not only the proportion of patients responding to bilateral adrenalectomy, but also the duration of tumour regression. There is no doubt also that tumour growth remissions after bilateral adrenalectomy are longer and more complete than those that occur after corticosteroid therapy.

HYPOPHYSEAL ABLATION

The site of metastasis affects the likelihood of response to hypophyseal ablation in that tumour regression is most likely in the case of metastases in bone, lung, pleura or soft tissue, and is less likely for those in the liver, brain or peritoneum. As in the case of bilateral adrenalectomy, pain relief after hypophyseal ablation is sometimes dramatic. In the majority of cases, however, it is of short duration, and only occasionally is it followed by evidence of recalcification of lytic bone metastases. For this reason it has been suggested that the relief of pain by hypophyseal ablation may be due to trauma to the diencephalon.

Objective evidence of favourable response to hypophyseal ablation may be achieved in a proportion of patients who have not responded previously either to the primary or secondary methods of endocrine therapy. This applies especially to the transnasal radioactive yttrium method of pituitary ablation, and its relatively minor morbidity recommends its use in such cases.

POST-ABLATION THERAPY

Localised radiation therapy is often useful for symptomatic relief in the presence of widespread breast cancer which has ceased to respond to endocrine methods. Relief of pain from bone metastases, healing of malignant skin ulceration, and relief of pressure symptoms from axillary, supraclavicular, cerebral or mediastinal metastases can usually be achieved by such therapy.

When the tumour reactivates after pituitary ablation, there may be evidence of pituitary secretion persisting after the operation. It is especially in such cases that a trial of additive hormone therapy may be considered. A trial of progestin and oestrogen in combination has led to a response in some cases, particularly those with soft tissue metastases. A course of the androgen fluoxymesterone may lead to a response in others, particularly those with bone metastases. Other hormonal methods of therapy have not proved of any value at this stage, apart from the use of large doses of corticosteroids, and further palliation is possible only from the use of radiation therapy or of cytotoxic agents (see Chapter 9).

Inadequate Hormonal Trials

It is tragically common to see case histories of patients with advanced breast cancer in whom several steroids and cytotoxic agents (often in various combinations) have been tried empirically and rejected, all within a period of a few months, and usually without adequate dosage or proper evaluation.

The writer reported on 170 women over 70 in whom a trial of oestrogen therapy was initiated for breast cancer (Stoll and Ackland, 1970). This is the age group where oestrogen therapy leads to the highest likelihood of tumour regression, and the longest examples of tumour control. In 92 patients the oestrogen was persisted with for an adequate period (longer than two months) and led to clearcut objective evidence of tumour regression in 49 per cent. In the remaining 78 patients, the hormone was prematurely discontinued and the inadequate trial declared a failure after periods varying from two weeks to two months. (Intolerance was the cause of suspending treatment in only 11 per cent.)

The reason for inadequate hormonal trials is the tendency to regard additive hormone therapy as a capricious and unpredictable modality worth a few weeks trial on a 'hit or miss' basis as long as there are no side-effects! It must be emphasised that all forms of additive hormone therapy (like all methods of endocrine ablation therapy) involve the acceptance of some degree of unwanted effects. A decision to attempt additive hormone therapy should be as carefully weighed and planned as a decision to carry out major endocrine ablation. If used selectively according to the principles mentioned in this chapter, the risks of aggravating tumour growth are very small, and the rewards may be high especially in the older age group.

The writer advises strongly that for the initiation of oestrogen, androgen or progestin therapy, the patient should be observed frequently during the first 7 to 14 days (and preferably hospitalised if the patient is in poor condition) for the following reasons:

Preliminary intolerance due to nausea or vomiting is common, especially with oestrogen administration, but can be overcome with administration of pyridoxine or antiemetics, and with encouragement of the patient.

Fluid retention, especially with oestrogen administration, may cause increase in existing symptoms of heart failure. This can be counteracted by adjustment of dosage and prescription of diuretics and potassium supplements.

General malaise or pyrexia occur not uncommonly in the first few days of therapy, but such cases often go on to tumour control if the patient is reassured and hormonal administration is persisted with.

Local symptomatic changes, such as aggravation of bone pains or increase in itching of skin nodules at the outset of hormonal therapy, may represent an immunological reaction in the tumour or its stroma, or may be evidence of tumour aggravation. The hormonal dosage should be cut for a week or so, and if symptoms persist, the aggravating hormone must be withdrawn and a short course of corticosteroid therapy substituted. The development of hypercalcaemia within two weeks of initiating therapy is also regarded by some as evidence of tumour aggravation.

Serial assessment of serum enzyme and calcium levels in the first two weeks after initiating hormonal therapy will help to elucidate the significance of symptomatic changes noted above, or may provide early prediction of a clinical response at a later date.

Breast Cancer in the Male

Endocrine therapy is necessary sooner or later in the management of the majority of male breast cancer patients because recurrence and metastases are so common. The prognosis of the disease is relatively worse than in the female, and it is likely that the disease is widely disseminated in the vast majority of patients, even before curative therapy is attempted.

HORMONAL CAUSATION OF MALE BREAST CANCER

The development of breast cancer probably reflects a hormonal imbalance between

androgens and oestrogens existing from 10 to 15 years before the clinical onset of the disease (Bulbrook, 1966). It could arise from:

Abnormal steroid production, induced by changes in anterior pituitary or adrenocortical activity.
Abnormal metabolism of steroids by the liver.
Abnormal susceptibility of breast tissue to normal concentrations of steroids.

Mammary cancer has been induced in male mice by castration and oestrogen administration (Lacassagne, 1936a). For this reason, long-continued oestrogen therapy has been suggested as a possible cause of male breast cancer, and the appearance of breast cancer after oestrogen therapy for prostatic cancer has been adduced as an example (Abramson and Warshawksy, 1948; Howard and Grosjean, 1949). Such an occurrence is however extremely rare considering the number of patients so treated, and, in addition, a high acid phosphatase level has been demonstrated in biopsies of such breast tumours (Campbell et al, 1962). This suggests that they are metastases of the prostatic cancer to breast tissue, which has become hyperplastic as a result of oestrogen therapy.

There is a recent report of the development of breast cancer in two males who underwent castration and subsequently took oestrogens orally, by implant and by breast inunction for a prolonged period (Symmers, 1968). It is important to establish the basic genetic and hormonal constitution in such cases, as an increased incidence of male breast cancer has been shown in association with Klinefelter's syndrome (Jackson et al, 1965). Diagnosis of this condition is suggested by the presence of gynaecomastia, aspermia and testicular hypoplasia and confirmed by increase in urinary gonadotropin excretion and the typical chromosome pattern in a buccal smear. The syndrome is associated with subnormal androgen excretion levels, although there is usually *hyperplasia* of the Leydig cells.

The Sertoli cells of the testis secrete oestrogens, while the Leydig cells secrete androgens, and hyperplasia of either group of cells can be associated with the development of gynaecomastia (Collins and Cameron, 1964; Collins and Symington, 1964). The presence of gynaecomastia and epithelial hyperplasia is reported in an abnormally high proportion of some male breast cancer series, although others find the association to be rare (Treves, 1959). In two major series (Gilbert, 1933; Liechty, Davis and Gleysteen, 1967) the proportion with associated gynaecomastia was 19 per cent and 12·5 per cent respectively, the gynaecomastia in these cases usually being unilateral.

There is a high incidence both of breast cancer and gynaecomastia in males of the Bantu race. The gynaecomastia in these cases is thought to be due to failure of oestrogen inactivation by a damaged liver, associated with vitamin B deficiency (Davies, 1949). The peak age incidence of male breast cancer is about 10 years later than that of gynaecomastia, and this time interval would be compatible with a causal relationship (Bonser, Dossett and Jull, 1961).

Oestriol production is said to be relatively high and oestrone production low in males who have developed breast cancer (Zumoff et al, 1966). Disturbed thyroid function is capable of causing such an abnormality, or alternatively it has been suggested that breast cancer is itself capable of secreting oestriol (Adams and Wong, 1968). It is, therefore, possible that the disturbance in the oestrogen component ratio is a result rather than a cause of male breast cancer.

RATIONALE OF ENDOCRINE THERAPY IN MALE BREAST CANCER

Whatever the hormonal imbalance responsible for the development of breast cancer in the male, it seems likely that once established, the continued growth of the tumour in some patients may require the presence of androgens (Burrows and Horning, 1952). The beneficial results of orchidectomy then follow from withdrawal of testicular androgens, and the exacerbating influence of androgens on the tumour, noted later, would also be explained on the basis of the 'androgen dependence' hypothesis (Figure 10.1). After a shorter or longer period, the initially hormone-sensitive tumour loses this androgen dependence and becomes autonomous.

The palliative effect which has been reported from oestrogen therapy in occasional cases has been explained on the basis of pituitary inhibition, or the less likely mechanism of direct antagonism to androgens at the target organ. A direct effect upon the metabolism of the tumour cells is, however, also possible (see Chapter 7). Whatever the mechanism, there is no doubt that oestrogen therapy is a relatively much less successful form of contrasexual hormone therapy in the male than is androgen therapy in the female.

may delay the onset of recurrence, thus giving the patient a longer period of physical and psychological well-being. The indication for prophylactic castration is greater in the male than in the female, because of the higher incidence of tumour recurrence and dissemination in the male.

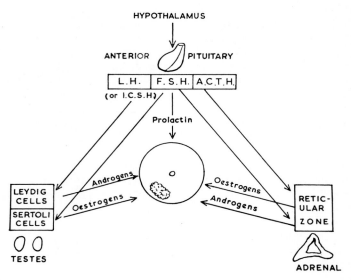

FIGURE 10.1. Diagrammatic representation of the hormonal factors which influence the growth of breast cancer in the male. (Modified from Valk and Owen, 1954. Figure reproduced from Stoll, 1969, by permission of Pitman Medical.)

It is possible that both forms of therapy act by upsetting the existing androgen-oestrogen balance in the body, the environment of which the tumour finds favourable for growth.

SEQUENTIAL ENDOCRINE THERAPY IN MALE BREAST CANCER

PROPHYLACTIC CASTRATION

Subcapsular orchidectomy as a prophylactic measure is advised at the time of mastectomy, especially in those patients with extensively invaded axillary nodes and aged over 65. Even if it does not actually prolong life, it

PRELIMINARY RADIOTHERAPY

Radiotherapy is always advisable as the first method of treatment for the control of soft tissue recurrences or metastases in nodes. The pain of bone metastases can also be relieved by radiotherapy within two weeks, and pressure symptoms from cerebral, mediastinal or soft tissue metastases may be temporarily alleviated.

PRIMARY ENDOCRINE THERAPY BY ORCHIDECTOMY

Objective evidence of tumour regression is seen in 68 per cent of male breast cancer patients following castration (Treves, 1959), approximately twice the proportion seen in the female. The average duration of such tumour growth remission is 30 months.

In the vast majority of patients with bone metastases, castration results in relief of pain which is not uncommonly maintained for two to five years. Healing of an ulcerated primary tumour and regression in either soft tissue or visceral metastases are also not uncommon, but rarely maintained for over two years. No relationship has been established between the histological grading of the cancer, and the likelihood of remission from castration. Nevertheless, as in the female, the longer the interval between mastectomy and recurrence, the longer the period of tumour growth remission following castration (Treves, 1959).

Subcapsular orchidectomy is widely practised but it is essential that it should ensure removal of *all* testicular tissue. This can be checked by the plasma testosterone level, as this steroid is almost completely synthesised in the testis. Persistent testosterone secretion has been reported in a high proportion of a group of patients treated by subcapsular orchidectomy, and in these cases the secretion was later abolished by total orchidectomy (O'Conor, Chiang and Grayhack, 1963).

Atrophy of the androgen-secreting Leydig cells of the testicular tissue will follow x-ray irradiation of the testis (Collins and Pugh, 1964), and irradiation is followed by marked decrease in the androgen excretion level. Complete suppression of androgen excretion requires very high dosage which would not be practicable, because the scrotal skin does not tolerate irradiation well.

SECONDARY ENDOCRINE THERAPY

Androgen administration is likely to cause exacerbation of pain in bone metastases from male breast cancer (Farrow and Adair, 1942; Huggins, 1954). Androgen-induced growth stimulation of visible lesions has not been described, but androgen provocation may be demonstrated biochemically, if testosterone propionate 100 mg is injected daily for three days. (The test is used in a similar way to the acid phosphatase stimulation test in prostatic cancer.) After control of the tumour growth has been lost from castration, an increase in the serum level of phosphohexose isomerase following androgen injection suggests persistent sensitivity of the breast cancer to sex hormones. Bilateral adrenalectomy, hypophyseal ablation or oestrogen therapy would then be indicated in preference to corticosteroid therapy under these circumstances.

MAJOR ENDOCRINE ABLATION

Major endocrine ablation has been recommended after castration has lost its control of tumour activity, but the reports of major ablation therapy are on very small groups of patients, and its place in management is, therefore, difficult to evaluate. From wide experience in the management of male breast cancer, Treves (1959) considers major endocrine ablation to be less useful than corticosteroid therapy. The majority of patients with tumour reactivation after castration are in any case too old or too ill for major surgery.

In a review of the literature, objective evidence of tumour regression has been shown following bilateral adrenalectomy in 9 out of 12 cases reported (McLaughlin et al, 1965). Temporary regression of lung or bone metastases has been noted in 5 out of 6 cases (Houttuin, van Prohaska and Taxman, 1967). All responding patients had previously responded to orchidectomy, and the average duration of control from the two procedures was 4·5 years. Of three patients in this series treated instead by hypophyseal ablation, there was not one who responded, although other authors have reported favourable response following hypophysectomy in occasional cases (Ray and Pearson, 1956; Luft et al, 1958). It is possible that the importance of pituitary prolactin in the control of female breast cancer is not paralleled by similar pituitary control in the case of male breast cancer.

CORTICOSTEROID THERAPY

The palliative results of corticosteroid therapy in male breast cancer are similar to those seen in the female and described in Chapter 8. This is the treatment advised in the majority of patients with male breast cancer reactivating after castration, but others might prefer to reserve corticosteroid therapy for such patients as are unfit for major endocrine ablation therapy.

Objective evidence of partial tumour regression is not uncommon, but complete healing of ulcerated breast tumour or sclerosis of lytic bone metastases is rarely seen from corticosteroid therapy. Subjective benefit with euphoria, increase in weight and appetite, and relief of pain are common. Palliation from corticosteroids, like that from castration, seems to be more prolonged in the male than in the female. Control of metastatic bone pain for two years or more is not uncommon in the male, in the writer's experience (Stoll, 1969).

The dosage of prednisolone recommended is 20 to 30 mg daily, and can be given as a single dose in the morning. The dose is increased to 100 mg daily in the presence of urgent symptoms from hypercalcaemia, brain or lung metastases, but is reduced once control of symptoms is established. It is commonly found necessary to increase the dose again later in order to maintain control over a prolonged period.

OESTROGEN THERAPY

Occasional benefit from oestrogen treatment is reported in advanced male breast cancer (Huggins and Taylor, 1955), although castration is always to be preferred as the primary method of endocrine treatment. Favourable response to oestrogen therapy was found in only 2 out of 14 patients treated by 15 mg

stilboestrol or 1·5 mg ethinyloestradiol daily (Treves, 1959). Corticosteroids are preferred to oestrogens as secondary therapy after loss of control from castration because, contrary to general belief, the results of oestrogen therapy in male breast cancer are poor and unpredictable.

There is no advantage to be gained from the addition of oestrogen therapy to castration, in the primary treatment of disseminated cancer of the breast in the male. Of 7 patients treated by diethylstilboestrol in combination with orchidectomy, temporary tumour regression resulted in only 3 cases (Keddie and Morris, 1967).

PROGESTIN THERAPY

A trial of progestins has been attempted with occasional success in male patients with breast cancer (Geller and Volk, 1961). The place of such therapy is not clear. Cyproterone acetate (a progestational steroid with antiandrogenic properties) has been used with occasional success in prostatic cancer and its use has been suggested also in male breast cancer.

CONCLUSION

There is no evidence that the expectation of life following early major endocrine ablation in breast cancer is any greater than that from surgery delayed after an attempt at conservative therapy. Thus, for each patient with breast cancer, the most suitable method of endocrine therapy is selected in a particular sequence, selecting less drastic forms of treatment first of all, and progressing with the advancing stages of the disease to more major methods. Such steps depend mainly on the age of the patient in relation to the menopause, the site and size of the major metastases, the urgency of the symptoms, the general condition of the patient, and the history of previous hormonal response.

Response to every form of endocrine therapy (apart from corticosteroid therapy) is more likely in the presence of a longer recurrence-free period after mastectomy and in the presence of smaller volumes of tumour. Corticosteroids are preferred in the very ill patients with large visceral metastases or hypercalcaemia. Both major endocrine ablation and additive therapy by sex hormones show their poorest results within five years of the menopause. Oestrogen and progestins show their best results in the older patient with soft tissue metastases, while androgen is more suitable for the patient with bone metastases. Combinations of steroids with cytotoxic agents also have their special indications, and yield more prolonged remissions than either method alone.

Specific biochemical aids to the selection of therapy are available. These include parameters of tumour activity, parameters of tumour sensitivity to hormones and parameters of the patient's hormonal profile.

References

Abramson, W. & Warshawsky, H. (1948) Cancer of the breast in the male, secondary to estrogenic administration; report of a case. *Journal of Urology*, **59,** 76.

Adams, J. B. & Wong, M. S. F. (1968) Paraendocrine behaviour of human breast carcinoma. *In vitro* transformation of steroids to physiologically active hormones. *Journal of Endocrinology*, **41,** 41.

Bonser, G. M., Dossett, J. A. & Jull, J. W. (1961) Selection of patients for hypophysectomy or adrenalectomy. In *Human and Experimental Breast Cancer*, p. 450. Springfield: Charles C. Thomas.

Bulbrook, R. D. (1966) Hormonal factors in the etiology and treatment of breast cancer. *Canadian Cancer Conference*, **6,** 36.

Burrows, H. & Horning, E. S. (1952) *Oestrogens and Neoplasia*. Oxford: Blackwell Scientific Publications.

Campbell, J. H., Cummins, S. D., Kirk, D. L. & Mathews, W. R. (1962) Secondary breast cancer of prostatic origin. *Journal of the American Medical Association*, **179,** 458.

Collins, D. H. & Cameron, K. M. (1964) Interstitial cell tumours. *British Journal of Urology Supplement* (The pathology of testicular tumours), **36,** 2, p. 62.

Collins, D. H. & Pugh, R. C. B. (1964) Classification and frequency of testicular tumours. *British Journal of Urology Supplement*. (The pathology of testicular tumours), **36,** 2, p. 1.

Collins, D. H. & Symington, T. (1964) Sertoli cell tumours. *British Journal of Urology Supplement* (The pathology of testicular tumours), **36,** 2, p. 52.

Cornil, L. (1949) The value of oestrogen treatment in postmenopausal epithelioma of the breast with late virilism. In *Excerpta Medica Section* 3 (1950), **4,** 389. English abstract.

Davies, J. N. P. (1949) Sex hormone upset in Africans. *British Medical Journal*, **ii,** 676.

Farrow, J. H. & Adair, F. E. (1942) Effect of orchidectomy on skeletal metastases from cancer of male breast. *Science*, **95,** 654.

Geller, J. & Volk, H. (1961) Objective remission of metastatic breast cancer in a male who received 17α hydroxyprogesterone caproate (Delalutin). *Cancer Chemotherapy Reports*, **14,** 77.

Gilbert, J. (1933) Carcinoma of the male breast. *Surgery, Gynecology and Obstetrics*, **57,** 451.

Green, A. (1966) General Discussion. In *The Value of Cytotoxic Agents and Anabolic Steroids in the Treatment of Advanced Malignant Disease*, p. 93, ed. Abrahamson, M. London: Parcener Press.

Houttuin, E., van Prohaska, J. & Taxman, P. (1967) Response of male mammary carcinoma metastases to bilateral adrenalectomy. *Surgery, Gynecology and Obstetrics*, **125,** 279.

Howard, R. R. & Grosjean, W. A. (1949) Bilateral mammary carcinoma in the male coincident with prolonged stilboestrol therapy. *Surgery*, **25,** 300.

Huggins, C. (1954) Endocrine methods of treatment of cancer of the breast. *Journal of the National Cancer Institute*, **15,** 1.

Huggins, C. & Taylor, G. W. (1955) Carcinoma of the male breast. *Archives of Surgery*, **70,** 303.

Jackson, A. W., Muldal, S., Ockey, C. H. & O'Connor, P. J. (1965) Carcinoma of male breast in association with the Klinefelter syndrome. *British Medical Journal*, **i,** 223.

Keddie, N. & Morris, P. J. (1967) Male breast tumours. *Surgery, Gynecology and Obstetrics*, **124,** 332.

Lacassagne, A. (1936a) Hormonal pathogenesis of adenocarcinoma of the breast. *American Journal of Cancer*, **27,** 217.

Liechty, R. D., Davis, J. & Gleysteen, J. (1967) Cancer of the male breast. *Cancer (Philadelphia)*, **20,** 1617.

Luft, R., Olivecrona, H., Ikkos, D., Nilsson, L. B. & Massberg, H. (1958) Hypophysectomy in the management of metastatic carcinoma of the breast. In *Endocrine Aspects of Breast Cancer*, p. 27, ed. Currie, A. R. and Illingsworth, C. F. W. Edinburgh: Livingstone.

McLaughlin, J. S., Hull, H. C., Oda, F. & Buxton, W. R. (1965) Metastatic carcinoma of the male breast: Remission by adrenalectomy. *Annals of Surgery*, **162,** 9.

Murad, T. M. (1971) A proposed histochemical and electromicroscopic classification of human breast cancer according to cell of origin. *Cancer (Philadelphia)*, **27,** 288.

O'Conor, V. J., Chiang, S. P. & Grayhack, J. T. (1963) Is subcapsular orchidectomy a definitive procedure? Studies of hormone excretion before and after orchidectomy. *Journal of Urology*, **89,** 236.

Ray, B. S. & Pearson, O. H. (1956) Hypophysectomy in the treatment of advanced cancer of breast. *Annals of Surgery*, **144,** 394.

Smithers, D. W. (1968) Clinical assessment of growth rate in human tumours. *Clinical Radiology*, **19,** 113.

Stewart, H. (1971) Oophorectomy response as an index to further endocrine ablation. In *Second Tenovus Workshop on Breast Cancer*, ed. Joslin, C. A. F. and Gleave, E. N. Cardiff: Tenovus Workshop.

Stoll, B. A. (1969) *Hormonal Management in Breast Cancer*. London: Pitman Medical.

Stoll, B. A. & Ackland, T. H. A. (1970) Management of breast cancer in old age. *British Medical Journal*, **iv,** 201.

Symmers, W. St C. (1968) Carcinoma of the breast in transexual individuals after surgical and hormonal interference with the primary and secondary sex characteristics. *British Medical Journal*, **i,** 83.

Treves, N. (1959) The treatment of cancer, especially inoperable cancer of the male breast by ablative surgery (orchidectomy, adrenalectomy, and hypophysectomy) and hormone therapy (estrogens and corticosteroids). *Cancer (Philadelphia)*, **12,** 820.

Zumoff, B., Fishman, J., Casaouto, J., Hellman, L. & Gallagher, T. F. (1966) Estradiol transformation in men with breast cancer. *Journal of Clinical Endocrinology and Metabolism*, **26,** 960.

Section III

Prostatic Cancer—Endocrine Therapy

Chapter 11

The Basis of Endocrine Therapy

J. D. FERGUSSON

It seems fair to say that a relationship between testicular function and prostatic disease had long been vaguely suspected prior to the experimental work of Huggins in 1939 and 1940 which first established it on a scientific basis. Formerly William Harvey in 1616 (Whitteridge, 1964) had noted simultaneous shrinkage of the testes and prostate in the hedgehog during hibernation and had also observed that the bull's prostate became smaller after castration.

Likewise, John Hunter in 1794 (Palmer, 1837) commented on the fact that the prostate failed to develop normally when the testes had been removed. Later, sporadic attempts were made by others to adapt this practice to the treatment of human prostatic disease and White (1893), on the evidence of animal experiments, advocated castration for the relief of prostatic obstruction.

A similar principle, perhaps, may be discerned in various techniques of vasoligation and oestrogen administration with a like objective during the earlier part of the present century (Steinach and Kun, 1926). It seems clear, however, that attention was mainly focused on benign enlargement of the gland and, with the possible exception of an inconclusive study reported by Randall (1942), the control of cancer was never seriously envisaged.

On this account full credit must be given to Huggins and his associates not only for demonstrating the functional and histological changes which take place in the dog's prostate after castration but more particularly for anticipating a similar response on the part of the disorderly epithelial proliferation which characterises human prostatic malignancy.

THE CONTRIBUTION OF HUGGINS

Huggins' original work (Huggins et al, 1939) was conducted on dogs, a species in which visible evidence of progressive prostatic swelling is not uncommon as age advances.

It was first confirmed that, as a result of castration, the gland diminished in size and further information was then sought as to the reason. Histological studies showed that senile enlargement of the canine prostate differed from that occurring in man on account of the prevalence of large cystic spaces containing prostatic secretion. These cavities appeared to represent distended acini whose ducts had become obstructed by epithelial hyperplasia.

The effect of castration was to promote shrinkage of the epithelium, thus allowing improved drainage of the retained secretion and, in turn, a decrease in the overall size of the gland. The significant feature was the response of the epithelial cells which underwent a variety of degenerative changes before being finally shed into the lumen of the ducts. For this reason it was assumed that their viability was, at least in some measure, connected with the presence of the testes and possibly dependent on the internal secretion of the latter.

This basic concept of androgen-dependence was carried a stage further by observing the histological changes in the prostate which followed the administration of male and female sex hormones respectively to the castrated animals (Huggins and Clark, 1940). Whereas injections of testosterone propionate brought about renewed epithelial growth and recurrent swelling of the gland, it was found that this effect could be reversed by the subsequent administration of oestrogens. Under such experimental conditions, therefore, the sensitivity of the prostatic epithelium to circulating sex hormones appeared to have been established.

This concept received further support from a series of animal experiments designed to investigate the *functional* response of the prostate to endocrine stimulation. By establishing a prostatic fistula in dogs it was shown that the rate of secretion of prostatic fluid, which normally proceeds at a constant level, was diminished or inhibited by oestrogens (or castration) and was resumed, at

least in part, if androgens were given (Huggins and Clark, 1940). It thus seemed beyond doubt that the epithelial component of the dogs' prostate was capable of reacting both structurally and functionally to sex hormone stimulation.

The next, and undoubtedly more far-reaching step, was to apply this knowledge to the treatment of human prostatic disease and particularly to that form in which epithelial activity was known to play a dominant role, namely prostatic cancer. To this end a number of patients with advanced metastatic cancer beyond the aid of current methods of therapy, were submitted to orchidectomy and kept under close clinical observation.

The results were encouraging in that not only was there a striking remission of symptoms but the subsequent periods of survival exceeded all expectation. In due course additional clinical studies, supplemented by biochemical and radiological methods of assessment, provided further opportunity for confirming the response of the disease (Huggins and Hodges, 1941; Huggins, Stevens and Hodges, 1941).

By a strange but fortunate coincidence the period during which Huggins' experimental studies were undertaken was also marked by a biochemical event of outstanding importance. This was the synthesis by Dodds and his colleagues (1938) of a diphenolic compound, diethylstilboestrol, which exhibited strong oestrogenic properties when given by mouth. It was this chemical in fact which was used by Huggins in the experiments already quoted on castrated dogs to reverse the stimulating effect of testosterone on the prostatic epithelium.

Little intuition was therefore required to suggest the hypothesis that its administration might exert a controlling influence on prostatic cancer similar to that induced by castration. This indeed proved to be the case and further studies clearly demonstrated the efficacy of synthetic oestrogens in retarding the activity of the disease. Thus, by their individual contributions to the introduction of oestrogen therapy for prostatic cancer, Huggins and Dodds may be said to share the honour of being the first to formulate a rational method of treating malignant disease by the oral route.

The foundations of what has now come to be termed 'endocrine-control therapy' having been laid in this manner, a brief attempt at recapitulation may not be out of place. Such treatment, based on animal studies demonstrating the sensitivity of prostatic epithelium to sex hormones, relies on an analogous relationship in the case of the human gland. It is further assumed that in cancer of the prostate some at least of the cells constituting the tumour retain their susceptibility to hormonal influence, and to this extent the disease remains endocrine-sensitive. Confirmation is afforded by a wide range of clinical observations and supplementary records indicating regression of the malignant process after the withdrawal of testicular androgens (castration) or, alternatively, the administration of oestrogens.

ENDOCRINE SENSITIVITY

The term 'endocrine-*sensitive*' as applied to prostatic cancer is preferred to 'endocrine-*dependent*' in that the latter implies an exclusive association, whereas the viability of the neoplastic process as a whole may well be partly contingent on other factors. The distinction is emphasised by the fact that some tumours are apparently uninfluenced by any form of endocrine therapy, while others, after showing an initial response subsequently become autonomous.

It may be accepted, however, that at the outset most cases of prostatic cancer retain some degree of hormone sensitivity and that their clinical behaviour is at least to some extent a reflection of androgenic stimulation. This does not of course imply that the disease is initiated in this manner (although prostatic cancer has never been recorded in a pre-pubertal castrate) but rather that, once

established, its activity may be thereby increased.

On this account ablation of the main sources of androgen production (castration) and the administration of oestrogens have both come to be regarded as conventional methods of conservative management. Their suitability for this purpose is enhanced by the fact that neither invokes the need for substitution therepy and, despite possible differences in their mode of action, the risks of troublesome sequelae are reasonably acceptable when compared with the natural hazards of the untreated disease. For these reasons, therefore, their use, either singly or in combination, has been widely acclaimed as a valuable aid in attempting to control the activity of the malignant process.

Nevertheless, in view of what has already been said, it can scarcely be expected that such measures will do more than affect those cells of the tumour which retain their sensitivity to hormones. No instances are in fact known where total elimination of the disease has been accomplished by endocrine therapy alone.

While many cases respond favourably at the outset some appear resistant, and others, after showing initial improvement, later relapse. In these it seems reasonable to suppose that a majority of the cells have ceased to be affected either by the withdrawal of testicular androgens or by the more comprehensive effect of oestrogen therapy. In some instances, no doubt, the disease simply becomes completely autonomous but in others the possibility remains that its renewed activity may be influenced by additional hormonal stimulation from extragenital sources.

In this respect considerable interest attaches to the adrenals whose presumed role in sustaining virility during the period of sexual decline has aptly led to their designation as, 'the gonads of old age'. The fact that compensatory androgen production takes place from these sources after castration, and that the glands may likewise undergo enlargement during oestrogen therapy, strongly supports their implication.

It is conceivable also that other endocrine organs play a part, either directly or indirectly, in promoting the elaboration of hormones which continue to affect the behaviour of the tumour. Speculation in this field has led to the suggestion of various measures to reduce or counteract any sustained stimulation of this nature. In the main, however, attention has been focused on the adrenals and the hypophysis—the former chiefly for reasons already mentioned and the latter on account of its gonadotropic and adrenotropic functions.

The complexity of endocrine interrelationship and the frequent need for substitution therapy when such endocrine glands are deliberately ablated or suppressed, place such measures outside the scope of conventional therapy and call for special experience and caution in their application.

RATIONALE OF ENDOCRINE THERAPY

Generally speaking, the procedures advocated have tended to fall into two categories, namely, attempts at functional suppression of the organs concerned by medical means, or their destruction by surgery, irradiation or other physical methods. While conservative treatment of the former type would naturally seem preferable, especially when dealing with frail and elderly patients, the results have unfortunately been somewhat discouraging.

As far as the adrenal is concerned, cortical-activity can be depressed to some extent by cortisone and its related hormones, but the effect is usually insufficient to modify the progress of the disease. Apart, therefore, from inducing a transient state of encouragement and euphoria, the use of such substances has so far proved of little value.

Surgical adrenalectomy on the other hand, while often temporarily capable of restoring a measure of control over a relapsing tumour, may well be accounted too severe a procedure to justify the unpredictability and duration of the response. Its success in the treatment of mammary cancer has not been matched in the case of the prostate, partly owing to the fact that operation is often delayed through over-reliance on castration and oestrogen therapy, and partly because of the greater age and debility of many of the patients involved.

On this account, and since other methods have recently shown greater promise, surgical interference with the adrenals has now been largely abandoned except in occasional younger cases. Instead, attention has become increasingly directed towards the hypophysis under whose influence it is now believed that the production of tumour-stimulating hormones is mainly sustained.

The full significance of the hypophysis in promoting the secretion of hormones which affect the activity of prostatic cancer remains unknown. Although a linkage with the testes and adrenals is well established its sphere of influence is probably wider, since it has been shown that even after removal of these organs hypophysectomy may still retard the progress of the disease.

Removal or destruction of the hypophysis would thus seem capable of affording a comprehensive method of endocrine control, which might well be more commonly applied were it not for certain practical considerations. Among these, the obscure situation of the gland imposes obvious difficulties and dangers as far as surgery is concerned, while on account of its manifold functions, ablation implies the need for substitution therapy.

Surgical hypophysectomy is thus open to the same objections as adrenalectomy in that the anticipated benefits, over and above what can be achieved by simpler methods of endocrine control, are seldom likely to compensate for the hazards involved. Removal of the hypophysis can thus only be considered in carefully selected patients in whom the disease is both rapidly progressive and incapable of suppression by other means.

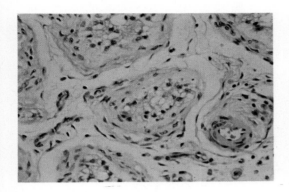

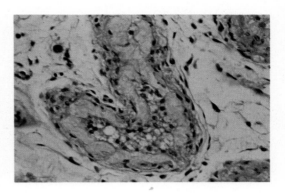

PLATE 12.1. Testis from a patient with oestrogen-treated carcinoma of the prostate. Note the absence of spermatogenesis and hyaline thickening of an interstitial arteriole.

PLATE 12.2. PAS stain to show the hyaline thickening in the region of the spermatic tubule basement membrane in oestrogen-treated carcinoma of the prostate.

Effect of oestrogens on the testis. (Reproduced by courtesy of Dr. R. C. B. Pugh, Institute of Urology, London.)

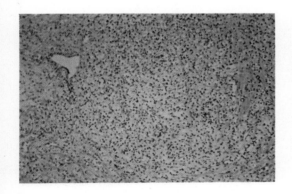

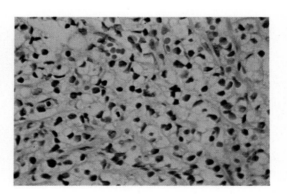

PLATE 14.1. Oestrogen-treated carcinoma of the prostate. Low power. Cytoplasmic vacuolation of tumour cells.

PLATE 14.2. High power of the same case. Many of the nuclei are hyperchromatic.

Effect of oestrogens on the prostate. (Reproduced by courtesy of Dr. R. C. B. Pugh, Institute of Urology, London.)

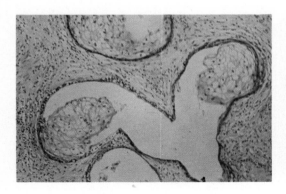

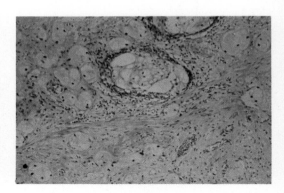

PLATE 14.3. Prostatic ducts showing squamous metaplasia of part of the lining epithelium.

PLATE 14.4. Oestrogen effect on prostatic ducts (squamous metaplasia) and tumour cells (pyknotic nuclei and vacuolated cytoplasm).

Effect of oestrogens on the prostate. (Reproduced by courtesy of Dr. R. C. B. Pugh, Institute of Urology, London.)

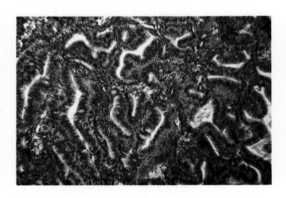

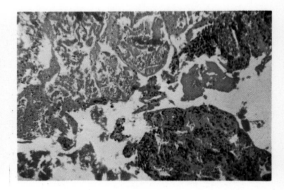

PLATE 17.1. Adenocarcinoma classified as Grade III in a 61-year-old patient (Kistner et al, 1965).

PLATE 17.2. Curettage specimen obtained one week after the instillation of 1200 mg medroxyprogesterone acetate into the uterine cavity. Note the extensive necrobiosis of tumour cells (Kistner et al, 1965).

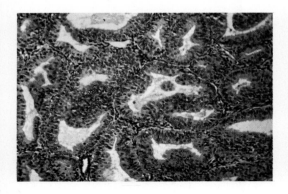

PLATE 17.3. Well-differentiated endometrial carcinoma prior to therapy (Kistner et al, 1965).

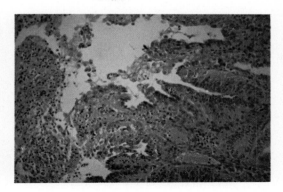

PLATE 17.4. Hysterectomy specimen in the same patient as shown in Plate 17.3 after four days of intrauterine medroxyprogesterone acetate (1·0 g). Note the surface necrobiosis and inflammatory exudate (Kistner et al, 1965).

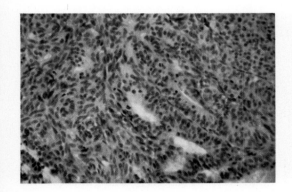

PLATE 17.5. Curettage specimen showing an undifferentiated adenocarcinoma prior to hysterectomy (Kistner et al, 1965).

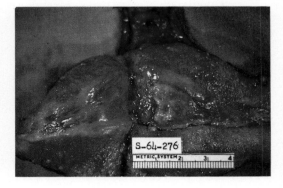

PLATE 17.6. Hysterectomy specimen obtained three weeks after intracavitary radium and parenteral administration of 5200 mg medroxyprogesterone acetate. Note the decidual cast in the cavity of the uterus (Kistner et al, 1965).

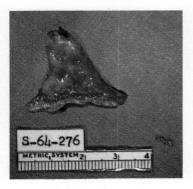

PLATE 17.7. High power view of decidual cast which was free floating in uterine cavity (Kistner et al, 1965).

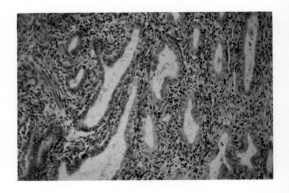

PLATE 17.8. Microscopic view of tissue in decidual cast. No viable tumour cells were found in the cast nor in the endometrium. The glands show typical progestational atrophy (Kistner et al, 1965).

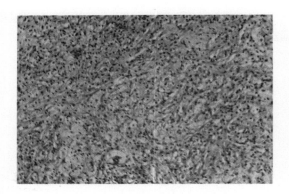

PLATE 18.1. Case J.A.D. Histology of residual nodule in Figure 18.5c showing partially degenerate renal cell carcinoma of lower grade malignancy than original primary growth (Plate 18.2) ($\times$160).

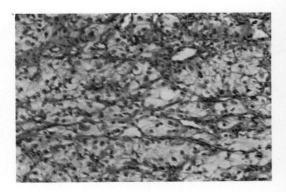

PLATE 18.2. Case J.A.D. Histology of original primary renal carcinoma: typical clear cell tumour of average grade malignancy ($\times$160).

Fortunately, however, a simpler alternative is available in the form of 'irradiation hypophysectomy', which is applicable with reasonable safety even in advanced and debilitated cases. This involves the introduction of a radioactive source into the gland, either by transnasal or transorbital puncture, with the object of inducing local pituitary necrosis. The hazards of open surgery are thus to a great extent avoided and, with suitable equipment and expertise, a substantial portion of the gland can be selectively destroyed.

Although destruction is seldom as complete as with surgical hypophysectomy, the resulting interference with function is usually sufficient to induce a demonstrable deficiency syndrome, often accompanied by dramatic symptomatic relief. Thus, despite the inevitable need for substitution therapy (cortisone), the simplicity and lesser risk of the irradiation procedure commend it as an eminently practicable measure in the treatment of the metastatic disease when simpler methods have failed.

Beyond the measures already referred to, the potential scope of endocrine-control therapy cannot as yet be finally assessed. There are, in fact, indications that further glands may well be implicated, including the thyroid and possibly even the pancreas. Nor is it known in what manner hormones basically affect the activity of prostatic cancer—whether by humoral, chemical or even physical action.

It is particularly remarkable that both the synthetic and naturally occurring oestrogens which differ considerably in their chemical constitution should be capable of exerting a similar effect on the disease; and also that androgens which normally stimulate activity should occasionally reverse their role. Furthermore, recent experimental work with compounds of a similar nature has suggested that some may have a capacity for suppressing the tumour without inducing any demonstrable endocrine side effects, thus suggesting that the two functions may be separable.

The inference that endocrine-control therapy merely represents an elaborate form of chemotherapy, however, is by no means acceptable since the response to purely ablative procedures such as castration and adrenalectomy suggests that a more complex or possibly dual mechanism may be involved.

PRINCIPLES OF ENDOCRINE MANAGEMENT

An attempt has been made in the foregoing presentation to outline the rationale of endocrine-control therapy and to give an introductory account of the place and scope of various methods in current use. Further details of their application and the results which can be expected are given in succeeding chapters. Before proceeding further, however, the following points should be borne in mind.

Endocrine-control therapy for prostatic cancer affords comprehensive means of suppressing the activity of the malignant process irrespective of its site and distribution. The measure of its success probably depends largely on how far the disease remains susceptible to hormonal influence, as well as on the quality and potency of the methods employed. Since none of these conditions is likely to be fully predictable, such treatment, despite its capacity for causing tumour regression, cannot be regarded as finally curative.

Some tumours are altogether resistant to treatment while others show only a transient response. Few are permanently suppressed but some, at least, may be amenable to adequate control throughout the lifetime of the patient. This applies particularly to elderly cases in which the disease is commonly less active and where, per contra, there is a greater liability to death from other causes.

Resistance to one form of endocrine-control therapy does not necessarily imply an inability to respond to others—and this also holds good for cases in relapse. While certain methods—for example, oestrogen

9

therapy and castration—may overlap in their effect and, indeed are frequently employed as alternatives, none should be regarded as exclusive.

It is customary to rely primarily on those forms of treatment which are simple to apply and which have become widely recognised as effective without entailing any disproportionate risk or inconvenience to the patient. The initial choice must likewise take account of the stage of the disease, the general clinical status and the competing claims of surgery, radiotherapy and other measures. More elaborate methods of endocrine-control therapy involving interference with the production of tumour-stimulating hormones from extragenital sources should be restricted to the treatment of advanced or relapsing cases, and then undertaken only when appropriate technical facilities and arrangements for substitution therapy are available.

All forms of endocrine-control therapy carry certain hazards many of which may be regarded as inconsiderable compared with the dangers of the untreated disease. Nevertheless, it is advisable that the diagnosis should always be reasonably assured before treatment is instituted and particularly that full histological confirmation should be obtained if ablative endocrine surgery is intended.

Finally, it must be remembered that endocrine-control therapy represents only one aspect of the management of prostatic cancer. While often effective in inducing tumour regression and promoting symptomatic relief, the response may be too slow or insufficient at the primary site to obviate the risks of established urinary obstruction. In this event, adjuvant surgery may well be required, particularly in those instances where prostatic cancer and benign hypertrophy happen to coexist. Likewise, failure to control the progress of the disease may determine the need for supplementary treatment either by palliative surgery, radiotherapy, or other means.

There is, indeed, nothing exclusive about endocrine-control therapy which restricts the application of other methods though it is noteworthy that with its wider adoption the need for such additional measures has become significantly reduced.

MODE OF ACTION OF OESTROGEN THERAPY IN PROSTATIC CANCER

Both from Huggins' experimental studies and from the clinical response of human prostatic cancer to castration and other forms of endocrine ablation, it has been widely assumed that the benefits of endocrine therapy depend on androgen suppression. In elaborating this concept it has seemed rational to seek to eliminate or neutralise all sources of male hormone in the body as required. While castration destroys the main source and adrenalectomy a second, hypophysectomy finally removes the controlling polypeptide hormones which may continue to activate androgen production from other extragonadal sites (Figure 11.1).

From the similarity of the initial clinical response, the therapeutic response to oestrogens in prostatic cancer has also been generally regarded as an anti-androgen effect. Speculation, however, continues as to the precise action involved and whether this is exerted directly on the target organ or is mediated through the pituitary gland. In the latter case the pituitary-gonadal relationship can be compared to a closed-cycle feed-back electrical circuit in which a rise in the oestrogen titre in the blood leads to a compensatory fall in circulating gonadotrophin (Figure 11.2). It is not yet clear, however, whether such a decline in gonadotrophic activity represents diminished production or a decreased release of hormone from the pituitary.

Apart from depending on a purely endocrine mechanism it remains conceivable that oestrogens act in other ways in modifying the activity and progress of prostatic cancer. The difference in chemical structure between the natural and synthetic 'female hormones' in fact suggests that the latter, in particular, may possibly exert an additional chemotherapeutic action. It has been suggested, indeed, that the ideal 'hormone' might be a 'non-oestrogenic oestrogen' capable of controlling the activity of the disease without

1961). The relative ratios of the steroidal concentration are of considerable importance. This antagonism should not be regarded as a chemical neutralisation, but rather as a blockage of activity at the target organ—possibly by competing at receptor molecules. Progestational agents with anti-androgenic

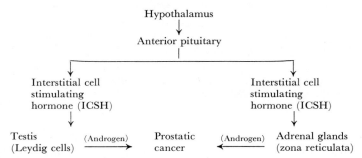

FIGURE 11.1. Androgen-dependent theory in the hormonal control of prostatic cancer.

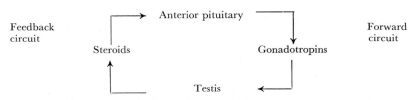

FIGURE 11.2. Closed-cycle system of pituitary-gonadal relationship (after Huggins, 1952).

inducing endocrine side-effects. Current clinical experience, however, continues to cast doubt on whether such substances as are at present available are ever fully effective.

Nevertheless, the possibility of some mechanism in addition to a strictly endocrine reaction remains conceivable and the following theories have been postulated (Table 11.1).

ANTI-ANDROGENIC EFFECT

Oestrogens may depress the growth of prostatic cancer by oestrogen-androgen antagonism at the tissue level. Such an antagonism has been shown in the prostate of castrated hypophysectomised dogs (Goodwin et al,

properties may also yield objective signs of regression of prostatic cancer (Geller et al, 1967).

Some evidence of direct inhibition has been adduced from culturing slices of human prostatic adenoma and carcinoma and noting the direct effect of added steroids. Prostatic adenoma shows stimulation of growth as a result of incubation with oestrone (Kallen and Roehl, 1960). Similar experiments with prostatic cancer have shown stimulation of growth by androsterone in small series (Roehl, 1958; Wojewski and Kaniewicz, 1965). There are, however, many difficulties in maintaining prostatic cancer in tissue culture and it would seem unwise to attach undue importance to such findings.

TABLE 11.1. *Oestrogen therapy—possible modes of action*

1. Disturbance of the androgen-oestrogen milieu:
   (a) Direct neutralisation of circulating androgens.
   (b) Androgen antagonism at the target organ—either on an extra- or intra-cellular basis.
   (c) Direct inhibition of androgen production at its major sites (i.e. the testes and adrenals).
   (d) Indirect suppression of androgenic activity via the pituitary.

2. Non-endocrine chemotherapeutic effect:
   Direct oncolytic action on the cancer cells—possibly by interfering with the synthesis of DNA.

3. Stimulation of natural body-defence mechanisms:
   (a) Enhancement of connective tissue reaction in the prostate.
   (b) Increased reticulo-endothelial response.

GONADOTROPIN SUPPRESSION

Although a direct action on the testes resulting in a depletion of androgen production can be envisaged it seems more likely that the effect of oestrogen, as in the case of the adrenals, is mediated by gonadotropin suppression via the pituitary. The hypophysis of patients receiving oestrogens shows reduced or absent gonadotropins (Dekker and Russfield, 1963), although corticotropin secretion is maintained. Following oestrogen therapy, there is a measurable decrease in the excretion of gonadotropins in the urine (Albert, 1956). This involves both the interstitial cell stimulating hormone (ICSH) which controls androgen secretion from the testis and adrenal cortex (Alder et al, 1968) and the follicle stimulating hormone (FSH).

Since ICSH holds the key to androgen secretion, whatever its source, it has been suggested that the reactivation of prostatic cancer after oestrogen therapy is due to 'escape' of ICSH secretion from control. This would lead to stimulation of androgen secretion both from the testes and adrenal cortex (hyperplasia of the adrenal cortex is known to occur both after oestrogen therapy and after orchidectomy). This theory would explain why a proportion of patients who have lost control from oestrogens are benefited by castration or adrenalectomy.

It has been reported that some patients with advanced prostatic cancer may respond to progesterone administration (Trunnell et al, 1951) or to cortisone (Hayward, 1953), and current developments in endocrine therapy are proceeding on these lines. Although the results at present remain inconclusive it may be noted that, like oestrogens, these steroids are capable of suppressing ICSH secretion.

Other anterior pituitary hormones apart from gonadotropins may also be involved in the control of prostatic cancer. Corticotropin can stimulate adrenal androgen secretion after castration (Burt, Finney and Scott, 1957) while growth hormone is reported to have a direct stimulating effect on the prostate (Kennedy, 1955). It appears that pituitary inhibition by oestrogen administration does not involve either of these two hormones (Alder et al, 1968).

Finally, mention should be made of the gonadotropin and corticotropin releasing centres in the hypothalamus. These regulate the secretory activities of the pituitary gland and may possibly be influenced by psychological factors among others.

BODY DEFENCE STIMULATION

Apart from the effect of oestrogenic compounds on the reproductive organs, these substances may stimulate the reticulo-endothelial system to raise body defences (Nicol et al, 1964). This applies to both males and females. Both natural and synthetic oestrogens may stimulate the activity of the phagocytic cells in animals and raise the level of the serum gamma globulins. There is no correlation between the degree of oestrogenicity of a compound as measured on the reproductive system, and the effect upon the reticulo-endothelial system.

While testosterone and progesterone have little effect on phagocytic activity, the corticosteroids, on the other hand, are strong depressants of this activity. This depressant effect of cortisone can be reversed by diethylstilboestrol (Nicol and Bilby, 1957).

An association between cancer growth and the immunological status of the patient has been suggested (Southam, 1965). It is possible therefore that non-specific stimulation of the reticulo-endothelial system by oestrogens leading to fibrosis may be one mode of their action in the treatment of prostatic or mammary cancer (Nicol and Helmy, 1951). It is interesting to note that in the few cases where successful immunisation against spontaneous tumours has been reported in animals, the effect was transient. The animals were able to control but not destroy disseminated tumour cells (Baldwin, 1967). This, so far, is also the case in the hormonal control of human cancer.

CONCLUSION

At least some of the cells of most prostatic cancers are susceptible to hormonal influence, as shown by tumour regression following withdrawal of testicular androgens or the administration of oestrogens. Tumour autonomy appears eventually and this is probably due either to increasing predominance of hormone-insensitive cells or to compensatory androgen production by the adrenal cortex.

The hypophysis probably influences the secretion of other hormones which control the activity of prostatic cancer, because hypophysectomy can still cause tumour regression even after orchidectomy and adrenalectomy. Nevertheless, although hypophyseal ablation appears to hold the key to the control of hormone-sensitive tumours, it is customary to rely primarily on the simpler effective methods, in order to avoid the hazards and substitution therapy associated with hypophyseal ablation. While the response to castration or to oestrogen therapy is temporary, it may provide adequate control of the tumour throughout the lifetime of the patient, particularly if the methods are used sequentially.

The effect of oestrogen therapy is thought to be exerted either by an anti-androgenic effect at the tissue level or by an indirect effect in suppressing gonadotropin production or release. Oestrogens may also play a part in the stimulation of the immune mechanism of the host, or it is conceivable that they have a non-endocrine, chemotherapeutic effect on the synthesis of DNA in the tumour cell.

References

Albert, A. (1956) Human urinary gonadotropin. *Recent Progress in Hormone Research*, **12**, 227–301.

Alder, A., Burger, H., Davis, J., Dulmanis, A., Hudson, B., Sarfaty, G. & Straffon, W. (1968) Carcinoma of prostate: response of plasma luteinizing hormone and testosterone to oestrogen therapy. *British Medical Journal*, **i**, 28–31.

Baldwin, R. W. (1967) Immunology of the cancer cell. *Clinical Radiology*, **18**, 261–267.

Burt, F. B., Finney, R. P. & Scott, W. W. (1957) Steroid response to therapy in prostatic cancer. *Journal of Urology*, **77**, 485–491.

Dekker, A. & Russfield, A. B. (1963) Pituitary tropic hormone studies and morphologic observations in carcinoma of the prostate. *Cancer*, **16**, 743–750.

Dodds, E. C., Goldberg, L., Lawson, W. & Robinson, R. (1938) Oestrogenic activity of certain synthetic compounds. *Nature*, **141**, 247–248.

Geller, J., Fruchtman, B., Newman, H., Roberts, T. & Silva, R. (1967) Effect of progestational agents on carcinoma of the prostate. *Cancer Chemotherapy Reports*, **51**, 41–46.

Goodwin, D. A., Rasmussen-Taxdal, D. S., Ferreira, A. A. & Scott, W. W. (1961) Estrogen inhibition of androgen maintained prostatic secretion in the hypophysectomized dog. *Journal of Urology*, **86**, 134–136.

Hayward, W. G. (1953) Treatment of late relapse in prostatic carcinoma by cortisone. *Journal of Urology*, **69**, 152–156.

Huggins, C. (1952) Endocrine factors in cancer. *Journal of Urology*, **68**, 875–884.

Huggins, C. & Clark, P. J. (1940) Quantitative studies of prostatic secretion: II. The effect of castration and of oestrogen injection on the normal and on the hyperplastic prostate glands of dogs. *Journal of Experimental Medicine*, **72**, 747–762.

Huggins, C. & Hodges, C. V. (1941) Studies on prostatic cancer; effect of castration, estrogen and of androgen injection on serum phosphates in metastatic carcinoma of the prostate. *Cancer Research*, **1**, 293–297.

Huggins, C., Masina, M. H., Eichelberger, L. & Wharton, J. D. (1939) Quantitative studies of prostatic secretion; characteristics of normal secretion; influence of thyroid, suprarenal, and testis extirpation and androgen substitution on prostatic output. *Journal of Experimental Medicine*, **70**, 543–556.

Huggins, C., Stevens, R. E. & Hodges, C. V. (1941) Studies on prostatic cancer; effects of castration on advanced carcinoma of the prostate gland. *Archives of Surgery*, **43**, 209–233.

Kallen, B. & Roehl, L. (1960) The fibrinolytic activity of human hyperplastic prostate studied in tissue culture. *Acta Chirurgica Scandinavica*, **118**, 240–245.

Kennedy, B. J. (1955) Effect of steroids in women with breast cancer. In *Hormones and the Ageing Process*, ed. Engle, E. T. and Pincus, G., pp. 253–272. London: Academic Press.

Nicol, T. & Bilbey, D. L. J. (1957) Reversal by diethylstilboestrol of the depressant effect of cortisone on the phagocytic activity of the reticulo-endothelial system. *Nature*, **179**, 1137–1138.

Nicol, T., Bilbey, D. L. J., Charles, L. M., Cordingley, J. L. & Vernon-Roberts, B. (1964) Oestrogen: the natural stimulant of body defence. *Journal of Endocrinology*, **30**, 277–291.

Nicol, T. & Helmy, I. D. (1951) Influence of oestrogenic hormones on reticulo-endothelial system in guinea pig. *Nature*, **167**, 321.

Palmer, J. F. (1837) Editor, *The Surgical Works of John Hunter F.R.C.S., With Notes*. London: Longmans.

Randall, A. (1942) Eight-year results of castration for cancer of the prostate. *Journal of Urology*, **48**, 706–709.

Roehl, L. (1958) Hormone dependency of prostatic cancer studied by cell culture technique. *British Journal of Urology*, **30**, 450–454.

Southam, C. M. (1965) Evidence of immunological reactions to autochthonous cancer in man. *European Journal of Cancer*, **1**, 173–181.

Steinach, E. & Kun, H. (1926) Antagonistiche Wirkungen der Keimdrüsen-Hormone. *Biologia generalis*, **2**, 815–834.

Trunnell, J. B., Duffy, B. J., Marshall, V., Whitmore, W. F. & Woodard, H. Q. (1951) Use of progesterone in treatment of cancer of prostate. *Journal of Clinical Endocrinology and Metabolism*, **11**, 663–676.

White, J. W. (1893) The surgery of the hypertrophied prostate. *Annals of Surgery*, **17**, 70–75.

Whitteridge, G. (1964) *The Anatomical Lectures of William Harvey*. London: Livingstones with the Royal College of Physicians.

Wojewski, A. & Kaniewicz, D. P. (1965) The influence of stilboestrol and testosterone on the growth of prostatic adenoma and carcinoma in tissue culture. *Journal of Urology*, **93**, 721–724.

Chapter 12

Castration and Oestrogen Therapy

J. D. FERGUSSON

The early enthusiasm which greeted the introduction of castration and oestrogen therapy as a dramatic advance in the management of prostatic cancer has now been somewhat tempered in the light of subsequent clinical experience. Despite the fact that many cases (probably about 80 per cent) respond initially, the duration of benefit remains unpredictable and no instances of complete cure have been reported. Furthermore, in the case of oestrogen therapy, it has recently been suggested that a potential liability to serious side-effects must be equated with the merits of sustained treatment.

At the same time the development of new radiotherapeutic techniques has introduced a practical alternative in the initial selection of treatment for the disease at its primary site. Thirty years ago, when oestrogen therapy was at its zenith, radiotherapy was hazardous and frequently unavailing, but with modern supervoltage apparatus the local complications of irradiation have now been minimised and recent results have been encouraging.

While there can be little doubt that endocrine therapy still affords the treatment of choice in disseminated prostatic cancer, opinions differ with regard to its role in the management of lesions which appear to be confined to the region of the gland itself. Furthermore, the question of timing also remains debatable—whether it is better to institute treatment at an early stage in the hope of curtailing the further spread of the disease or, in anticipation of a temporary response, to withhold its benefits until serious obstructive symptoms threaten. Each case undoubtedly has to be assessed on its own merits and reviewed in clinical perspective where, not only the medical and social circumstances, but also the need and availability of other forms of treatment (such as surgery and radiotherapy) are taken into account.

INDICATIONS FOR ENDOCRINE THERAPY

Much of the information relating to the effect of castration and oestrogen therapy has emanated from urological clinics where patients have been referred primarily on account of urinary disability. In a majority of cases, the symptoms have already progressed to the extent of requiring early relief and, if improvement cannot be effected by other means (palliative surgery or radiotherapy), the question of postponing endocrine therapy may well be largely academic. There can be little doubt in the minds of those who witnessed the inexorable advance of the disease before the days of hormonal control that, even though the results are apt to prove impermanent, a worthwhile period of suppression can often be achieved. The same clearly applies in most symptomatic cases of the disseminated disease, in which, after simple palliative measures have failed, endocrine-control therapy offers the only feasible alternative.

Nevertheless, some cases are encountered in which either the symptoms remain unobtrusive or are due, at least in part, to other causes. Some are brought to light virtually by chance, as during routine or casual rectal examination, others in the course of more detailed investigation for differing reasons. For example, it is by no means unusual for prostatic cancer to coexist with benign prostatic hyperplasia and for clinical examination—instituted on a suspicion of the latter—to lead to its discovery. Such complicated cases raise special problems in endocrine management which can only be resolved in relation to the probable extent and activity of the malignant process. In a few, extended surgery alone may offer a prospect of total cure but, in most, palliative resection or prostatectomy with the choice of subsequent irradiation or endocrine therapy will be required.

Likewise, the fortuitous detection of typical bone deposits during radiological investigation for other reasons may occasion doubt as to the need or otherwise for instituting endocrine control. In such instances the disease has clearly already disseminated and any theoretical prospect of preventing this process by hormone therapy has been lost. Provided therefore that the secondary lesions remain asymptomatic, there may be good grounds for withholding treatment until they become troublesome.

It is not, perhaps, sufficiently appreciated that in general hospital practice a significant number of cases of prostatic cancer (probably about 20 per cent) are first detected solely on account of symptoms due to metastatic spread. Such patients, who admit to little or nothing in the way of urinary disability, have generally accepted the onset of bone pains and other disturbances as the natural accompaniment of old age and seek advice only when their discomfort becomes intolerable. It is in these circumstances that the relief afforded by oestrogen therapy or castration is often most dramatic, and there can be little justification for withholding treatment at this stage of the disease.

TIMING OF TREATMENT

From the foregoing it will be understood that general and unequivocal statements on the optimum timing of endocrine-control therapy should be treated with some reserve. Nevertheless, as might be expected, various views have been expressed representing individual and collective experience. An early report (Flocks et al, 1951) suggested that postponing stilboestrol therapy until pain appeared resulted in a better survival rate than if oestrogens were prescribed at the time the patient was first seen. However, the author (Fergusson, 1963) claimed that from his experience the high mortality rate seen in the first 12 months after the diagnosis of prostatic cancer could be decreased if endocrine therapy were instituted early. Moreover, those patients who survived 12 months appeared to have an improved likelihood of five-year survival.

The issue has been further confused by numerous reports relating to the individual advantages of different oestrogens and to the effect of various dosages and methods of administration. Others have commented on the respective merits of oestrogen therapy and castration as well as on their use in combination (Nesbit and Plumb, 1946). Regarding castration, it is perhaps natural that the operation should sometimes be deferred for emotional reasons and it is thus difficult to assess the true value of the time factor in its performance. This is, unfortunately, often the case with younger patients in whom the disease is commonly more active and in need of early treatment but who may understandably express a greater reluctance to accept emasculation.

At the other extreme of age there appears to be a tendency for the disease to develop more slowly and to metastasise less frequently when it occurs in later life (Franks, Fergusson and Murnaghan, 1958), and in these circumstances the need for early operation is less compelling. Likewise, since elderly patients normally incur a greater risk of dying from other causes, there may be added grounds also for withholding oestrogen therapy for as long as possible, in view of the increased liability to cardiovascular and cerebrovascular complications suggested in the report of the Veterans Administration Cooperative Urological Research Group (1967). Whether this policy should also apply in intermediate cases with progressive symptoms remains a matter for speculation, though it is notable that since the publication of the Veterans report increased attention has been focused on the theoretical hazards of prolonged treatment, and the indiscriminate use of oestrogens in the early stages has consequently declined.

To summarise briefly, the ability of castration and oestrogen therapy to suppress malignant activity in a high proportion of cases of prostatic cancer remains incontestable.

Unfortunately the effect is variable in duration and current opinion tends to favour a delay in their application until they are most likely to exert their maximum benefit. This policy disregards any potential advantage which may accrue from earlier treatment in retarding metastatic spread, but takes full account of the occasional risks now believed to be associated with prolonged oestrogen administration. Some modification of timing, however, may be indicated when such factors as age, malignant activity and the availability of alternative methods of treatment are taken into consideration.

CHOICE OF TREATMENT

Both methods are capable of inducing early symptomatic relief and the ensuing survival rates, when either is used independently, appear to be closely similar. Fundamentally, castration, although involving a minor surgical procedure, commends itself as a direct and obvious method of eliminating testicular androgen production. By comparison, the mechanism of oestrogen therapy which aims, inter alia, at hormonal 'castration' is probably more comprehensive but remains somewhat obscure. Both measures, however, evoke a similar response and, disregarding the side-effects of oestrogen administration, there is no doubt that their functions overlap considerably. On this account and for other reasons referred to later, they are often employed individually although on theoretical grounds there may be something to favour their use in combination.

CLINICAL EVIDENCE OF PALLIATION

Evidence of symptomatic improvement may be expected within a few days of instituting treatment. In some cases the response is dramatic and may take place, particularly after castration, within 24 to 48 hours. Such rapid relief is difficult to explain solely on the basis of tumour regression, although it may be partly accounted for by decrease in tissue oedema around the tumour and its metastases. The response to oestrogens usually takes a little longer but, nevertheless, corresponding histological changes are often discernible within a few days of commencing treatment.

Characteristically, the effect on the primary tumour is shown by a reduction of urinary disability and accompanying changes in the contours and consistency of the gland. Improved voiding leads to diminished frequency and a gradual lessening of the general signs of pre-existing urinary obstruction. Intravenous administration of oestrogens, in particular, is claimed to accelerate these changes and may obviate the need for surgical relief in some cases. Rectal palpation shows the gland to become smaller and softer and any irregularity of outline dissolves as the tumour regresses. In many cases the local characteristics of malignancy entirely disappear and subsequent examination may arouse little suspicion of continuing disease.

Even more dramatic is the relief of metastatic symptoms, particularly those related to widespread skeletal involvement. In some cases the relief of pain is absolute though in others it may return on attempts to exercise. There are, however, numerous reports of patients previously immobilised on account of metastatic pain who have been restored to ambulant activity. In this context, perhaps, it should be mentioned that pain from bone metastases can also sometimes be relieved by corticosteroid therapy and even from testosterone administration, although in these cases the disease is found to progress clinically.

In this vein also it may be noted that in the series of cases collected by the Veterans Administration the use of a placebo instead of stilboestrol yielded an *overall* response in 21 per cent cases (VACURG, 1964). As measured by pain control, no difference was found between the placebo-treated patients and those who received hormones although, as gauged by decrease in the size of the prostate and by serum acid phosphatase estimation. the placebo was inferior (VACURG, 1967), All that can be said in this connection is that any resulting impression that oestrogens are devoid of merit in relieving metastatic pain runs entirely contrary to the general clinical experience of others. Further allusion will be made to this later as well as to the altered appearances of the bone deposits in patients who have received endocrine therapy (see Chapter 14).

With relief of pain is often associated general clinical improvement with increased mobility and performance ability, and gain in weight. Such improvement, however, may sometimes also be observed with the use of anabolic androgens, corticosteroids and progestational agents and, moreover, the gain in weight may be illusory if in part due to increased water retention. Nevertheless, the obvious beneficial response to oestrogen therapy and castration needs no additional emphasis on account of comparisons or qualifications of this nature.

Further evidence of the clinical effect is afforded by the behaviour of soft part metastases. Extension by lymphatic spread is a common feature of the disease which, in the later stages, may promote solid oedema of the lower extremities through blockage of the intrapelvic nodes. When due to this cause the swelling can often be reduced by oestrogen or castration. Similarly, in rare cases where the superficial lymph nodes have become involved, visible and tangible signs of regression rapidly follow the institution of treatment. Further examples of the objective response will be found in Chapter 14.

Castration

Castration implies the removal or destruction of all functional testicular tissue with the object of preventing the continued secretion of tumour-stimulating androgens. Attempts to achieve this by local irradiation (Munger, 1941) have in general proved unreliable and, moreover, are only followed by a slow decrease in the urinary androgen excretion and relief of symptoms. Such relief is less dramatic than that following orchidectomy (Moore, 1947) and a further disadvantage is that the scrotal skin does not tolerate radiation well.

Surgical ablation is thus to be preferred but may be resented by some on aesthetic as well as sexual grounds. To counteract any emotional objection, subcapsular orchidectomy is now widely practised—the operation cavity eventually filling with organised blood clot thus restoring to the patient a semblance of scrotal dignity, albeit usually with impotence. It is essential that all testicular tissue should be removed and that complete evisceration should be ensured by thorough swabbing of the lining of the tunica albuginea before the capsule is resutured.

Persistent androgen secretion in response to chorionic gonadotropin stimulation has, in fact, been reported in some cases submitted to subcapsular orchidectomy and could only be abolished by complete removal of the testes (O'Conor, Chiang and Grayhack, 1963). In most instances, however, a satisfactory clearance is obtained, and, in a series of patients so treated by the author, ultimate histological studies at autopsy failed to define any residual testicular tissue.

THE OPERATION

Subcapsular or 'evisceration' orchidectomy is conveniently performed through a single horizontal scrotal incision exposing both testes. The scrotum is firmly grasped so as to stretch the skin and the incision is deepened through the investing layers until each testis is exposed. A vertical incision through the tunica albuginea from pole to pole then exposes the testicular substance which is readily separated by blunt dissection and swabbing and removed after ligation and division of the rete testis. Attempts to preserve the contours of the eviscerated organ by the insertion of an inert plastic prosthesis have in general often proved unsatisfactory owing to the subsequent tendency for dislocation or extrusion. All that is necessary is to resuture the tunica, whereupon the dead-space becomes filled with exudate and clot which is later replaced by fibrous tissue. In this way a psychologically acceptable appearance of masculinity can be preserved.

Whether performed in this manner or by radical orchidectomy, the great merit of castration as opposed to oestrogen therapy is that it provides a permanent means of abolishing testicular function without any troublesome side-effects or serious sequelae. Sterility must of course be accepted as inevitable, but impotence is not invariably absolute.

INDICATIONS FOR CASTRATION

Excluding emotional factors, the choice of castration as opposed to oestrogen therapy is often a matter of individual preference and is sometimes eluded by employing both methods in combination. Theoretically, at least, the most compelling reason for its adoption would seem to be in younger patients in whom the disease is commonly more active and, consequently, in more urgent need of suppression. Conversely in elderly cases an equivalent period of symptomatic relief sometimes extending throughout the lifetime of the patient can be obtained from oestrogen therapy alone. Nevertheless there are certain positive indications for its use as follows:

Intolerance of oestrogens. Some patients are unable to tolerate oestrogens on account of their side-effects (notably nausea and vomiting) and in such cases castration affords an appropriate alternative. This applies similarly to those in whom the presence of cardiac decompensation or hepatic disease contra-indicates sustained hormonal therapy.

Inability to sustain oestrogen therapy. Some patients are unreliable as far as continuing oral medication is concerned and may well be adjudged incapable of sustaining regular treatment. In these, castration may provide a better alternative than parenteral administration or depot therapy.

Malabsorption of oestrogens. Impaired absorption from the alimentary tract may reduce the effectiveness of oral oestrogen therapy. Chronic intestinal disease and the regular use of oily purgatives are often responsible factors. Inability or failure to correct these may support the need for adopting other methods of administration or, alternatively, castration.

Lack of response to oestrogens. Despite the usual similarity of the clinical response to oestrogen therapy and castration, there are some cases in which one may succeed where the other fails. Failure with oestrogens generally implies inadequate treatment but

if this possibility can be excluded castration should be undertaken. Although the relationship of tumour suppression and the development of oestrogenic side-effects remains uncertain the non-appearance of the latter (particularly genital shrinkage) during sustained treatment should favour the adoption of castration if the activity of the disease remains uncontrolled. On the other hand, in cases relapsing after prolonged oestrogen therapy, little benefit can usually be expected from supplementary castration if the testes have already become small.

CONTRAINDICATIONS TO CASTRATION

Castration should never be performed unless the diagnosis of prostatic cancer is fully assured. Clinical evidence alone is seldom sufficient and confirmation by other methods of investigation is usually required. In this respect castration may appear at some disadvantage with oestrogen therapy since the latter can, if necessary, be employed speculatively in unproven cases with comparatively little risk. Nevertheless, it is a good rule never to apply any form of endocrine-control therapy without reasonable proof of active malignant disease. Apart from such considerations the only major contraindications to castration comprise general unsuitability for surgical treatment or the refusal of the patient to consent to operation.

Oestrogen Therapy

The experimental basis for oestrogen therapy has already been discussed (Chapter 11) but the full mechanism of its effect on prostatic cancer remains obscure. It is generally assumed that in the intact subject the response stems mainly from a suppression of testicular

function mediated through lack of gonadotropic stimulation by the pituitary. Characteristic histological changes in the latter gland resemble those following castration, and consist of hyperplasia of the basophilic cells of the anterior lobe with vacuolation of the cytoplasm (Plates 12.1 and 12.2, facing p. 240).

At the same time the possibility of a direct effect on the testicular tissue itself has been investigated by some observers but reports on the degree and quality of any structural changes have varied considerably. Clinical experience, however, indicates that in most patients receiving oestrogen the testes diminish in size and become atrophic, although there are some in whom, despite a favourable response on the part of the disease, little alteration can be noted. In general it seems to be agreed that the main effect is on the spermatogenic tissues and that later when the connective tissue degenerates the interstitial cells become isolated and surrounded by fibrous tissue.

It is possible that the varying histological changes described may be related to the type and dosage of the oestrogen employed, and indeed current observations on the rapidity of the decline of circulating androgen in response to individual preparations would seem to accord with this view. On the other hand, such structural and functional changes may be purely secondary to the lack of pituitary influence. It should be mentioned, however, that the concept of local action on the testis has appealed to some to the extent of advising direct implantation of oestrogen into the testis (Darget, 1958).

Finally the possibility of an additional chemotherapeutic action on the tumour cells themselves must be taken into account, and evidence has been adduced from biological research to support the view that certain oestrogens at least may compromise the synthesis of DNA and other metabolic mechanisms in the rapidly dividing cells which characterise the malignant process. The histological changes both in the prostatic tumour and its metastases are referred to later in Chapter 14.

CHOICE OF OESTROGENS

Oestrogen therapy offers the great advantage, as compared with castration, of avoiding surgical intervention and there is at present little convincing evidence that it is any the less effective. Indeed, it seems likely that its action may even be more comprehensive and, when appropriately employed, the need for supplementary castration often becomes redundant. Moreover, the attraction of oral administration, in particular, in preference to a minor operative procedure is especially noteworthy.

On the other hand, sustained treatment carries the disadvantage of inducing certain side-effects, some of which in minor degree are reasonably acceptable, while others in the long term, according to recent suggestions, may be seriously incapacitating or lethal. Much undoubtedly may be gained by appropriate timing as well as by the suitable choice of preparation and dosage to minimise the risks involved.

Effective therapy primarily depends on the selection of an active preparation which is readily absorbed and well tolerated. It is perhaps unfortunate that there are too few clinicians with sufficient biochemical expertise to discriminate among the wide variety of oestrogenic compounds preferred by the pharmaceutical industry. Nevertheless, considerable credit is due to the latter for much painstaking research directed towards the elaboration of new compounds immune from the liability of causing troublesome sequelae.

Fundamentally, it remains uncertain whether the cancer-suppressant effect of oestrogens can be fully divorced from their oestrogenic activity; and, from a purely clinical aspect, the non-appearance of feminising changes may still cast doubt on the efficacy of a particular preparation. Conversely, certain substances which appear pre-eminently capable of inducing oestrous changes in animals would seem to have little therapeutic value. Likewise others, which are capable of exercising a direct suppressant action on cellular metabolism in the laboratory, are either ineffective or unsuitable in clinical use. Reliance has thus to be placed at the present time on a relatively restricted range of preparations which, from extended experience, have been adjudged both active and reasonably safe.

CLASSIFICATION OF OESTROGENS

Basically, oestrogens may be classed in two main groups according to their derivation. Those prepared or extracted from natural or animal sources are termed 'natural' oestrogens while those formulated by chemical processes are referred to as 'synthetic' oestrogens. In addition, the seemingly paradoxical term 'non-oestrogenic oestrogen' has been applied to a number of steroid compounds which, it is claimed, exert a tumour-suppressive effect without inducing feminising changes.

Many of the naturally occurring oestrogens, unless modified by chemical substitution, have little or no potency on oral administration. Moreover, they are comparatively expensive to extract and prepare for therapeutic purposes. The use of substituted preparations, however, finds limited scope either by the parenteral route or, occasionally, as an alternative by mouth in cases where synthetic oestrogens are poorly tolerated. It has not, as yet, been shown whether their prolonged administration carries any significant difference in the incidence of thrombotic or cardiovascular complications.

Most of the synthetic oestrogens, on the other hand, are highly active by mouth and the clinical effect of their administration may be noted within a few days. Although superficially differing in their chemical structure from the naturally occurring hormones, in some instances a rearrangement in spatial relationship suggests a degree of resemblance. In general, therefore, on the grounds of potency, expense and ease of administration, synthetic oestrogens are widely preferred. Moreover in the event of oral intolerance (nausea or vomiting) they can also be administered in modified form parenterally, either by the intravenous route (Honvan) or by subcutaneous implantation.

MODES OF ADMINISTRATION OF OESTROGENS

While there are obvious advantages in employing the oral route, the success of this method depends not only on the efficacy of the ingested preparation, but on the capacity of the patient to cooperate. Some patients cannot be relied upon to sustain regular treatment and in many it may be necessary to divulge something of the serious nature of their disease to ensure continuity. Others may be unable to conform on account of side-effects or gastrointestinal intolerance.

Furthermore, the rate and amount of absorption from the alimentary tract may be modified by intrinsic bowel disease or by the use of oily purgatives. To meet these difficulties other methods of administration may sometimes have to be considered, as for example the intravenous, intramuscular or subcutaneous routes. Table 12.1, which in no way claims to be comprehensive, may be taken as illustrative of the possibilities.

In general, most patients tolerate stilboestrol well by the oral route and there is at present little clinical evidence to suggest that any of its related synthetic preparations is superior in the long-term control of prostatic cancer. There are, however, occasions when, irrespective of dosage, the onset of nausea and side-effects precludes its continued use. In these circumstances, as also in cases of relapse where the disease is no longer responding, there is usually nothing to be gained by substituting an alternative synthetic product. On the other hand, a change to one of the natural oestrogens may overcome the disadvantage of gastric intolerance although the tumour-suppressive effect is unlikely to be enhanced. Failure to obtain control for any of these reasons supports the need for considering other methods of administration, or, alternatively, castration.

The main indication for intravenous administration is where, on account of the severity of the symptoms and particularly in cases of impending urinary obstruction, a rapid response is desired. In this respect, the use of a water-soluble synthetic oestrogen (Honvan) may bring about a dramatic improvement and, on occasions, obviate the need for catheterisation or palliative surgery. The obvious disadvantage of the intravenous route, however, lies in the inconvenience of its continued use and for this reason regular injections are usually restricted to a period of from 5 to 10 days.

natural oestrogen Estradurin at 2 to 4-week intervals may afford a reliable and effective means of controlling the disease, and in refractory cases there may be no objection to simultaneous treatment with synthetic preparations given by the oral route.

The use of subcutaneously implanted oestrogen pellets has found little favour in the treatment of malignant prostatic disease mainly because a constant rate of absorption cannot be guaranteed. Introduction demands

TABLE 12.1. *Some oestrogens and their modes of administration*

Type of oestrogen	Mode of administration: Oral	Intravenous	Intramuscular	Subcutaneous
Natural	Ethinyl-oestradiol Premarin		Oestradiol phosphate (Estradurin)	Oestradiol
Synthetic	Stilboestrol Dienoestrol Hexoestrol Chlorotrianisene (TACE)	Stilboestrol diphosphate (Honvan)		Stilboestrol

Whereas full dosage can be ensured for this period, there is some risk if treatment is continued longer that the over-accumulation of oestrogen metabolites in the liver may lead to serious consequences.

The same objection applies in some degree to other methods of parenteral and depot administration. It should always be borne in mind that the advantage of being able to deliver a prescribed, and often large, dose of oestrogen by such means may be offset by difficulty in counteracting its continuing action if serious complications develop. The chief risks stem from water retention which may lead to additional cardiac embarrassment in patients already suffering from incipient heart disease and, as mentioned above, from the hepatotoxic effect of accumulated metabolites in the liver.

Nevertheless, in selected patients, regular intramuscular injections of the substituted

the use of a large-bore cannula or a small surgical procedure under full asepsis and carries both the risks of fragmentation of the pellets and subsequent extrusion. The rate of absorption depends not only on the composition and method of preparation of the pellet but also on its naturally diminishing speed of decay as well as on the reaction of the surrounding tissues.

USEFUL OESTROGENS AND THEIR DOSAGE

No attempt is made to provide a comprehensive list but attention is directed towards a number of preparations in common use of which the author has had personal clinical experience.

ORALLY ACTIVE OESTROGENS

As previously mentioned, general opinion inclines to the use of *synthetic* preparations but their dosage still remains arbitrary. Initially the latter was based partly on the quantity required to induce oestrus changes in laboratory animals and partly on experience of the results of treatment of endocrine deficiencies in gynaecological practice. In both instances emphasis was laid on the hormonal effect and caution dictated a conservative attitude.

Despite the fact that the symptomatic manifestations of prostatic cancer were often relieved by the small doses then currently prescribed, the appearance of early relapse soon led to larger quantities being given in the hope of being able to extend the period of control. At the same time, the suggestion that oestrogens might also exert a direct effect on the tumour cells gave added impetus to this practice. Since neither premise has received unqualified scientific support it is perhaps hardly surprising that widely differing amounts continue to be prescribed.

Diethylstilboestrol which is often favoured as a relatively cheap and orally potent compound remains the treatment of choice for prostatic cancer, and *hexoestrol* or *dienoestrol* have no proven advantage over it. Although the dosage advocated has varied between 1 mg and 100 mg (or even 1000 mg) in different hands, it is usually given in the ranges of 5 to 15 mg or of 50 to 100 mg daily according to individual preference. The former level takes account of the fact that such quantities are usually sufficient to induce definable endocrine changes thus indicating that they are at least effective in this respect.

The case for employing larger amounts rests mainly on the presumption of an additional direct oncolytic or chemotherapeutic action on the tumour. Added support for their use comes from clinical experience in some series in which more effective control of symptoms and a reduction of the early mortality rate have been found to follow initial high dosage (Fergusson, 1958). Moreover, in cases relapsing after treatment at the lower level, some measure of renewed control can sometimes be achieved by more intensive therapy. At the same time, repeated biopsies have shown histological evidence of further tumour regression (Fergusson and Franks, 1953).

As far as tolerance and the incidence of endocrine side-effects are concerned there seems to be little difference between the use of low and high dosage, but the potential risk of cardiovascular complications calls for some caution in continuing the latter indefinitely. It is now the author's practice to prescribe 50 mg stilboestrol b.d. initially and to reduce this to a maintenance dose of 25 mg b.d. after the first three months if a favourable clinical response has been shown. In elderly cases, where the disease is less active, correspondingly smaller quantities may suffice.

Alternation with other allied synthetic compounds, for example dienoestrol or hexoestrol, has no advantage and any claim for these substances based on their possibly greater oestrogenic activity has not been reflected in their clinical effect.

There are some observers, however, who have declared a preference for phosphorylated diethyl stilboestrol (*Honvan*), based presumably on the view that active stilboestrol is liberated from this compound at the tumour sites (see intravenous administration). The oral dose ranges between 100 and 300 mg daily and at the latter level has been claimed to yield benefit in occasional patients in whom conventional stilboestrol therapy has lost its effect (Trafford, 1965). Dosage starting as high as 15 000 mg daily has also been stated to give a response in a majority of patients not responding to or relapsing after orchidectomy or oestrogen administration (Colapinto and Aberhart, 1961). Long-term results *are not* quoted.

A somewhat structurally different prooestrogen *chlorotrianisine* (TACE) has also been widely used on the grounds that it appears less likely to induce compensatory hyperplasia of the adrenals (hence increased androgen secretion) as commonly occurs after the employment of other oestrogens or castration. However, in the author's experience this compound has shown no therapeutic superiority and the additional claim that it also protects against mammary enlargement has not been substantiated. It is given in doses of 24 mg daily but larger amounts up to 180 mg a day are well tolerated (Carroll and Brennan, 1954). It is also claimed to be effective in occasional patients when stilboestrol fails (Mortensen, 1953).

In most cases when synthetic oestrogens in sufficient dosage fail to induce a symptomatic response, it may be inferred that the tumour has already become altogether resistant to oestrogen therapy and little or no improvement can be expected from a change to natural hormones. There are, however, some patients who are initially intolerant of the synthetic preparations and who may respond to the latter without disturbance.

In these circumstances both *ethinyloestradiol* and *Premarin* are suitable preparations, each capable of promoting an endocrine response even though a direct effect on tumour-cell metabolism remains unproven. The former is given in the dosage of one-fiftieth to one-tenth of that of stilboestrol while the latter is usually employed in the range of 5 to 15 mg daily. It has been stated that after two to three weeks' administration of Premarin the patient will often tolerate stilboestrol without difficulty.

INTRAVENOUS THERAPY

The intravenous administration of oestrogens should be restricted to those cases with acute symptoms in whom a rapid response is required pending the establishment of regular treatment by the oral route. Stilboestrol itself is relatively insoluble in water and thus unsuitable, but by a process of phosphorylation it can be modified to produce a soluble though inert compound *Honvan*. This is commonly administered in doses of 250 to 500 mg daily either by immediate injection or rapid-drip infusion.

The circulating compound is said to be converted to active stilboestrol by a process of 'dephosphorylation' at the sites of phosphatase activity in the body (notably the tumour cells) and thus to induce an enhanced effect by local concentration (Druckrey and Raabe, 1952). Much of the earlier work on this compound was based on biological research which suggested direct interference with cellular metabolism. Furthermore, its subsequent application to the treatment of prostatic cancer in man was encouraged by reports of the occurrence of perineal and sacral pain immediately following injection which were construed as due to the concentration of liberated stilboestrol at the site of the primary tumour. This, however, would seem to be a misconception since a similar effect has been recorded in female patients in whom it has been used for the treatment of cancer of the breast. Moreover, in other patients the distribution of local discomfort has been found to vary widely and, in one case of the author's—an observant surgeon—it was limited to the shaving area of the face.

There is some evidence from trials with radioactively labelled Honvan that a selective concentration of free stilboestrol may be achieved at least temporarily at the tumour sites (Segal, Marberger and Flocks, 1959; Fergusson, 1961). This, however, is not entirely in accordance with the experience of others (Twombly and Schoenewaldt, 1951; Bozoky et al, 1957) who found little evidence of any therapeutically significant local activity. It seems, likely, indeed, that any liberated 'free' stilboestrol soon passes into the general circulation and thus has comparatively little opportunity for exerting an enhanced antimitotic effect on the tumour.

INTRAMUSCULAR THERAPY

This method is favoured by some for patients who are likely to require long-term maintenance therapy. It should be used with caution as side-effects once established take longer to reverse. Various esters such as the valerianate or undecyclate may be used for this purpose. Probably more effective is *Estradurin* (polyoestradiol phosphate) which is given in doses ranging from 80 to 200 mg monthly or more often (Goodhope, 1957).

Gynaecomastia and dyspepsia are said to be less troublesome from this agent than from therapy with oral oestrogens. Palliation of symptoms may be slower but occurs after two to three doses, and like other newer oestrogenic preparations it is claimed to be useful occasionally when stilboestrol resistance develops. Likewise, there is no particular contraindication to its use in combination with synthetic hormones.

Because of the relatively small reduction in androgen excretion which follows its use, it has been suggested by Jonsson (1965) that the major part of its effect is directly upon the prostatic cancer cells. This author now uses it in combination with an oncolytic agent.

IMPLANTED OESTROGENS

Theoretically, subcutaneously implanted pellets should yield the slowest absorption and therefore the greatest biological effectiveness per dose. Unfortunately their rate of absorption is inconstant and may be significantly affected by the reaction of the surrounding tissue. Nevertheless, there are some who favour this route and pellets of α-oestradiol 25 mg or hexoestrol 100 mg can be implanted at six to eight week intervals.

The bilateral intratesticular implant of diethylstilboestrol, 125 mg on each side, has already been referred to and has been described in the French literature as an 'elegant' method of combining 'medical castration' with oestrogen therapy.

SIDE-EFFECTS OF OESTROGENS

These may be conveniently subdivided into toxic, 'feminising', systemic and psychological.

TOXIC EFFECTS

Nausea and vomiting. These symptoms of oestrogen intolerance are comparatively rare in the male, and when they occur the disturbance is often only transient. The evening dose of oestrogen is usually well tolerated and dosage can then be slowly increased or antiemetics can be prescribed during the first few weeks of treatment. As an alternative, intravenous therapy can be given although an initial period of anorexia is common. In susceptible cases the factor of dosage appears unimportant and large amounts seem no more likely to cause nausea and vomiting than when small quantities are given.

Hepatotoxic effect. Many steroids are apt to induce hepatic damage and cholestasis when the agent is given in sufficient dosage for prolonged periods (Sherlock, 1968). Tracer experiments with labelled oestrogens have demonstrated an accumulation of metabolites in the liver and this is likely to be accentuated after high dosage by the parenteral route (Fergusson, 1963). *Jaundice* and rapidly progressive *liver failure* have been reported on a number of occasions mainly after excessive therapy by the intravenous route. Emphasis is laid on the need for caution in patients already suffering from cirrhosis or allied biliary disorders.

Skin rashes are relatively infrequent but, when severe, may sometimes prompt the need for stopping treatment.

FEMINISING EFFECTS

These are possibly better termed 'sex-neutralising' effects and consist mainly of a reversal of the normal masculine characteristics. *Shrinkage of the genitalia* is not confined to the testes and both scrotum and penis are affected. *Loss of libido, impotence* and *azoospermia* are to be expected but are not necessarily absolute. Nevertheless, they may be ponderable factors when selecting treatment especially in the case of younger patients.

Breast changes. Some degree of *mammary*

enlargement accompanied by increased sensitivity of the nipples takes place in a majority of cases (Moore, Wattenberg and Rose, 1945). This is often evident within a week or two of commencing treatment and, if oral therapy has been adopted, affords some indication of the patient's cooperation. It is usually wise to warn the patient in advance, otherwise such changes are apt to be alarming, or alternatively, to institute a course of local prophylactic radiotherapy before commencing treatment. Gynaecomastia can usually be prevented by giving an erythema dose of x-ray therapy to both breasts on the first day of steroid therapy. It reduces the number of ducts in the mammary tissue and thus decreases proliferation (Larson and Sundbom, 1962). After gynaecomastia has developed, however, regression is not caused by this dose of irradiation (Alfthan and Kettunen, 1965).

It is a peculiar feature that when breast changes become noticeable during the early stages of treatment they may subsequently vary in intensity and even regress despite continuation of the same dosage. Rarely, excessive enlargement may lead to serious psychological embarrassment and prompt the need for local mastectomy. At an earlier stage surgical excision of the potentially hyperplastic ductal tissue (periareolar incision) has been advocated (Amelar, 1962).

The incidence of *breast cancer* is said to be higher than normal in patients receiving oestrogen therapy. About 20 case reports have been published and it appears likely in most instances that this tumour represented a metastasis from the prostate rather than a primary breast lesion (Benson, 1957). Differentiation may be aided by staining the histological preparations for acid phosphatase.

Pigmentation often occurs in the enlarged nipples and less frequently in the periareolar zone. The anoscrotal raphe may also be affected and, likewise, the midline in the lower abdomen and cutaneous scar tissue.

Changes in the complexion and a *reduction of hair growth* are further examples of the 'feminising' effect and a characteristic facies often develops which enables the patient receiving oestrogen to be recognised at a glance. In a few cases vasomotor attacks resembling menopausal 'flushings' may be experienced.

SYSTEMIC EFFECTS

These may arise from disturbances in the water and electrolyte balance or result from changes in the coagulability of the blood and interference with the haemopoietic system.

Some degree of salt and water retention predisposing to *oedema* is an inevitable sequel to oestrogen administration. In most cases the accumulation is insignificant and may do little more than create the illusion of a healthy gain in weight. In others the appearance of oedema of the lower extremities is more alarming and suggests the possibility of cardiac embarrassment resulting from the excessive water load. Difficulty may sometimes arise in distinguishing oedema due to this cause, from that occurring as the result of lymphatic spread of the disease in the pelvis, although the latter is more likely to be predominantly unilateral.

Treatment of fluid retention may be attempted with diuretics or a low sodium diet, but, if prolonged, potassium supplements may be necessary. It is imperative, however, that diuretics should be used with caution, as rapid over-filling of the bladder in patients with impending urinary obstruction may precipitate retention. In serious cases of congestive cardiac failure, oestrogen therapy may have to be abandoned and other alternatives (such as castration) sought.

Disturbances of blood clotting and a liability to *thrombotic complication*. Reports of defective blood coagulation are by no means uncommon in untreated prostatic cancer and are usually ascribable to excessive fibrinolysis due to an enzyme present in the prostatic cells (Tagnon et al, 1953; Aboulker, Soulier and Larrieu, 1955). Rare instances of bleeding after the institution of oestrogen therapy have been recorded (Schwerdtfeger, 1954;

Balogh, 1960) but this complication has been denied by others (Cottier, Leupold and Scheitlin, 1955). Of far greater significance is the suggestion that oestrogens may promote a thrombotic tendency even in low dosage corresponding with 5 mg of stilboestrol daily (VACURG, 1967), and caution is therefore advisable in all patients with a suspicion of cardiovascular or cerebrovascular disease.

Evidence of an increased risk, however, has failed to secure support from other quarters, and it would seem manifestly difficult to arrive at a reliable conclusion in the patients under review. All that can be said, at the present, is that any potential liability to thrombosis should be viewed in perspective against the notable benefits which sustained oestrogen therapy can confer.

It has also been stated that sustained treatment may in rare instances lead to impairment of the haemopoietic system (Balogh and Szendroi, 1968) and result in a failure of bone-marrow function. This, however, must clearly be difficult to differentiate from the destructive effect of metastastic osseous involvement.

PSYCHOLOGICAL EFFECTS

Serious mental disturbances are uncommon with the exception of those occasionally arising in younger patients from the contemplation of their diminished potency and probable sterility. Most of the manifestations reported in more elderly cases are somewhat nebulous and little more than would normally be expected at this age. Most patients adapt themselves well to the circumstances which generally include some inkling of the nature of their complaint and, while occasional 'flushings' may be experienced, the usual tenor of life remains unchanged.

It should also be borne in mind that attempts have been made to define the psychological status of those who are prone to the development of prostatic cancer (Trunnell et al, 1951) and it is thus remotely possible that those at risk would show some subsequent tendency to instability. This to the author's knowledge has never been recorded.

CONCLUSION

The ability of castration or oestrogen therapy to suppress the activity of prostatic cancer is undoubted, but variable in duration. Castration, usually in the form of subcapsular orchidectomy, is indicated in patients where an urgent response is required, where tolerance or absorption of oestrogens is low, or where oestrogens fail to control the disease. Because of the occasional risks associated with prolonged oestrogen administration, its use should be deferred when alternative treatment is available, until such time as its maximum benefit is required.

The mechanism of oestrogen action in prostatic cancer is either by suppression of pituitary gonadotropin or by a direct action on the tumour cells. Oral administration of the synthetic oestrogen diethylstilboestrol is satisfactory in the vast majority of patients. High dosage levels may lead to more effective control of symptoms when used as initial treatment, or renewed control when used for relapse after low dose therapy. Ethinyloestradiol or Premarin may be tolerated orally when stilboestrol is not. Intravenous administration of Honvan is useful in cases of urgency or intramuscular administration of Estradurin when oral administration is uncertain.

Some degree of feminisation is inevitable from oestrogen therapy, but the cardiovascular, hepatotoxic or thrombotic hazards of oestrogen administration should be viewed in perspective against the notable benefits it can confer in prostatic cancer.

References

Aboulker, P., Soulier, J. P. & Larrieu, M. J. (1955) Syndrome hemorrhagique avec fibrinolyse associe au cancer de la prostate. *Presse Médicale*, **63**, 353–354.

Alfthan, O. & Kettunen, K. (1965) The effect of roentgen ray treatment of gynecomastia in patients with prostatic carcinoma treated with estrogenic hormones: a preliminary communication. *Journal of Urology*, **94**, 604–606.

Amelar, R. D. (1962) Subareolar mastectomy to prevent estrogen-induced male breast enlargement: a new procedure for use in patients with carcinoma of the prostate. *Journal of Urology*, **87**, 479–484.

Balogh, F. (1960) On a rare complication following treatment with Honvan. *Zeitschrift für Urologie*, **53**, 505–508.

Balogh, F. & Szendroi, Z. (1968) *Cancer of the prostate*. Budapest: Akademiai Kiado.

Benson, W. R. (1957) Carcinoma of the prostate with metastases to breasts and testis; critical review of the literature and report of a case. *Cancer*, **10**, 1235–1245.

Bozoky, L., Szendroi, Z., Fejes, P. & Magasi, P. (1957) Szervspecifikus izotop terapia lehetosege prostataraknal. (Therapeutic use of organ specific isotopes in prostatic cancer.) *Kiserletes Orvostudomany*, **9**, 130–132.

Carroll, G. & Brennan, R. V. (1954) TACE in prostatic cancer. Clinical and biochemical considerations. *Journal of Urology*, **72**, 497–503.

Colapinto, V. & Aberhart, C. (1961) Clinical trial of massive stilboestrol diphosphate therapy in advanced carcinoma of the prostate. *British Journal of Urology*, **33**, 171–177.

Cottier, P., Leupold, R. & Scheitlin, W. (1955) Die Hämorrhagische Diathese bei Prostatakarzinom und ihne Behandlung. *Schweizerische medizinische Wochenschrift*, **85**, 781–786.

Darget, R. (1958) Le cancer de la prostate, son diagnostic, son traitement radiumtherapeutique. Paris: Masson.

Druckrey, H. & Raabe, S. (1952) Organspecifische des Krebs (Prostata-Karzinom). *Klinische Wochenschrift*, **30**, 882–884.

Fergusson, J. D. (1958) Endocrine control therapy in prostatic cancer. *British Journal of Urology*, **30**, 397–406.

Fergusson, J. D. (1961) Advances in urology. *Practitioner*, **185**, 517–523.

Fergusson, J. D. (1963) Some aspects of the conservative management of prostatic cancer. *Proceedings of the Royal Society of Medicine*, **56**, 81–88.

Fergusson, J. D. & Franks, L. M. (1953) Response of prostatic carcinoma to oestrogen treatment. *British Journal of Surgery*, **40**, 422–428.

Flocks, R. H., Harness, W. N., Tudor, J. M. & Prendergast, L. (1951) Treatment of carcinoma of prostate. *Journal of Urology*, **66**, 393–407.

Franks, L. M., Fergusson, J. D. & Murnaghan, G. F. (1958) An assessment of factors influencing survival in prostatic cancer: the absence of reliable prognostic features. *British Journal of Cancer*, **12**, 321–326.

Goodhope, C. D. (1957) Polyestradiol phosphate for carcinoma of the prostate: a clinical study. *Journal of Urology*, **77**, 312–314.

Jonsson, G. (1965) Estradurin (polyoestradiol phosphate) in the treatment of prostatic carcinoma. A clinical and steroid metabolic study. *Urologia Internationalis*, **19**, 11–18.

Larsson, L. G. & Sundbom, C. M. (1962) Roentgen irradiation of the male breast. *Acta Radiologica*, **58**, 253–256.

Moore, G. F., Wattenberg, C. A. & Rose, D. K. (1945) Breast changes due to diethylstilboestrol during treatment of cancer of the prostate gland. *Journal of the American Medical Association*, **127**, 60–62.

Moore, R. A. (1947) Benign hypertrophy and carcinoma of the prostate. In *Endocrinology of Neoplastic Diseases*, ed. Twombly, G. H. and Pack, G. T., pp. 194–212. New York: Oxford University Press.

Mortensen, H. (1953) Treatment of carcinoma of prostate with new oestrogen "TACE". *Medical Journal of Australia*, **1**, 728–730.

Munger, A. D. (1941) Experiences in treatment of carcinoma of prostate with irradiation of testicles. *Journal of Urology*, **46**, 1007–1011.

Nesbit, R. M. & Plumb, R. T. (1946) Prostatic carcinoma; follow up on 795 patients treated prior to endocrine era and comparison of survival rates between these and patients treated by endocrine therapy. *Surgery*, **20**, 263–272.

O'Conor, V. J., Chiang, S. P. & Grayhack, J. T. (1963) Is subcapsular orchiectomy a definitive procedure? Studies of hormone excretion before and after orchiectomy. *Journal of Urology*, **89**, 236–240.

Schwerdtfeger, K. (1954) Bedeutet das Präparat ST52 Asta einen Fortschritt in der Behandlung des Prostatacarcinoms? *Medizinische Klinik*, **49**, 1290–1293.

Segal, S. J., Marberger, H. & Flocks, R. H. (1959) Tissue distribution of stilboestrol diphosphate: concentration in prostatic tissue. *Journal of Urology*, **81**, 474–478.

Sherlock, S. (1968) Drugs and the liver. *British Medical Journal*, **1**, 227–229.

Tagnon, H. G., Schulman, P., Whitmore, W. F. &
   Leone, A. (1953) Prostatic fibrinolysin. Study of a
   case illustrating the role in hemorrhagic diathesis of
   cancer of the prostate. *American Journal of Medicine*,
   15, 875–884.
Trafford, H. S. (1965) The place of Honvan (diethylstilboestrol diphosphate) in the treatment of prostatic cancer; a review of 24 cases. *British Journal of
   Urology*, **37**, 317–319.
Trunnell, J. B., Duffy, B. J., Marshall, V., Whitmore,
   W. F. & Woodard, H. Q. (1951) Use of progesterone
   in treatment of cancer of prostate. *Journal of Clinical
   Endocrinology and Metabolism*, **11**, 663–676.

Twombly, G. H. & Schoenewaldt, E. F. (1951)
   Tissue localisation and excretion routes of radio-
   active diethylstilboestrol. *Cancer*, **4**, 296–302.
Veterans Administration Co-operative Urological
   Research Group (1964) Carcinoma of the prostate:
   analysis of patient morbidity at 6 month, 12 month
   and 18 month follow up examinations. *Journal of
   Chronic diseases*, **17**, 207–223.
Veterans Administration Co-operative Urological
   Research Group (1967) Treatment and survival of
   patients with cancer of the prostate. *Surgery, Gynecology and Obstetrics*, **124**, 1011–1017.

Chapter 13

Secondary Endocrine Therapy

J. D. FERGUSSON

To a large extent the need for secondary endocrine therapy has been prompted by the occurrence of relapse after an initial response to oestrogens and castration. At the same time the fact that some tumours fail to respond to such measures from the outset has lead to a search for alternative methods of hormonal suppression. The whole matter has been further complicated by the introduction of new endocrine substances designed primarily for the treatment of *benign* prostatic hyperplasia (such as progestins).

Broadly speaking the measures under review comprise:

1. The use of alternative hormones known to have an effect on the pituitary and possibly also exerting a direct action on the tumour (for example, androgens and progestins).
2. The use of cortical suppressants to diminish the compensatory secretion of androgens by the adrenals known to occur after oestrogen therapy and castration (corticosteroid therapy).
3. Ablative surgery designed to suppress or eliminate the continuing elaboration of tumour-stimulating hormones from extragonadal sources (adrenalectomy and hypophyseal destruction).

At first sight, the variety of methods advocated might appear to cast some doubt on their efficacy and, in some instances, this may well be true. In view of the complications noted with oestrogen therapy, recent research into the formulation of alternative compounds has tended to concentrate rather more on their tumour-inhibiting properties than on their endocrine qualities. Additional considerations have also included the need to avoid toxicity and thrombotic sequelae. In consequence some of the preparations put forward under the guise of being tumour-suppressing hormones or 'non-oestrogenic oestrogens' would seem to qualify mainly from their *chemo*-therapeutic effect. It is on this account that attention is here directed solely towards certain agents which are known on physiological grounds to induce an endocrine response.

Androgens in Prostatic Cancer

Although seemingly paradoxical, it has been noted that in rare instances cases of prostatic cancer which fail to respond to oestrogens may react favourably, though possibly temporarily, to androgen administration. In other circumstances the more usual effect of stimulating tumour activity may be put to advantage either in combination with other forms of treatment (for example, radioactive phosphorus—see below) or as a measure of 'reculer pour mieux sauter' to enhance the response to a further trial of conventional therapy. The use of androgens has been suggested as follows:

STIMULATION OF THE ACID PHOSPHATASE LEVEL

The administration of 25 mg testosterone propionate intramuscularly daily has been reported to lead to the relief of pain from bone metastases in some cases (Brendler, Chase and Scott, 1950; Pearson, 1957; Prout and Brewer, 1967). This relief of pain is difficult to explain except on the basis of a placebo effect and other authors have reported an increase in bone pain following androgen administration of 100 mg daily (Parsons, Campbell and Thomley, 1962; Donati, Ellis and Gallagher, 1966). The use of androgens has been said to cause a rise in the serum acid phosphatase level in all patients with prostatic cancer (Huggins and Hodges, 1941; Brendler et al, 1950) but this claim is not confirmed by Prout and Brewer (1967). The observation originally formed the basis of the 'provocation test' in patients where the diagnosis of prostatic cancer remained obscure.

COMBINATION WITH RADIO-ACTIVE COMPOUNDS

Malignant tissue will take up and retain radioactive phosphorus to a greater degree than normal tissues. It has been shown that pretreatment of patients with androgen or oestrogen will increase the concentration of ^{32}P in various types of tumour, by a factor of 5 to 10 times that of normal tissue (Hertz, 1950). For these reasons a combination of ^{32}P and androgens has been suggested for the treatment of bone metastases in patients with prostatic cancer, especially if the pain has not responded to oestrogen therapy, castration or corticosteroid therapy (Parsons et al, 1962). Androgen pretreatment may also be useful because of its stimulant effect on erythropoiesis in the bone marrow (Gardner and Pringle, 1961).

The regime involves the administration of testosterone propionate intramuscularly in doses of 100 mg daily for five days before, during and five days after the course of ^{32}P. The dosage of the latter is 1·8 mCi orally, daily for seven days. Oestrogen therapy is then resumed one week after ceasing androgen therapy (Parsons et al, 1962; Donati et al, 1966). Relief of pain is stated to occur in the majority of patients so treated but the effect on the serum acid phosphatase level is not constant.

Relief of pain from bone metastases is also said to follow the administration of ^{32}P in combination with the pro-oestrogen TACE (Kaplan et al, 1960) but it remains doubtful whether this may not be due mainly to the latter. Nevertheless the combination of oestrogen with the radioactive substance would seem safer if less logical than using an androgen.

HORMONAL 'SHOCK' THERAPY

The use of androgens in patients with prostatic cancer has been suggested in those who have become clinically resistant to oestrogen therapy (Pedrotti and Frizzi, 1966). Daily intramuscular injections of testosterone propionate 25 mg for a week are suggested, followed by a resumption of oestrogens. It is claimed that some degree of responsiveness to oestrogens is restored in a majority of patients.

The action of androgens in such cases may be similar to that postulated by others who have advocated alternation in hormonal therapy (Desberg, 1960). It has sometimes been observed that in non-orchidectomised patients showing new spread of the disease or a rising serum acid phosphatase level, a change in the form of oestrogen administered may lead to a renewed response and a fall in the serum enzyme level. It is, therefore, possible that there is a direct action of steroids on malignant tissue, whereby enzymatic pathways which have adapted to the presence of an individual hormone may still be inhibited by others.

Progestin Therapy

The administration of progesterone in doses of 25 to 300 mg intramuscularly daily has been reported to yield both objective and subjective benefit in advanced prostatic cancer (Trunnell et al, 1951), both in previously untreated patients and those in relapse. Progesterone has, however, the disadvantage of causing painful induration at the site of injection. More recently the use of 17 α-hydroxyprogesterone caproate (Delalutin) has been reported in prostatic cancer (Brendler and Prout, 1962; Geller et al, 1967). According to the former authors 250 mg intramuscularly weekly is well tolerated but larger or more frequent doses involve the risk of making the tumour more active. The latter authors, however, report on the use of 3 g weekly, with reduction of the acid phosphatase level to normal in the third week in all cases, and rapid relief of bone pain. Gain in weight and improvement in appetite were maintained in some for longer than one year. The patients were not castrated and all showed a fall in the plasma testosterone level as a result of progestin therapy but without reduction of the plasma luteinising hormone (LH) level.

Latterly, megestrol acetate, 20 to 30 mg orally daily, has also been reported to yield objective benefit in advanced prostatic cancer (Lebech, 1967). The progestins of the 17α-hydroxyprogesterone group (of which Delalutin and megestrol are members) are said to possess no inherent oestrogenicity or androgenicity. They are well tolerated and unlikely to cause liver damage even at high dosage.

The mode of action of progestins on prostatic cancer may be through one or more of the following mechanisms:

1. Depressing LH secretion by the anterior pituitary.

2. Competitive blocking of androgen action at the target organ.

3. Direct effect on the testis (Geller et al, 1967).

4. Synergistically to another hormone. Such an action has been suggested in breast carcinoma (Stoll, 1967) and in endometrial carcinoma (Sherman and Woolf, 1959).

Corticosteroid Therapy

The basis of this form of treatment relies on the fact that following castration there is an increased output of gonadotropins by the pituitary which in turn increases the activity of the adrenal cortex. The resultant adrenal hyperplasia, which is also apparent after sustained oestrogen therapy, leads to a compensatory secretion of androgens and a consequent change in the hormonal milieu which is favourable to the continuing activity of prostatic cancer. Corticosteroid therapy aims at antagonising the pituitary and, by so doing, reducing the stimulus to gonadotropin secretion and its consequent effect on the adrenals. As a result cortical activity is diminished and the elaboration of tumour-stimulating androgens by the adrenals becomes significantly reduced.

This concept of extragonadal androgen activity had previously occurred to Huggins and his co-workers before the synthesis of cortisone and led to a courageous though premature attempt at bilateral total adrenalectomy (Huggins and Scott, 1945). Following the availability of cortisone, surgical treatment of this nature was placed on a practical footing and has since achieved considerable success in the case of mammary cancer if only on a lesser scale in prostatic malignancy. It will be obvious, indeed, that in dealing with the higher age group involved with prostatic cancer and its attendant hazards of intercurrent disease, an operation of this calibre can only be considered in exceptional circumstances. The idea of promoting a similar effect by endocrine therapy (medical adrenalectomy) would thus seem highly commendable.

Sprague and his co-workers (1950) suggested that as corticosteroid administration leads to atrophy of the adrenal cortex, effects similar to those of adrenalectomy might well be achieved by its use in advanced hormone-sensitive cancers. Corticosteroid administration depresses ACTH secretion which, together with LH secretion, controls the release of androgens from the adrenal cortex. It has the added advantage of increasing weight and appetite and inducing a sense of euphoria in advanced cases—features which have to be taken into account in the assessment of any benefit which may result from tumour suppression. On the other hand, sustained therapy involves a high incidence of adverse side-effects, most of which appear after high and prolonged dosage.

Varying degrees of improvement have been reported from cortisone or prednisolone administration in advanced prostatic cancer (Hayward, 1953; Valk and Owens, 1954; Burt, Finney and Scott, 1957; Grayhack, 1959; Mellinger, 1965). However, the papers published to date are on small series, and do not agree on such vital points as the proportion of cases responding, the most effective compounds, the optimum dose level and the relation between benefit from corticosteroids and that from other endocrine manipulation. Also unestablished is the selection of cases likely to respond to such therapy.

It has been suggested at one extreme that corticosteroid therapy is as effective as adrenalectomy in prostatic cancer (Miller and Hinman, 1954) while, at the other, its benefits have appeared transient and purely symptomatic (Fergusson, 1963). Indeed it is not uncommon to see temporary subjective improvement while radiographic studies show spread of the tumour.

Benefit from corticosteroid therapy in prostatic cancer may be considered from four aspects: benefit in relation to dosage, benefit in relation to that from anti-androgen therapy, benefit in relation to that from adrenalectomy and benefit in relation to the excretion level of androgenic 17-ketosteroids.

BENEFIT IN RELATION TO THE DOSAGE OF CORTICOSTEROIDS

An early report (Valk and Owens, 1954) suggested the rather massive dose of 300 mg cortisone daily for two months in combination with oestrogens, gradually decreasing to a maintenance dose of 25 to 50 mg daily. The purpose of the added oestrogen was to inhibit the hypophysis in addition to the adrenal cortex. Given for two months this high dosage would seem likely to cause considerable sodium retention and tissue oedema and these complications would be aggravated by the addition of the oestrogen. Other side-effects such as gastric irritation, hypertension, glycosuria and osteoporosis might also be feared particularly if treatment was further prolonged.

Relief of bone pain, gain in energy and weight and an increase in appetite and mobility are seen in the majority of patients treated even by 100 mg cortisone daily, but on average these effects last only for about three months (Harrison, Thorn and Jenkins, 1953; Miller and Hinman, 1954; Burt et al, 1957). There may either be a fall or a rise in the serum acid phosphatase levels. Radiological evidence of repair of involved bone or regression of visceral lesions is rarely seen although the primary lesion may appear to regress for several months (Miller and Hinman, 1954).

A dose level of 100 mg cortisone daily (equivalent to 20 mg prednisolone) is the minimum effective, and doses below these levels are of doubtful value in the relief of metastatic pain (Burt et al, 1957). On the other hand, except in cases of urgency, there is no proven advantage in using more than 30 mg prednisolone daily, particularly since higher dosage involves a considerable increase in side-effects. Elderly patients with cardiac disease often tolerate 20 mg daily only with difficulty. Higher dose levels may, however, be necessary in emergencies such as orthopnoea due to mediastinal or pulmonary metastases or coma resulting from cerebral deposits. In these cases the dosage should be reduced to 60 mg daily as soon as symptoms improve and to 40 mg a day when the patient becomes ambulant.

BENEFIT IN RELATION TO THAT FROM ANTI-ANDROGEN THERAPY

There is no correlation between response to corticosteroid therapy and the previous response of the patient to anti-androgen therapy. It seems likely that from its euphoric effect the response to corticosteroid therapy in prostatic cancer is related to a local anti-inflammatory action on the tumour bed. In the case of the primary lesion as well as its pulmonary, cerebral and other soft tissue deposits it is suggested that treatment may inhibit stromal reaction by an anti-inflammatory effect which can decrease vascular permeability and oedema around the growing edge of the tumour. This may account for the common observation of reduction in size of soft tissue or pulmonary metastases but almost never complete regression. The efficacy of corticosteroids in cancer seems to run parallel with their anti-inflammatory effect, and is just as transient.

COMPARISON WITH ADRENALECTOMY

Some confusion has been caused in this context by the use of the term 'medical adrenalectomy'. Some take this to mean corticosteroid therapy alone, even if castration has not previously been carried out, whereas surgical adrenalectomy is nearly always practised following or in combination with orchidectomy. A true comparison therefore is seldom practicable.

It has been suggested that the beneficial effects of adrenalectomy may be due to the cortisone replacement therapy used after the operation. This seems unlikely as in cases of mammary cancer when adrenalectomy often leads to extended survival the response is far more prolonged and complete than that following cortisone administration alone. Furthermore, when the operation is conducted in two stages some degree of objective improvement, as shown by calcium balance studies in cases with active bone metastases, may be demonstrable after the removal of one adrenal and before any substitution therapy is employed. There may be a fall or a rise in the serum acid phosphatase level after adrenalectomy, just as after corticosteroid therapy (Miller and Hinman, 1954).

It is sometimes held that a good clinical response by prostatic cancer to corticosteroids predicts a good subsequent response to bilateral adrenalectomy. This is not always true, nor is the reverse true. Adrenalectomy may lead to a response after failure of previous corticosteroid therapy (Miller and Hinman, 1954). Nevertheless, corticosteroid administration may be valuable in causing subjective improvement in patients who are seriously ill, enabling them to withstand an operative procedure such as total adrenalectomy or hypophyseal ablation. Adrenalectomy may lead to a second remission after a temporary response to corticosteroid therapy and in such cases the previous administration of corticosteroids does not appear to increase the difficulties of post-surgical management.

BENEFIT IN RELATION TO ANDROGENIC 17-KETOSTEROID LEVEL

Cortisone administration at 100 mg daily usually abolishes androgenic 17-ketosteroid excretion (Birke, Franksson and Plantin, 1955; Burt et al, 1957). In this respect it has been claimed to be on a par with bilateral adrenalectomy and superior to orchidectomy or oestrogen therapy (Birke et al, 1955). There is, however, no evidence of correlation between the degree of reduction of 17-ketosteroid excretion and the subjective or objective response of the patient. Anabolic steroids such as norethandrolone (Nilevar) cause a marked decline in the excretion of androgenic 17-ketosteroids but appear to induce little clinical benefit in cases of prostatic cancer (Brendler et al, 1960).

It seems fair to add that until recently hormone assays on a large scale have seldom proved practicable partly on account of the use of unreliable techniques and partly from their time-consuming nature. Further confusion has been caused by difficulty in differentiating the end products of steroid therapy from those of the naturally occurring hormones which it is desired to assess.

To summarise, objective benefit from corticosteroids is, in general, not as prolonged or as complete as that following adrenalectomy, but temporary subjective improvement may be noted in a considerable proportion of cases. It is suggested that this benefit in cases of prostatic cancer may have a different mechanism from that due to anti-androgenic therapy.

Major Ablative Surgery

Although their technical consideration is not strictly included in the subject of this work, the place of surgical adrenalectomy and pituitary ablation must be discussed.

ADRENALECTOMY

Adrenalectomy aims at the removal of an important extragonadal source of tumour-stimulating androgens, particularly when their compensatory production has been stimulated by previous castration or oestrogen therapy. The operation may be carried out either in one or two stages, but prior to the removal of the second adrenal it is advisable that substitution therapy with cortisone should be commenced and this must subsequently be continued indefinitely in maintenance dosage usually ranging between 25 and 50 mg daily.

The selection of cases should be confined to those in relapse after previous oestrogen therapy and if castration has not already been performed it should be incorporated in the operation. It is important that patients should be made aware of the subsequent need for continuing substitution therapy and if there is any doubt about their capacity for this they should be excluded.

The symptomatic response, particularly in patients suffering from metastatic bone pain, is often immediate and dramatic but difficult to explain on a purely pathological basis. Nevertheless, in some cases, the reversal of a previously negative calcium balance would indicate that metastatic bone destruction had been halted. It has been suggested that the corticosteroid-replacement therapy used after operation might account for this (see above) but the dosage commonly used for this purpose has seldom proved availing in non-adrenalectomised cases. Other objective evidence of the response may include a fall in the serum acid phosphatase level, particularly if simultaneous castration has been performed, but in previously castrated patients the reduction is often less evident.

Dissociation between subjective and objective improvement is common (as after corticosteroid therapy) and frequently masked by the euphoric effect of cortisone replacement. Moreover the relief of symptoms may be transient and often associated with slow progression of bone metastases as demonstrated radiologically. In a series of 20 cases operated on by the author the average period of survival amounted to only a few

months although exceptional patients continued in comfort for up to three years. These results bear poor comparison with some of those achieved in mammary cancer but it must be remembered that the average age of patients with relapsing prostatic cancer is considerably higher and their life expectation is correspondingly reduced.

In general, the long-term effect of total adrenalectomy for advanced prostatic cancer has been disappointing and it has now been superseded by hypophyseal ablation.

HYPOPHYSECTOMY OR PITUITARY DESTRUCTION

These procedures aim at the suppression of pituitary gonadotropic activity and the elimination of other hormones possibly associated with the stimulation of prostatic cancer. In general, surgical hypophysectomy, as in the case of adrenalectomy, may be accounted too severe an operation in frail and elderly patients to warrant its attendant risks and the ensuing need for substitution therapy. Fortunately, however, 'irradiation hypophysectomy' provides a relatively safe alternative although the need for cortisone replacement is still involved (Figure 13.1). The operation, which demands a short general anaesthetic, consists of the introduction of two to three sources of radioactive yttrium-90 (approximately 3·5–4 mCi strength) into the substance of the gland by means of a fine cannula inserted by the transnasal or transethmoid route under radiological control. With the aid of an x-ray image intensifier and with reasonable expertise the procedure can be completed within a few minutes (Fergusson and Stevenson, 1960). The isotope liberates only beta-irradiation which is confined to the vicinity of the source, and with careful distribution a substantial area of pituitary destruction can be achieved without endangering the adjacent nervous structures.

This relatively simple technique is far more suitable for the typical frail elderly patient with metastatic cancer and carries far less risk of morbidity and mortality than does surgical ablation. Destruction of the pituitary may not always be complete by this method but the symptomatic response is usually dramatic and substantial, and the need for substitution therapy with cortisone (25 to 50 mg daily) is apparent within two to three days. Again the rapidity of the response, at least in terms of the relief of metastatic pain, is difficult to account for on

unaffected. Many of the latter group were in the penultimate stages of the disease and could hardly be expected to respond. Similar results in a smaller series have been reported by Straffon et al (1968) and Morales, Blair and Steyn (1971).

CONCLUSION

In the absence of response to castration or oestrogens, or in the presence of relapse after

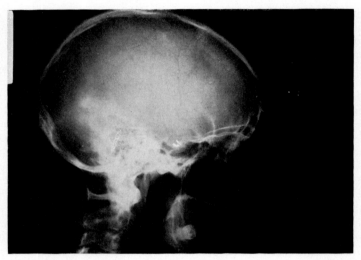

FIGURE 13.1. Irradiation hypophysectomy. X-ray of skull showing radioactive sources of yttrium-90 deposited in the pituitary by transnasal inoculation. (Reproduced from Fergusson, 1970, by permission of the Editor, *British Medical Journal*.)

pathological grounds, but recent hormone assays have shown a striking fall of the plasma testosterone value to zero within 48 hours of operation.

The selection of cases is again mainly confined to patients in relapse after oestrogen therapy with continuing or aggravated metastatic bone pain. On this basis, in a series of over 100 cases (Fergusson and Hendry, 1971) about one third have been completely relieved for a substantial period extending up to two to three years, one third has benefited temporarily for several months and the remainder have been

such initial therapy, secondary endocrine therapy may provide temporary control of prostatic cancer. Androgens may have a direct action on the tumour cells which may sensitise them to the effect of oestrogens or radioactive phosphorus. Progestational compounds have been recently introduced into therapy, but their value is not yet clear. They have the advantage of being well tolerated and of providing subjective benefits in a high proportion of patients.

Objective benefit from corticosteroid therapy is in general, not as prolonged or as complete as that following castration or oestrogen therapy. Its local mechanism is probably by an anti-inflammatory effect on the tumour bed, but subjective benefit and euphoria are common, following its use. To avoid severe side-effects, dosage should be kept between 20 and 30 mg of prednisone or prednisolone daily.

The results of bilateral adrenalectomy are disappointing and it is rarely indicated in patients of advanced age. The use of pituitary ablation by radioactive yttrium implant is far more suitable in such patients, carrying as it does, minimal morbidity and mortality risks. Immediate but temporary pain relief in bone metastases is common from both procedures. It is usually not associated with objective evidence of tumour regression and difficult to explain on a pathological basis.

References

Birke, G., Franksson, G. & Plantin, L. O. (1955) Carcinoma of the prostate; a clinical and steroid metabolic study. *Acta Chirurgica Scandinavica*, **109**, 129–149.

Brendler, H., Chase, W. E. & Scott, W. W. (1950) Prostatic cancer; further investigation of hormonal relationships. *Archives of Surgery*, **61**, 433–440.

Brendler, H. & Prout, G. (1962) A co-operative group study of prostatic cancer: stilboestrol versus placebo in advanced progressive disease. *Cancer Chemotherapy Reports*, **16**, 323–328.

Brendler, H., Werner, S., Baker, W. & Hodges, S. (1960) Therapy of certain endocrine and endocrine sensitive tumors. *National Cancer Institute Monograph*, **3**, 229–251.

Burt, F. B., Finney, R. P. & Scott, W. W. (1957) Steroid response to therapy in prostatic cancer. *Journal of Urology*, **77**, 485–491.

Desberg, D. (1960) Alteration of estrogen therapy in advanced carcinoma of the prostate. *Journal of Urology*, **83**, 463–467.

Donati, R. M., Ellis, H., & Gallagher, N. I. (1966) Testosterone potentiated ^{32}P therapy in prostatic carcinoma. *Cancer*, **19**, 1088–1090.

Fergusson, J. D. (1963) Some aspects of the conservative management of prostatic cancer. *Proceedings of the Royal Society of Medicine*, **56**, 81–88.

Fergusson, J. D. (1970) Cancer of the prostate. II. *British Medical Journal*, **iv**, 539.

Fergusson, J. D. & Hendry, W. F. (1971) Pituitary irradiation in advanced carcinoma of the prostate: analysis of 100 cases. *British Journal of Urology*, **43**, 514–519.

Fergusson, J. D. & Stevenson, J. J. (1960) X-ray television in urology. *British Journal of Urology*, **32**, 484–490.

Gardner, F. H. & Pringle, J. C. (1961) Androgens and erythropoiesis. I. Preliminary clinical observations. *Archives of Internal Medicine*, **107**, 846–862.

Geller, J., Fruchtman, B., Newman, H., Roberts, T. & Silva, R. (1967) Effect of progestational agents on carcinoma of the prostate. *Cancer Chemotherapy Reports*, **51**, 41–46.

Grayhack, J. T. (1959) Hormonal treatment of prostatic cancer. *Surgical Clinics of North America*, **39** (1), 13–30.

Harrison, J. H., Thorn, G. W. & Jenkins, D. (1953) Total adrenalectomy for reactivated carcinoma of prostate. *New England Journal of Medicine*, **248**, 86–92.

Hayward, W. G. (1953) Treatment of late relapse in prostatic carcinoma by cortisone. *Journal of Urology*, **69**, 152–156.

Hertz, S. (1950) The modifying effects of steroid therapy on human neoplastic tissue as judged by radio-active phosphorus. (P-32 studies.) *Journal of Clinical Investigation*, **29**, 821.

Huggins, C. & Hodges, C. V. (1941) Studies on prostatic cancer; effect of castration, estrogen and of androgen injection on serum phosphates in metastatic carcinoma of the prostate. *Cancer Research*, **1**, 293–297.

Huggins, C. & Scott, W. W. (1945) Bilateral adrenalectomy in prostatic cancer, clinical features and urinary excretion of 17-ketosteroids and estrogen. *Annals of Surgery*, **122**, 1031–1041.

Kaplan, E., Fels, I. G., Kotlowski, B. R., Greco, J. & Walsh, W. S. (1960) Therapy of carcinoma of prostate metastatic to bone with ^{32}P labelled condensed phosphate. *Journal of Nuclear Medicine*, **1**, 1–13.

Lebech, P. E. (1967) Personal communication.

Mellinger, G. T. (1965) Carcinoma of the prostate. *Surgical Clinics of North America*, **45**, 1413–1426.

Miller, G. M. & Hinman, F. (1954) Cortisone treatment in advanced carcinoma of prostate. *Journal of Urology*, **72**, 485–496.

Morales, A., Blair, D. W. & Steyn, J. (1971) Yttrium-90 pituitary ablation in advanced cancer of the prostate. *British Journal of Urology*, **43**, 520–522.

Parsons, R., Campbell, J. L. & Thomley, M. W. (1962) Experiences with P-32 in the treatment of metastatic carcinoma of the prostate: a follow up report. *Journal of Urology*, **88**, 812–813.

Pearson, O. H. (1957) Discussion of Dr Huggin's paper "Control of cancers of man by endocrinological methods". *Cancer Research*, **17**, 473–479.

Pedrotti, R. & Frizzi, V. (1966) Treatment of prostatic carcinoma by hormonal shock as suggested by Mayor. *Cancer Chemotherapy Abstracts*, **7**, 100.

Prout, G. R. & Brewer, W. R. (1967) Response of men with advanced prostatic carcinoma to exogenous administration of testosterone. *Cancer*, **20**, 1871–1878.

Sherman, A. I. & Woolf, R. B. (1959) An endocrine basis for endometrial carcinoma. *American Journal of Obstetrics and Gynecology*, **77**, 233–242.

Sprague, R., Power, M. H., Mason, H. L., Albert, A., Mathieson, D. R., Hench, P. S., Kendall, E. C.,

Slocumb, C. H. & Polley, H. F. (1950) Observations on the physiologic effects of cortisone and ACTH in man. *Archives of Internal Medicine*, **85**, 199–258.

Stoll, B. A. (1967) Progestin therapy of breast cancer: comparison of agents. *British Medical Journal*, **3**, 338–341.

Straffon, R. A., Kiser, W. S., Robitaille, M. & Dohn, D. F. (1968) 90-yttrium hypophysectomy of metastatic carcinoma of the prostate gland in 13 patients. *Journal of Urology*, **99**, 102–105.

Trunnell, J. B., Duffy, B. J., Marshall, V., Whitmore, W. F. & Woodard, H. Q. (1951) Use of progesterone in treatment of cancer of prostate. *Journal of Clinical Endocrinology*, **11**, 663–676.

Valk, W. L. & Owens, R. H. (1954) Effect of cortisone on patients with carcinoma of the prostate. *Journal of Urology*, **71**, 219–225.

Chapter 14

Indices of Hormone Responsiveness

J. D. FERGUSSON

About 80 per cent of prostatic cancers are hormone sensitive in the sense that they appear to respond clinically to endocrine therapy. After varying periods of control the tumour enters a further phase of activity during which it becomes more resistant and eventually autonomous. If there were a parameter for predicting hormone sensitivity with certainty, patients could be selected for, and others spared, the inconvenience of steroid or surgical endocrine therapy.

Although about 20 per cent of prostatic cancer patients fail to show any evidence of a clinical response to hormones, it is possible that in the life history of every prostatic tumour there is a phase when it is hormone dependent. This phase may be so short-lived that it is not clinically discernible. After a shorter or longer period, all prostatic cancers probably become independent of hormone control if, in the meantime, the patient does not die of intercurrent disease.

CLINICAL RESPONSE

Evidence of the clinical response may be gauged subjectively by the relief of symptoms due, either directly or remotely, to the primary tumour and its metastases. Thus, improved voiding and a reduction of urinary frequency reflect a response at the primary site, while the relief of pain due to the suppression of osseous metastatic activity or associated nerve involvement may also be striking. Objectively, the effect may be appreciated by digital palpation of the prostatic tumour which characteristically becomes smaller and softer and, in some cases, imperceptible. At the same time oedema due to intrapelvic lymphatic obstruction may be felt to diminish and any affected superficial lymph nodes may shrink and disappear.

These features, indicative of the local response of the disease, are often matched by general evidence of clinical improvement due partly to recovery from anaemia (caused by bone marrow involvement) and also from 'uraemia' occasioned by previous urinary obstruction. A variety of simple tests, including estimation of the sedimentation rate, haemoglobin, and BUN, may be employed to substantiate the clinical impression, while other more specific and sophisticated methods of investigation are referred to later.

HISTOLOGICAL RESPONSE

Degenerative changes in the prostatic tumour may be visible as early as 24 hours after commencing stilboestrol administration (Fergusson and Franks, 1953). Similar changes after castration may be a little more delayed. Among the first reports were those of Schenken, Burns and Kahle (1942) and Fergusson and Pagel (1945) in which the following changes were described. The epithelial cells constituting the tumour become swollen and the cytoplasm undergoes vacuolar degeneration. At the same time the nuclei show chromatin fragmentation, disappearance of mitotic figures and finally pyknosis.

The cells ultimately disintegrate and their debris is shed into the prostatic ducts. These changes may be patchy, sometimes occurring in the primary growth but not in the metastases (Franks, 1963) or involving only some parts of the tumour. After long-term oestrogen administration, there usually follows atrophy of the normal prostatic tissue with decrease in the proportion of glandular acini and proliferation of fibrous tissue around them (Plates 14.1–4, facing p. 240).

By the use of suitable staining techniques (Gomori, 1941) the presence of acid phosphatase in the cells can be demonstrated and quantitative assays can also be made. A decrease in the amount of enzyme following stilboestrol administration has been reported (Bainborough, 1952; Fergusson and Franks, 1953), but Rothauge and Gieshake (1959) observed a high concentration remaining after the use of stilboestrol diphosphate (Honvan), from which they concluded that

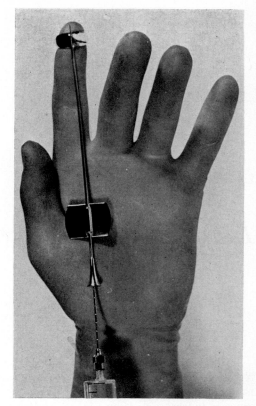

FIGURE 14.1. The modified Franzen needle used for transrectal aspiration biopsy. (Reproduced from Fergusson, 1970, by permission of the Editor, *British Medical Journal*.)

the latter did not act by inactivating the enzyme in the cells.

It is generally accepted that tumours in which the structure is predominantly adenocarcinomatous in type respond best to endocrine therapy. Histological changes as outlined above have been well demonstrated in serial biopsy material obtained at intervals over a period of several months (Fergusson and Franks, 1953). The value of such observations in indicating a response must, however, be qualified by the obvious difficulty in obtaining representative material from the same part of the tumour on successive occasions. Furthermore, the need or opportunity for repeated surgical interference is relatively infrequent, thus limiting the scope of the method in practice. However, with the advent of fine-needle transrectal aspiration biopsy (Franzen, Giertz and Zajicek, 1960; Figure 14.1) which can be painlessly performed without an anaesthetic, the potentialities of serial tissue examination may merit further consideration as a means of interpreting the biochemical or enzymatic reaction to treatment.

RADIOLOGICAL CHANGES AND SCINTIGRAPHY

Conventional radiological studies can seldom do more than corroborate the impressions gained from clinical examination. Applied to the urinary tract, excretion urography may show better voiding of the bladder and improvement in the structure and function of the upper urinary tract coincident with the symptomatic response. In some cases the relief of ureteric obstruction (due to local extension of the primary growth) and restoration of renal function may be demonstrated. Other methods, such as vasoseminal vesiculography for demonstrating the local extent of the primary neoplasm, have no application in serial form.

As applied to the behaviour of metastases, the information gained from repeated radiological examination is likewise somewhat crude. Apart from defining the extent of pulmonary and mediastinal deposits (Figures 14.2A, B), it has little value in showing the

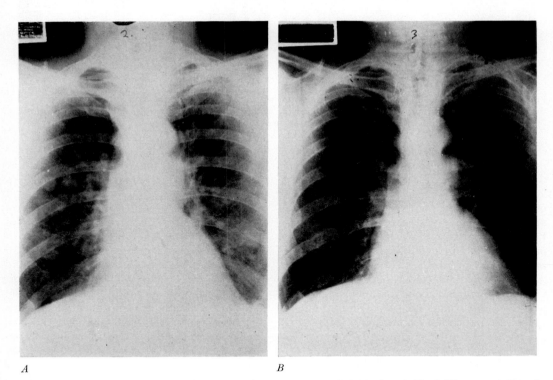

A B

FIGURE 14.2. *A*, X-ray of chest showing well-defined metastatic deposits in the lung fields. *B*, The same patient after treatment with stilboestrol for three weeks, showing disappearance of deposits. (Reproduced from Fergusson, 1970, by permission of the Editor, *British Medical Journal*.)

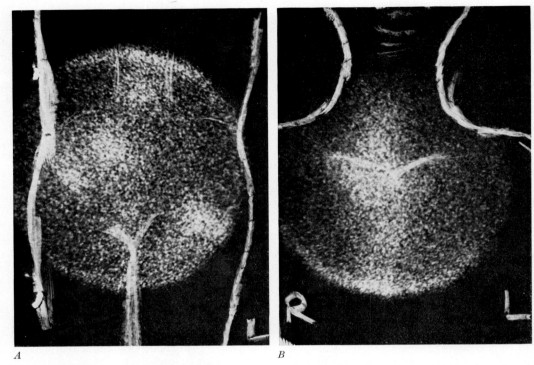

A   *B*

FIGURE 14.3. Scintigram (using [87]Sr) showing concentration of the isotope (indicative of metastatic deposits): *A*, in the lumbar spine, right ilium, and left ischium, and, *B*, at inner end of right clavicle (subsequently confirmed by biopsy). (Reproduced from Fergusson, 1970, by permission of the Editor, *British Medical Journal*.)

reaction of soft-tissue lesions elsewhere. Its main importance undoubtedly lies in assessing the response or progress of secondary bone lesions, and in this respect the results may often seem disappointing through their apparent variance with the clinical features. For example, it is not altogether unusual for patients, in whom a satisfactory symptomatic response has occurred, to show radiological evidence of further osseous metastatic spread. On the other hand, bone deposits which are well controlled and already sclerotic may show little indication of change.

Characteristically, in prostatic cancer, the secondary bone lesions vary in type. Many appear sclerotic with increase in bone density, while others are osteolytic, with decreased density, and combinations of the two are common. After successful endocrine therapy little change is usually demonstrable in the sclerotic deposits, but lytic lesions often show a ring of sclerosis around the affected area which denotes healing at the junction of malignant and normal tissue. The centre of the lytic area then fills in and usually assumes a sclerotic appearance before proceeding in *rare* cases to apparently normal bone.

This sclerotic reaction denotes healing and explains the seemingly paradoxical report often given in successfully treated cases: 'healing of old lesions, but appearance of new sclerotic areas'. The explanation is that the detection of discrete sclerotic areas, in what earlier appeared to be normal bone, may well represent the healing of previously unsuspected metastases and is not a manifestation of spreading disease.

The recent introduction of bone scanning

with strontium and fluorine isotopes gives promise of a new parameter for assessing the response of bone lesions. This method, however, is still only in its trial stages and further standardisation of the methods with computerisation of the results will be required before it can be considered reliable. Nevertheless, in some instances this technique is capable of detecting bone involvement (Figures 14.3A, B) in advance of radiography and a comparison of the findings on serial examination may in due course provide useful information on the endocrine response.

Apart from the methods referred to above, the indices of responsiveness of prostatic cancer to endocrines can conveniently be considered under two headings:

Indices reflecting tumour activity.

Indices reflecting the hormonal environment of the tumour.

Indices Reflecting Tumour Activity

Most methods of assessing changes in tumour activity are based on serial estimation of the serum or plasma content of substances thought to be elaborated by the prostatic tumour cells. Of these, acid phosphatase continues to afford the most reliable guide to the response to endocrine treatment provided that the level is initially raised. Conversely, a rising value from a previously normal level indicates that the disease is inadequately controlled.

SERUM ACID PHOSPHATASE

A study of serum enzyme levels before and after initiating therapy can well lead to a more rational programme of treatment for the individual patient with prostatic cancer. About two-thirds of those who qualify for endocrine therapy are found to have a raised serum 'prostatic' acid phosphatase value, thus giving opportunity for measuring the response.

ESTIMATION

Phosphatase is the enzyme concerned in the splitting off of phosphoric acid from phosphoric esters and its estimation depends on measurement of this reaction when incubated under prescribed conditions of dilution and temperature with a suitable substrate. In the King and Armstrong method, which is widely employed, the substrate used is phenylphosphate and the quantity of free phenol liberated by the reaction is estimated colorimetrically. The resulting value indicates the total quantity of phosphatase in the serum, but by the use of suitable buffer solutions the acid and alkaline components can be differentiated. The further addition of certain substances (for example L-tartrate or copper solutions) may allow a more precise estimate of the amount of enzyme derived from the prostatic epithelial cells, that is, the 'prostatic fraction' (Fishman, Bonner and Homburger, 1956).

It is of interest that the acid phosphatase content of malignant prostatic tissue is on average somewhat less than that of the normal adult prostate. This would seem to indicate that some, at least, of the neoplastic cells appear to lose their capacity for elaborating the enzyme. However, the reason for the raised serum levels commonly encountered in prostatic cancer probably lies in damage to the normal cellular barrier which ordinarily prevents the entry of the enzyme into the blood. Thus, elevation of the serum enzyme value may partly depend on the increased permeability of the cell membrane or surrounding tissues, as well as on the extent of local or metastatic spread of the disease.

SIGNIFICANCE OF RAISED LEVEL

In clinical practice the serum level is raised only in about one quarter of patients in whom no metastases are evident but in about three quarters if they are present. As a result, the presence of a high serum 'prostatic' acid phosphatase value, even in the absence of detectable metastases, is a bad prognostic sign and most of such cases develop demonstrable secondary spread within two years (Ganem, 1956).

Raised enzyme levels are just as common with soft-tissue metastases as with bone involvement and, indeed, it has been claimed that they correlate better with the extent of the disease than with its site (Woodard, 1959). Nevertheless, it is well recognised that in some cases the serum acid phosphatase may remain low even in the presence of widespread dissemination. This may result either from progressive inability of the tumour cells to produce the enzyme or alternatively from failure of the enzyme to enter the circulation, from its having a very rapid turnover or from the development of a serum acid phosphatase inhibitor.

The interpretation of the serum acid phosphatase values may require further qualification in the light of certain circumstances and pathological conditions in which abnormal results may be encountered. Firstly, circadian variation has been shown in the total serum acid phosphatase, but this is said to be accounted for by the tartrate inhibited portion, that is, the non-prostatic fraction (Doe and Mellinger, 1964). Nevertheless, it is advisable that serum estimations should always be made at the same time of day. Secondly, it is common experience that raised values are liable to occur after manipulation of the primary lesion either by rectal palpation or even following an enema. A period of at least 24 hours should be allowed to elapse before serum samples are taken. Thirdly, slow deterioration of the enzyme content may take place over two or three days if examination of the sample is postponed. In this respect, if delay is unavoidable, plasma samples are considered superior to serum and should be kept at a cool temperature (Daniel, 1954).

A number of pathological states have been implicated as liable to cause 'false positive' values. Many of these, however, relate to the *total* serum acid phosphatase and can be excluded by fractional estimation, while others are either rare or unlikely to occur in the age group of prostatic cancer. Among those which occasionally obtrude are hepatic dysfunction and certain bone afflictions including Paget's disease (osteitis deformans).

EFFECT OF ENDOCRINE THERAPY

When due allowance is made for the foregoing considerations it becomes possible to evaluate the significance of serial serum acid phosphatase estimation in relation to the endocrine response. Both orchidectomy and oestrogen administration will reduce a raised enzyme level—within 3 to 4 days in the case of the former but after 7 to 14 days for the latter. If there is no significant fall within these periods there is usually no satisfactory clinical response. The readings tend to remain low for as long as the remission continues, but when relapse occurs the acid phosphatase value in the serum usually rises, although rarely to the original high level. In some relapsing cases it has been shown that a renewed decline in the serum acid phosphatase content may temporarily follow an increase in oestrogen dosage, while in others which have failed initially to respond to hormones, castration may promote a similar effect (Gutman, Sproul and Gutman, 1936).

Progestin administration affects a raised enzyme level similarly to oestrogens, but after corticosteroid therapy the enzyme value often remains high even though the pain from bone metastases has been relieved (Miller and Hinman, 1954).

Androgen administration usually causes a sharp rise in the serum acid phosphatase (Huggins and Hodges, 1941) even in the occasional case where the steroid appears to abolish metastatic pain (Brendler, Chase and Scott, 1950). This is the basis of the androgen provocation test which has been suggested when the diagnosis of prostatic cancer is in doubt (Wray, 1956; Emerson and Jessiman, 1956). It is especially useful if oestrogens have previously been prescribed speculatively and the serum enzyme level is normal. Testosterone propionate 100 mg injected intramuscularly daily for three days may cause a temporary rise in the serum acid phosphatase level. The test, which involves certain ethical considerations, is positive only in a small minority of cases but, when so, appears diagnostic of prostatic cancer.

To summarise, serial acid phosphatase levels in the serum may be used to reflect the efficacy of endocrine therapy. They may also indicate increasing tumour activity and rising values often occur well in advance of pain recurrence or other clinical indications of relapse. The serum enzyme level correlates more closely with malignant activity early in the disease than in patients surviving five years or more. By serial enzyme estimations, tumour activators such as testosterone can be recognised, as can new tumour inhibitors such as the progestational agents.

SERUM ALKALINE PHOSPHATASE

About 90 per cent of all patients with untreated bone metastases from prostatic cancer show a significantly raised serum *alkaline* phosphatase level when first seen (Woodard, 1959). This is considerably greater than in the case of secondary bone involvement from other primary tumours and serial studies might thus be expected to yield useful information on the effects of endocrine therapy.

When prostatic cancer metastasises to bone it provokes osteoblastic activity which releases increased quantities of alkaline phosphatase into the blood. After the institution of endocrine therapy, serial enzyme estimations show a *further* rise in the serum level in most cases. The rise appears within a month, reaching a peak after two to three months, but is apparently independent of whether treatment is successful or not. Temporary elevations of this nature tend to occur with any change in hormone therapy, both at the institution and after the cessation of treatment (Woodard, 1959). They presumably represent an attempt at bone regeneration which may or may not be successful in controlling the tumour depending on its malignant activity. It has been suggested that any steroid not causing a 'flare' in the serum alkaline phosphatase level is unlikely to yield clinical benefit (Wray, 1956).

If clinical remission occurs following hormone therapy, the serum alkaline phosphatase value begins to fall after three months, and then declines to normal as bone healing takes place. This fall in enzyme level may therefore be regarded as a delayed indicator of the bone response and usually occurs at the same time as the first radiological signs of bone healing appear. A subsequent elevation can likewise be interpreted as a warning of reactivation of the disease, and may be especially significant in the later stages when serum *acid* phosphatase levels tend to become unreliable. Note should be taken, however, that as alkaline phosphatase is metabolised in the liver its serum level may also be affected by the presence of hepatic disease. This should be confirmed, if necessary, by other tests of liver insufficiency.

SERUM PHOSPHOHEXOSE ISOMERASE

The serum level of phosphohexose isomerase is stated to be raised in a high proportion of patients with metastatic cancer of the prostate (Bodansky, 1954). In a small series of patients the values given for this enzyme and for isocitric dehydrogenase were reported to be better correlated with alterations in the clinical status than were the serum acid and alkaline phosphatase levels (Schwartz, Greenberg and Bodansky, 1963). It is suggested that swelling of the tumour cells consequent on endocrine therapy may cause disruption in the normal contiguous tissue with liberation of large amounts of the isomerase into the circulation.

If estimations of isomerase are used as an index of tumour activity it must be remembered that both major surgery and liver disease will cause a rise in the serum enzyme level. Also that all blood specimens must be taken on a fasting stomach, as the serum values are affected by food ingestion (Griffith and Beck, 1963).

SERUM LACTIC DEHYDROGENASE

There is a relatively higher lactic dehydrogenase content in malignant tissues, presumably associated with a high degree of anaerobic glycolysis. Raised enzyme levels in the serum have been reported in a large proportion of cancer patients, especially in the presence of enhanced mitotic activity (Hill and Levi, 1954; Goldman, Kaplan and Hall, 1964). A marked degree of correlation has been shown between variations in the enzyme level and changes in the size of the tumour during therapy in a series embracing patients with various types of malignant disease (Brindley and Francis, 1963).

In a group of patients with prostatic cancer the initial level of the enzyme was not found to be raised in the majority and an attempt to correlate clinical progress with serial enzyme estimations was unsuccessful (King and Holland, 1963). However, it has been suggested that differential estimation of the constituent isoenzymes might better reflect the effect of hormone administration (Goodfriend and Kaplan, 1964). Elevation of specific LDH isozymes in the serum was found in 17 out of 28 patients with prostatic cancer and the raised levels returned to normal in all cases within two weeks of instituting castration or oestrogen therapy (Prout et al, 1965).

SERUM FIBRINOLYSIN

Many prostatic tumours elaborate a fibrinolysin and the serum level of this substance has been claimed as an index of malignant activity in prostatic cancer (Tagnon, Whitmore and Shulman, 1952). When raised, the quantity of enzyme is said to fall to normal after orchidectomy or oestrogen therapy. Subsequent administration of androgens causes the level to rise again.

Indices Reflecting the Hormonal Environment of the Tumour

Numerous attempts have been made to define the alterations in the hormonal milieu which result from endocrine therapy, and to correlate these with the clinical response. Such investigations have, for obvious reasons, been mainly concerned with the androgen-oestrogen ratio and, in addition to serum assays have included studies of the urinary excretion of these hormones or their metabolites. Many of the techniques used are both complicated and time-consuming and thus difficult to adapt to routine serial use. Nevertheless, despite earlier confusion in interpreting some of the results, considerable information has been gained to illustrate the effect of hormone therapy.

ANDROGEN EXCRETION

A study of the urinary 17-ketosteroid output before and after initiating treatment can lead to a rational control of therapy for the individual patient with prostatic cancer. The 17-ketosteroids excreted in the urine are of two types:

(a) 17-keto-11-desoxysteroids (i.e. no oxygen atom at position 11). These have an adrenocortical or testicular origin and are *androgen* metabolites, mainly aetiocholanolone and androsterone.

(b) 17-keto-11-oxysteroids (i.e. oxygen atom at position 11). These have an adrenocortical origin only and are *corticoid* metabolites.

The value of serial studies in the control of prostatic cancer therapy has until recently been somewhat confused because most workers assayed the *combination* of androgen and corticoid metabolites in their 17-ketosteroid estimations.

EFFECT OF ENDOCRINE THERAPY

Following castration for prostatic cancer, there is a fall in the level of the androgenic 17-ketosteroid excretion within about two weeks (Scott and Vermeulen, 1942; Burt, Finney and Scott, 1957; Bulbrook, Franks and Greenwood, 1959). Early reports suggested that the 17-ketosteroid excretion returned to normal after three months but with the separation of androgenic and corticoid metabolites it is now considered that a rise in androgenic 17-ketosteroid output heralds the advent of clinical relapse. This is presumably due to hypersecretion of androgens by the adrenal cortex (Burt et al, 1957) as after bilateral adrenalectomy there is again a rapid fall in the excretion level.

Stilboestrol therapy causes a fall both in the corticoid and in the androgenic 17-ketosteroid level both in the intact and the castrated patient. The effect of stilboestrol is presumably by inhibition of pituitary LH secretion, and not directly on the adrenal cortex, as it does not interfere with the androgenic response of the adrenal to ACTH stimulation (Burt et al, 1957).

It is interesting to note that secretion of androgenic and corticoid 17-ketosteroids from the adrenal cortex is controlled by ACTH as well as by LH secretion. This suggests that non-specific stress or anxiety may cause an outpouring of androgen (Gallagher et al, 1963) and possibly an increase in malignant activity in some patients.

CORRELATION WITH TUMOUR ACTIVITY

Within the first two years after treatment there is in general a correlation in the *individual* patient between changes in the androgenic 17-ketosteroid excretion level and the degree of tumour activity (Bulbrook et al, 1959) and this correlation can be used to control treatment. Thus it has been shown that 30 mg stilboestrol daily is twice as effective as 5 mg daily in reducing the androgenic 17-ketosteroid excretion (Burt et al, 1957). This does not apply, however, to all forms of therapy, as although the administration of 100 mg of cortisone daily after orchidectomy will abolish a persistently high level of androgenic 17-ketosteroid excretion in practically all cases (Burt et al, 1957), this is not usually associated with objective evidence of clinical benefit.

Signs of tumour reactivation associated with rising androgenic 17-ketosteroid level would suggest (though not all would agree) that the relapse is more likely due to steroid stimulation than to the development of tumour autonomy (Gallagher et al, 1963). Thus, in a patient relapsing after castration or stilboestrol therapy and showing a rising level of ketosteroid excretion, an increase in the stilboestrol dosage or a course of progestins should be considered as an alternative to the more formidable procedures of bilateral adrenalectomy or pituitary ablation.

Nevertheless, as previously noted for cortisone therapy, a decrease in the androgenic 17-ketosteroid output does not automatically indicate a reduction of malignant activity. Anabolic steroids, such as norethandrolone (Nilevar) at 100 mg daily, also cause a marked reduction in androgenic 17-ketosteroid excretion by interfering with the breakdown of testosterone into its metabolites, but have little objective effect upon the growth of prostatic cancer (Brendler et al, 1960).

Furthermore, in a given group of patients with prostatic cancer there is no correlation between the degree of fall in androgenic 17-ketosteroid excretion and the measure of clinical response, either after orchidectomy (Gallagher et al, 1963) or after 15 mg stilboestrol daily (Bradshaw et al, 1964). This according to Bulbrook and his co-workers (1959) is because of the wide range in the pretreatment levels of steroid excretion and also because the level after treatment varies individually according to the delay before response occurs.

A suggestion that the ratio of the *constituent* androgenic 17-ketosteroids (mainly androsterone and aetiocholanolone) excreted in the urine before treatment might indicate the likelihood of response, or that a similar study during treatment might define the risk of relapse (Scott, 1964) has received little support.

To summarise, it is more accurate to compare serial changes in the excretion level of androgenic 17-ketosteroids in the individual patient than to predict results from isolated assays. If the former is done it is found that for the first two years after castration or oestrogen therapy, rising levels generally precede clinical relapse. This does not apply, however, to those patients surviving five years or more, when steroid levels sometimes remain low even in relapse (see similar observation for serum acid phosphatase levels).

PLASMA TESTOSTERONE LEVEL

Techniques for the accurate estimation of testosterone in the plasma are both complicated and time consuming and it is only comparatively recently that reliable methods have been devised. Furthermore, account has to be taken of the possibility of natural and diurnal variations in the hormone level and, on this account, in serial studies, regular timing is advisable.

In non-castrated patients, changes in the plasma testosterone level can be used to measure the anti-androgenic quality of steroid therapy and may correlate with its tumour-controlling ability (Geller et al, 1967). It has been suggested that by this means non-oestrogenic steroids might be selected for the treatment of advanced prostatic cancer and feminising side-effects avoided. Current studies by the author and his associates have been directed towards explaining the dramatic relief of metastatic pain often observed *immediately* after hypophyseal ablation. In these cases the plasma testosterone levels show a striking decline to near zero within one to two days following operation.

OESTROGEN EXCRETION

It has been shown that there is no evidence of any increase in the total oestrogen production in patients with carcinoma of the prostate (Bulbrook et al, 1959). However, it has been observed that the oestrogen excretion level falls both after castration and after oestrogen administration (parallel with the androgenic 17-ketosteroid level). It is interesting to note that the return of oestrogen excretion to previous levels in such cases may be more closely associated with a relapse than the similar change in the androgenic 17-ketosteroid levels. If confirmed, this observation is difficult to explain on the androgen-dependent theory of prostatic cancer activity.

URETHRAL CORNIFICATION

A further indication of changes in the hormonal (androgen/oestrogen) milieu may be afforded by cytological studies of the urethral epithelium as demonstrated by direct smears or the examination of exfoliated cells in the urine. The urethral cytology during oestrogen therapy is a biological indicator of the balance between oestrogens and androgens in the individual patient. The urethral epithelium of the fossa navicularis normally mirrors the endogenous testicular and adrenal secretion, but is also influenced by exogenous hormone administration. The principal exfoliated epithelial cells are: cornified (superficial) cells, precornified (intermediate) cells and parabasal cells. The karyopyknotic index (KPI) measures the percentage of cornified cells and thereby reflects oestrogen concentration at the target tissue. The administration of stilboestrol in doses of 5 mg or more, daily, usually leads to a KPI of over 50 per cent.

As androgens tend to increase the proportion of parabasal and intermediate cells, the KPI level reflects the *anti*-androgenic efficacy of oestrogen therapy. A fall in the KPI level during prolonged treatment thus suggests an inadequate effect (Gotthardt, 1965). An increase in oestrogen dosage is then indicated or, if this is not successful, intravenous or intramuscular therapy may be tried because of a possible failure of oral absorption. If this still does not raise the KPI level the form of oestrogen may be changed or other methods of hormonal control adopted. Higher LPI readings are said to correlate with improvement of the clinical response by prostatic cancer to oestrogen therapy.

As urethral cytology demonstrates the balance between androgen secretion and anti-androgen therapy as mirrored in a target organ it provides more evidence than the androgen 17-ketosteroid level by itself. It has been shown that folic acid is necessary for oestrogens to exert many of their characteristic effects upon the tissues (Hertz and Tullner, 1950). Folic acid deficiency may, thus, sometimes account for low degrees of cornification in the urethral epithelium during oestrogen therapy and may possibly also influence the response by prostatic cancer.

Other indices of the response to hormonal therapy have been suggested with varying degrees of confidence and success. Among these it has not escaped attention that other hormones apart from oestrogens and androgens, might be affected by treatment. Studies of thyroid iodine uptake, for example, after pituitary ablation have in some instances confirmed the presence of thyroid depression but the accuracy of repeated measurements has been insufficient to provide reliable information as to the continuing effect.

Current interest in the immune defence mechanism as a factor in controlling the spread of cancer has likewise suggested a new field for exploration. Lymphocyte transformation studies during various forms of endocrine-control therapy are at present proceeding and may possibly afford a new parameter for gauging the response.

CONCLUSION

Clinical observations on the primary tumour provide the best assessment of response to endocrine therapy. While both serial biopsy and serial x-ray examinations may provide useful information, they have some inherent disadvantages. Serial acid phosphatase estimations correlate better with the tumour activity in the early stages of the disease than in the later stages. On the other hand, serum alkaline phosphatase estimations correlate better with the clinical activity of bone metastases, later in the course of the disease. The value of other enzyme estimations, such as phosphohexose isomerase and lactic dehydrogenase levels in the blood, is not as well established.

Parameters of the tumour environment may assist in deciding the progress of treatment. Thus, serial measurements of androgen excretion have been shown useful in predicting relapse in the first few years after treatment is initiated. A fall in plasma testosterone level may explain the immediate relief of metastatic pain after hypophyseal ablation. Measurement of oestrogen excretion, either biochemically, or in the urethral smear, may provide further information as to the balance between oestrogen and androgen in the individual patient.

References

Bainborough, A. R. (1952) Squamous metaplasia of prostate following oestrogen therapy. *Journal of Urology*, **68,** 329–336.

Bodansky, O. (1954) Serum phosphohexose isomerase in cancer; an index of tumour growth in metastatic carcinoma of breast. *Cancer*, **7,** 1200–1226.

Bradshaw, L. R. A., Bagness, J. E., Pyrah, L. N. & Raper, F. P. (1964) A study of steroid excretion in patients with prostatic cancer. *Investigative Urology*, **1,** 466–476.

Brendler, H., Werner, S., Baker, W. & Hodges, C. V. (1960) Therapy of certain endocrine and endocrine sensitive tumours. *National Cancer Institute Monograph*, **3,** 229–255.

Brendler, H., Chase, W. E. & Scott, W. W. (1950) Prostatic cancer; further investigation of hormonal relationships. *Archives of Surgery*, **61,** 433–440.

Brindley, C. O. & Francis, F. L. (1963) Serum lactic dehydrogenase and glutamic oxalacetic transaminase correlation with measurements of tumour masses during therapy. *Cancer Research*, **23,** 112–117.

Bulbrook, L. D., Franks, L. M. & Greenwood, F. C. (1959) Hormone excretion in prostatic cancer: the early and late effects of endocrine treatment on urinary oestrogens, 17-ketosteroids and 17-ketogenic steroids. *Acta Endocrinologia*, **31,** 481–499.

Burt, F. B., Finney, R. P. & Scott, W. W. (1957) Steroid response to therapy in prostatic cancer. *Journal of Urology*, **77,** 485–491.

Daniel, O. (1954) The stability of acid phosphatase in blood and other fluids. *British Journal of Urology*, **26,** 153–159.

Doe, R. P. & Mellinger, G. T. (1964) Circadian variation of serum acid phosphatase in prostatic cancer. *Metabolism*, **13,** 445–452.

Emerson, K. & Jessiman, A. G. (1956) Hormonal influences on growth and progression of cancer; tests for hormone dependency in mammary and prostatic cancer. *New England Journal of Medicine*, **254,** 252–258.

Fergusson, J. D. (1970) Cancer of the prostate. I. *British Medical Journal*, **iv,** 475.

Fergusson, J. D. & Franks, L. M. (1953) Response of prostatic carcinoma to oestrogen treatment. *British Journal of Surgery*, **40,** 422–428.

Fergusson, J. D. & Pagel, W. (1945) Some observations on carcinoma of the prostate treated with oestrogens—as demonstrated by serial biopsies. *British Journal of Surgery*, **33,** 122–130.

Fishman, W. H., Bonner, C. D. & Homburger, F. (1956) Serum "prostatic" acid phosphatase and cancer of the prostate. *New England Journal of Medicine*, **255,** 925–933.

Franks, L. M. (1963) Nutritional and other factors influencing the balance between function and proliferation in organ culture. *National Cancer Institute Monograph*, **11,** 83–94.

Franzen, S., Giertz, G. & Zajicek, J. (1960) Cytological diagnosis of prostatic tumours by transrectal aspiration biopsy: a preliminary report. *British Journal of Urology*, **32,** 193–196.

Gallagher, T. F., Whitmore, W. F., Zumoff, B. & Hellman, L. (1963) Steroid hormone metabolites before and after orchidectomy for prostatic cancer. *Journal of Clinical Endocrinology*, **23,** 523–532.

Ganem, E. J. (1956) Prognostic significance of elevated serum acid phosphatase level in advanced prostatic carcinoma. *Journal of Urology*, **76,** 179–181.

Geller, J., Fruchtman, B., Newman, H., Roberts, T. & Silva, R. (1967) Effect of progestational agents on carcinoma of the prostate. *Cancer Chemotherapy Reports*, **51,** 41–46.

Goldman, R. D., Kaplan, N. O. & Hall, T. C. (1964) Lactic dehydrogenase in human neoplastic tissues. *Cancer Research*, **24,** 389–399.

Gomori, G. (1941) Distribution of acid phosphatase in tissues under normal and pathologic conditions. *Archives of Pathology*, **32,** 189–199.

Goodfriend, T. & Kaplan, N. O. (1964) Effects of hormone administration on lactic dehydrogenase. *Journal of Biological Chemistry*, **239,** 130–135.

Gotthardt, E. (1965) Cytologic investigations during hormonal therapy of prostate carcinoma. *Cancer Chemotherapy Abstracts*, **6,** 427.

Griffith, M. M. & Beck, J. C. (1963) The value of serum phosphohexose isomerase as an index of metastatic breast carcinoma activity. *Cancer*, **16,** 1032–1041.

Gutman, E. B., Sproul, E. E. & Gutman, A. B. (1936) Significance of increased phosphatase activity of bone at the site of osteoplastic metastase secondary to carcinoma of the prostate gland. *American Journal of Cancer*, **28**, 485–495.

Hertz, R. & Tullner, W. W. (1950) Interference with hormonal effects by anti-vitamins and competition between structurally similar steroid hormones. *Annals of the New York Academy of Sciences*, **52**, 1260–1273.

Hill, B. R. & Levi, C. (1954) Elevation of serum component in neoplastic disease. *Cancer Research*, **14**, 513–515.

Huggins, C. & Hodges, C. V. (1941) Studies on prostatic cancer; effect of castration, estrogen and of androgen injection on serum phosphates in metastatic carcinoma of the prostate. *Cancer Research*, **1**, 293–297.

King, L. R. & Holland, J. M. (1963) Serum lactic acid dehydrogenase (LDH) level in patients with prostatic cancer. *Journal of Urology*, **89**, 472–474.

Miller, G. M. & Hinman, F. (1954) Cortisone treatment in advanced carcinoma of prostate. *Journal of Urology*, **72**, 485–496.

Prout, G. R., Macalalag, E. V., Denis, L. J. & Preston, L. W. (1965) Alterations in serum lactate dehydrogenase and its fourth and fifth isozymes in patients with prostatic carcinoma. *Journal of Urology*, **94**, 451–461.

Rothauge, C. F. & Gieshake, F. W. (1959) Vergleichende Untersuchung der sauren Blutund Gewebsphosphatase bei Prostata-Carcinomen unter besonderer Berücksichtigung der Behandlung mit phosphoryliertem Diathyl stilbostrol. *Urologia Internationalis*, **8**, 55–64.

Schenken, J. R., Burns, E. L. & Kahle, P. J. (1942) The effect of diethylstilbestrol and diethylstilbestrol propionate on carcinoma of the prostate gland. II. Cytological changes following treatment. *Journal of Urology*, **48**, 99–112.

Schwartz, M. K., Greenberg, E. & Bodansky, O. (1963) Comparative values of phosphatases and other serum enzymes in following patients with prostatic carcinoma. Consideration of phosphohexose isomerase, glutamic oxalacetic transaminase, isocitric dehydrogenase, and acid and alkaline phosphatases. *Cancer*, **16**, 583–589.

Scott, W. W. (1964) An evaluation of endocrine therapy plus radical perineal prostatectomy in the treatment of advanced carcinoma of the prostate. *Journal of Urology*, **91**, 97–102.

Scott, W. W. & Vermeulen, C. (1942) Studies on prostatic cancer; excretion of 17-ketosteroids, estrogens and gonadotropins before and after castration. *Journal of Clinical Endocrinology*, **2**, 450–456.

Tagnon, H. J., Whitmore, W. F. & Shulman, N. R. (1952) Fibrinolysis in metastatic cancer of prostate. *Cancer*, **5**, 9–12.

Woodard, H. Q. (1959) The clinical significance of serum acid phosphatase. *American Journal of Medicine*, **27**, 849.

Wray, S. (1956) Significance of blood acid and alkaline phosphatase values in cancer of prostate. *Journal of Clinical Pathology*, **9**, 341–346.

Chapter 15

Sequential Management in Advanced Disease

J. D. FERGUSSON

Before formulating any plan of management it may be appropriate to reflect on certain aspects of the natural history of the disease and to review some of the therapeutic experiences of others. Particularly relevant in the first instance, is the wide range of activity evinced by the malignant process and the disparity often observed between its extent and the quality and intensity of the clinical manifestations.

FACTORS INFLUENCING CHOICE OF TREATMENT

At one end of the scale it may be difficult to assess the malignant potential of an isolated asymptomatic primary nodule, especially since statistical evidence suggests that many of these fail to progress to morbid significance (Hudson et al, 1954); while, at the other, the radiological demonstration of diffuse osteosclerotic reaction may do little more than suggest that the disease, though widely disseminated, is reasonably well controlled. Such considerations are clearly of importance not only in deciding on the need or otherwise for treatment, but in determining the timing and character of its application.

Factors of age and current physical fitness must likewise be taken into account, together with such practical aspects as the liability to side-effects incurred with certain forms of therapy, the psychological implications of others and finally the availability of more sophisticated techniques. In these respects treatment which might ordinarily be dictated by the clinical stage of the disease may often have to be adjusted to meet the circumstances of the individual patient.

On this account it is sometimes difficult to evaluate the results quoted in some large

series, especially when cases have been
derived from several sources and various
methods and combinations of therapy have
been employed. On the other hand, data
accruing from smaller individual series,
although often better documented, may also
be deemed uncritical if representative of
personal enthusiasm for a particular therapeutic approach. Nevertheless, it may be
profitable to refer briefly to a selection of
published reports which illustrate some of the
problems involved, so that management of
the advanced disease can be planned in
proper perspective.

EFFECT OF TREATMENT ON
NATURAL COURSE OF DISEASE

Among earlier reports relating to the natural
course of the disease, the collective series of
1000 cases recorded by Bumpus (1926)
deserves special mention. This report, com-
piled well before the advent of endocrine
treatment or effective radiotherapy, emphasised the almost uniformly poor prognosis
when once a diagnosis of prostatic cancer had
been made. This was especially so if metastases
were already present when the patient was
first seen, and few cases of this type survived
for more than nine months.

Since then, despite a growing awareness
of the disease, fostered by the development of
new confirmatory techniques, mortality statistics have suggested only a moderate increase in its overall incidence. From this it
may be surmised that any subsequent improvement in the prognosis is unlikely to represent the diluting effect of additional early
cases but rather to reflect the response to
more effective methods of management. This
is clearly an important concept in evaluating
the merits of specific forms of treatment and
one which is liable to be overlooked by those
unfamiliar with the commonly distressing
course of the disease before endocrine
therapy became available.

As might be expected, the wide adoption
of anti-androgen therapy soon led to a

series of comparisons between treated and
untreated cases. Apart from earlier accounts
dealing with the symptomatic and objective
response to oestrogens and castration, it
was some years before sufficient data were
available to evaluate their influence on
survival.

In 1946 Nesbit and Plumb, in a preliminary
review, were able to compare the survival
rates of 795 patients treated prior to the
endocrine era with a small series of cases
treated by endocrine therapy, and, later
(Nesbit and Baum, 1950) to adduce similar
statistics on 947 patients treated by orchidectomy and/or oestrogens. In the earlier
group of patients (untreated by endocrine
methods) the average period of survival from
diagnosis to death amounted to 21 months
while in those who presented with metastases
the average interval declined to 17 months.
Regarding the cause of death, 83 per cent
patients were classed as dying from prostatic
cancer, 9 per cent from other causes (including cardiac disease 29 cases, cerebral haemorrhage 9 cases) and 8 per cent from surgical
misadventure.

The fate of these cases was compared in
the subsequent report (Nesbit and Baum,
1950) with the three and five-year survival
rates of a large series of patients who received
anti-androgen therapy. Of the latter, 947
were available for three-year review and 587
at five years. Detailed analysis included
a distinction between those with or without
metastases when first seen and a further sub-
division according to whether they were
treated with oestrogens or by castration, or
both.

At three years the control (untreated)
group showed a mortality rate of 78 per cent
(without initial metastases) and 89 per cent
(with metastases), contrasted with 34 per
cent and 64·8 per cent in the corresponding groups where a combination of castration and stilboestrol had been employed.
The comparable rates when orchidectomy
and oestrogens were employed separately
amounted to 46·6 per cent and 63·6 per

cent (orchidectomy) and 50·3 per cent and 74 per cent (stilboestrol).

At five years the control (untreated) group showed a mortality rate of 90 per cent (without initial metastases) and 94 per cent (with metastases) contrasted with 56 per cent and 79 per cent respectively in the cases treated by a combination of oestrogens and castration. Those treated by castration alone showed a death rate of 69 per cent and 79 per cent according to the presence or absence of metastases when first diagnosed, and those receiving oestrogens alone 71 per cent and 90 per cent respectively.

Chief among the conclusions drawn was that a significant improvement in the survival rates occurred in all groups in which anti-androgenic therapy was employed and that this, coupled with the symptomatic benefit which commonly ensued, certainly rendered such treatment worthwhile. It was evident, however, that the maximum response, particularly in cases with established metastases, occurred during the first three years and appeared marginally better when both castration and oestrogens were used in combination. Beyond this period the survival rates for patients treated either independently with oestrogens or by orchidectomy, or with the two in combination, showed a closer approximation. Unfortunately, the data for treated cases were not qualified by the ages of the patients nor by any reference to the eventual cause of death.

EARLY OR DELAYED ENDOCRINE THERAPY

At this time the liability of the disease to relapse during sustained endocrine therapy had already become recognised and led to the view in some quarters that anti-androgen therapy should be withheld until troublesome metastatic symptoms had developed. Nesbit and Baum, however, concluded from their studies that although the presence of metastases adversely affected survival, even when castration and oestrogen therapy were employed, there was some evidence to indicate that androgen independence occurred more often early than late. On these grounds they felt it logical to treat all patients at the time of first diagnosis.

Further support for this view was adduced by the present author from a study of survival in a personal series of 150 patients treated with oestrogens compared with a control group of 48 untreated cases (Fergusson, 1958). From this it appeared that while a small proportion (about 20 per cent) of the former were totally unresponsive (presumably autonomous) when first seen, the average survival of the remainder seemed to be significantly improved if early treatment were instituted. Moreover, in relation to oestrogen dosage, it was noted that the immediate mortality rate was reduced when larger doses of stilboestrol were given, although after a period of three years this factor became less important.

At the same time, an enquiry into the eventual causes of death showed an interesting correlation with the ages of the patient concerned. Whereas in patients encountered below the age of 60 a majority (approximately 90 per cent) eventually died directly from the effect of their prostatic cancer, in succeeding age groups a growing proportion succumbed to intercurrent disease. This outcome applied to both treated and untreated cases, the ratio between death attributable to cancer and death from intercurrent illness declining from 3 to 1 in the seventh decade to an almost equal distribution in the ninth.

In summary, all the control series of untreated patients died within three years of diagnosis, while of those receiving oestrogens 40 per cent were surviving at this period and 20 per cent were alive at five years.

Among other reviews at this period dealing with the general effect of endocrine therapy on survival, the series of 1101 cases, reported by Emmett, Greene and Papantonioa (1960) showed a similar trend. In this series, which included both early and late cases the five year survival for treated patients amounted to 32 per cent compared with 15 per cent for those who received no treatment.

Subsequent findings, however, in a more recent collective series of 2052 cases organised by the Veterans Administration Co-operative Urological Research Group (VACURG, 1967) have tended to detract from the value of anti-androgenic therapy by suggesting an increased liability to complications and, in some groups, a higher mortality. This report claimed that, 'patients assigned to treatment regimes including oestrogen alone, with orchidectomy or with radical prostatectomy, have a substantially higher overall mortality rate than those assigned to treatments not including oestrogen. Although oestrogen therapy does cause a modest decrease in the mortality level from *prostatic cancer*, this decrease is outweighed by a substantial elevation in the mortality rate from other causes, primarily heart disease and cerebro-vascular accident.'

It was further concluded that 'the average patient with prostatic carcinoma did not derive much clinical benefit from immediate treatment with either orchidectomy or a daily 5 mg orally administered dose of stilboestrol unless the cancer was causing serious problems' and that 'the excess number of mortalities associated with oestrogen therapy, the psychological trauma of orchidectomy, etc. . . . all combine to suggest that therapy by oestrogens or orchidectomy should be withheld until the symptoms are so severe that they require relief.' While recognising the role of oestrogens and castration in the treatment of metastatic cancer of the prostate with symptoms, the immediate use of such measures in the earlier phases of the disease was therefore discouraged.

The validity of this policy however, must remain open to doubt. In the first place, in ordinary circumstances, comparatively few patients seek advice before their symptoms have become sufficiently troublesome as to warrant early relief. In view, however, of the suggested liability to cardiovascular

complications it would seem reasonable to avoid oestrogens initially in those in whom the distribution and activity of the disease are such as to make it amenable to other measures (for example, local surgery or radio-therapy). Failing a satisfactory response to the latter there should then be no hesitation in advising endocrine therapy.

At the same time it must be stated that the conclusions drawn from the VACURG report have not been universally accepted. Coming at a time when attention was dramatically focused on the risk of thromboembolic sequelae following hormonal methods of contraception, it was perhaps inevitable that this facet of endocrine administration should have received prominence. Little mention, however, has been made of the incidence of such complications which might be expected to occur naturally at the advanced age of many of the patients under review.

It is, indeed, unfortunate that the mortality rate from cardiovascular and cerebrovascular accidents in the Veterans' series was not correlated with age, and also that the implied dosage of 5 mg stilboestrol daily was not qualified by details of its duration nor by reference to the additional methods of treatment which three quarters of the patients were stated to have received. Nevertheless, with regard to the latter, a final conclusion was expressed that 'either oestrogen alone or orchidectomy alone seems to provide all of the clinical benefits of both techniques combined'.

Whatever the pros and cons of early or delayed endocrine therapy in the management of prostatic cancer as a whole, there would appear to be little disagreement about its role in the treatment of advanced metastatic symptoms. Currently, at this stage of the disease there is no alternative which can be expected to induce comparable benefit in proportion to the safety and ease of its application. Moreover, when simpler measures such as oestrogen and castration cease to be effective there may be a further prospect of gaining renewed control by the use of more sophisticated endocrine techniques (for example, hypophysectomy). Failing this it must be assumed that the disease has become totally endocrine-resistant and resort must ultimately be made to the use of cytotoxic agents which are non-specific in their action and often poorly tolerated.

With this brief review of some of the natural features of the disease and the virtues and drawbacks of endocrine therapy it may now be easier to consider the selection of treatment appropriate to the various stages of the disease.

Cancer of the prostate can be divided into 4 stages according to its extent at the time of diagnosis:

Stage 1. Occult carcinoma discovered at operation for benign disease.
Stage 2. Localised tumour with no invasion of seminal vesicles or bladder.
Stage 3. Extension to seminal vesicles or bladder but no other clinical evidence of metastases.
Stage 4. Metastases present.

THE PLACE OF SURGERY IN MANAGEMENT

STAGE 1

The results of treatment in this stage must be considered in relation to the natural expectation of life for a man in the affected age group.

The expected 10-year survival rate for the general population for this category has been calculated as 48·7 per cent (Greene and Simon, 1955). Apart from the general clinical status of the patient, two other factors would appear to affect the prognosis, namely, the degree of differentiation of the tumour and its position relative to the plane of enucleation or resection.

In Greene and Simons' review of 83 cases with Stage 1 prostatic cancer, the overall survival rate at five years was 70·7 per cent declining to 39·4 per cent at the end of 10 years. Bauer, McGarvan and Carlin (1960), however, showed that if histological examination disclosed a well-differentiated tumour the prognosis was almost identical with that of the general population (Table 15.1). This would suggest that no treatment other than the initial enucleation or resection is required in such cases. If, however, the tumour is less well differentiated, the outlook would appear distinctly unfavourable and there may be a case for secondary radical prostatectomy if on general grounds a life expectancy of over 10 years would otherwise seem likely.

Not only the site of the occult tumour in relation to the plane of enucleation or resection, but, possibly also, the presence of a surrounding lymphocytic reaction may have a bearing on the prognosis. Tumours which extend to the edge of the operated material can be adjudged to have been incompletely removed, and irrespective of any histological

TABLE 15.1. *Survival in Stage 1 prostatic cancer*

| Author | Cases | Percentage survival: | | Histology |
		5 years	10 years	
Bauer et al, 1960	55	75	47	Well differentiated
		33	14	Less well differentiated
Greene and Simon, 1955	83	70·7	39·4	

indication of their potential activity, carry a worse prognosis than those which are completely insulated.

In a comparative series studied by the author, 27 cases of the latter type (insulated) were followed for five years without additional treatment: 22 survived this period without further evidence of the disease and of the 5 deaths, none was from cancer. In a further 22 instances where the tumour abutted on the plane of enucleation, all save one showed progression of the malignant process, and 7 died within a year (Fergusson, 1965).

Recent studies of the immune defence

both radiotherapy and endocrine methods can be held in reserve.

STAGE 2

Overemphasis on staging without qualification by allusion to symptomatology and age has undoubtedly contributed to some of the high survival rates quoted following radical prostatectomy for this stage of the disease. An obvious distinction exists between the small asymptomatic nodule of dubious activity randomly detected on casual rectal examination and a more extensive area of local

TABLE 15.2. *Survival in Stage 2 prostatic cancer (radical prostatectomy)*

| Author | Cases | Percentage survival: | |
		5 years	10 years
Jewett, 1954	127	61	37
Turner and Belt, 1957	229	55	34

mechanism in relation to tumour spread have suggested that the lymphocytic response may also afford some guidance as to the risk of extension of the disease. In a current investigation by one of the author's colleagues (Robinson, Nakhla and Whitaker, 1971) a consistently high lymphocyte transformation rate (on incubation of the patients lymphocytes with a stimulating agent) has been observed in cases remaining free from metastases, while in those showing extension of the disease the rate has been significantly lower.

Similarly, as in the case of breast cancer, a local concentration of lymphocytes around the tumour would appear to indicate that the liability to dissemination is reduced. In such cases, as also in those where the tumour remains contained within the tissue removed at operation, there is probably little need to consider further immediate treatment and

induration to which attention is drawn by the presence of urological symptoms. Nevertheless, both are conventionally included in this category.

The fact that many small nodules appear to remain quiescent for an indefinite period while most of the more extensive lesions have already spread beyond the range of operative removal, would seem to argue against the case for radical surgery and this view is held by many observers. At the same time, 10-year survival figures have been adduced by some which closely approximate to those obtained in Stage 1 (Table 15.2).

It must also be remembered that some of the more favourable results derive from cases in which local symptoms due to coincident benign prostatic hypertrophy or other factors have fortuitously drawn attention to the disease at a time appropriate to its removal, and that figures comparable to those given above may thus relate to a selected group. It remains, therefore, difficult to define how far radical surgery should be advised, particularly when it is remembered that in inexpert hands the postoperative morbidity from incontinence may not be inconsiderable.

Although current opinion has veered from the early use of endocrine therapy for this stage of the disease, it may be interesting in comparison to note that one small series (Barnes and Emery, 1959) has disclosed the remarkable 10-year survival figure of 50 per cent for a group of patients with tumours staged 1 or 2, treated by endocrine methods only. This is remarkably similar to the expected 10-year survival in the general population mentioned above. At the same time, the greatly improved results of current methods of radiotherapy as applied to the primary site (see below) would now seem to offer an attractive alternative either to radical surgery or endocrine therapy.

Irrespective, however, of whatever method is employed it is important that preoccupation with the treatment of the malignant process should not obscure the need for dealing with the dangerous consequences of continuing urinary obstruction. Palliative resection, as distinct from radical surgery, may therefore sometimes be required in this and subsequent stages of the disease and would not seem to lead to any increased risk of dissemination.

STAGES 3 AND 4

Primary treatment in these late stages is by endocrine therapy although, as mentioned above, palliative endoscopic resection may also be needed to relieve persistent urinary obstruction. Sporadic attempts, however, have been made at radical prostatectomy in Stage 3 in selected cases when maximum regression has been obtained with endocrine therapy (Scott, 1964; Chute and Fox, 1966) but the ultimate results have not been encouraging. Since prostatic cancer varies so greatly in its degree of malignancy, only the results of a large series can establish the final value of this manoeuvre.

THE PLACE OF RADIOTHERAPY IN MANAGEMENT

A general survey in present circumstances suggests that nearly 50 per cent of patients show evidence of blood-borne metastases when first seen, a further small proportion (less than 5 per cent) may be candidates for radical resection, and the remainder have locally advanced disease. Since the recent report (VACURG, 1967) incriminating oestrogen therapy as a cause of increased mortality from vascular complications, members of this last group have been referred more often for radical radiation therapy. This trend has been supported by the encouraging results now being obtained by the use of supervoltage and cobalt teletherapy (Bagshaw, Kaplan and Sagerman, 1965; del Regato, 1967).

Adenocarcinoma of the prostate is often a slow growing tumour and tends to respond *slowly* to radiotherapy if the tumour is well differentiated. For this reason it used to be considered relatively radioresistant, but it is now believed that tumours of this type have a high likelihood of cure from radiotherapy. Many of the earlier radiotherapeutic techniques for this purpose depended on interstitial radiation, rather than external radiation, because of the severe reaction in the moist skin of the perineum and anus which followed the latter.

Radon seeds were inserted at open operation via the bladder (Barringer, 1924) or radium needles via the perineum, rectum or urethra (Silverstone, 1940) or by the ischiorectal route (Darget, 1955). These techniques involved difficulty in securing a uniform distribution of radiation throughout the volume of potential invasion and thus were liable to lead to necrosis in overdosed areas and persistent tumour in others. To obviate this, Flocks (Flocks et al, 1952; Flocks, 1953) introduced a technique of interstitial injection of radioactive gold into the prostate and seminal vesicles in the hope of obtaining better distribution. The results certainly showed improvement in the control of the local disease, but problems still remain in achieving uniform dosage, and possible spread to lymph nodes is not included in the scope of the radiation.

SUPERVOLTAGE AND COBALT TELETHERAPY

The advantage of external radiation therapy is that extraprostatic structures such as the seminal vesicles are easily included, and a wide area of potential involvement in the pelvis can be raised to a uniformly high dose of radiation. The added advantage of cobalt and supervoltage sources is that the aim can be achieved with minimal skin reaction. Cases suitable for radical radiation therapy are selected from those where the primary lesion is too large for prostatectomy to be considered, and the tumour is still localised to the capsule and periprostatic tissue with no evidence of blood-borne metastasis. A raised serum acid phosphatase level is not necessarily considered a contraindication to such treatment.

The supervoltage technique described by Bagshaw et al (1965) involves a rotating beam and a 4·7 meV linear accelerator, aiming at a maximum tumour dose of 7000 rads in six weeks, and a minimum of 3500 rads throughout the pelvis. The cobalt teletherapy technique described by del Regato (1967) uses pelvic and perineal fields, and aims at a maximum tumour dose of 7500 rads in five to six weeks and 6000 rads throughout most of the volume of potential invasion. In the former series, 13 of 30 patients survived five years, the majority of deaths being due to blood-borne metastases.

Complications of such treatment include diarrhoea due to oedema of the bowel wall which commonly appears two to three weeks after starting therapy, but which should not lead to cessation of treatment. Some measure of alleviation may be afforded by the oral use of codeine phosphate. In rare cases a necrotic rectal ulcer may develop subsequently, and a resultant anal stricture may require dilatation. Dysuria is not uncommon during treatment, and urethral stricturing may occur later, though this has been observed mainly in patients who have undergone repeated perurethral resection. The skin reaction is usually moderate and there is apparently little effect on libido or potency in the majority of patients treated.

One of the assets of radical radiotherapy is that it does not preclude the subsequent use of endocrine methods, if such become indicated by local recurrence or metastatic spread. It is advisable, however, that the two methods of treatment should not be used in combination in order that the tumour cells should remain maximally sensitive to the radiation. On the other hand radiotherapy temporarily reduces the body defence mechanism to the tumour and it may be wise not to withhold oestrogens for too long.

PALLIATIVE RADIOTHERAPY

Palliative radiotherapy can be used to shrink soft tissue and lymphatic deposits and will almost invariably relieve the pain of bone metastases within two to three weeks of radiation. Its scope in this respect is obviously limited by the extent of the disease and its application cannot be more than strictly local. Lung and liver metastases are better treated by endocrine methods.

Initial Endocrine Therapy

DECISIONS IN SELECTION

Initial endocrine therapy offers a choice between oestrogens and castration or, alternatively, the two in combination. In making a selection, due regard must be paid, not only to the timing of its application in relation to other forms of treatment but also to the benefits likely to accrue. Endocrine therapy will not cure prostatic cancer but can be expected to control the activity of the disease in a majority of cases, at least for a time.

It is important to realise, however, that duration of survival is not the only parameter by which its success can be gauged and, in many instances, the symptomatic relief which it induces, albeit with gradual extension of the disease, may be of greater merit. In fact, in certain circumstances, particularly in the aged, the aim of promoting survival in comfort may seem preferable, and equally acceptable ethically, to striving for survival alone.

As has already been mentioned, a majority of patients only seek advice when symptoms have already become troublesome. In the early stages of the disease, failing relief from surgery or radiotherapy (if suitable facilities are available), endocrine therapy offers the best prospect of alleviation. Similarly in Stage 4 of the disease, when symptomatic metastases are present, such treatment would appear paramount as a means of affording relief. The main problem is therefore to decide whether the initial attack should take the form of castration or oestrogen therapy.

Some guidance in this respect has already been given in Chapter 12 from which it will be inferred that, in the absence of pre-existing cardiac or vascular disease, the results of either form of treatment would seem closely similar. Indeed, the main objection to castration, as involving a minor but impalatable operative procedure, would appear reasonably balanced by the inconvenience and possible sequelae of sustained oestrogen therapy. It has been suggested, however (Nesbit and Baum, 1950), that combined therapy may yield better results than either method alone.

A recent review (Badenoch, 1966) describes the lack of agreement as to the initial form of endocrine treatment in cases with inoperable prostatic cancer as follows: 'Most urologists give a dose of 45–60 mg (stilboestrol) daily in divided doses until the primary, and if present, secondary lesions are clinically under control. . . . There is another school which uses a much higher dosage, giving 100–300 mg daily and continuing this indefinitely. . . . Another school prefers to treat the patient by castration in the first instance, and only gives oestrogen when the lesion ceases to be controlled. . . . It is said that when both treatments are given from the start, survival is longer.'

The latter suggestion is refuted by the VACURG (1967) report which concluded that orchidectomy combined with 5 mg stilboestrol daily, yielded a *lower* overall survival rate than orchidectomy combined with a placebo, both in early and late cases of prostatic cancer. Although deaths from cancer appeared to be lower, the stilboestrol series had a higher mortality from cerebrovascular and cardiovascular complications. Whether the latter was due to sodium retention or alteration in blood clotting factors remains uncertain, but even with this small dose of oestrogens the death rate from infarction seemed to be substantially increased.

The same report also endorsed the view

that orchidectomy and oestrogen therapy are of virtually equal value as measured by relief of pain, decrease in size of the prostatic tumour and fall in the serum acid phosphatase level. Furthermore, that either method alone provided all the clinical benefits of both methods combined.

From this it was suggested that since oestrogen therapy early in the course of the disease may be harmful, such therapy should be delayed until symptoms are so severe that they cannot be relieved by any other method. This conclusion has been criticised on the grounds that most of the excess deaths in the VACURG series fell within the first five months after beginning oestrogen treatment. This observation may be correlated with another (Bennett, Dowd and Harrison, 1970), that the danger of oestrogen therapy in increasing the mortality from vascular disease lies almost wholly in patients with significant pre-existing cardiovascular disorders.

Although the relationship between oestrogen therapy and infarction remains confused, some evidence of dose dependency has been suggested in the literature. Thus, while large doses are said to increase the risk of thrombosis (Stamler et al, 1963), very small doses may protect against further episodes of myocardial or cerebral infarction (Marmorston et al, 1962). According to Furman et al (1958) either castration or the administration of stilboestrol, 5 to 75 mg daily, to males is likely to protect against the development of atherosclerosis.

INDIVIDUALISATION OF INITIAL THERAPY

Most reports agree that castration and oestrogen therapy afford similar degrees of palliation in advanced prostatic cancer and the respective merits of these two forms of treatment have already been referred to (Chapter 12). It should be stressed, however, that even if two methods yield similar overall results in a large heterogenous group of patients, this does not make them equally suitable for the management of a particular case. Individual consideration has to be taken into account, such as aversion to castration for sexual or psychological reasons, capacity for sustaining oral therapy with oestrogens, and the ability to compete with any ensuing complications.

In addition, the palliative role of surgery and radiotherapy, even in the advanced disease, has to be remembered and the need for additional endocrine treatment should be based as far as possible on the biological potential of the disease. This will depend on the age group, the rate of tumour growth, its histological characteristics, the site and extent of metastases and the presence of other disease.

It is established that in the younger patient prostatic cancer is more rapidly growing, and the majority of cases succumb directly from tumour spread. In older patients, on the other hand, the disease progresses more slowly and there is a higher proportion of deaths from intercurrent disease (Fergusson, 1958; Franks, Fergusson and Murnaghan, 1958). In some older patients, therefore, the progress of the disease can be watched for a time before undertaking active treatment.

A comparison between hormone-sensitive and hormone-resistant tumours is said to show no difference in histological grading (Franks et al, 1958). Nevertheless, according to Emmett et al (1960) the palliative results of oestrogen therapy in prostatic cancer are better if the tumour histology is of a higher grade, and this is the generally accepted clinical impression.

Because of the frequency of bone metastases in the late stages of the disease, pain is often the most prominent symptom and has been widely used as an indicator of the response to endocrine therapy. Although the report of the VACURG (1967) purported to show that placebo tablets had the same degree of efficacy as stilboestrol in promoting relief, this would seem contrary to general experience. It is, however, advisable that a decision to institute or change endocrine therapy in cases with metastases should be based as far as possible on objective evidence of progressing disease.

As an example of active progression Brendler and Prout (1962) quote increasing size of the primary growth or metastases, *or* elevation of the serum acid phosphatase level above normal *or* at least two of the following manifestations of cancer: pain, neurological deficit, dilation of the upper urinary tract, pathological fracture, anaemia and weight loss.

Individualisation of therapy is also helped by the use of indices reflecting the hormonal environment of the tumour. Thus the efficacy of anti-androgen therapy can be assessed by the effect on the plasma testosterone level and the androgenic 17-ketosteroid level, and also by the urethral cytology if oestrogen therapy is being administered.

Secondary Endocrine Therapy

DECISIONS IN SELECTION

Secondary endocrine therapy relates to the further treatment of cases resistant to, or in relapse after initial treatment with oestrogens or castration. The basis of such treatment has already been discussed in Chapter 13.

The practice of endocrine manipulation in prostatic cancer is largely empirical because the existence of hormone dependence in the tumour cannot be predicted before treatment is instituted. This applies especially when relapse occurs after the initial treatment, although an earlier response has been viewed by some as a favourable indication. Relapse may be due either to the development of true autonomy, *or* to a rise in the threshold of response to oestrogen therapy *or* to the development of a rising androgen level.

The assessment of certain indices may help to identify the cause.

IDENTIFYING THE CAUSE OF RELAPSE

DEVELOPMENT OF TUMOUR AUTONOMY

The metabolic processes of the tumour may become independent of the hormone environment, either by enzymatic adaption to the changed conditions, or by the natural selection of cell types which can grow without androgens (Foulds, 1954). It has been suggested that failure of the serum acid phosphatase to rise when clinical evidence of relapse occurs, is a sign of tumour autonomy (Woodard and Dean, 1947). This is likely only if the enzyme level cannot be stimulated by a provocative test dose of testosterone (see Chapter 14) which in such circumstances of doubt may seem justifiable.

RISE IN THE THRESHOLD OF RESPONSE TO STEROID THERAPY

It has been noted in the case of oestrogen therapy that a fall in the KPI level (see urethral cytology, Chapter 13) during prolonged treatment may indicate an inadequate anti-oestrogenic effect. If this is associated with clinical relapse and a rise in the serum acid phosphatase level, then an increase in dose or a change in the form of oestrogen therapy may lead to renewed control of tumour activity. A similar conclusion based on the examination of serial biopsy material showing evidence of a renewed response to increased doses of stilboestrol was reached by Fergusson and Franks (1953).

RISING ANDROGEN LEVEL

Androgen secretion is mediated by LH (and also by ACTH) secretion from the anterior pituitary, and relapse may occur when oestrogen therapy no longer controls LH secretion. A rising androgen level may originate in the adrenal cortex or from the interstitial cells of the testis, which may remain capable of androgen secretion even after some years of continuous oestrogen therapy (Dekker and Russfield, 1963). Such a change would be suggested by signs of tumour reactivation associated with a rising trend in serial androgenic 17-ketosteroid excretion levels.

EFFECT OF STEROIDS ON THE TUMOUR IN VITRO

Attempts to assess the direct effect of sex hormones on the growth of prostatic cancer in organ culture have been largely frustrated by difficulties in maintaining cultures in representative form. However, a few successes are reported but certain qualifications are required.

Such bioassay ignores the influence of other endogenous hormones upon the tumour tissue, and measures the effect of the individual hormone itself and not its metabolites. It also ignores the indirect effect which such administered hormones might have *in vivo* on the endocrine system. With these qualifications studies of a biopsy specimen *in vitro* may possibly be able to predict tumour sensitivity in the patient to an administered hormone.

The effect of androgens on prostatic cancer biopsy material in organ culture has been examined in small series (Roehl, 1958; Jonsson et al, 1963; Wojewski and Kaniewicz, 1965). Stimulation of growth by androsterone has been shown, especially with highly differentiated adenocarcinoma (Roehl, 1958). The degree of growth stimulation by androsterone in organ culture is said to be proportional to the degree of clinical palliation from oestrogen therapy given previously (Jonsson et al, 1963).

Although stimulation of tumour growth by androgens in organ culture may indicate hormone sensitivity as against autonomy, the observation of tumour growth *depression* by oestrogens or other steroids in organ culture might suggest their selection for individual therapy. This has so far not been attempted for prostatic cancer although biochemical and histochemical evidence of growth depression by steroids has been shown in organ cultures of breast cancer (Stoll, 1970; Chayen et al, 1970).

MANAGEMENT OF THE RELAPSE

RELAPSE AFTER OESTROGEN THERAPY

Tumour reactivation often occurs after one to two years of control by oestrogen therapy. In such cases the cessation of oestrogen therapy may itself yield a 'withdrawal response' in a proportion of cases, and this may account for some of the responses reported from placebo administration at this stage. An observation period of at least one month (and preferably two) should be allowed after discontinuing oestrogen therapy, in order to ensure that both clinical and biochemical parameters indicate advancing disease.

Castration is occasionally worth a trial following loss of control from initial oestrogen therapy. The degree of testicular atrophy following such therapy varies according to the dose and duration of oestrogen therapy but, as mentioned above, Dekker and Russfield (1963) suggest that the interstitial cells of the testis may secrete androgen in response to LH stimulation, even after continuous oestrogen administration for several years. Testicular shrinkage does not necessarily indicate complete loss of ability to secrete androgen, and estimation of the plasma testosterone level (Kliman and Peterson, 1960) may assist in the decision to castrate in such cases.

RELAPSE AFTER CASTRATION

A trial of oestrogen therapy after loss of control from castration may sometimes yield significant clinical benefit in this disease, and a fall in the serum acid phosphatase level is occasionally observed. The prescription of a placebo instead of oestrogen in such cases has been noted (VACURG, 1967) to lead to clinical improvement in the same proportion (40 per cent) of cases. However, no distinction is made in this report between subjective and objective improvement.

In a patient who has not responded to castration, corticosteroid therapy may be used in preference to oestrogens, as response to corticosteroids is not confined to androgen-dependent tumours. At a later stage hypophyseal ablation by yttrium (see Chapter 13) may be tried in such cases, particularly when pain from bone metastases becomes disabling.

RELAPSE AFTER BOTH OESTROGEN AND CASTRATION

In the case of a tumour which has manifested hormone sensitivity, a trial of a progestational agent may be considered at this stage. The advantage of this group of agents is their relative freedom from side-effects, so that even if not effective in controlling the tumour, no harm is done. As an alternative, the use of androgens may be considered as hormonal 'shock' therapy, with the addition of ^{32}P if bone metastases are present. After 7 to 14 days' administration of testosterone propionate 25 mg daily, oestrogens are recommenced. Neither of these measures, however, has proved of much avail in the author's hands and if the patient's general condition justifies it, hypophyseal ablation by yttrium is to be preferred (see Chapter 13).

Place of Cytotoxic Therapy in Management

The reports in the literature on the treatment of prostatic cancer by cytotoxic agents are scanty, and some authorities believe that no form of chemotherapy has been shown to control the disease effectively. Whereas Murphy (1966) states that neither 5-fluorouracil nor nitrogen mustard are of significant value in prostatic cancer, Flocks (1969) reports that a combination of the two agents caused subjective benefit in 11 of 12 patients and a fall in the serum acid phosphatase level in 5 of those with previous elevation. The difference in opinion probably reflects different criteria of improvement.

ALKYLATING AGENTS

There is no basic difference in the mechanism of action of the different alkylating agents used. Most are derived from the basic nitrogen mustard structure, and have been modified either to permit oral administration or a longer half-life in the blood.

NITROGEN MUSTARD

Given intravenously at a dose of 0·4 mg/kg, pain relief and temporary remission of the disease was achieved in 50 per cent of 12 patients with widely disseminated cancer of the prostate (Flocks, 1969). The disadvantage of the agent is its marked irritant effect upon the tissues, but this can be turned to advantage if given intrapleurally, when it causes adhesive pleuritis in the presence of malignant effusion.

THIOTEPA

This is administered at a dose of 0·5 mg/kg at fortnightly intervals either intravenously, intramuscularly, intraperitoneally or directly into the tumour. It is non-irritating and well tolerated systemically, although a sudden inexplicable fall in the leucocyte or platelet counts occasionally takes place. Its use in prostatic cancer has been reported to yield significant remissions in some cases (Weyrauch and Nesbit, 1959).

CYCLOPHOSPHAMIDE

This is probably the most widely used alkylating agent for this disease. It is recommended for the treatment of prostatic cancer which is no longer hormone sensitive, and has been claimed to yield a remission in 17 out of 28 patients in relapse after previous oestrogen response (Chauvin, 1967). The dose given was 200 mg daily intravenously for about three weeks, but another report of benefit in prostatic cancer has referred to doses of from 400 to 500 mg daily for a shorter period (Fox, 1965). On the other hand, oral administration is also possible at a dose of 100 to 150 mg daily for prolonged periods. An interesting observation by Chauvin (1967) is that there was not a single remission among 9 patients who had *not* previously responded to oestrogen therapy. Alopecia and cystitis may result from high dosage of cyclophosphamide, but marrow depression is usually readily foreseen.

FLUORINATED PYRIMIDINES

5-Fluorouracil is a substituted form of the pyrimidine uracil, and, when taken up in the synthesis of tumour RNA, prevents proper coding of the RNA. 5-Fluorodeoxyuridine when given as a rapid injection, is converted to 5-fluorouracil and has the same degree of activity. Used in the treatment of prostatic cancer, the former is reported to have achieved remission of the disease in 3 out of 8 cases (Wilson et al, 1967). Intolerance to these drugs is mainly gastrointestinal and haemopoietic.

The cytotoxic agents mentioned are capable of inducing remission in approximately 20 per cent of patients with widely disseminated prostatic cancer, with temporary regression of the primary growth, metastatic soft tissue tumour or pulmonary metastases. The average duration of such remission is, unfortunately, only about six months, and this has to be set against the haemopoietic and gastrointestinal toxicity of these agents. Their administration, too, is rarely associated with the subjective feeling of well-being which is often noted with steroid administration whether or not objective evidence of remission is achieved. Nevertheless, given with caution, agents such as cyclophosphamide may be useful in relieving the pain of bone metastases from prostatic cancer, when hormonal therapy or hypophyseal ablation have lost their effect.

CONCLUSIONS

The endocrine management of the patient with prostatic cancer must be individualised, as every form of hormonal control carries certain hazards which must be weighed against the dangers of the untreated disease. Treatment is carried through in sequential stages, and it is customary to rely primarily on the simplest effective method, taking account of the stage of the disease and the general clinical status of the patient.

Orchidectomy and oestrogen therapy have been demonstrated to have virtually equivalent ability to decrease the size of the primary tumour or to control the manifestations of the metastases. Either method alone provides all the clinical benefit of both methods combined. The choice between the methods depends on psychological factors, the age of the patient, the capacity to sustain oestrogen therapy and its complications. The recent report of increased liability of oestrogen-treated patients to cardiovascular complications suggests that it is reasonable to delay the administration of oestrogens in those patients where the disease is amenable to local surgery or radiotherapy.

In the presence of relapse after either orchidectomy or oestrogen therapy, the alternative form of therapy can be used depending on the results of biochemical estimations of the hormonal environment of the tumour. More elaborate methods of endocrine ablation therapy, such as adrenalectomy or hypophyseal ablation, are restricted to the treatment of advanced or relapsing cases when appropriate technical facilities and arrangements for substitution therapy are available. Corticosteroid therapy or cytotoxic therapy may be useful as palliative alternatives in patients who are not suitable for major surgery of this type. Finally, it must be stressed that supplementary treatment by palliative surgery or radiotherapy must be considered at any stage.

References

Badenoch, A. W. (1966) The management of cancer of the prostate. *Practitioner*, **196**, 60–64.

Bagshaw, M. A., Kaplan, H. S. & Sagerman, R. H. (1965) Linear accelerator super voltage radiotherapy. VII. Cancer of the prostate. *Radiology*, **85**, 121–129.

Barnes, R. W. & Emery, D. S. (1959) Management of early prostatic carcinoma. *California Medical Journal*, **91**, 57–61.

Barringer, B. S. (1924) Radium in the treatment of prostatic carcinoma. *Annals of Surgery*, **80**, 881–884.

Bauer, W. C., McGarvan, M. H. & Carlin, M. R. (1960) Unsuspected carcinoma of the prostate in suprapubic prostatectomy specimens. *Cancer*, **13**, 370–378.

Bennett, A. H., Dowd, J. B. & Harrison, J. H. (1970) Estrogen and survival data in carcinoma of the prostate. *Surgery, Gynecology and Obstetrics*, **130**, 505–508.

Brendler, H. & Prout, G. (1962) A co-operative group study of prostatic cancer: stilboestrol versus placebo in advanced progressive disease. *Cancer Chemotherapy Reports*, **16**, 323–328.

Bumpus, H. C. (1926) Carcinoma of prostate; clinical study of one thousand cases. *Surgery, Gynecology and Obstetrics*, **43**, 150–155.

Chauvin, H. F. (1967) Hormone independent cancer of the prostate. *Cancer Chemotherapy Abstracts*, **8**, 543.

Chayen, J., Altmann, F. P., Bitensky, L. & Daly, J. R. (1970) Response of human breast-cancer tissue to steroid hormones in vitro. *Lancet*, **1**, 868–870.

Chute, R. & Fox, B. M. (1966) Non-resectable carcinoma of the prostate rendered resectable by endocrine therapy. *Journal of Urology*, **95**, 577–579.

Darget, R. (1955) Implantation par voie ischiorectale d'aguilles de radium dans certain cas de cancers prostatiques. *Bordeaux Chirurgical*, **2**, 109–110.

Dekker, A. & Russfield, A. B. (1963) Pituitary tropic hormone studies and morphologic observations in carcinoma of the prostate. *Cancer*, **16**, 743–750.

Emmett, J. L., Greene, L. F. & Papantoniou, A. (1960) Endocrine therapy in carcinoma of the prostate gland: 10-year survival studies. *Journal of Urology*, **83**, 471–484.

Fergusson, J. D. (1958) Endocrine control therapy in prostatic cancer. *British Journal of Urology*, **30**, 397–406.

Fergusson, J. D. (1965) The doubtfully malignant prostate. *British Journal of Surgery*, **52**, 746–750.

Fergusson, J. D. & Franks, L. M. (1953) Response of prostatic carcinoma to oestrogen treatment. *British Journal of Surgery*, **40**, 422–428.

Flocks, R. H. (1953) Treatment of carcinoma of prostate. *Journal of Urology*, **70**, 491–498.

Flocks, R. H. (1969) Carcinoma of the prostate. *Journal of Urology*, **101**, 741–749.

Flocks, R. H., Kerr, H. D., Elkins, H. B. & Culp, D. (1952) Treatment of carcinoma of prostate with interstitial radiation with radioactive gold (Au 98): a preliminary report. *Journal of Urology*, **68**, 510–522.

Fox, M. (1965) The effect of cyclophosphamide on some urinary tract tumours. *British Journal of Urology*, **37**, 399–409.

Foulds, L. (1954) The experimental study of tumour progression: a review. *Cancer Research*, **14**, 327–339.

Franks, L. M., Fergusson, J. D. & Murnaghan, G. F. (1958) An assessment of factors influencing survival in prostatic cancer: the absence of reliable prognostic features. *British Journal of Cancer*, **12**, 321–326.

Furman, R. H., Howard, R. P., Norcia, L. N. & Keaty, E. C. (1958) The influence of androgens, estrogens and related steroids on serum lipoids and lipo-proteins. *American Journal of Medicine*, **24**, 80–97.

Greene, L. F. & Simon, H. B. (1955) Occult carcinoma of the prostate. *Journal of the American Medical Association*, **158**, 1494–1498.

Hudson, P. B., Finkle, A. L., Trifilio, A., Jost, H. M., Sproul, E. E. & Stout, A. P. (1954) Prostatic cancer. VIII. Detection of unsuspected adenocarcinoma in the aging male population. *Journal of the American Medical Association*, **155**, 426–429.

Jewett, H. J. (1954) Radical perineal prostatectomy for carcinoma, an analysis of cases at Johns Hopkins Hospital, 1904–1954. *Journal of the American Medical Association*, **156**, 139–141.

Jonsson, G., Dicfalusy, E., Plantin, L. O., Rohl, L. & Birke, G. (1963) Estradurin (polyestradiol phosphate) in the treatment of prostatic carcinoma. A clinical and steroid metabolic study. *Acta Endocrinologica*, **44**, Supplement 83, 3–41.

Kliman, B. & Peterson, R. E. (1960) Double isotope derivative assay of aldosterone in biological extracts. *Journal of Biological Chemistry*, **235**, 1803–1808.

Marmorston, J., Moore, F. J., Hopkins, C. E., Kuzma, O. T. & Weiner, J. (1962) Clinical studies of long term estrogen therapy in men with myocardial infarction. *Proceedings of the Society of Experimental Biology and Medicine*, **110**, 400–408.

Murphy, J. J. (1966) Carcinoma of the urinary tract. In *Current Perspectives in Cancer Therapy*, ed. Bakemore, W. S. and Ravdin, I. S., pp. 211–217. New York and London: Hoeber.

Nesbit, R. M. & Baum, W. C. (1950) Endocrine control of prostatic carcinoma; clinical and statistical survey of 1818 cases. *Journal of the American Medical Association*, **143**, 1317–1320.

Nesbit, R. M. & Plumb, R. T. (1946) Prostatic carcinoma; follow up on 795 patients treated prior to endocrine era and comparison of survival rates between these and patients treated by endocrine therapy. *Surgery*, **20**, 263–272.

del Regato, J. A. (1967) Radiotherapy in the conservative treatment of operable and locally inoperable carcinoma of the prostate. *Radiology*, **88**, 761–766.

Robinson, M. R. G., Nakhla, L. S. & Whitaker, R. H. (1971) Lymphocyte transformation in carcinoma of the prostate. *British Journal of Urology*, **43**, 480–486.

Roehl, L. (1958) Hormone dependency of prostatic cancer studied by cell culture technique. *British Journal of Urology*, **30**, 450–454.

Scott, W. W. (1964) An evaluation of endocrine therapy plus radical perineal prostatectomy in the treatment of advanced carcinoma of the prostate. *Journal of Urology*, **91**, 97–102.

Silverstone, M. (1940) Radium in treatment of carcinoma of the prostate. *British Journal of Surgery*, **27**, 498–505.

Stamler, J., Pick, R., Katz, L. N., Pick, A., Kaplan, B. M., Berkson, D. M. & Century, D. (1963) Effectiveness of estrogens for therapy of myocardial infarction in middle-age men. *Journal of the American Medical Association*, **183**, 632–638.

Stoll, B. A. (1970) Investigation of organ culture as an aid to the hormonal management of breast cancer. *Cancer*, **25**, 1228–1233.

Turner, R. D. & Belt, E. (1957) A study of 229 consecutive cases of total perineal prostatectomy for cancer of the prostate. *Journal of Urology*, **77**, 62–77.

Veterans Administration Co-operative Urological Research Group (1967) Treatment and survival of patients with cancer of the prostate. *Surgery, Gynecology and Obstetrics*, **124**, 1011–1017.

Weyrauch, H. M. & Nesbet, J. D. (1959) Use of triethylene thio-phosphoramide (thiotepa) in treatment of advanced carcinoma of prostate. *Journal of Urology*, **81**, 185–193.

Wilson, W. L., Bisel, H. F., Krementz, E. T., Lien, R. C. & Prohaska, J. V. (1967) Further clinical evaluation of 2′-deoxy-5-fluorouridine (NSC-27640)[1,2]. *Cancer Chemotherapy Reports*, **51**, 85–90.

Wojewski, A. & Kaniewicz, D. P. (1965) The influence of stilboestrol and testosterone on the growth of prostatic adenoma and carcinoma in tissue culture. *Journal of Urology*, **93**, 721–724.

Woodard, H. Q. & Dean, A. L. (1947) The significance of phosphatase findings in carcinoma of the prostate. *Journal of Urology*, **57**, 158–171.

Other Tumours—Endocrine Aspects

Chapter 16

Endometrial Hyperplasia and Carcinoma in situ

ROBERT W. KISTNER

Critical evaluation of the data concerning the histogenesis of endometrial hyperplasia suggests that prolonged episodes of anovulation, and unopposed oestrogen stimulation, predispose to its development. Correction of this deficiency will result in increased fertility and may also serve as a prophylactic measure against the development of endometrial carcinoma.

ENDOCRINE ROLE IN INITIATION AND PROGRESSION OF ENDOMETRIAL CANCER

The basic postulate mentioned above is of singular importance but its acceptance depends upon our ability to answer specific questions regarding the natural history of this disease. First, may patients with atypical adenomatous hyperplasia (carcinoma in situ) of the endometrium develop invasive carcinoma? If so, how frequent is this occurrence? Second, is this progression reversible at a specific point, and what is the incidence of spontaneous disappearance of the lesion? If the lesion is capable of being arrested or reversed spontaneously, how may this be accomplished therapeutically? Third, what are the factors that permit areas of cellular atypia to become locally invasive?

Patients with certain types of endometrial hyperplasia are more likely to develop carcinoma than are patients with normal cyclic or senescent endometrial patterns. Although the exact incidence of carcinoma of the endometrium developing in patients with endometrial hyperplasia of all types is difficult to determine, several prospective studies have indicated that it may be expected to occur in between 5 and 12 per cent of patients with atypical adenomatous hyperplasia (carcinoma in situ). This process is often relatively slow and progression from hyperplasia to carcinoma may take five or more years. It should be remembered, however, that various hyperplastic patterns may be found in the non-malignant endometrium of patients with endometrial carcinoma.

The answer to the second question is now definite. Not only have potent progestational agents been shown to cause marked changes in endometrial hyperplasia and carcinoma in situ, but they have also a marked morphologic and histochemical effect on invasive carcinoma of the endometrium, both in its intrauterine site and in metastatic foci. In selected patients having atypical endometrial patterns associated with the Stein–Leventhal syndrome, wedge resection has been followed by ovulation, secretion of progesterone, and reversion of the hyperplastic process.

Fifteen years ago I suggested that the ideal treatment for the young patient who was found to have endometrial hyperplasia was to secure ovulation and conception. Prior to 1960 this was not accomplished easily except in an occasional patient with surgically corrected Stein–Leventhal syndrome. In 1957 Younge speculated that carcinoma of the cervix might be a preventable disease if adequate therapy was instituted during the premalignant phase. Similar therapy applied energetically to endometrial hyperplasia may result in similar prophylaxis.

Prolonged periods of anovulation occur most often during the postmenarchal and premenopausal periods in the human female. In the young female the causes may be multiple, involving abnormal function of the pituitary, thyroid, adrenal or ovary. In the premenopausal female it is the result of an inability of the ageing ovary to respond to sequential gonadotropic stimulation. Prolonged periods of unopposed oestrogen stimulation of the endometrium may produce cystic and adenomatous hyperplasia and, in certain patients, carcinoma in situ. The cause for this variation in response is unknown.

ENDOMETRIAL HYPERPLASIA AND CARCINOMA OF THE ENDOMETRIUM

An association between endometrial hyperplasia and subsequent carcinoma was first noted by Bäcker in 1904. The review by Taylor (1932) and that by Novak and Yui (1936) suggested that a definite correlation between these entities did exist and, furthermore, that oestrogenic substances might, under favourable circumstances, be carcinogenic. Larson (1954) reviewed the literature relative to the relationship of oestrogens to endometrial carcinoma, and was able to formulate five distinctly different points of view held by various groups of investigators. Briefly, these are as follows:

First, endometrial hyperplasia does not have any tendency toward malignant change in the reproductive years, but when it occurs as a result of *post*menopausal oestrogenic stimulation of the endometrium, it may predispose toward malignant disease.

Second, endometrial hyperplasia (and hence excess oestrogen stimulation) predisposes to carcinoma at any age.

Third, endometrial hyperplasia and cancer are not associated but 'the unopposed action of oestrin, with its resultant effect on the endometrium, is the basic principle at work in the development of malignancy of the endometrium of those individuals who possess the genetic factor necessary for the development of cancer'.

Fourth, endometrial hyperplasia may be followed by anaplasia, carcinoma in situ, and adenocarcinoma of the uterus but: 'No convincing studies are available to show that oestrogen stimulation alone will produce this picture, and many excellent oestrogen studies fail to mention such histological changes.'

Fifth, neither hyperplasia nor prolonged oestrogen stimulation is associated with endometrial cancer other than on a chance basis.

The available data from human material would suggest that:

There is little, if any, evidence that oestrogenic substances are carcinogenic in the premenopausal woman.

Only meagre evidence is available to indicate that cystic ('Swiss-cheese') hyperplasia is causally related to endometrial carcinoma.

In *predisposed individuals*, the unopposed action of oestrogenic substances for considerable periods of time will result in endometrial adenomatous hyperplasia, anaplasia, carcinoma in situ, and, eventually, carcinoma.

Kistner, Duncan and Mansell (1956) produced varying degrees of hyperplasia and anaplasia in young, normally menstruating women by the administration of an oestrogen for 45 to 100 days. Thirty-four patients were so treated and, at the time of biopsy or curettage, 15 showed proliferative endometrium, 5 had cystic hyperplasia, 10 had cystic and adenomatous hyperplasia, and 4 had lesions that were termed anaplasia. After oestrogen administration was stopped, all patients subsequently had normal menstrual periods and normal endometrium as determined by biopsy.

Figure 16.1 illustrates in diagrammatic fashion the sequence of progressive changes in the endometrium leading to the development of invasive carcinoma. This diagram is based on the work of Sommers, Hertig and Bengaloff (1949) and although this was a retrospective study, several important conclusions may be made. In the first place, it

indicates that women who are destined to develop endometrial carcinoma demonstrate progressive phases of glandular stimulation which, up to a point, are dependent upon oestrogen. Removal of oestrogen results in glandular regression. The critical turning point is the stage known as atypical adenomatous hyperplasia or, in Boston, carcinoma in situ. According to prospective studies, approximately 10 per cent of patients having this lesion subsequently develop invasive carcinoma. Undoubtedly cellular autonomy occurs in these individuals and, according to Wagner, Richart and Terner (1967) the cells of these truly pre-malignant lesions demonstrate abnormal DNA distribution and aneuploidy. Thus some degree of predictability is now available by specialised studies, but not on the basis of routine morphological examination.

A fair summation of the data seems to be that *in predisposed individuals, the unopposed action of oestrogenic substances for considerable periods of time will result in endometrial adenomatous hyperplasia, carcinoma in situ and, eventually, carcinoma.* Recent studies have suggested an endocrine basis in patients with endometrial carcinoma, because of the high incidence of prolonged anovulation, dysfunctional uterine bleeding and infertility in these patients. A suggested method of prophylaxis against this progressive 'unrest' of the endometrial epithelium has been to secure ovulation, menstruation, and pregnancy. In the past this has been an unattainable goal.

Although the specific morphologic changes preceding carcinoma of the endometrium are not adequately documented, some

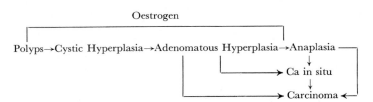

FIGURE 16.1. Concept of the histogenesis of endometrial carcinoma.

suggestive evidence has been advanced by Hertig and Sommers (1949) to indicate that adenomatous hyperplasia precedes carcinoma. This study was based on a retrospective examination of prior curettings in women known to have endometrial cancer. However, several prospective experiments have been carried out which support the premise that adenomatous hyperplasia does not always proceed relentlessly toward unequivocal carcinoma; at present it is impossible to predict which type of hyperplasia will, and which will not, develop a malignant potential. Gusberg and Kaplan (1963) have classified 'atypical' hyperplasia as being histologically identical with adenomatous hyperplasia, carcinoma in situ, and Stage O cancer. They state that approximately 12 per cent of patients having this particular lesion subsequently develop invasive carcinoma of the endometrium if no treatment except curettage is performed. They conclude that adenomatous hyperplasia may be present in the same endometrium with adenocarcinoma, or it might be a cancer precursor.

The relationship of oestrogens to the development of endometrial hyperplasia is clear; the relationship of oestrogens to invasive carcinoma is clouded by assumptions based on individual case reports, retrospective reasoning, and uncontrolled experimentation. Although we have been able to produce invasive carcinoma of the endometrium in the rabbit by the insertion of a cotton string impregnated with 3-methylcholanthrene, it takes almost one year to do so, and the ovaries must be present. The administration of synthetic progestins to these animals significantly inhibits carcinogenesis in the endometrium and will cause regression of established carcinoma.

RATIONALE FOR ENDOCRINE THERAPY

An important clinical question arises as a result of these studies. What is the optimum therapeutic approach in patients demonstrating atypical adenomatous hyperplasia? The answer depends, in part, on the age of the individual and on the reversibility of the lesion. In the postmenopausal patient the obvious treatment is surgical extirpation of the uterus whereas in young women desirous of childbearing, uterine preservation is desirable. During the premenopausal years the answer is not so clear-cut. Several clinical studies have shown that endometrial hyperplasia, including that of the atypical type, may undergo spontaneous regression.

Recent reports have indicated that the administration of progestational agents effects a rapid regression and even atrophy of the hyperplastic process. Data are not available to indicate the incidence of endometrial hyperplasia in premenopausal women since the majority of these individuals are not subjected to curettage. I suspect, however, that the majority of women who fail to ovulate regularly during the early menopause and whose endometrium is chronically stimulated by oestrogen would show hyperplasia if the endometrium were sampled by biopsy or curettage.

What is the life history of this endometrial abnormality subsequent to its appearance in the premenopausal female? Unfortunately we do not know. Several years ago I reviewed the slides of 220 patients at the Boston Hospital for Women in whom a diagnosis of carcinoma in situ of the endometrium had been made. All of these patients were premenopausal, all had presented with abnormal bleeding and the diagnosis had been made in each case by curettage. Unfortunately, a prospective study was not possible since 200 were treated by hysterectomy, and 10 were lost to follow-up. Only 10 without definitive therapy were followed up, and none of these has, as yet, developed invasive endometrial carcinoma in a follow-up period of five years. Furthermore, there was no evidence of invasive carcinoma in any of the hysterectomy specimens.

In a study by Buehl et al (1964) of 31 patients with carcinoma in situ, 23 had immediate hysterectomy, and of these, 7 received radium application preoperatively. There was no residual lesion in the 7 radiated, and only 8 of the other 16 uteri showed residual in situ lesions. Only 4 unoperated patients were followed and 3 were alive and well without evidence of disease at five years without further therapy except curettage (one patient was lost to follow-up). Obviously, it is not sufficient to study endomyometrial tissue obtained at hysterectomy after progestational therapy, since the lesion may have been removed by the initial curettage.

The complexity of the problem of following the progress of the disease is accentuated by the difficulty in obtaining patients who are not subjected to immediate extirpative procedures. This is exemplified by the treatment of three recent patients at the Boston Hospital for Women. Each of these individuals had received continuous daily doses of oestrogen for the relief of menopausal symptoms and each had a diagnosis of invasive endometrial cancer made on the curettings. The first patient received intracavitary radium prior to hysterectomy and the extirpated uterus showed no evidence of carcinoma, carcinoma in situ or even hyperplasia. The second patient had a hysterectomy three weeks following the curettage during which time no oestrogen was given. The endometrium showed only a few cystically dilated glands. The third patient also was operated on after an interval of three weeks and carcinoma in situ was found in only one microscopic focus.

Perplexing questions arise as a result of these findings. Was the original lesion really invasive carcinoma or was this morphologic abnormality produced by the exogenous oestrogen? If this lesion is an induced *adenoma malignum* will it disappear following cessation of oestrogen administration? Is it possible to remove the only area of invasive carcinoma by curettage? Is it safe to observe these patients prospectively and follow the progression or regression of the lesion by sequential curettages? Can these patients be treated by the administration of potent progestational agents which possess anti-oestrogenic activity? Only properly planned prospective studies will answer these questions but it is difficult to programme such a study.

The reasons for surgical approach are obvious and salutary:

First, the procedure is not difficult and carries minimal risk to a healthy patient.

Second, the results are excellent—the patient is cured.

Third, both patient and surgeon are relieved of apprehension.

Only patients having serious medical disorders contraindicating surgery seem suitable for a conservative approach at the present time. We have treated six such patients during the last 10 years by the administration of progestational agents and then performed diagnostic curettage at regular intervals. None of these patients has subsequently shown evidence of recurrent invasive carcinoma although that was the original diagnosis at the time of the initial curettage.

Observations in the human female have indicated that endogenous progesterone, or synthetic progestins are capable of reversing endometrial hyperplasia or carcinoma in situ.

ENDOCRINE THERAPY OF ENDOMETRIAL HYPERPLASIA AND CARCINOMA IN SITU

In 1953 Wellenbach and Rakoff demonstrated in oophorectomised hamsters that induced endometrial hyperplasia underwent rapid regression when progesterone was given. They further showed that if progesterone was administered with oestrogen, hyperplastic endometrial changes were virtually prevented.

In 1956, potent synthetic progestational agents were made available for clinical investigation. In 1959 and 1962 we reported our results of treatment of nine patients having either endometrial hyperplasia or carcinoma in situ (Kistner, 1959, 1962).

Seven of these patients were treated by hysterectomy following administration of these agents, permitting extensive morphologic study of the specimen. Prolonged therapy with these progestogens resulted in a decidual reaction of the stroma and a state of glandular 'regression'.

Kaufman, Abbot and Wall (1959) reported that endometrial hyperplasia of varying degrees could be reversed by the subsequent cyclic action of endogenous progesterone induced by ovarian wedge resection. Another method for the induction of ovulation in patients having this syndrome was reported by Kistner and Smith (1959) using a non-steroidal oestrogen antagonist, ethamoxytriphenol (MER-25). They reported ovulation occurring in four patients with Stein–Leventhal syndrome following the administration of this agent. Three of these patients subsequently became pregnant; and the fourth, not married but having a diagnosis of early invasive carcinoma, has been followed for twelve years without a recurrence of endometrial atypia. Further interest in the effects of progesterone on abnormalities of the endometrium was stimulated by the report of Kelley and Baker (1960) describing the effects of 17α-hydroxyprogesterone caproate on metastatic endometrial cancer.

We have recently analysed a group of 117 patients seen at the Boston Hospital for Women whose complaints were either primary amenorrhoea, secondary oligomenorrhoea, irregular bleeding or infertility. These patients varied in age from 14 to 30 years, and all had a diagnosis of either hyperplasia or carcinoma in situ of the endometrium. Sixty-one of these patients were treated prior to 1957 by the methods available at that time in order to stimulate ovulation. The majority of these patients were treated by ovarian wedge resection; but other therapeutic measures included the use of progesterone, ethinyl testosterone, and cortisone. Subsequent ovulation was obtained in 17 of the 61 patients, but term pregnancy in only 11. Sixteen patients were subsequently treated by hysterectomy, three of these eventually developing invasive carcinoma.

A further group of 76 patients have been treated since 1958 by ovarian wedge resection, cortisone, cyclic administration of synthetic progestogens, continuous administration of synthetic progestogens, ethamoxytriphenol (MER-25) or clomiphene citrate (Clomid) (Kistner, 1965a, b). Subsequent ovulation was obtained in 52 patients, and term pregnancies have occurred in 33. Hysterectomy has been required in only one patient, and this was for a suspicious curettage specimen which was not confirmed as invasive carcinoma at the time of hysterectomy (Table 16.1).

Case reports are presented to illustrate the management of endometrial hyperplasia and carcinoma in situ in three different circumstances:

Management in patients desiring children
Management prior to hysterectomy
Management in patients inoperable due to serious medical disease.

ILLUSTRATIVE CASE REPORTS

Figure 16.2A illustrates the endometrium of a 26-year-old female, a Stein–Leventhal type, who had three previous curettages for abnormal bleeding. Each of the three previous specimens showed atypical endometrial hyperplasia. A wedge resection of the ovaries was performed at the time of the fourth curettage. The specimen illustrated was called early invasive carcinoma by Dr Arthur T. Hertig* and the patient was advised to have a hysterectomy but this was refused. Subsequent to the wedge resection, ovulation occurred only sporadically. Clomiphene citrate was then administered and the patient became pregnant during the third cycle of treatment (Figure 16.2B). This pregnancy resulted in the birth of a stillborn infant during the seventh month of

---

* Shattuck Professor of Pathology Emeritus, Harvard Medical School.

TABLE 16.1. *Comparison of results obtained in the induction of ovulation and incidence of pregnancy during two periods of study (1950–1957 and 1958–1962)*

Therapy	No.	Ovulation	Pregnancy	Cancer
1950–1957				
Wedge resection	22	12	8 (Ab. 2)	0
Hormonal	39	5	3	3
Total	61	17	11	3
Hysterectomy	16	—	—	3
1958–1970				
Wedge resection	26	20	16	0
Cyclic progestins or cortisone	24	14	6	0
Constant progestins	6	0	0	0
MER-25	4	4	3*	0
MER-25 and Clomid	2	2	2	0
Clomid	14	12	6†	0
Total	76	52	33	0
Hysterectomy	1	—	—	1?

* One patient in this group (Miss M. B.) is not married.
† One patient in this group (Miss J. O'B) is not married; one patient in the group (Mrs R. G.) has other reasons for infertility.

gestation. The patient again became amenorrhoeic following delivery and this was followed by irregular bleeding episodes. Clomiphene citrate was again administered and pregnancy occurred during the third month of therapy. The patient was subsequently delivered of normal, dizygotic twins. The original therapeutic measures with clomiphene were carried out in 1962 and, since that time, this patient has had two additional normal pregnancies and has delivered two normal children. Following the last delivery the patient was placed on an oral contraceptive containing a potent anti-oestrogenic progestin. Withdrawal bleeding episodes have been scanty and two curettages, performed as

precautionary measures, produced typical 'progestin-type' endometrial tissue.

This case history exemplifies an ideal approach to the problem of management of hyperplasia or carcinoma *in situ* in the woman desirous of having children. I have successfully treated 16 additional patients in this category during the last 10 years. The optimum method, therefore, of eliminating endometrial hyperplasia is to secure ovulation and pregnancy. Unfortunately, methods for accomplishing this goal did not become available until 1958 when we initiated clinical studies with MER-25 (a substance closely related to clomiphene citrate) to induce ovulation. In 1960 we substituted clomiphene

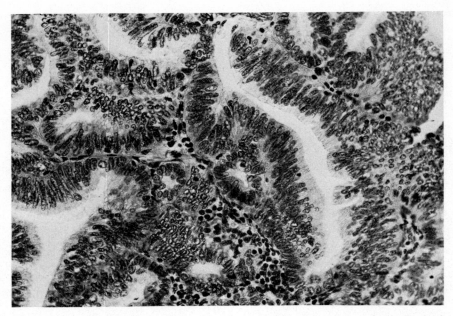

FIGURE 16.2A. Curettage specimen from a 26-year-old patient with Stein–Leventhal syndrome obtained at the time of ovarian wedge resection.

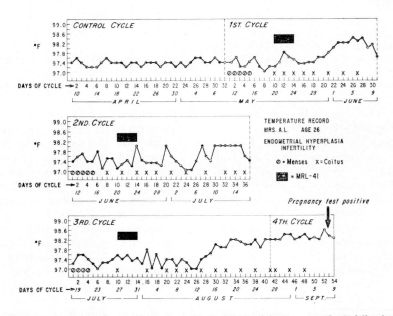

FIGURE 16.2B. Basal body temperature graph of the patient described in FIGURE 16.2A following treatment with clomiphene citrate (MRL-41). Pregnancy occurred during the third cycle of treatment.

for MER-25 and in 1966 reported our results of 10 patients with endometrial abnormalities in Stein–Leventhal syndrome treated with MER-25 and clomiphene citrate (Kistner, Lewis and Steiner, 1966). None of these patients has subsequently developed endometrial cancer and the original therapy occurred between 1957 and 1963.

to two months. The endomyometrium was then subjected to special processing: 10 blocks from the anterior wall, 10 blocks from the posterior wall; six slides were then made from each block.

Residual adenomatous hyperplasia showing progestin effect was noted in only two patients and one demonstrated residual carcinoma in situ with progestin effect.

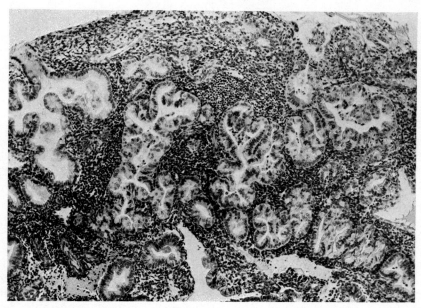

FIGURE 16.3. Curettage specimen obtained from a 55-year-old patient who had noticed hypermenorrhoea for six months. The glands are back-to-back, pale, eosinophilic staining, and show many mitotic figures. This is a typical example of carcinoma in situ. The stroma is compact and contains numerous lymphocytes. Figures 16.3–7 are by courtesy of J. B. Lippincott Co., Philadelphia, publishers of *Cancer* (Kistner, 1959).

The next series of figures illustrate the results of treatment of carcinoma in situ of the endometrium with progestational agents given prior to hysterectomy. Ten patients were selected for this study on the basis of tissue obtained at currettage. Six patients were treated with varying doses of 17α-ethinyl-17-hydroxy-5(10)-oestren-3-one (Enovid) for 24 to 80 days prior to hysterectomy. Two patients were treated by medroxyprogesterone acetate (Depo-Provera). The duration of preoperative therapy varied from three weeks

The residual carcinoma in situ was restricted to the basal layer of the endometrium and, although carcinoma in situ may originate in the basalis, its occurrence in the superficial zone indicates that the same gland may be involved in all endometrial stratas.

Figure 16.3 illustrates the curettings obtained from a 55-year-old patient who had noticed hypermenorrhoea for six months. The glands are back-to-back, pale, eosinophilic staining and show many mitotic figures. It is a typical example of carcinoma

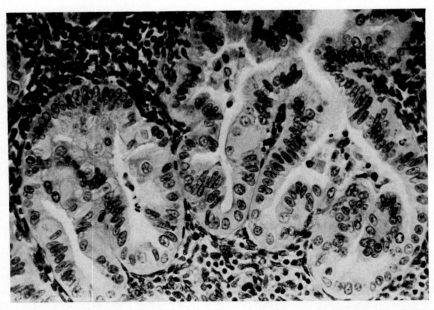

FIGURE 16.4. Higher power magnification of the specimen seen in Figure 16.3 showing the detailed morphology of the glands.

in situ. The stroma is compact and contains numerous lymphocytes. Figure 16.4 shows a higher-power magnification of the lesion shown in Figure 16.3. Note the dyspolarity and vesicular appearance of the nuclei.

Figure 16.5 illustrates the effect on the endometrium after 80 days of Enovid. The compact superficial layer shows well-preserved decidua. Two inactive glands are seen in the spongiosa layer below and to the left of a dilated blood vessel.

Figure 16.6 shows another section from the same uterus showing an extremely thin layer of endometrium with decidual effect. A thinned out basal gland with some evidence of secretion is seen under the surface decidua. An area of adenomyosis is seen amid the myometrial fibres at the lower right.

Figure 16.7 illustrates the progestin effect on the glands of the basalis. The cells lining the dilated glands are of low cuboidal type and there is evidence of intraluminal glycogen. Apparently these glands have proceeded

through the stage of glycogen secretion and are now in 'resting' phase.

The next series of figures illustrate the results of treatment of eight patients with carcinoma in situ and two patients with 'early invasive' carcinoma of the endometrium deemed inoperable because of serious medical disease. One patient, age 35, was treated because of her refusal to permit surgery. The others were postmenopausal, obese, hypertensive and gave past histories of cardiac failure, uncontrolled diabetes, pulmonary and myocardial infarctions and inadequate pulmonary function. The progestins used were 17α-hydroxyprogesterone caproate (Delalutin) and medroxyprogesterone acetate (Depo-Provera). The duration of therapy varied from three to six months and the usual dosage regimen was 1 g of Delalutin weekly or 400 mg of Depo-Provera monthly. Initial heavy leading was utilised in most patients giving 3·5 g of Delalutin and 2 to 3 g of Depo-Provera

during the first week of treatment. Figure
16.8A illustrates the endometrium obtained
at the time of curettage from a 65-year-old
patient. There is extensive cystic and adenomatous hyperplasia with a focus of carcinoma
in situ.

Figure 16.8B shows a higher power view
of the endometrium shown in Figure 16.8A.
Note that the glands are back-to-back and
show numerous mitoses, cytoplasmic pallor
and glandular 'intussusception'.

Figure 16.9 illustrates the curettage specimen obtained after six months of hydroxyprogesterone caproate. Atrophic glands with
focal decidua and chronic endometritis
are noted with no evidence of carcinoma
in situ or adenomatous hyperplasia. This
illustration contains all of the endometrium
recovered at the time of curettage.

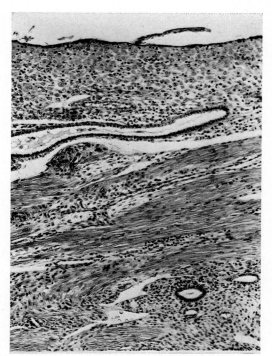

FIGURE 16.6. Section taken from an adjacent area
showing an extremely thin layer of endometrium with
decidual effect. Under the surface decidua is a thinned
out basal gland with some evidence of secretion. An
area of adenomyosis is seen amid the myometrial
fibres at the lower right.

A complete resolution of the abnormal
endometrial process occurred following the
initial therapy in all patients. A recurrence
of hyperplasia, but not carcinoma in situ,
occurred in two patients but in each instance
secondary regression was obtained by retreat-
ment with a progestational agent. The length
of follow-up on this group of patients has
varied from 10 years in one patient, 7 years
in two patients to 3 years in the most recently
treated group. In order to provide adequate
tissue for study we have not relied on
endometrial biopsies, but have admitted the
patients to the hospital for a thorough
curettage on an annual basis. In all individuals the last series of curettages revealed
either no tissue or scraps of senescent glands
and stroma (Kistner, 1970).

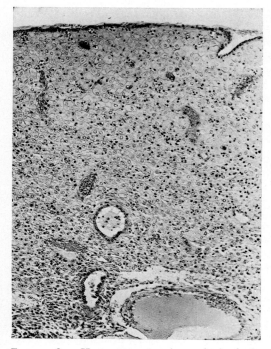

FIGURE 16.5. Hysterectomy specimen obtained after
80 days of continuous Enovid therapy. The compact
layer shows well-preserved decidua. Two inactive
glands are seen in the spongiosa layer below and to the
left of a dilated blood vessel.

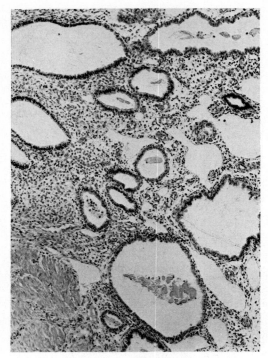

FIGURE 16.7. Section taken from another area to show the effect of Enovid on cystically dilated basal glands. The myometrium is at lower left.

RÉSUMÉ OF THERAPEUTIC REGIMEN

Active therapeutic measures should be instituted without delay in the treatment of the adolescent female whose endometrium shows evidence of hyperplasia, anaplasia or carcinoma in situ. An effort should be made to secure ovulation and cyclic secretory differentiation of the endometrium followed by shedding. It is important to ascertain the precise aetiology of the anovulatory process by a complete diagnostic survey.

Subsequent therapy with cortisone, clomiphene, wedge resection of the ovaries or progestins should be selected based upon the diagnosis. Ovarian wedge resection should be the last, not the first, therapeutic measure employed, particularly, since the ovary characteristic of Stein–Leventhal syndrome seems unusually responsive to clomiphene. If ovulation cannot be established, or if the patient is not desirous of pregnancy, substitutional therapy may be administered in the form of cyclic synthetic progestins. Any one of the oral contraceptives may be utilised for this purpose. Such therapy will produce regular bleeding episodes, diminish the size of the sclerocystic ovary and effect a reversion of the hyperplastic endometrium.

The clinician should realise that the situation is not acute and that immediate hysterectomy is neither necessary nor indicated. This is of particular importance in the young, infertile female. It is imperative, however, that a thorough uterine curettage be performed in all patients prior to therapy in order to exclude the presence of simultaneously occurring invasive carcinoma. Although the progestational agents are able to effect rather striking changes in the morphology of the endometrial glands, they should not be regarded as a panacea and in no way should be construed by the clinician as a substitute for usual medical diagnostic procedures and appropriate therapy.

Since it is impossible for the pathologist to predict the malignant potential of atypical endometrium, it is necessary that the clinician select the optimum method of therapy on the basis of other factors. The presence of specific pathologic processes involving the internal genitalia or the inability to follow the patient adequately are valid indications for hysterectomy. In the young, the infertile, or the very old patient with serious medical disease, a more conservative approach is now possible.

Although the patient most likely to benefit from the therapeutic regimens outlined previously is the young female with the problem of irregular or absent ovulation, it should also be recommended that the hyperplastic process may occur in women approaching the menopause as a result of constant oestrogen stimulation. I have previously reported (Kistner, 1968) the results

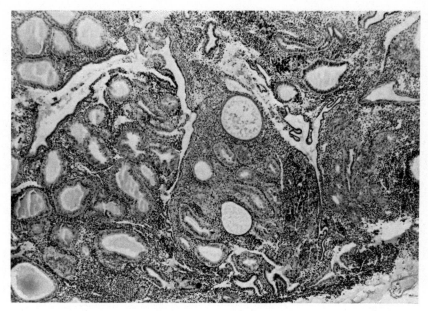

FIGURE 16.8A. Curettage specimen showing cystic and adenomatous hyperplasia and a focus of carcinoma in situ at the left. Figures 16.8–16.9 are by courtesy of Grune and Stratton, publishers of Metabolism (Steiner, Kistner and Craig, 1965).

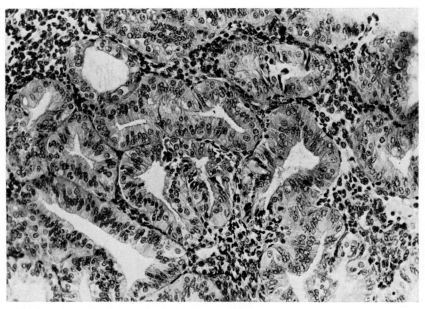

FIGURE 16.8B. Higher power of Figure 16.8A, delineating details of the area of carcinoma in situ. Note back-to-back glands, numerous mitoses, cytoplasmic pallor and dyspolarity of nuclei.

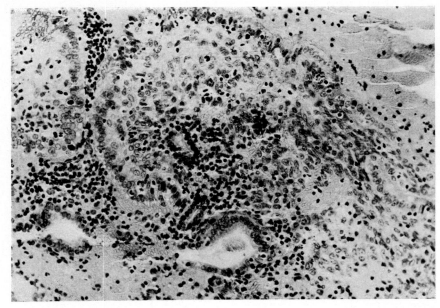

FIGURE 16.9. Curettage specimen obtained after 6 months of hydroxyprogesterone caproate. Atrophic glands with focal decidua and chronic endometritis are noted with no evidence of carcinoma in situ or adenomatous hyperplasia. This illustration contains all of the endometrium recovered at the time of curettage.

of treatment of 35 patients with premenopausal endometrial hyperplasia by the administration of oestrogen-progestin combinations given orally in 21-day cycles for 6 to 12 months. The oral contraceptive agents have been utilised for this purpose. In each patient the hyperplastic process was replaced by an atrophic endometrium.

The following recommendations for treatment of the premenopausal patient with endometrial hyperplasia can be made. After invasive carcinoma has been excluded by uterine curettage, cyclic progestins or oestrogen-progestins may be given for 6 to 12 months or until the patient reaches the menopause. The optimum medications are ones which employ a potent anti-oestrogenic progestin such as norethindrone or norgestrel. In lesions diagnosed as carcinoma in situ of the endometrium, we have employed constant parenteral progestational therapy for a minimum of six months. Hysterectomy may

be performed subsequently depending upon the age of the patient, her medical status, and the histologic response noted at the time of follow-up curettage. The medications used for constant therapy are: Depo-Provera, 100 mg weekly for four weeks, followed by 400 mg monthly for the next five months; Delalutin, 500 mg weekly for four weeks, followed by 1 g weekly for five months.

In the postmenopausal patient hysterectomy is indicated for any degree of endometrial hyperplasia. If the patient is considered inoperable because of medical contraindications, either Depo-Provera or Delalutin should be administered as suggested above, but the length of treatment should be increased to one year.

I have suggested that carcinoma of the endometrium may be a preventable disease if appropriate therapeutic measures are taken to secure ovulation (and secretion of progesterone) in younger women, or if an oestrogen-progestin combination is supplied cyclically to patients approaching the menopause. The potent synthetic progestins in the combined oral contraceptives result eventually in diminished bleeding due to endometrial atrophy. This is true in patients

In the latter patients, however, the constant anti-oestrogenic effect of the progestin was not available.

Table 16.2 summarises the regimens utilised by the author in the management of endometrial hyperplasia and carcinoma in situ.

TABLE 16.2. *Therapeutic regimens employed in the management of endometrial hyperplasia and carcinoma in situ*

Age group	Therapeutic regimen
Postpubescent	Oestrogen-progestin artificial cycles for 6 months; secure ovulation
Childbearing	1. Secure ovulation—cortisone, clomiphene or wedge resection of ovaries or 2. Oestrogen-progestin artificial cycles for 6 to 12 months.
Premenopausal	1. Oestrogen-progestin artificial cycles until age 50–52. 2. Hysterectomy in uncontrolled cases.
Postmenopausal	1. Hysterectomy. 2. If inoperable, constant intramuscular progestins (Depo-provera or Delalutin) for one year.

having normal or hyperplastic endometria at the onset of use. Since most, if not all, cancers of the endometrium in the premenopausal female develop in or from atypical hyperplastic glands, I have stated that, 'it is impossible for endometrial cancer to develop in or from hyperplasia if such hyperplasia is not permitted to develop or is forced into "regression".' Obviously, this statement does not pertain to the redevelopment of hyperplasia after the oestrogen-progestin combination has been discontinued. I have not seen endometrial carcinoma develop in any women during the administration of a combined oral contraceptive since our original report in 1959. However, I have seen two patients who developed early endometrial adenocarcinoma while they were taking sequential oral contraceptives.

CONCLUSION

Prolonged stimulation of the endometrium by endogenous or exogenous oestrogen results in the development of endometrial hyperplasia. Intermittent secretory differentiation of endometrial glands, either by progesterone or synthetic progestins, prevents the development of hyperplasia. Retrospective studies of patients having endometrial cancer suggest a progression of abnormal endometrial glandular patterns from cystic to adenomatous hyperplasia, then to atypical hyperplasia (carcinoma in situ). Hysterectomy specimens indicate that carcinoma in situ and invasive carcinoma of the endometrium frequently occur simultaneously and suggest that carcinoma may arise, in or from, the atypical endometrial glands.

Prospective studies in the human have shown that approximately 10 per cent of patients having atypical endometrial hyperplasia will eventually develop invasive carcinoma if untreated. Although the precise factors which convert pre-malignant to malignant epithelium are unknown, recent studies indicate that the cells in glands which subsequently become malignant demonstrate abnormal DNA distribution and aneuploidy.

Both progesterone and synthetic progestins have been shown to be capable of producing reversion of adenomatous and atypical adenomatous hyperplasia to an atrophic pattern. In women desirous of pregnancy this may be effected by induction of ovulation. During the premenopausal years the administration of synthetic oestrogen-progestin combinations, as found in the combined oral contraceptives, produce reversion of adenomatous hyperplasia. In this age group, atypical adenomatous hyperplasia has been converted into atrophic endometrium by the parenteral administration of synthetic progestins. In the postmenopausal patient, hysterectomy is indicated for any degree of endometrial hyperplasia. However, if the patient is considered to be inoperable, synthetic progestins may be given parenterally but the length of therapy should be for at least one year.

Although the progestational agents are able to produce striking changes in the morphology of the endometrial glands, they should not be regarded as a panacea and in no way should be construed by the clinician as a substitute for usual diagnostic procedures and appropriate therapy.

References

Bäcker, J. (1904) Zwei fälle von carcinoma corporis uteri. *Zentralblatt fur Gynäkologie*, **28**, 735.

Buehl, I. A., Vellios, F., Carter, J. E. & Huber, C. P. (1964) Carcinoma in situ of the endometrium. *American Journal of Clinical Pathology*, **42**, 594.

Gusberg, S. B. & Kaplan, A. L. (1963) Precursors of corpus cancer: IV. Adenomatous hyperplasia as Stage O carcinoma of the endometrium. *American Journal of Obstetrics and Gynecology*, **87**, 662.

Hertig, A. T. & Sommers, S. C. (1949) Genesis of endometrial carcinoma: 1. Study of prior biopsies. *Cancer*, **2**, 946.

Kaufman, R. H., Abbott, W. P. & Wall, J. A. (1959). The endometrium before and after wedge resection of the ovaries for Stein–Leventhal syndrome. *American Journal of Obstetrics and Gynecology*, **77**, 1271.

Kelley, R. M. & Baker, W. H. (1960) Effects of 17-alpha-hydroxyprogesterone caproate on metastatic endometrial cancer. Conference on Experimental Clinical Cancer Chemotherapy. Monograph 9, p. 235. Bethesda, Md: National Cancer Institute.

Kistner, R. W. (1959) Histological effects of progestins on hyperplasia and carcinoma in situ of the endometrium. *Cancer*, **12**, 1106.

Kistner, R. W. (1962) Premalignant lesions of the female genital tract and breast. Treatment of carcinoma in situ of the endometrium. *Clinical Obstetrics and Gynecology*, **5**, 1166.

Kistner, R. W. (1965a) Further observations on the use of clomiphene citrate for the induction of ovulation. *American Journal of Obstetrics and Gynecology*, **92**, 380.

Kistner, R. W. (1965b) Induction of ovulation with clomiphene citrate—a review. *Obstetrical and Gynecological Survey*, **20** (6), 873.

Kistner, R. W. (1968) Further observations on the effects of progestational agents on hyperplasia and carcinoma in situ of the endometrium. *Clinical Trials Journal*, Special Issue, **5**, 57.

Kistner, R. W. (1970) The effects of progestational agents on hyperplasia and carcinoma in situ of the endometrium. *International Journal of Obstetrics and Gynaecology*, (Part 2) **8**, 561.

Kistner, R. W., Duncan, C. J. & Mansell, H. (1956) Suppression of ovulation by Tri-p-anisyl chloroethylene (TACE). *Obstetrics and Gynecology*, **8**, 399.

Kistner, R. W., Lewis, J. L. & Steiner, C. J. (1966) Effects of clomiphene citrate on endometrial hyperplasia in the premenopausal female. *Cancer*, **19**, 115.

Kistner, R. W. & Smith, O. W. (1959) Observations on the use of a non-steroidal estrogen antagonist: MER-25. *Surgical Forum*, **10**, 725.

Larson, J. A. (1954) Estrogens and endometrial carcinoma. *Obstetrics and Gynecology*, **3**, 551.

Novak, E. & Yui, E. (1936) Relation of endometrial hyperplasia to adenocarcinoma of uterus. *American Journal of Obstetrics and Gynecology*, **32,** 674.

Sommers, S. C., Hertig, A. T. & Bengaloff, H. (1949) Genesis of endometrial carcinoma: II. Cases 19–35 years old. *Cancer*, **2,** 957.

Steiner, G. J., Kistner, R. W. & Craig, J. M. (1965) Histological effects of progestins on hyperplasia and carcinoma in situ of the endometrium. Further observations. *Metabolism*, **14** (2), 356.

Taylor, H. C., Jr (1932) Endometrial hyperplasia and carcinoma of body of uterus. *American Journal of Obstetrics and Gynecology*, **23,** 309.

Wellenbach, B. L. & Rakoff, A. E. (1953) Hyperplasia of the endometrium. *Journal of the Albert Einstein Medical Center*, **2,** 3.

Wagner, D., Richart, R. M. & Terner, J. Y. (1967) Deoxyribonucleic acid content of presumed precursors of endometrial carcinoma. *Cancer*, **20,** 2067.

Younge, P. A. (1957) Cancer of the uterine cervix, a preventable disease. *Obstetrics and Gynecology*, **10,** 469.

Chapter 17

Endometrial and Cervical Cancer

ROBERT W. KISTNER

Carcinoma of the endometrium, when confined to the uterus, responds well to standard surgical and radiation therapy, with 60 to 70 per cent five-year cure rates having been reported in Stage 1. However, many patients when first seen, have extensive disease beyond local control, or widespread distant metastases with the lung the most common site of such dissemination.

Endocrine Therapy in Advanced Endometrial Cancer

Following the success reported for hormonal therapy in the treatment of cancer of the breast and prostate, similar approaches have been applied to endometrial cancer. Although the precise aetiology of endometrial cancer is unknown, considerable evidence from clinical, endocrinologic and pathologic studies has accumulated which indicates that this lesion develops in certain patients as a result of long-continued oestrogen stimulation in the absence of the cyclic action of progesterone.

An attempt to modify the course of disseminated or inoperable uterine cancer was, therefore, a logical sequel to the demonstration that the growth of certain malignant tumours arising in organs under endocrine control could be altered by hormonal manipulation of the host. It is well recognised that endometrial carcinoma is frequently a well-differentiated tumour retaining marked histological similarity to the parent tissue. In postmenopausal women such tumours

323

may even show evidence of secretory activity with foci of squamous metaplasia, suggesting an atypical response to a progesterone-like substance. In premenopausal patients, secretory activity in the carcinoma may actually resemble that noted in the adjacent normal endometrial tissue. The profound effect of progesterone on the maturation of normal endometrium, and the apparent sensitivity of this tissue and its well differentiated neoplastic counterpart to hormonal stimuli, suggested a therapeutic trial of progestational agents in disseminated endometrial cancer.

CHOICE OF PROGESTATIONAL AGENT

17α-HYDROXYPROGESTERONE CAPROATE

In 1960, Kelley and Baker reported objective signs of remission of metastatic endometrial carcinoma in 7 of 22 patients following treatment with this progestational agent. Factors favouring a good response include a long hiatus between the original treatment and the appearance of cancer recurrence, well-differentiated adenocarcinoma or adenoacanthoma histologically, and the presence of pulmonary metastases. In favourable cases, pulmonary metastases were noted to regress within two months of the initiation of therapy and to disappear within four to six months. Kelley and Baker have reported such lesions to remain in abeyance for as long as four-and-a-half years.

Pelvic recurrences were much less impressive in their response, although a diminution in size of the tumour masses for periods of months have been described. Kelley and Baker (1960) have also described regression of extensive hepatic metastases causing obstructive jaundice, with marked clinical and biochemical improvement and, in a few patients, osteolytic lesions have been observed to calcify. Symptomatic relief of pain and debility has occasionally been striking and sustained even in the absence of demonstrable tumour regression.

The results of 50 investigators who treated 165 patients having disseminated endometrial cancer with 17α-hydroxyprogesterone caproate were reported by Kelley and Baker in 1970. Response rates for different sites of metastases were: local 28 per cent; pulmonary 37 per cent; abdominal 20 per cent; osseous and pulmonary 50 per cent. Summation of all patients with adenocarcinoma of the endometrium with metastases treated with 17α-hydroxyprogesterone caproate has shown an objective remission in 85 of 247 patients (34·4 per cent) (Reifenstein, 1968).

Kennedy (1963) reported on 27 patients treated for advanced endometrial carcinoma with 17α-hydroxyprogesterone caproate, and noted objective improvement in 8 patients. A comparison of the patients in the responding group with those in the non-responding (refractory) group showed an apparent biologic difference in the cancer with respect to the natural pattern of growth. The disease in the responders was of long duration and slow growth, whereas the disease in the non-responders appeared to be of short duration and exhibited rapid growth. Varga and Henriksen (1961) reported their observations on the clinical and histopathologic effects of this progestational agent in endometrial carcinoma and noted results similar to those quoted above.

DIMETHISTERONE

Wentz (1964) reported 10 patients with primary endometrial cancer treated by oral and intracavitary administration of dimethisterone. Subsequent curettage, preceding radium therapy or hysterectomy, showed no evidence of residual carcinoma in 7 patients. The remaining 3 patients were treated solely with dimethisterone, and at subsequent hysterectomy the uteri were found free of cancer in each case. Wentz also described objective as well as subjective response in 6 patients with advanced endometrial carcinoma and distant metastases.

Fluid accumulation diminished greatly in 2 of these patients with ascites.

Hayakawa (1969) has recently reported the histological effects of dimethisterone on adenocarcinoma of the endometrium as examined by electron microscopy. Specimens were examined from 7 patients both before and after treatment to determine cellular response to this progestin and for comparison, 10 cases of normal luteal phase endometrium were examined.

Prominent ultrastructural changes were noted in well-differentiated areas. These changes were: an increased number of organelles, large aggregations of glycogen particles in the subapical area, and the occasional coexistence of lipid droplets; an increase in endoplasmic reticulum and lysosomal elements including large autophagic vacuoles. These changes resembled those observed in the normal, non-malignant endometrial glandular cells obtained during the luteal phase and, to a certain extent, seemed to represent a retrogressive process.

MEDROXYPROGESTERONE

Anderson (1965) has reported on 20 patients with metastatic carcinoma treated by oral medroxyprogesterone acetate. Eight of the 20 patients responded to the progestin with complete or partial tumour regression and a marked reduction in symptoms. Serial biopsies of the neoplasm in 4 patients demonstrated the following histologic changes which were interpreted as being the result of the progestational agent: increased amounts of cytoplasm, often becoming more granular and eosinophilic, with a marked reduction in mitotic figures. Anderson also noted a decrease in the degree of secondary infection and necrosis of the lesions, a diminution in vaginal discharge or bleeding and a reduction in regional induration and thickening. Nine of the 12 patients who failed to respond to the administration of medroxyprogesterone acetate had undifferentiated or poorly differentiated neoplasms, while 7 of the 8

patients with remissions had well-differentiated lesions. The longest remission noted in this series was 42 months.

Kistner, Griffiths and Craig (1965) reported 3 complete remissions and 2 partial remissions in 6 patients treated with medroxyprogesterone acetate. The 3 patients with complete tumour regression are still alive and well at the time of writing, without evidence of carcinoma for periods of 91, 82 and 66 months respectively. Kistner and Griffiths (1968), in a study of dose-response relationships, emphasised the importance of the loading dose in producing a remission. Of those patients who responded, all received a minimum of 2 g medroxyprogesterone acetate within the first eight weeks of therapy.

Bonte (1969) treated 65 patients with disseminated or recurrent endometrial carcinoma by the administration of medroxyprogesterone acetate, either by intramuscular injection or orally. He utilised an average dose of 1 g per week, considerably higher than that used by American investigators. Bonte noted complete, or almost complete, regression in 35 of the 65 patients treated by means of medroxyprogesterone therapy alone, regression persisting up to five years in some cases.

ETHYNODIOL DIACETATE

Cox and Kirkland (1964) have reported the effect of ethynodiol diacetate in 3 patients with recurrent endometrial carcinoma and noted regression of the tumour in each patient. They also administered ethynodiol diacetate to 6 patients prior to hysterectomy instead of intracavitary cobalt-60. In very high dosage, parenteral administration of this compound produced secretory changes in the carcinoma. In 1 patient, a repeat curettage after administration of ethynodiol diacetate failed to reveal residual carcinoma.

Truscott (1964) described his observations on the treatment of endometrial carcinoma by the intracavitary instillation of ethynodiol diacetate. Using the method described by

Kistner et al (1962), Truscott injected 3 ml (300 mg) of ethynodiol diacetate into the uterine cavity of 2 patients with endometrial carcinoma. Daily injections of 10 mg were then given subsequently into the cavity of the uterus for one week and hysterectomy was then performed. The appearance of the endometrial cavity at the time of hysterectomy was described as being ulcerated with a surface necrotic exudate. The microscopic report revealed that the cavity was haemorrhagic and necrotic but no residual carcinoma was present. Kistner et al (1965) described a similar morphologic pattern following the intracavitary administration of medroxyprogesterone acetate.

MECHANISM OF DRUG ACTION

The mechanism of action of progestational agents in effecting remissions in patients with endometrial carcinoma has not been precisely defined. There is evidence to favour a local effect as shown by the marked changes noted after the direct instillation of these agents into the endometrial cavity. Although an effect on the tumour cells via the pituitary has been suggested, conflicting data have been reported on the effect of progestin administration on gonadotropin excretion.

EFFECT VIA PITUITARY GLAND

The variation in results reported may represent differences in techniques of measuring gonadotropin. Whereas Sherman and Woolf (1959) reported that luteinising hormone (LH) levels in urine were elevated in all of 31 patients with primary endometrial carcinoma, Varga and Henriksen (1963) reported that only 5 of 18 patients had elevated levels. Sherman and Woolf (1959) also reported that elevated LH levels were suppressed to normal range by administration of 17α-hydroxyprogesterone caproate in each of 4 patients with primary endometrial carcinoma. On the other hand, of the 5

patients with elevated LH levels reported by Varga and Henriksen (1963) only 2 were suppressed to normal range and 2 remained elevated; valid determinations could not be made in the fifth patient.

From several studies of patients with metastatic disease, there is no evidence that the administration of 17α-hydroxyprogesterone caproate produced significant change in blood chemistry, or in the excretion of oestrogens, androgens or adrenal corticoids. It appears that there are no specific contraindications to the use of progestational agents in patients having disseminated endometrial carcinoma, but further studies of calcium metabolism and gonadotropin excretion seem indicated.

LOCAL EFFECT OF PROGESTATIONAL AGENTS

Evidence favouring the local effect of progestational agents on endometrial cancer is available from two groups of clinical observations. We have observed metastatic lesions in the vagina to diminish markedly in size and eventually disappear, subsequent to the direct injection of progestational agents into tumour masses. Sequential biopsy of the lesions has shown a preliminary secretory effect followed by glandular atrophy and replacement of the glands and stroma by fibrous connective tissue. We have also studied the effect of several progestational agents (Depo-Provera, Delalutin and ethynodiol diacetate) on normal, hyperplastic and malignant endometria by direct injection of the agent into the cavity of the uterus (Plates 17.1–4, following p. 240). In the majority of patients, subsequent endometrial biopsies and curettage have shown both a secretory effect in normally proliferative and hyperplastic endometrium and also marked necrobiosis of the endometrial cancer. In several patients so treated, viable tumour was not identified in the hysterectomy specimen subsequent to repeated administration of these agents into the cavity of the uterus.

Added support for a local effect of progesterone on the tumour cell has been furnished by the report of Nordqvist (1969). In this experiment, specimens from 11 uterine adenocarcinomas, obtained by curettage, were grown in organ culture. One culture from each specimen served as a control, and to other cultures oestrone, progesterone (at a concentration of either 8 or 80 µg/ml) or androsterone were added. After one week, there was excellent survival of all control cultures, but there was advanced or total necrosis in 9 of 11 tumours treated with the stronger solution of progesterone. Androsterone was less effective: there was excellent survival in 5 of 11 tumours. The cultures treated with oestrogen or weak progesterone solution demonstrated only slightly altered survival.

Bonte (1969) agrees that the mechanism of action of medroxyprogesterone acetate on uterine adenocarcinoma is likely to include a direct effect on the cancer tissue, provoking differentiation, maturation, epithelial metaplasia, atrophy and finally disappearance of neoplastic structures. Repeated endometrial biopsies during treatment have demonstrated that anaplastic adenocarcinoma assumed a more glandular appearance, papillary lesions developed endopapillary acinus formation, and well-differentiated adenocarcinoma was transformed into adenoacanthoma.

Bonte (1969) reproduced the same histological transformations by adding medroxyprogesterone acetate to organ cultures of these different types of uterine adenocarcinoma. He was able to induce dedifferentiation by adding oestrogen to the culture medium, and to neutralise this oestrogenic effect by simultaneously adding medroxyprogesterone acetate. As a clinical corollary of this observation, Bonte noted complete regression of uterine adenocarcinoma only in postmenopausal patients whose oestrogenic vaginal smear became atrophic subsequent to medroxyprogesterone acetate therapy.

Nordqvist (1969) has described a method for short-term incubation in vitro of malignant endometrial tissue for the study of nucleic acid synthesis. Different carcinomas showed a marked variation in the synthesis of both DNA and RNA. A specific effect of progesterone, leading to a reduction of the synthesis of both nucleic acids, was obtained when this hormone was added to the incubation medium in a concentration of 40 to 80 µg/ml. In 13 women treated with progestogens, comparisons were made of the nucleic acid synthesis in curettage specimens before and after the treatment. The relative response in DNA and RNA synthesis to progesterone in vitro, and to progestogens in vivo was significantly correlated. In approximately two-thirds of the cases, a correlation was also possibly present in the quantitative response in nucleic acid synthesis in vitro and in vivo.

In all systems used, a hormonal response was recorded in approximately 70 per cent of the carcinomas studied. Thus, Nordqvist (1969) presents strong evidence in support of the view that the action of progesterone and progestogens on endometrial carcinomas is directly on the cancer cells and their nucleic acid synthesis. Although not yet suitable for routine clinical use, the short-term incubation procedure devised by Nordqvist is a promising tool as an objective and quantitative method for prediction of the hormonal responsiveness in vivo of individual endometrial carcinomas.

Normal human endometrial cells have a propensity for binding oestrogen. A specific receptor molecule is found in the cytoplasm and another receptor protein exists in the nucleus. Oestrogen is transferred from the cytoplasmic receptor to the nuclear receptor before specific stimulation of the endometrial cell occurs. Brush, Taylor and King (1967a, b) showed that human endometrium takes up administered oestrogen during both the proliferative and secretory phases of the menstrual cycle, but during the latter phase, the proportion of oestrogen which gains access to the nucleus is diminished. This is an important effect of endogenous progesterone, and may be reproduced by the administration of synthetic progestins.

Taylor et al (1971) studied the binding of intravenous oestrogen by the cells of various gynaecologic cancers. Squamous carcinoma of the vagina, adenocarcinoma of the cervix and endometrium all bound oestrogen avidly and transferred a significant proportion to the nuclear fraction. The degree of differentiation of the endometrial carcinoma did not affect the uptake of administered oestrogen

DOSE-RESPONSE RELATIONSHIPS

In the treatment of metastatic endometrial carcinomas, the optimum dosage of 17α-hydroxyprogesterone caproate seems to be in the range of 3–5 g intramuscularly per week. Patients with either well-differentiated lesions or a long hiatus between original treatment and the discovery of the metastases, will respond to lower doses, whereas maximum amounts should be given to other patients.

TABLE 17.1. *Dose-response intervals. The relationship of loading dose of medroxyprogesterone acetate to time before response*

Patient	Grams/week before response	Weeks before response	Total dose before response in grams
N.C.	1·65	4	6·6
G.R.	0·6	5	3·0
L.C.	0·6	6	3·6
E.P.	0·35	7	2·4
V.D.	0·2	13	2·5
A.N.	0·2	15	2·7
J.O.	0·1	36	3·6

nor its intracellular distribution. Furthermore, preoperative radiotherapy did not affect the ability of the malignant cell to take up oestrogen nor to permit its nuclear binding.

These investigators reported that the proportion of radioactivity within the nuclear fraction of the cells, in 18 patients with well-differentiated adenocarcinoma of the endometrium, was markedly increased after administration of 100 mg medroxyprogesterone daily, but decreased after 100 mg norgestrel daily. In spite of the ability of the cancer cells to bind oestradiol to the cell nucleus, clinical regression of the tumour was noted in two of the patients. This suggests that progestational agents may not exert a simple anti-oestrogenic effect, but are effective in endometrial cancer by altering intracellular metabolism or by depressing other potentially tumour-stimulating compounds.

Kistner and Griffiths (1968), in studying dose-response relationships, emphasised the importance of a 'loading-dose' in producing a remission. Table 17.1 illustrates the correlation between dosage in grams per week, total dosage and the number of weeks to obtain an objective remission using medroxyprogesterone acetate. The table indicates details of therapy of the first seven responders. It is apparent that a dose of 0·1 g/week necessitated 36 weeks to obtain a response, whereas this interval was halved if the dose was doubled. Two patients responded in five to six weeks when the dose was 0·6 g/week and one patient responded in four weeks when the weekly dose was increased to 1·65 g/week. No response occurred in patients who received less than 2·4 g of the progestin.

After these early observations, Kistner and Griffiths suggested that a minimal 'loading-dose' of 3·5 g of medroxyprogesterone acetate be given during the first three weeks of therapy. Using the 400 mg/ml preparation, several regimens may be utilised, for example:

400 mg 3 times weekly for 3 weeks (3·6 g)
or   400 mg daily   for 5 days ⎫
then 400 mg twice weekly for 2 weeks⎭ 3·6 g

Recently I have increased the dose as follows:

400 mg daily   for 7 days ⎫
then 400 mg 3 times weekly for 2 weeks⎭ 5·2 g

Therapy should be administered for at least 12 weeks before regarding treatment as having failed. If tumour regression is obtained, dosage is maintained at a level of 400–1000 mg monthly. If a remission of objective type is obtained with one of the progestational agents, it should be continued *indefinitely* and not diminished in dosage or discontinued.

In most reported series, 30 to 35 per cent of patients treated with progestational agents have shown objective diminution in or disappearance of measurable lesions, with a considerably higher subjective response rate. Even patients not showing measurable tumour regression may enjoy sustained periods of subjective relief of pain and debility, and there is often failure of lesions to advance. The type of patients demonstrating the most favourable objective response are those with a histologic pattern of well-differentiated adenocarcinoma or adenoacanthoma, with a long free interval between the treatment of the primary tumour and its first metastasis. This observation suggests the presence of a heightened host resistance.

Pulmonary metastases have been found to be the most responsive, but osseous, hepatic, intra-abdominal and pelvic metastases have also shown regression, particularly if they have not been subjected to prior radiotherapy. Evidence of objective regression is usually detectable within 8 to 12 weeks of initiation of therapy and such regressions are usually maintained for 12 to 18 months. One of the striking features of this mode of therapy is the occasional very prolonged remission observed in patients with pulmonary lesions as the main site of recurrence. Several of these patients have remissions in the range of 2 to 8 years, and are still living and well without evidence of disease.

PROLONGATION OF SURVIVAL IN RESPONDING CASES

Kelley and Baker (1970) reported a personal series of 58 unselected patients, treating all cases referred with metastatic endometrial carcinoma by means of 17α-hydroxyprogesterone caproate. They observed tumour regression in 18 patients, a remission rate of 32 per cent. Of the 18 patients who responded, 11 died an average of 31·3 months after initiation of therapy, the range being from 7 to 165 months. Seven patients were still alive an average of 55 months, the range being from 19 to 93 months. The nonresponders, on the other hand, averaged only 5 months survival after initiation of therapy, with a range of 3 to 21 months.

Reifenstein (1971) reviewed 314 women with advanced progressing adenocarcinoma of the uterine corpus no longer responding to established anticancer measures. Hydroxyprogesterone caproate (1·0 or more g/week intramuscularly for 4 or more weeks) induced an objective response (averaging 20 months in duration) consisting of regression in 30·2 per cent or arrest of the disease in 6·8 per cent. These responders survived an average of 27 months, four times as long as the nonresponders. The incidence of responders was significantly greater in patients with slowly growing tumours and in those treated for 12 or more weeks. Neither the objective response rate nor the duration of survival was influenced significantly by the age of the patient, the amount of hydroxyprogesterone per week, the site of neoplastic recurrence or metastasis, the type of previous cancer therapy, or presence of concomitant established anticancer therapy. Hydroxyprogesterone caproate (up to 7·0 g/week) was safe and well tolerated. Undesirable manifestations occurred infrequently.

It would thus appear from these reports that survival is prolonged in those patients who show an objective remission to progestational agents. Another possible explanation is that response to therapy is more likely to occur in slowly growing types of tumour, as has been suggested also for breast cancer.

'PROPHYLACTIC' POSTOPERATIVE THERAPY IN ENDOMETRIAL CANCER

On the basis of the morphologic changes effected by progestins on endometrial carcinoma, and the objective remissions observed in metastatic lesions, we have elected to treat certain patients with progestins subsequent to hysterectomy. Unfortunately, the number of patients treated to date has been small and definitive conclusions regarding the degree of 'prophylaxis' provided cannot be made.

If the extirpated specimen showed extension of carcinoma beyond the outer third of the myometrium, or if the disease process involved the tubes, ovaries or adjacent structures, we have administered a total of 2·5 to 3 g of medroxyprogesterone acetate during the first three weeks postoperatively. This is given as adjunctive therapy to radiation. Although continuation of the progestin beyond this three-week period has been suggested, no objective end-point is available to guide the length of therapy. However, in certain patients, we have given a maintenance dose of 1 g per month during the first year following surgery.

TREATMENT OF REACTIVATION AFTER HORMONAL THERAPY

Reactivation of metastatic endometrial carcinoma during the administration of progestational agents has been noted to occur sooner if the original treatment dose was low. In such cases treatment should be continued with the same progestational agent but instituting the loading dose described earlier in this chapter. In a few patients the substitution of hydroxyprogesterone caproate for medroxyprogesterone acetate may prove beneficial, while those patients who develop recurrence while on hydroxyprogesterone caproate therapy should be given large doses of medroxyprogesterone acetate, ethynodiol diacetate or dimethisterone.

The Mayo Clinic has reported a favourable response in 8 out of 21 patients with advanced disease who received 5-fluorouracil, and this cytotoxic agent can be tried in cases of recurrent disease not responding to progestational therapy. Response in endometrial cancer has not been obtained from treatment by chlorambucil but about 20 per cent of patients treated with cyclophosphamide were reported to demonstrate remission. The administration of such alkylating agents *in combination* with progestational agents may secure remission in tumours showing resistance to progestin therapy alone.

The vinca alkaloids have been tried in the treatment of endometrial carcinoma but, in a small series, neither vincristine nor vinblastine have been reported as having achieved remissions. Mitomycin C is reported to have induced an objective remission in one patient with this disease. Combinations of chemotherapeutic agents such as those utilised in the treatment of choriocarcinoma or malignant teratoma seem to have little advantage over single agents in the treatment of endometrial cancer.

It is interesting to note that we have observed objective response subsequent to the administration of large doses of oestrogen in two patients who showed reactivation of endometrial cancer while receiving progestational agents. Although this hormonal agent would seem to be poorly chosen for the treatment of this disease, there is no doubt about the objective nature of the response observed in these cases. The mechanism of action of oestrogen in these patients is unknown.

SEQUENTIAL MANAGEMENT IN ADVANCED ENDOMETRIAL CANCER

The basic treatment of carcinoma of the endometrium is surgical, but various combinations of external irradiation and radium are used as adjunctive measures by most gynaecologists. Several clinics, however, have continued to utilise surgery alone whenever this is possible, and report five-year cure rates from 47 to 66 per cent. If a particular clinic is fortunate enough to have most of their patients in Stage I or Stage II the cure rate by surgery alone should approach 60 to 70 per cent.

With newer techniques of radium and external irradiation followed by hysterectomy and bilateral salpingo-oophorectomy, five-year salvage rates from 75 to 94 per cent have been reported. It is important to realise that, because of the commonly complicating factors of obesity, hypertension, diabetes and heart disease, death due to causes unrelated to the malignancy will occur in about 15 to 20 per cent of patients in any series.

During the years 1955 through 1960 at the Boston Hospital for Women nine different treatment methods were utilised in the management of patients with endometrial carcinoma. It is difficult to standardise treatment in a disease of this type, but if the diagnosis is made at the time of curettage, our generally accepted plan has been to insert intracavitary radium at this time, and to carry out a total hysterectomy and bilateral salpingo-oophorectomy approximately three weeks later. During this interval the patient receives from 3 to 5 g of Depo-Provera, as described later.

Beginning in 1945 a so-called 'modified' radical hysterectomy was introduced. This consists of removal of the external iliac, hypogastric, obturator and periureteral lymph nodes together with the adjacent areolar tissue. If the excised lymph nodes contain tumour or if there is extension of tumour to the oviduct, ovaries, outer portion of the myometrium or uterine area, postoperative external irradiation is administered.

There has been an effort to treat endometrial carcinoma by a radical surgical approach in a similar manner to that in which cervical cancer is treated. Unfortunately, endometrial cancer occurs during the later decades when obesity and cardiorenal disease are common and these factors reduce the total number which can be treated by such radical surgery. Furthermore, several studies have indicated that the operative and postoperative mortality rates are higher, so that at the Boston Hospital for Women, radical hysterectomy and pelvic lymphadenectomy is not utilised in the treatment of endometrial cancer unless the cervix is involved.

It has been suggested that if the uterus is small and the contained tumour minute, intracavitary radium need not be administered. However, it is impossible to judge the full extent of the tumour by curettage and it is further believed that irradiation decreases the size of the tumour, reduces vascularity and probably devitalises a proportion of cells. Thus there is less risk of spreading viable tumour cells during operation. Previous studies have indicated that residual carcinoma is found in approximately 50 per cent of uteri at hysterectomy after at least 3600 mg/h of radium, but with the use of Heyman capsules the incidence of tumour in removed uteri has been reduced to approximately 25 per cent.

A further reduction in the incidence of residual tumour may be obtained by the adjunctive use of progestational steroids in addition to radium. For the last 10 years it has been my policy to administer medroxyprogesterone acetate intramuscularly for three weeks prior to surgery, beginning at the time radium is inserted. The following regimen is used: 400 mg intramuscularly daily for seven days (2800 mg); then 400 mg three times weekly for two weeks (2400 mg) (see Plates 17.5–8, following p. 240). Progestational steroids may be used also after surgery if the excised specimen shows viable tumour beyond the inner third of the myometrium. Medroxyprogesterone acetate is given along with external radiation therapy in the following regimen: 400 mg daily for seven days; then 400 mg three times weekly as long as radiation therapy is given.

When surgery is contraindicated, the patient is usually given two applications of intracavitary radium followed by full external irradiation. Since 1960 I have treated patients in the inoperable group also by adding medroxyprogesterone acetate to the radiation plan. There is evidence, although not as yet conclusive, that the progestin may increase sensitivity of the tumour cell to radiation. The progestin is given in the following regimen: 400 mg intramuscularly for seven days beginning at the time of the first radium insertion; then 400 mg is given three times weekly during the next two weeks, giving a total 'loading dose' of 5200 mg during the first three weeks. During the period of external irradiation, progestin is continued at a dose of 400 mg weekly. If a repeat curettage fails to reveal viable tumour, progestin therapy is discontinued. However, if tumour remains or if there is evidence of distant metastases, the progestin is continued indefinitely at a dose of 400 mg monthly.

If radium and external irradiation are used without surgery, it is essential to perform a thorough curettage about 6 months following the first treatment to determine the presence of persistent disease. If disease is present, the patient may have become operable either by reduction in the size of the pelvic tumour or by an improvement in her general condition.

RESULTS OF THERAPY

Austin and MacMahon (1969) reviewed all cases of carcinoma of the endometrium admitted to the Boston Hospital for Women between 1920 and 1959. Cases of in situ carcinoma were not included. During this interval 941 patients were classified as having invasive carcinoma but 180 were excluded because of prior treatment, lack of histological confirmation, mixed tumours, and lack of follow-up. A total of 761 patients were then available for analysis. For the series as a whole, the crude five-year survival rate was 67·3 per cent, and the relative survival rate was 75·1 per cent. Among patients in Stage I, the assignment of nuclear grade appeared to have considerable prognostic value since the survival was 93·3 per cent in Grade I tumours but only 39·8 per cent in Grade IV. This differential was maintained in patients not classified in Stage I.

The crude cumulative survival rate for the 761 patients diminished from 67·3 per cent at five years to 36·5 per cent at 20 years, but the *relative* cumulative survival rate dropped only from 76·5 per cent at five years to 70·8 per cent at 20 years.

During the interval 1960–1968, 61 patients with varying stages of endometrial carcinoma were treated with progestational agents at the Boston Hospital for Women. These patients were divided into four groups:

Group I includes patients with apparently localised disease. They received the progestin either intramuscularly combined with intracavitary radium or by instillation of the progestin into the uterine cavity prior to hysterectomy.

Group II includes patients whose uterus showed extension of tumour beyond the outer third of the myometrium. Medroxyprogesterone acetate (Depo-Provera) plus external radiation therapy was administered to these patients after surgery.

Group III patients had evidence of extrapelvic tumour, usually pulmonary. In these patients treatment consisted of intramuscular medroxyprogesterone, hydroxyprogesterone caproate or ethynodiol diacetate. Neither surgery nor radiation was utilised.

Group IV includes patients whose disease appeared confined to the pelvis but in whom surgery was contraindicated because of medical disease. In these patients therapy consisted of intracavitary radium, external cobalt or super-voltage radiation and progestin therapy.

RESULTS OF PROGESTIN THERAPY

Group I. Fifteen patients were treated with intramuscular medroxyprogesterone acetate prior to surgery. In 10 of these, intracavitary radium was also administered. Residual carcinoma was present in only one patient, who had cervical involvement necessitating radical hysterectomy and pelvic lymph-adenectomy. Although all nodes were negative and the lines of surgical excision were free of tumour, the patient died of disseminated metastases seven months after surgery. Nine patients are living and well without evidence of disease.

Five patients received intracavitary medroxyprogesterone acetate without radium prior to surgery, the length of preoperative therapy varying from one to three weeks. Residual carcinoma was present in one uterus. Four patients are living and well without evidence of disease—all over five years post surgery. No vaginal metastases occurred in this group. One patient died of pulmonary and cerebral metastases 39 months postoperatively.

Group II. Twenty-two patients, showing extension of carcinoma beyond the outer third of the myometrium were treated with postoperative external radiation plus medroxyprogesterone acetate. Five-year follow-up is available on only eight patients—five are living and well without evidence of disease, two are dead of disease and one is living with disease.

Group III. Eighteen patients with extra-pelvic dissemination of carcinoma were treated by various progestational agents. Most of these patients had already received standard surgical and radiation therapy for their disease. An objective response (a reduction in tumour volume by 50 per cent for three months or longer) occurred in seven patients, a response rate of 38 per cent. The survival time for responders varied from 9 to 91 months. Two patients are living and well without evidence of disease at 91 and 82 months respectively.

Group IV. Six patients with tumour apparently localised to the pelvis, but inoperable because of medical contraindications, received intracavitary radium and external cobalt or supervoltage radiation. In addition, medroxyprogesterone acetate was given during the course of radiation therapy and was continued if post-therapy curettage demonstrated active tumour. Four patients are living without evidence of disease but no five-year survivals are available as yet. One patient died of intercurrent disease and one died of widespread metastases within 30 days of the conclusion of therapy.

Hormones and Cancer of the Cervix

Statistically valid evidence does not exist to implicate hormonal abnormalities as aetiologic factors in cancer of the uterine cervix in the human female. Furthermore, favourable response to hormonal regimens has not been proven in women having this disease.

Cervical carcinoma is probably caused by a viral agent transmitted by coitus and contained in the smegma or seminal fluid. However, since this tumour develops during the childbearing period (the average age being 47 years at the Boston Hospital for Women), it is impossible to exclude the role of oestrogen and progesterone in providing a milieu suitable for tumour growth. Carcinoma of the cervix has been reported to occur in the surgical castrate but most of these patients had received exogenous oestrogen subsequent to oophorectomy.

RELATION TO OESTROGEN

Experimentally, Taki and Iijima (1963) induced cervical cancer in spayed mice by a chemical carcinogen, methylcholanthrene, but noted that carcinogenesis was accelerated by the addition of oestradiol. Progesterone and testosterone, given at a level which inhibits the biological effect of oestrogen, markedly suppressed carcinogenesis in such cases. The technique used by these investigators was similar to that reported by Kistner et al (1962) for the induction of endometrial cancer in the rabbit. The results reported by Taki and Iijima (1963) are also similar to those reported by us in the rabbit.

The epithelial changes of cervix and corpus cancer which have been induced by methylcholanthrene are, for a limited time, strongly influenced also by oestradiol given *after removal* of carcinogen application. The advance of atypical changes is enhanced resulting in an increased incidence of invasive carcinoma both in cervix and corpus uteri. *On the other hand, castration and administration of progesterone suppress this increased cancer incidence.*

The results of these experiments suggest that the progression of in situ cervical carcinoma into invasive cancer depends upon specific hormonal influences, and may be reversible under certain conditions. The results also suggest the possibility that the anti-oestrogenic progestins in oral contraceptives might act as an anticancer agent in cervical neoplasia, much as they do in endometrial carcinoma.

Ebner and Sandritter (1968) applied a chemical carcinogen to the cervical canal of 75 mice but simultaneously treated half of these animals with a norprogestin. Carcinoma of the cervix developed in 50 per cent of the untreated mice, while *no* cancer developed in the progestin-treated mice. If the progestin was administered at a later period of anaplastic activity, no inhibitory influence was manifested and these authors concluded that the potential and actual cancer cells were no longer responsive to the hormone. They suggested that the progestin might act by protecting the cell from the carcinogen. Ebner and Sandritter suggested that normal cervical cells possess a 'receptor' which in progestin-treated animals is occupied by the progestin, with the result that the carcinogen cannot attach itself to the cell, or only in insufficient amounts. Cancer cells seem to have lost this 'hormone receptor'.

Kaminetzky and Swerdlow (1968), in a study of experimental dysplasia of the rhesus monkey cervix, produced advanced cervical dysplasia in 4 of 8 monkeys by topical methylcholanthrene application and parenteral oestrogen administration. The squamous epithelium of the cervix was hyperplastic in oestrogen-treated animals and epithelial pegs were found deeper in the stroma of these animals than in the physiologically menstruating animals.

Exogenous oestrogen has thus been shown to be carcinogenic or cocarcinogenic in experimental animals but not in man. There is speculation that unopposed endogenous oestrogen may predispose to endometrial cancer but there is no evidence of such a relationship to cervical cancer in the human.

RELATION TO ORAL CONTRACEPTIVES

Ayre and co-workers (1969) reported an intensive study of the effects of the oral progestins on cervical cells during a six-year period. They screened 1020 women who attended a Planned Parenthood Clinic at regular intervals. Twenty-seven of these women having dysplasia of carcinoma in situ were suitable for study and available for prolonged research investigation. Of the 27 women, almost two-thirds had persistence of atypical changes, without alteration, following the use of Enovid as an oral contraceptive.

However, one-third of the group showed regression of cervical lesions on Enovid. No biopsy or other anticancer treatment was administered during the period of investigation.

Ayre and co-workers (1969) concluded that the pill does not initiate or accelerate precancerous lesions of the cervix. Indeed, they suggested that the very opposite seemed to be true since Enovid, especially at high-dosage levels, demonstrated certain cancer-inhibitory or regressive influences. A similar effect of Enovid on advanced endometrial cancer was reported by Stoll in 1961. He noted regression of metastatic lesions in the vagina subsequent to the administration of Enovid in doses of 20 to 30 mg daily.

There is no doubt that oestrogens and progestins affect cervical mucus, cellular morphology and vascularity of the cervix. Carbia, Alvardo-Duran and Lopez-Llera (1968) have reported the result of periodic colposcopic examinations in patients given 1 mg ethynodiol diacetate with 0·1 mg mestranol for up to two years. They found that users of oral contraceptives containing this oestrogen-progestin combination, showed an increase in ectopia, ectropion and vascular congestion of the cervix and changes in the character of the cervical mucus. These effects enhance the efficacy of the contraceptive, but they also may contribute to the higher incidence of chronic cervicitis if the cervix is not treated properly and regularly.

Women attending Planned Parenthood or birth control clinics are being subjected to more aggressive and frequent cytologic testing than perhaps any other population group in the United States today. New evidence of coital viral transmission implies that promiscuity by either partner increases the risk of viral infection and cervical cancer. Women attending birth control clinics are perhaps more active sexually than the average. Single girls attending such clinics in increasing numbers signify premarital sexual activity often starting in their teens and continuing with a multiplicity of partners. It is,

therefore, to be expected that this population group will show a high incidence of carcinoma in situ and dysplasia of the cervix when an efficient cytologic screening is applied.

Cervical cancer has a developmental period extending over many years, whereas most women found to have cancer in situ or dysplasia in Planned Parenthood screening programme have been taking the pill for a relatively short period of time. Ayre and co-workers (1969) therefore suggest that the existence of dysplasia or cancer in situ of the cervix of women attending such clinics antedates the taking of the pill perhaps by several years. They further suggest that 'there is no known evidence that the oral progestins initiate carcinoma in situ or dysplasia in normal cervical cells and tissues'. Their findings substantiate the view that the high incidence of dysplasia and carcinoma in situ among women who attend birth control clinics is *not* a result of the pill usage, but rather is attributable to sexual performance.

The first long-range cancer prospective study comparing users and non-users of oral contraceptives has recently been reported. Dr Herbert F. Sandmire reported in 1970 the findings in a homogeneous group of white, middle-class women in Greenbay, Wisconsin. Twenty-eight cancers of the cervix were found among 12 000 Papanicolaou smears from women not on oral contraceptives, a rate of 1 per 428. Six cancers were found among pill users from whom 3000 Papanicolaou smears were taken, a rate of 1 per 500. These findings contradict a New York study which indicated that the incidence of cancer of the cervix was higher among pill users than non-users. Sandmire suggests that the New York study was probably invalid because of the type of women who selected the pill at the family planning centre used for the investigation. These women, he noted, were of a type who probably had sexual intercourse early in life with a variety of partners.

Prevention of cervical carcinoma depends

on regular pelvic examination, serial cytologic study and biopsy and treatment of cervical abnormalities. If the use of oral contraceptives necessitates the regular appearance of the patient in the physician's office, much may be accomplished in the field of preventive medicine. Careful and regular pelvic examination together with properly timed cytological studies and cervical biopsies may indeed make carcinoma of the cervix a preventable disease.

CONCLUSION

On the basis of the studies reported here, the following conclusions regarding the use of progestational agents in metastatic endometrial carcinoma seem valid:

1. Despite the reported catabolic action of the progestational agents used, subjective improvement may be expected in about 70 per cent of patients.
2. Objective remissions may be expected in 30 to 35 per cent of the patients if adequate therapy is administered.

3. Pulmonary and osseous lesions respond better to the progestational agents than those confined to the pelvis and abdomen.
4. Objective responses are seen more frequently in patients with slowly growing tumours which are often well differentiated morphologically.

The dose administered to the patient is variable, depending on the growth rate and differentiation of the tumour. It seems important, however, to initiate therapy with a high 'loading' dose.

Although carcinoma of the cervix has been induced in certain test animals by known carcinogens, there is no statistically valid evidence to implicate hormonal factors in the histogenesis of this neoplasm in the human female. Furthermore, objective remissions have not been obtained in patients having disseminated cervical carcinoma by the administration of hormonal agents. Recent observations in women utilising oestrogen-progestin combinations for conception control have not indicated an increase in either pre-malignant or malignant lesions of the cervix.

References

Anderson, D. G. (1965) Management of advanced endometrial adenocarcinoma with medroxyprogesterone acetate. *American Journal of Obstetrics and Gynecology*, **92**, 87.

Austin, J. H. & MacMahon, B. (1969) Indicators of prognosis in carcinoma of the corpus uteri. *Surgery, Gynecology and Obstetrics*, **128**, 1247.

Ayre, J. E., Reyner, F. C., Fagundes, W. B. & Leguerrier, J. M. (1969) Oral progestins and regression of carcinoma in situ and cervical dysplasia. *Obstetrics and Gynecology*, **34**, 545.

Bonte, J. (1969) Recent advances in medroxyprogesterone therapy and its possible mechanism of action in the treatment of uterine adenocarcinoma. Presented at the Upjohn conference on medroxyprogesterone acetate, Brussels, Belgium.

Brush, M. G., Taylor, R. W. & King, R. J. B. (1967a) The uptake of (6,7³H) oestradiol by human endometrium after subcutaneous and intravenous injection. *Journal of Endocrinology*, **38**, 20.

Brush, M. G., Taylor, R. W. & King, R. J. B. (1967b) The uptake of (6,7³H) oestradiol by the normal human female reproductive tract. *Journal of Endocrinology*, **39**, 599.

Carbia, E., Alvardo-Duran, A. & Lopez-Llera, M. (1968) Colposcopic study of the uterine cervix during administration of ethynodiol diacetate with mestranol. *American Journal of Obstetrics and Gynecology*, **102**, 1023.

Cox, L. W. & Kirkland, J. A. (1964) Effect of ethynodiol diacetate on endometrial carcinoma. Symposium on recent advances in ovarian and synthetic steroids, Sydney, Australia.

Ebner, W. & Sandritter, W. (1968) The effects of norprogesterone on experimental cancer of the cervix. *German Medical Monthly*, **13**, 41.

Hayakawa, K. (1969) Effects of dimethysterone on endometrial adenocarcinoma; electron microscopic study. *Acta Obstetrica Gynaecologica Japonica (Tokyo)*, **16**, 285.

Kaminetsky, H. A. & Swerdlow, M. (1968) Experimental cervical dysplasia in Rhesus monkeys: estrogen a cofactor with methylcholanthrene. *American Journal of Obstetrics and Gynecology*, **102**, 404.

Kelley, R. M. & Baker, W. H. (1960) Effects of 17-alpha-hydroxyprogesterone caproate on metastatic endometrial cancer. Conference on Experimental Clinical Cancer Chemotherapy. *Monograph* 9, p. 235. Bethesda, Md: National Cancer Institute.

Kelley, R. M. & Baker, W. H. (1970) Progestational agents in the treatment of carcinoma of the genitourinary tract. In *Progress in Gynecology*, ed. Sturgis, S. H. and Taymor, M. L., p. 362. New York: Grune and Stratton.

Kennedy, B. J. (1963) Progestogen for the treatment of advanced endometrial cancer. *Journal of the American Medical Association*, **184**, 758.

Kistner, R. W., Baginsky, S., Craig, J. M. & Bigler, P. (1962) Effective progestins on induced endometrial cancer in the rabbit. *Surgical Forum*, **13**, 410.

Kistner, R. W., Griffiths, C. T. & Craig, J. M. (1965) The use of progestational agents in the management of endometrial cancer. *Cancer*, **18**, 1563.

Kistner, R. W. & Griffiths, C. T. (1968) Use of progestational agents in the management of metastatic carcinoma of the endometrium. *Clinical Obstetrics and Gynecology*, **11**, 439.

Nordqvist, R. S. B. (1969) *Hormonal Responsiveness of Human Endometrial Carcinoma Studied in Vitro and in Vivo*. Lund, Sweden: Studenlitteratur.

Reifenstein, E. C., Jr (1968) Personal communication. The Squibb Institute for Medical Research, New Brunswick, N.J.

Reifenstein, E. C. (1971) Hydroxyprogesterone caproate therapy in advanced endometrial cancer. *Cancer*, 485.

Sandmire, H. F. (1970) Presentation before A.C.O.G., District VI.

Sherman, A. I. & Woolf, R. B. (1959) Endocrine basis for endometrial carcinoma. *American Journal of Obstetrics and Gynecology*, **77**, 233.

Stoll, B. A. (1961) A new progestational steroid in the therapy of endometrial carcinoma—a preliminary report. *Cancer Chemotherapy Reports*, **14**, 83.

Taki, I. & Iijima, H. (1963) A new method of producing endometrial cancer in mice. *American Journal of Obstetrics and Gynecology*, **87**, 926.

Taylor, R. W., Brush, M. G., King, R. J. B. & Witt, M. (1971) The uptake of oestrogen by endometrial carcinoma. *Proceedings of the Royal Society of Medicine*, **64**, 407.

Truscott, I. D. (1964) Treatment of endometrial cancer by the instillation of a progestational agent. Presented at a Symposium on Recent Advances in Ovarian and Synthetic Steroids. Sydney, Australia.

Varga, A. & Henriksen, E. (1961) Clinical and histopathologic evaluation of effect of 17-alpha-hydroxyprogesterone caproate on endometrial cancer. *Obstetrics and Gynecology*, **18**, 658.

Varga, A. & Henriksen, E. (1963) Urinary excretion assays of pituitary luteinizing hormone (LH) related to endometrial carcinoma. *Obstetrics and Gynecology*, **22**, 120.

Wentz, W. B. (1964) Effect of a progestational agent on endometrial hyperplasia and endometrial cancer. *Obstetrics and Gynecology*, **24**, 370.

Chapter 18

Renal Cancer

H. J. G. BLOOM

The treatment of advanced carcinoma of the kidney with cytotoxic agents has been disappointing with regard to both subjective and objective improvement. In 1967 the literature was reviewed by Woodruff and his colleagues. Of a total of 243 collected cases treated with some 33 different drugs only 10 per cent showed signs of objective improvement, and in most instances this was slight or of brief duration. Talley et al (1969) reported their own experience with 57 patients treated with 15 different agents, chiefly alkylating drugs, antimetabolites and vinblastine: objective improvement was seen in only two cases (3·5 per cent). In 17 cases of metastatic renal carcinoma treated with cytotoxic agents by Jelliffe (1964) there was no objective remission and subjective responses were unconvincing. Apart from giving poor results, the agents employed in these studies are highly toxic and have a relatively small margin of safety.

Over the past decade attention has been drawn to the concept of an endocrine background to the progress and perhaps the development of carcinoma of the kidney, and to the possible benefit of hormone treatment in a proportion of very advanced cases (Bloom, 1964, 1967a, b, 1971; Bloom and Wallace, 1964; Bloom et al, 1963a,). Hormones now appear to be not only more effective than cytotoxic drugs for this disease, but also remarkably free from serious side-effects.

Hormones and Renal Neoplasia

ENDOCRINE FACTORS AND THE NORMAL KIDNEY

The relationship of the kidney to the endocrine glands appears to be greater than perhaps generally appreciated. Thus, the normal kidney is a target organ for hormones from the pituitary, adrenal cortex and parathyroids, and also appears to fulfil the role of an endocrine gland itself by producing such substances as erythropoietin and renin. Sex hormones are known to influence renal structure, at least in experimental animals. In mice and rats castration reduces renal hypertrophy. Oestrogens produce degenerative changes and a reduction in renal weight, an effect which is antagonised by progesterone.

SEX FACTOR IN RENAL CANCER

A sex factor may be involved in the development and progress of renal tumours in man. Thus, small renal cortical adenomas are found more frequently in males than in females, and the incidence of adenocarcinoma in men is twice as great as in women. It is interesting that renal carcinoma occurs with equal frequency in men and women up to about the time of the female menopause, after which the incidence in males increases to three to four times that found in women (Bloom, 1964). Spontaneous regression in renal cancer occurs predominantly in males: of 34 cases reported in the literature only 7 (21 per cent) were females. Generally speaking, survival rates are comparable for male and female patients with carcinoma of the kidney, but in some reports the prognosis seems better for women (Swanson and Holmes, 1970; Mostofi, 1967; Glenn, 1967).

A direct relationship between sex hormones and renal neoplasia has been firmly established in the experimental field. Multiple adenomas and adenocarcinomas of the kidney can be produced in the hamster by prolonged administration of oestrogen. Under normal conditions this occurs only in males (Kirkman, 1959), and it is interesting that tritium-labelled stilboestrol administered to hamsters has a significantly greater renal concentration in males compared with females (Ghaleb, 1961). The sex factor in renal neoplasia together with the effects of sex hormones on the normal kidney suggest that, if there is a hormonal background to the development and progress of human renal cancer, it may be of gonadal origin.

OESTROGEN-INDUCED RENAL TUMOURS IN THE HAMSTER

In 1947 Matthews, Kirkman and Bacon described an adenomatous tumour of the kidney in the Syrian hamster following continuous prolonged oestrogen administration. This observation was extended by Kirkman (1959) at Stanford University, and also by Horning (1956) at the Institute of Cancer Research, London.

Following subcutaneous implantations of stilboestrol pellets in male hamsters, multiple tumours develop in both kidneys. The tumours are adenomas and adenocarcinomas, and probably arise from the proximal tubular epithelium. They appear as small cortical nodules in about 7 months, and become palpable in the flank by 9 to 12 months in approximately 75 per cent of treated animals.

Primary renal tumour-induction of the hamster by oestrogen can be prevented by the simultaneous administration of testosterone or progesterone (Kirkman, 1959; Horning, 1956). Oestrogen-induced renal tumours can be produced in females only after certain endocrine manipulations such as oophorectomy (Kirkman, 1959).

The hamster renal tumour has been successfully transplanted but, initially, the graft was dependent upon pretreatment of the host with oestrogen. After some five years of serial transfer at the Institute of Cancer Research, the tumour ceased to be dependent upon administered oestrogen and grew more rapidly. Experiments in our laboratories have shown that after several years of serial transfer this tumour can still be influenced by endocrine manipulation. Thus, tumour growth rate was reduced by cortisone administration, the effect being proportional to the dose, and totally suppressed by a combination of cortisone and the progestin medroxyprogesterone acetate (Bloom et al, 1963a). Neither medroxyprogesterone acetate alone nor testosterone, in the doses we used, had any inhibitory effect on the tumour. The suppression brought about by cortisone, and by cortisone plus medroxyprogesterone acetate, has some degree of specificity for the hamster renal neoplasm, since these hormones had no such influence on two nonrenal transplanted tumours acting as controls (Bloom, Dukes and Mitchley, 1963a).

Bilateral adrenalectomy caused some delay in tumour growth. Orchidectomy resulted in complete inhibition and ultimate regression of early tumour grafts, and brought well-established transplants to a standstill for nearly 100 days (Bloom et al, 1963b). The marked anti-tumour effect of orchidectomy was completely overcome by the administration of oestradiol or testosterone. In further experiments it was shown that the administration of an oestrogen-antagonist caused marked inhibition of tumour transplant growth, and that this effect could also be neutralised by the administration of oestradiol (Bloom, Roe and Mitchley, 1967).

OTHER EXPERIMENTAL RENAL TUMOURS

The susceptibility to develop hormone-dependent adenocarcinomas of the kidney following prolonged treatment with stilboestrol is peculiar to the hamster, although a 2 per cent incidence of renal tumours was reported in oestrogen-treated mice by Richardson (1957). The occurrence and type of renal tumour induced by dimethylnitrosamine and dimethylbenzanthracene in Sprague–Dawley rats is influenced by sex and by oophorectomy (Jasmin and Riopelle, 1964, 1970). Attempts in our laboratory to modify the development and growth of dimethyldimethylnitrosamine-induced renal tumours (carcinoma and nephroblastoma) in Wister rats by prolonged administration of various hormones, commencing four weeks after treatment with the carcinogen, were unsuccessful, although a slight inhibitory effect was observed with testosterone (Bloom and Stephens, 1968).

It is clear that the hamster renal tumour should be classified as a hormone-dependent neoplasm and placed in the same category as other dependent growths in laboratory animals, such as those arising in the thyroid, ovary and mammary gland. This is an especially interesting concept as the kidney is not a secondary sex organ, nor at present generally regarded as a member of the endocrine system.

Caution is of course necessary when trying to extrapolate from observations in laboratory animals to clinical practice, but because the principal actions of hormonal agents are fundamentally alike in most species, it is tempting to apply knowledge derived from endocrine-dependent tumours in animals to possibly analogous tumours in man.

HORMONAL ACTIVITY AND RENAL CANCER IN MAN

A direct link between endocrine activity and human renal cancer exists in the rare but well-established association of renal cell carcinoma and polycythaemia or hypercalcaemia. In such cases, the tumours secrete excessive amounts of erythropoietin and a parathormone-like substance. Such chemical abnormalities can be corrected by nephrectomy but may recur with the appearance of metastases. An increased incidence of endocrine gland hyperplasia (adrenal cortex, pancreatic islets, parathyroid and pituitary) has been reported in patients with renal cell carcinoma (Whisenand, Kostas and Sommers, 1962), but the controls in this study were patients without malignant disease.

The sex factor in renal neoplasia and the known effect of sex hormones on the normal kidney in experimental animals, encouraged us to embark on a clinical trial to test the value of gonadal hormones, chiefly the progestin medroxyprogesterone acetate, and testosterone, in patients with far-advanced renal cancer. Our interest in the use of progestins for this tumour was subsequently heightened by knowledge of their value in endometrial and breast cancer, two human tumours with a known oestrogen relationship.

The possible relationship between oestrogens derived from the environment and the development of renal cancer in man has been discussed elsewhere (Bloom, 1967b). Is the stilboestrol used to increase meat production in cattle and to caponise poultry, and the oestrogen taken for gynaecological disorders or in contraceptive pills, renocarcinogenic in the human? Although an unusually high incidence of second primary malignant tumours has been reported in patients coming to autopsy with renal cell carcinoma (Hajdu and Thomas, 1967), there appears to be no correlation with any specific tumour. The occurrence of renal tumours does not seem to be increased in men treated with oestrogens over a number of years for prostatic cancer, nor do statistics in the South-West Metropolitan Region suggest that the incidence of renal tumours is greater among women with breast or endometrial cancer, both of which may be related to oestrogen imbalance (Bloom, 1970).

Hormonal Therapy

HORMONES USED IN THE TREATMENT OF EXPERIMENTAL AND HUMAN RENAL CELL TUMOURS

MEDROXYPROGESTERONE ACETATE

Progesterone inhibits the development of oestrogen-induced neoplasms in experimental animals, including renal adenocarcinoma in hamsters (Kirkman, 1959). Progestins may induce regression of recurrent or metastatic endometrial and breast cancer (Briggs, Caldwell and Pitchford, 1967), tumours long thought to be related to the presence of excess oestrogen.

It was decided to use a progestational compound as the main agent with which to treat human renal cell carcinoma, and medroxyprogesterone acetate (Figure 18.1), a powerful synthetic progestin, was chosen because of its high oral efficiency and freedom from oestrogenic and androgenic activity. Prolonged administration, even in high dosage (300 to 400 mg daily), appears to be virtually free from toxic effects. Treatment in all cases of the present author's series (Bloom, 1971) was initiated with a progestin, medroxyprogesterone acetate, in 79 cases and 17α-hydroxyprogesterone caproate in one case. The dose of the former was 100 mg orally tds and of the latter, 250 mg intra-muscularly thrice weekly. Medroxyproges-terone acetate has also been used for renal carcinoma by Samuels, Sullivan and Howe (1968), Paine, Wright and Ellis (1970) and Talley et al (1969). The last authors also used hydroxyprogesterone caproate in some cases.

von Schreeb (1967) used a progestin and testosterone together for their cases.

CORTICOSTEROIDS

The induction of primary renal tumours in hamsters by stilboestrol can also be inhibited by desoxycorticosterone acetate. On the other hand, cortisone appeared to increase

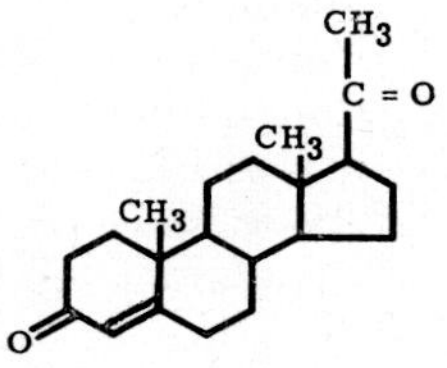

PROGESTERONE

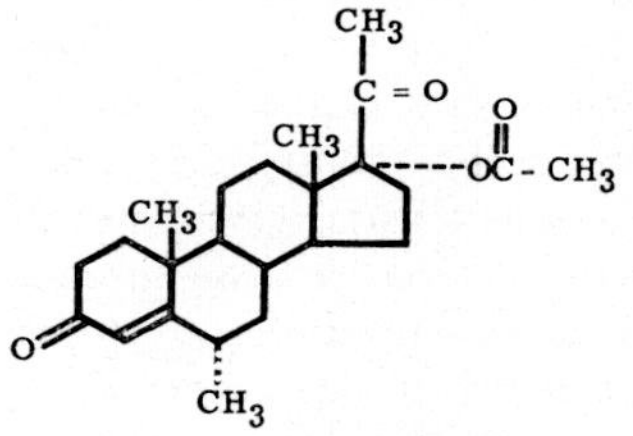

PROVERA
6 α - methyl - 17 α - hydroxyprogesterone acetate

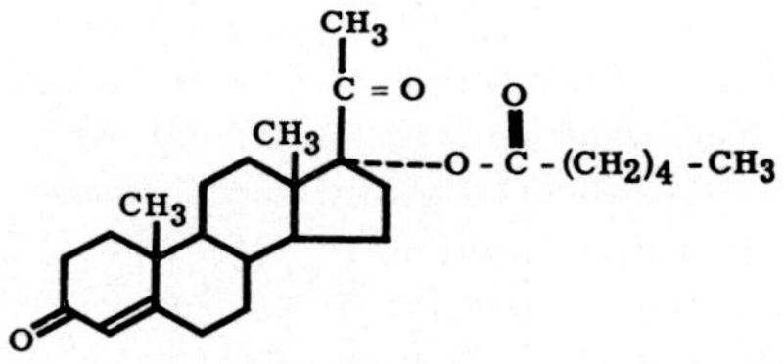

DELALUTIN
17 - α - hydroxy-progesterone
17 - N - caproate

FIGURE 18.1. The comparative structure of progesterone, medroxyprogesterone acetate and hydroxyprogesterone caproate.

TESTOSTERONE PROPIONATE

The development of primary renal tumours in oestrogen-treated hamsters is also inhibited by testosterone (Horning, 1956; Kirkman, 1959). This effect, however, was not observed with tumour transplants (Kirkman, 1959; Bloom et al, 1963a). We have used testo-sterone propionate, 100 mg intramuscularly daily, later reduced to thrice weekly, for patients who fail to respond to medroxy-progesterone acetate. This policy was also adopted by Samuels et al (1968), but Jenkin (1967) chose to treat his cases from the start with androgens. Melander, Notter and

the incidence of such tumours (Kirkman, 1959). Working with a strain of renal tumour transplant, independent of adminis-tered oestrogen, we found that large doses of cortisone inhibited tumour growth and that this effect was dose-dependent (Bloom et al, 1963a). In these experiments medroxypro-gesterone acetate alone had no effect on tumour growth rate but, when combined with cortisone, caused virtually complete tumour inhibition—a far greater effect than was produced with the same dose of cortisone alone.

A few patients in our series who failed to respond to medroxyprogesterone acetate or to testosterone propionate were treated with prednisone, initially 30 to 40 mg daily in divided doses, either alone or with medroxyprogesterone acetate. Talley et al (1969) are the only other authors who have reported experience with corticosteroids for renal cancer cases.

STILBOESTROL

More recent experiments in our laboratories have shown that a later generation of hamster renal transplant can be inhibited by large doses of stilboestrol. Thus, we have an interesting cycle of tumour behaviour whereby the renal neoplasm was induced by oestrogen, and was initially fully dependent on this hormone for sustained primary growth and, for a time, as a serial transplant. After several transfers it gained independence from stilboestrol but was still dependent upon endogenous oestrogen derived from the adrenal gland and testis (Bloom et al, 1963b; Bloom et al, 1967). Finally, the tumour was inhibited by stilboestrol, the hormone which caused its development.

Stilboestrol was given as a final resort to a few patients in whom there was no response to either medroxyprogesterone acetate or to testosterone, or if tumour-stimulation appeared to occur with testosterone.

It should be noted that neither medroxyprogesterone acetate nor testosterone inhibited the growth of the strain of transplanted hamster tumour (independent of administered oestrogen) used in our experiments (Bloom et al, 1963a). Although Kirkman (1959) found that progesterone and also testosterone prevented the development of primary renal tumours in stilboestrol-treated hamsters, he observed no such effect in animals bearing oestrogen-dependent tumour transplants. Nevertheless, we decided to use initially medroxyprogesterone acetate and testosterone as the principal agents for patients with advanced renal carcinoma,

chiefly because of their known inhibitory effect on experimental oestrogen-dependent tumours in general, including the hamster primary renal tumour.

RESULTS OF HORMONE TREATMENT IN A PERSONAL SERIES OF 80 CASES

Between 1959 and 1969, 80 patients with incurable adenocarcinoma of the kidney were treated with hormones (Bloom, 1971). Only patients with clear evidence of advancing disease for whom no other treatment, apart from cytotoxic drugs, was feasible were accepted for a trial of hormones. In this category, no case was refused treatment, no matter how near death appeared to be. Thus, 38 patients (47 per cent) were seriously ill or considered to be terminal when hormone treatment was started, and 20 died within six weeks (that is, 25 per cent of the total series). Cases with operable solitary metastases, such as may occur in the lung or brain, were not treated with hormones in the first instance but were referred for surgery. Patients with localised inoperable metastases in the spine or pelvis were treated with irradiation.

The series consisted of 54 men and 26 women (Table 18.1) Nephrectomy had been

TABLE 18.1. *Advanced renal adenocarcinoma treated by hormones (1959–1969)*

Total cases	80
Males	54
Females	26
Nephrectomy	67
Histology	73 (91%)

performed in 67 cases. Histological confirmation of the diagnosis of renal cell carcinoma was obtained, sooner or later, in

TABLE 18.2. *Cases of advanced renal adenocarcinoma treated with hormones. 80 cases (1959–1969)*

Site of tumour	Cases	%
Multiple metastases	75	*94*
Multiple different organs involved	61	*76*
Lungs, mediastinum	57	*71*
Skeleton	23	*29*
Hepatomegaly*	19	*24*
Brain	7	*9*
Inoperable primary†	10	*12*
Other abdominal masses‡	17	*21*
Seriously ill or terminal	38	*47*
Presented primary + metastases	32	*40*

* Umbilical level in 8
† Laparotomy in 7
‡ >12 cm in 9

91 per cent of the total series. Ninety-four per cent of the 80 cases had multiple metastases, and more than one organ was involved in 76 per cent (Table 18.2).

Significant subjective improvement following the administration of one or more hormone preparations was experienced by at least 44 patients (55 per cent) (Table 18.3). Attention will be focused only on those cases with objective signs of tumour regression, or where the tumour remained stationary for more than one year. Ten cases, showing minor or doubtful changes which have been of interest to the observer but of no great moment to the patient, are mentioned but excluded from the final consideration.

TABLE 18.3. *Advanced renal adenocarcinoma. Results of hormone treatment in 80 cases*

Response	Cases	
	No.	%
Subjective	44	*55*
Objective		
Marked tumour regression	11*	*14*
Tumour stationary >1 year	2†	*2·5*
Slight tumour regression	10	*12*
Total objective	*23*	*28·5*

* For 2, 2, 3, 3, 3, 9, 13, 20, 24, 24, 35 months
† For 21, 20+ months

In 11 cases (14 per cent) there was undeniable improvement in the radiological or clinical signs of tumour within a short time of commencing treatment or changing to a different hormone: this lasted for 2 to 35 months (Tables 18.3 and 18.4). There were two additional cases in whom marked improvement in general condition was associated with stationary tumour for 20 to 21 months (Table 18.5). Histological confirmation of the diagnosis was obtained in all of 13 cases, and in 5 of 11 dead cases an

TABLE 18.4. *Hormone therapy for metastatic renal cancer. Marked objective response*

Case	Sex age	Extent prior to hormones	Successful hormone	Duration of response (months)	Survival from start of hormones (months)
A.P.	♂ 70	*Lung*, bone	MPA	20	32
D.W.	♂ 58	*Lung, bone, brain*	T	35	41
G.D.	♂ 64	*Lung*	MPA	9	13
W.D.	♂ 59	Liver, *lung, inop. primary*	MPA	3	3
A.J.	♀ 69	*Abdominal masses*	MPA	3	7
F.H.	♂ 49	*Abdomen, suprac. nodes*	HPC T	22	24
J.A.D.	♂ 78	*Lung, scar*	MPA	24	37
B.S.	♀ 58	*Inop. primary, liver*	MPA	2	3
A.G.	♂ 82	*Scar, abdomen*	MPA	3	14
E.G.	♂ 58	Lungs, *abdomen*	MPA T	9 4	20
Y.A.	♂ 65	*Scar, abdomen*	MPA	2·5	Untraced

MPA = medroxyprogesterone acetate
HPC = 17α-hydroxyprogesterone caproate
T = testosterone propionate

The organs in which tumour regression occurred are in italic type. Note that in some cases not all tumour sites responded to treatment.

TABLE 18.5. *Disease stationary for >12 months*

Case	Sex Age	Extent prior to hormones	Hormone	Response	Survival
A.D.	♂ 71	*Bone, lung*	MPA T	Multiple bone metastases stationary 21 months. Regression lung metastases 15 months	Died 22 months: lung and spinal metastases active
W.G.	♀ 62	*Mediastinum*	MPA	Mass stationary 20+ months	Alive and well 20 months

MPA = medroxyprogesterone acetate
T = testosterone propionate

autopsy was performed. A significant objective response was therefore observed in 13 of the 80 cases (16 per cent). If the seriously ill patients who died shortly after commencing treatment are excluded (a practice endorsed by several authors reporting results of hormonal or cytotoxic agents) the overall response rate in the present series is 22 per cent (Table 18.9). Paine et al (1970) excluded 10 cases from their series of 35 patients with various tumours treated with medroxyprogesterone acetate because of early death or because of insufficient data.

ILLUSTRATIVE CASE SUMMARIES

Partial Selective Regression—Case A.P., male aged 70 (Bloom, 1964)

Metastases in left lung (Figure 18.2A) and lower femur, 4 years after nephrectomy. Medroxyprogesterone acetate, 300 mg daily, and irradiation to femoral deposit because of pain and fracture-risk. After 6 weeks lung deposit smaller but the femoral lesion larger. By 4 months, mid-thigh amputation for

pathological fracture. Pulmonary metastasis continued to regress (Figure 18.2B) and finally became stationary for 20 months. Progressive destruction of femoral stump eventually required hip disarticulation. Intrathoracic metastases recurred which proved resistant to larger doses of medroxyprogesterone acetate, prednisone, medroxyprogesterone acetate plus prednisone and, finally, testosterone propionate. Death with widespread metastases 32 months after starting hormone therapy.

Partial Selective Regression—Case B.S., female aged 58 (Bloom, 1967a)

General condition very poor, massive tumour in solitary kidney and hard irregular liver to umbilicus. Nephrectomy for tuberculosis 32 years previously. Thyroid mass recently excised which showed metastatic clear cell adenocarcinoma. Nephrotomogram: small cap of residual functioning renal tissue above large kidney tumour. Medroxyprogesterone acetate 300 mg daily started. After 10 days, improved general condition, increased appetite, more physical activity and renal mass smaller; hepatomegaly unchanged. After 6 weeks, discharged from hospital with renal tumour approximately one-third its original size, but liver size unchanged (Figure 18.3A). General improvement and response of primary tumour maintained for 2 months after which readmitted to hospital having

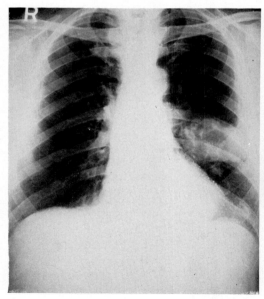
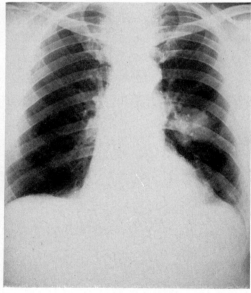

A   *B*

FIGURES 18.2A and B. *Case A.P.* Partial regression of a pulmonary metastasis. Condition 3 months after commencing medroxyprogesterone acetate. Maintained for 20 months (Bloom, 1964).

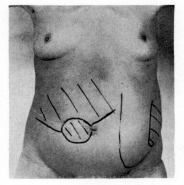

FIGURE 18.3A. *Case B.S.* Rapid partial response of primary tumour in solitary kidney, but hepatic metastases resistant. Shaded areas show condition 5 weeks after commencing medroxyprogesterone acetate (Bloom, 1967a).

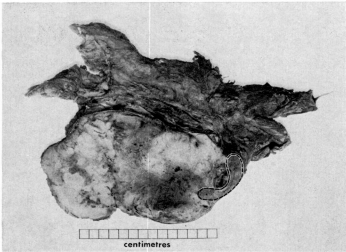

FIGURE 18.3B. Autopsy 3 months after commencing medroxyprogesterone acetate: huge renal cell carcinoma (2100 g) replacing kidney and showing extensive necrosis and calcification. Small cap of residual normal renal tissue outlined.

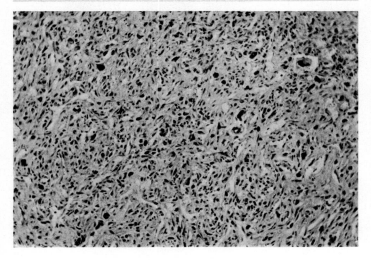

FIGURE 18.3C. Residual area of viable-looking anaplastic carcinoma of high grade malignancy in primary renal tumour shown in Figure 18.3B (× 160).

deteriorated with increasing hepatomegaly. No response to testosterone. Death 3 months after commencing hormone therapy. Autopsy: large renal tumour showing extensive necrosis and calcification (Figure 18.3B). Histology: residual clear cell adenocarcinoma and extensive areas of anaplastic tumour (Figure 18.3C) with marked pleomorphism and hyperchromatism.

Total Regression—Case J.A.D., male aged 78 (Bloom, 1971)

General weakness, chest and abdominal symptoms 9 months after nephrectomy. Abdominal mass, 15 × 12 cm, involving nephrectomy scar; second more superficial mass, 8 × 6 cm, in drain scar. Multiple small bilateral lung metastases. Marked subjective and objective response within 2 weeks of

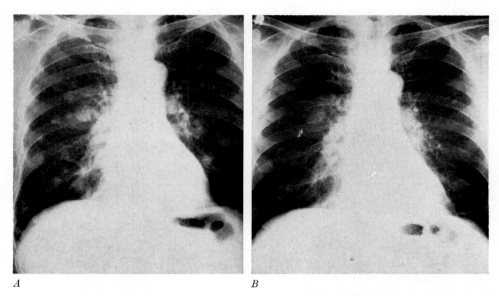

A   B

FIGURES 18.4A and B. *Case G.D.* Multiple bilateral pulmonary metastases, 2 months after nephrectomy. Second radiograph shows disappearance of all but two metastases in right lung, 2 months after starting medroxyprogesterone acetate (Bloom, 1964).

Total Selective Regression—Case G.D., male aged 64 (Bloom, 1964)

Presented with renal tumour and solitary pulmonary shadow. Preoperative irradiation for primary tumour during which pulmonary lesion increased. Nephrectomy performed. Two months later, numerous bilateral lung lesions (Figure 18.4A). Medroxyprogesterone acetate 300 mg daily started. After 5 weeks' treatment pulmonary deposits reduced in size and number, and after 2 months all but two had disappeared (Figure 18.4B). These remained stationary for 8 months during which time patient was well and active. Metastases then advanced with no response to prednisone or testosterone. Haematuria, suggesting metastases in remaining kidney. Died at home 12 months after starting hormone therapy.

commencing medroxyprogesterone acetate 300 mg daily. By 4 weeks larger abdominal tumour reduced to 6 × 6 cm, and smaller to 2·5 cm (Figure 18.5A). At 8 weeks chest clear and total regression of smaller abdominal recurrence. Larger abdominal tumour now a superficial lump, 3·5 cm (Figure 18.5B). General condition good, symptom-free, able to walk two miles daily.

At 3 months, excision of residual abdominal tumour 2·5 cm (Figure 18.5C). Histology: secondary renal cell carcinoma (Plate 18.1, facing p. 241), appearance suggesting lower grade activity than original primary (Plate 18.2, facing p. 241).

Patient passed 80th birthday in good health (Figure 18.5D) and remained well for 25 months. Then further abdominal recurrence with slow progression over the next 12 months and no responses to larger doses of

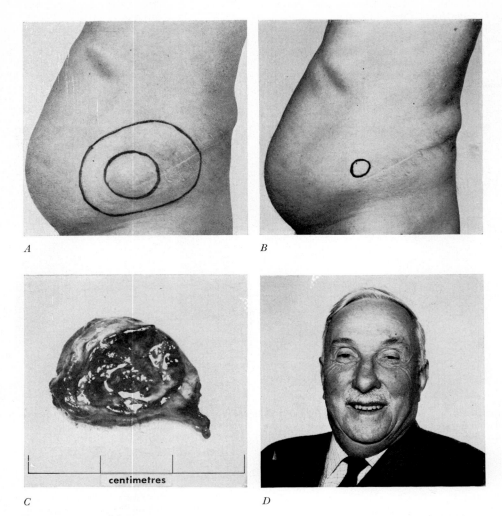

A

B

C

D

FIGURES 18.5A and B. *Case J.A.D.* Outer ring showing recurrent abdominal mass (12 × 15 cm) 9 months after nephrectomy in man aged 78. Inner ring outlines tumour 4 weeks after commencing medroxyprogesterone acetate. Second photograph shows residual superficial tumour (3·5 cm) after 2 months treatment with medroxyprogesterone acetate.

FIGURE 18.5C. Excision of residual tumour (2·5 cm), 3 months after starting medroxyprogesterone acetate (Bloom, 1971).

FIGURE 18.5D. *Case J.A.D.* Aged 80. Continuous medroxyprogesterone acetate treatment for 15 months. Clinically and radiologically free from recurrence. Excellent response maintained for 2 years.

medroxyprogesterone acetate (400 mg daily), an anti-oestrogen (U-11, 100A) and testosterone propionate. Death at 81, three years after commencing hormone therapy.

Tumour Acceleration with Medroxyprogesterone Acetate: Total Regression with Testosterone—Case D.W., male aged 58 (Bloom and Wallace, 1964)

Presented with renal tumour and metastases in tibia, chest, and skull (Figure 18.6A). Nephrectomy (D. M. Wallace). Because of pain and risk of fracture, large osteolytic deposit upper tibia treated by irradiation, curettage, bone-chip replacement and insertion of intramedullary nail (G. R. Fisk). While receiving medroxyprogesterone acetate 300 mg daily over 2 months, marked general deterioration, onset of hemiparesis and increase in all metastases (Figure 18.6B). Medroxyprogesterone acetate replaced by 100 mg testosterone propionate i.m. daily, 5 days weekly. Within 4 weeks, striking improvement in general health; by 8 weeks, a 'new man'.

After 18 months on testosterone propionate, in good health and full employment. Weight gain 23 kg. Recovery from hemiparesis. Radiological regression of metastases in chest, tibia (unirradiated area) and skull (Figure 18.6C). Tibial metastasis, treated by surgery and irradiation, healed. Continued in good health with no recurrence for 3 years. Then sudden deterioration and collapse with hemiplegia. Skeletal lesions inactive but new advancing soft tissue metastases. Stilboestrol, prednisone and further testosterone propionate all tried in turn without effect. Death with visceral metastases 41 months after starting hormone therapy. At autopsy previous large skull defect covered by fibrous membrane with no evidence of residual tumour (Figure 18.6D).

HORMONE-RESPONSE INTERVAL

This is the time between commencing or changing a hormone preparation and observing signs of clinical improvement. In our 11 cases showing undoubted tumour regression this interval varied between 2 and 6 weeks (Table 18.6). These patients often felt and looked better within a few days of starting treatment. The first discernible signs of tumour regression were seen within 2 weeks in six patients, and within 4 to 6 weeks in the remaining five patients. If a hormone preparation fails to bring about improvement in a patient with renal cancer, it would seem from this experience, unnecessary to delay the trial of an alternative preparation beyond, say, 6 to 8 weeks. If seriously ill

TABLE 18.6. *Hormone-response interval*

Case			Hormone	Response interval in weeks	
				Subjective	Objective
A.P.	♂	70	MPA	5	5
D.W.	♂	58	T	4	6
G.D.	♂	64	MPA	5	5
W.D.	♂	59	MPA	1	2
A.J.	♀	69	MPA	2	2
F.H.	♂	49	HPC	4	4
J.A.D.	♂	78	MPA	2	2
B.S.	♀	58	MPA	2	2
A.G.	♂	82	MPA	2	2
E.G.	♂	58	MPA	3	3
			T	4	4
Y.A.	♂	65	MPA	2	2

MPA = medroxyprogesterone acetate
T = testosterone
HPC = 17α-hydroxyprogesterone caproate

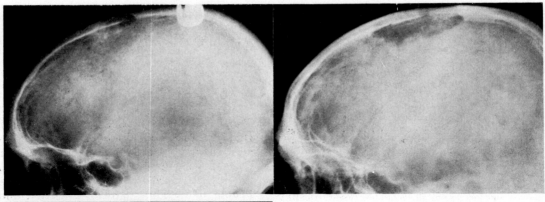

A & B

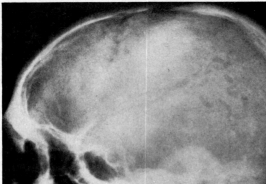

FIGURES 18.6A, B. C. *Case D.W.* Small osteolytic skull metastasis (A) which increased rapidly during treatment with medroxyprogesterone acetate (B). Progressive healing after changing to testosterone: radiograph 38 months after starting testosterone (C) (Bloom and Wallace, 1964).

FIGURE 18.6D. *Case D.W.* Skull section (autopsy specimen) showing fibrous tissue bridging bone defect: no trace of residual tumour (Bloom and Wallace, 1964).

C

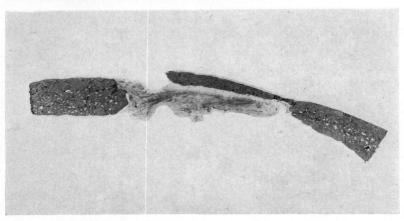

D

patients continue to deteriorate rapidly in spite of treatment it has been our practice to effect this change after only 2 to 4 weeks.

Experience elsewhere suggests that signs of improvement in cases of renal cancer may be delayed for longer than 6 weeks. Thus, Samuels et al (1968) and also Paine et al (1970) reported objective responses at 2 months, while Talley et al (1969) had to wait for as long as 5 and 8 months before seeing regression in two of their cases. With this in mind it would seem reasonable not to interrupt the initial hormone treatment as long as the patient's general condition remains satisfactorily and the disease stationary. A change in treatment may also be postponed for some time if the tumour advances only slowly.

DURATION OF LIFE IN HORMONE-TREATED CASES

The average duration of life from onset of hormone treatment in 78 of the 80 cases in the present series was 7·2 months. Of the remaining two cases, one is still alive and the other is lost to follow-up. This average figure is comparable to that reported by Royce and Tormey (1955) for 16 non-hormone-treated cases presenting preoperatively with metastases (6·7 months), and to that for 27 patients with local tumour extension outside the kidney at operation (5·7 months). The average survival of our 11 patients (13, less one untraced and one still alive) showing a well-marked objective response to hormone treatment was 19·6 months, which is substantially longer than the 5·2 months for our 67 non-responding cases (Table 18.7).

Compared with advanced cases not treated with hormones these are conservative figures, since the duration of life in the present series has been measured from the onset of hormone treatment which, in many instances, was introduced some time after the initial appearance of recurrent tumour. Nearly half our cases were seriously ill or terminal at the onset of hormone therapy, 25 per cent of the total

TABLE 18.7. *Average survival of patients with advanced renal carcinoma treated by hormones*

Objective response	Cases	Average survival (months)
Present	11*	19·6
Absent	67	5·2
Total	78	7·2

* Excluding 1 untraced case and 1 still alive

series dying within six weeks. Objective improvement during hormone therapy in patients with renal carcinoma appears to be associated with prolongation of life. A similar conclusion was reached by Samuels et al (1968).

OTHER REPORTED SERIES

Since our first reports on hormone therapy for advanced renal cancer (Bloom et al, 1963a; Bloom, 1964; Bloom and Wallace, 1964) six other groups of workers have described their experience in this field (Table 18.8). Apart from the cases reported by Jenkin (1967) and by Talley et al (1969) in which objective improvement occurred in only 7 per cent of cases, the overall picture is of one in five or six cases responding to hormone therapy. Of the total of 184 collected cases, including the present series, 15 per cent showed a significant objective response (Table 18.8). The results are more optimistic when selected case-groups are examined. In the present series, if only males are considered and deaths within six weeks excluded, the response rate is 27 per cent (Table 18.9).

Jenkin (1967) at the Princess Margaret Hospital, Toronto, treated 15 male cases of metastatic renal cancer with testosterone propionate, 150 mg i.m. twice weekly for up to three months. If continuation of androgen therapy seemed warranted, this was followed by oral fluoxymesterone 5 mg q.d. Subjective

TABLE 18.8. *Objective response to hormone treatment in advanced cases of renal carcinoma reported in the literature. Some overlap of cases exists in the medroxyprogesterone acetate and testosterone-treated groups of Talley et al (1969)*

Author	Hormones used	Cases	Objective response No.	%	Successful hormone P	A
Woodruff et al (1967)	P	4	1	25	1	–
Melander et al (1967)	P + A	20	4	20	P + A	
Jenkin (1967)	A	15	1	7	—	1
Samuels et al (1968)	P/A*	23	4	17	3	1
Talley et al (1969)	P	16	2	12	2	–
	A	11	0		—	0
Paine et al (1970)	P	15	3	20	3	–
Bloom (1971)	P/A*	80	13	16	12	1
Total		184	28	15		

P = Progestin
A = Androgen
* = Androgen used for progestin failures

TABLE 18.9. *Advanced renal adenocarcinoma. Hormone response in selected groups*

Author	Group	Response No.	%
Melander et al (1967)	T + P for at least 12 weeks	4/13	31
Paine et al (1970)	P in males	3/12	25
Bloom (1971)	Excluding deaths ≤6 weeks	13/60	22
	Males, excluding deaths ≤6 weeks	11/41	27

P = Progestin
T = Testosterone

improvement, often to a marked degree, occurred in approximately 50 per cent of cases but a significant objective response was observed in only one (7 per cent). It is interesting that regrowth of pulmonary metastases in this case coincided with a change of hormone preparation (fluoxymesterone in place of testosterone).

Melander et al (1967) at the Radiumhemmet, Stockholm, treated 20 cases of metastatic renal cancer with testosterone or/and a depot-progestin. In 13 cases receiving 100 mg of testosterone propionate on alternate days, together with daily progestin for at least three months, regression of metastases was seen in four cases (31 per cent, or 20 per cent of the entire series).

Samuels et al (1968) at the M. D. Anderson Hospital, Houston, treated 23 cases with medroxyprogesterone acetate. Seven cases received 300 mg daily orally, and 16 had a depot-preparation of the same hormone, either 400 mg once weekly, or 100 mg daily i.m. No response was observed with the oral preparation. Three cases responded to the parenteral treatment. Eleven patients who failed to respond to medroxyprogesterone acetate were subsequently treated with testosterone, 100 mg i.m. daily, and one of these showed a response. An objective response therefore occurred in 4 of 23 cases (17 per cent), and in 3 of 16 cases (19 per cent) treated initially with parenteral medroxyprogesterone acetate. In 3 cases there was partial regression of pulmonary metastases; in one case a mass in the loin disappeared. The interval from starting treatment to observing more than 50 per cent regression varied from 67 to 107 days. Responses lasted from 4 to more than 30 months. The mean survival time of responding cases was greater than 18 months (2 cases still alive), compared with 7·7 months for those showing no such response (8 still alive).

Talley et al (1969) from Detroit reported their experience with a wide variety of cyto-toxic compounds in a series of 72 patients with metastatic renal carcinoma. These authors also used corticosteroids, androgens and progestins. Various corticosteroid preparations were administered to 38 cases with subjective improvement in 10 (26 per cent), but no objective responses were observed. An excellent response was seen in 1 of 8 cases treated with medroxyprogesterone acetate, and in 1 of 8 cases receiving 17α-hydroxyprogesterone caproate. Thus, 2 of 16 cases (12 per cent) treated with progestins showed a good objective response. In 1 case there was disappearance of pulmonary metastases. In the other, marked regression of pulmonary metastases occurred together with healing of an osteolytic bone deposit. It is interesting that the hormone-response interval in these two cases was as long as 5 and 13 months, respectively: no tumour progression occurred during the latent period and an earlier subjective improvement was

noted. Androgens were administered to 11 cases with no improvement.

Woodruff et al (1967) from Roswell Park Memorial Institute, Buffalo, reviewed the current status of chemotherapy for advanced renal cancer, and referred to 1 of 4 personal cases which showed partial regression of pulmonary metastases during treatment with medroxyprogesterone acetate.

Paine et al (1970) from Oxford reported results of treatment with medroxyprogesterone acetate in advanced cases of renal and endometrial cancer. Three of 15 cases (20 per cent) of renal carcinoma showed an objective response to treatment. In all three cases there was regression of intrathoracic disease commencing within two months of treatment and lasting for approximately one year. In one case, bilateral pulmonary metastases, so numerous that almost no normal lung could be seen, virtually disappeared.

RELATION OF SEX AND AGE TO HORMONE RESPONSE

SEX

Under normal circumstances only male hamsters develop oestrogen-induced renal tumours. It requires certain artificial conditions before such tumours will appear in females (Kirkman, 1959). On the clinical side, the incidence of carcinoma of the kidney and of spontaneous regression of this tumour is much greater in men.

Marked objective improvement in the present series of cases was seen more often in hormone-treated men (11 of 54 cases, 20 per cent) than in women (2 of 26 cases, 8 per cent) (Bloom, 1971). Furthermore, in each of the two female cases the response was limited. In our experience, the best results have been confined to men (Table 18.10). Only Samuels et al (1968) have reported an excellent response in a woman who had complete regression of an abdominal recurrence for 30+ months during treatment

TABLE 18.10. *Advanced renal adenocarcinoma. Hormone response according to sex*

Objective Tumour response	Male No.	%	Female No.	%
Marked reduction	9/54	17	2/26	8
Stationary for >1 year	2/54	4	0/26	0
Slight reduction	8/54	15	2/26	8
Total	19/54	35	4/26	15

with medroxyprogesterone acetate. When all cases showing some degree of objective improvement during hormone treatment in the present author's series are considered, the response rate for men is 35 per cent (19 of 54 cases) and for women 15 per cent (4 of 26) (Table 18.10). If the 20 extremely ill patients who died within six weeks of starting hormone treatment (8 within 16 days) are excluded on the grounds that there may not have been sufficient time for a response to

occur, then the proportion of cases showing a well-marked objective response to treatment is increased to 27 per cent for men, but remains at only 10 per cent for women (Table 18.11).

AGE

The mean age of our patients showing a well-marked objective response to hormone therapy was greater by a decade than in hormone-resistant cases (Table 18.12). Complete

TABLE 18.11. *Advanced renal adenocarcinoma. Response to hormones excluding 20 cases dying ≤6 weeks*

Sex	Cases	Marked tumour inhibition No.	%
♂	41	11	27
♀	19	2	10
Total	60	13	22

TABLE 18.12. *Advanced renal adenocarcinoma. Mean age by hormone response*

Objective response	Cases	Mean age (years)
Marked	13	64·6
Slight	10	59·6
None	57	54·3

tumour regression may occur even in old age; one of our most impressive responses, lasting two years, was seen in a man aged 78 (Case J.A.D.). Samuels et al (1968) found no significant age difference between their responsive and resistant cases.

TUMOUR ACCELERATION DURING HORMONE THERAPY

It is well known that the growth of prostatic cancer can be accelerated during the administration of androgens, and that the tempo of breast carcinoma in premenopausal women is sometimes increased by oestrogen. Clinical acceleration of tumour growth during hormone treatment of renal cancer seemed to occur in 5 of our 80 cases. In 2 of these, however, the increase in tumour size was probably the result of an inflammatory reaction, perhaps associated with acute necrosis, since the swelling subsided spontaneously within a few hours or days while the patient continued on the same hormone. In the remaining 3 cases, the changes were progressive and associated with deterioration of general health: in one, this was so rapid as to demand emergency admission to the local hospital within 48 hours of commencing hormone treatment.

Acceleration of tumour growth with serious consequences during hormone therapy occurred in 3 of our 80 cases, an incidence of 4 per cent. The hormone in 2 patients was medroxyprogesterone acetate and in the third, testosterone. Clinical improvement in all 3 patients soon followed upon a change of hormone preparation. In 1 patient, skeletal and intrathoracic deposits increased rapidly during medroxyprogesterone acetate treatment; manifestations of intracranial metastases appeared and the patient's general condition quickly deteriorated. When testosterone propionate was substituted for the progestin, the patient improved quite dramatically, returning to good health without evidence of active disease for 3 years (Case D.W., Bloom and Wallace, 1964).

Exacerbation of the disease which might be ascribed to hormone treatment has not been reported in other series of renal cancer. However, Bergsjö (1965) observed tumour acceleration in 1 of 15 cases of endometrial cancer treated with progestins. Patients receiving hormones for advanced renal cancer should be watched at frequent intervals during the early stages of treatment for signs of significant tumour advance associated with general deterioration. In such cases, which appear to be rare, the preparation should be promptly changed (for example, testosterone propionate for medroxyprogesterone acetate as in case D.W.).

In some cases small changes in tumour growth rate can be detected only by careful measurement of metastases in serial x-rays. This approach in one of our patients revealed interesting features which were not obvious on routine examination of the films (Bloom, 1967a). The pretreatment growth rate of three pulmonary deposits was identical, while the fourth lesion remained unchanged. During treatment with medroxyprogesterone acetate, the first three lesions continued to increase at the same rate, whereas the tumour, previously stationary, began to grow at a rate comparable to that of the other deposits. After nine weeks, testosterone propionate was substituted for medroxyprogesterone acetate and, approximately six weeks later, all the metastases were showing a reduced growth rate: this was associated with distinct clinical improvement. In spite of continued treatment with large doses of testosterone propionate the metastases soon resumed their original growth rate. The changes in the pulmonary deposits were not evident on cursory examination of the x-ray films, and this patient is not included among the cases showing objective signs of regression.

The possible stimulation of renal cancer during hormone treatment is a further reason why we wait for clear evidence of advancing disease before embarking on endocrine therapy. Renal cancer metastases may occasionally remain latent for a time, or progress only very slowly, and in such patients no treatment at all may be preferable to a treatment which may disturb a satisfactory tumour-host relationship. This concept takes on special significance if hormone administration is ever contemplated in a prophylactic role, in conjunction with surgery and radiotherapy, for the primary treatment of the disease.

The variable response of advanced renal cancer to hormone treatment is in keeping with the capricious behaviour of other hormone-dependent tumours to endocrine therapy.

MODE OF HORMONE ACTION IN RENAL CANCER

Available evidence suggests that the hamster renal tumour is induced by the direct action of oestrogen on the kidney cells. Firstly, these cell tumours have been successfully induced in stilboestrol-treated hypophysectomised animals (Kirkman, 1959). Ghaleb (1961) found that tritium-labelled stilboestrol was concentrated in the renal tubular epithelium to a greater degree in the male than the female: only the former sex is normally susceptible to renal tumour induction by oestrogens. Second, the observations of Algard (1960) indicate that the hamster renal tumour can grow in dispersed cell culture without oestrogen in the medium, whereas the presence of this hormone is necessary for successful growth in organ culture. Third, the growth of the transplanted renal tumour can be greatly reduced in vivo by an anti-oestrogen, and this action is neutralised by the simultaneous administration of oestradiol (Bloom et al, 1967).

Studies of the effects of different hormones against human renal carcinoma in organ culture indicate that the action of such agents as medroxyprogesterone acetate is probably also at the cellular level (Tchao et al, 1968). It was of special interest to note that in these in vitro experiments no toxic effects were observed on normal renal tissue controls. This makes hormone administration a potentially far more attractive treatment for renal cancer than the use of cytotoxic drugs.

We have found no clinical evidence to support an indirect hormonal action via the pituitary in the patients we have treated. Tests of thyroid and adrenal function remain within normal limits in cases receiving large doses of medroxyprogesterone acetate for many months.

SIDE-EFFECTS AND POSSIBLE COMPLICATIONS OF PROGESTIN THERAPY

Increased appetite, weight gain, and improved well-being are often seen in patients with advanced cancer receiving medroxyprogesterone acetate, even in the absence of tumour regression. Patients treated with large doses of progestins may experience headache, and a tendency to oedema may be aggravated. The majority of patients taking medroxyprogesterone acetate 300 mg daily regularly for many months, even up to two to three years, appear to remain in good general health. Treatment of cancer with medroxyprogesterone acetate and similar agents is particularly encouraging since, unlike cytotoxic drugs, they are exceptionally free from serious side-effects.

Liver and thyroid function tests carried out at intervals in some of our long-term patients receiving medroxyprogesterone acetate remained normal. Glucose tolerance and plasma cortisol levels, and urinary 17-hydroxyketosteroid excretion were not significantly reduced. On the other hand, Macdonald (1970) has reported a reduced adrenal response to metyrapone stimulation tests during treatment with medroxyprogesterone acetate. Logothetopoulos, Sharma and Kraicer (1961) studied the effects of administering medroxyprogesterone acetate to rats from soon after birth to maturity (up to 110 days) and found this caused hypoplasia of the adrenal glands and gonads, comparable to changes seen following hypophysectomy. The pituitary itself was decreased in size with absence of delta cells ('gonadotrophs') and the authors concluded that medroxyprogesterone acetate acts at the hypothalamic–hypophyseal level. The thyroid and pancreas were not affected. The undeveloped gonads and adrenals reacted promptly to administration of their trophic hormones. In a further report, thyroid function tests were shown to be normal in rats treated by medroxyprogesterone acetate (Kraicer and Logothetopoulos, 1962).

It is advisable to watch for evidence of endocrine insufficiency and of biochemical disturbance in patients receiving long-term, high-dose progestin therapy. Stoll, Andrews and Motteram (1966) found raised serum transaminase levels together with histological evidence of hepatocellular damage in patients receiving the progestin lynoestrenol, but this may be peculiar to the group of 19 nortestosterone derivatives of which this agent is a member.

Since progestins may contribute to the thromboembolic risk of oestrogen-progestin contraceptives (Inman et al, 1970) there may be an increased incidence of this complication in patients receiving large doses of medroxyprogesterone acetate or 17α-hydroxyprogesterone caproate over many months. Vascular thrombosis, however, does not appear to be a special hazard of progestin therapy in cases of renal, endometrial or breast cancer. Recently, we have reported ruptures of the aorta in hamsters treated with large doses of megestrol or melengestrol acetate, progestational compounds structurally closely related to medroxyprogesterone acetate (Cobb et al, 1971). The aortic ruptures may be due to exacerbation of a pre-existing pathological change seen in the tunica adventitia of control hamsters by the anti-inflammatory activity of the steroids used. Fortunately, this disaster has not been observed in any of our patients treated with medroxyprogesterone acetate.

Prognosis in Advanced Renal Cancer

When trying to assess the value of hormonal and cytotoxic agents in cases of advanced cancer it is important to take account of the variable natural history of the disease. Growth of metastases may be exceptionally slow; recurrence following nephrectomy may be delayed for a decade or more, and prolonged survival in good health may occur after incomplete excision of an extensive primary tumour. Following removal of a solitary metastasis, a patient may be cured, or further recurrence delayed for several years. Very rarely, one may be fortunate enough to observe the phenomenon of spontaneous regression.

Although most centres can recall examples of unexpectedly prolonged survival after palliative treatment for metastatic or locally advanced renal cancer, for the majority of patients the appearance of advancing distant metastases heralds death within a year or so. In a series of cases reported by Flocks and Kadesky (1958) the five-year survival rate for 116 patients presenting with distant metastases was 3·5 per cent: at 10 years only 1 of 79 cases was still alive (1·3 per cent). In the American Urological Association Series, all but 2 of 500 cases with metastases at the time of admission to hospital were dead within two years (Mostofi, 1967). Of 131 cases presenting with distant metastases in addition to the primary renal tumour studied by Middleton (1967), adequate follow-up information was available in 98 of which 91 (93 per cent) failed to survive one year; all patients were dead by two years. Nephrectomy, which was performed on one third of these cases, made no difference to the prognosis. Kay (1968) refers to 13 cases with known metastases in whom nephrectomy was performed: approximately half of these patients were dead by five months and none were alive beyond 17 months.

Mims et al (1966) reported a more hopeful experience in the treatment of cases with locally advanced or metastatic renal carcinoma. These authors reviewed 145 cases of which 48 were excluded because of inadequate follow-up. Of the remaining 97 cases, 57 had distant metastases, 27 had renal vein involvement, 33 had gross extension beyond the capsule, and 12 had lymph node metastases. Nephrectomy was carried out in all cases, with an operative mortality of 6 per cent. Irradiation was given to the renal bed in 25 cases and to distant metastases in 23. Cytotoxic drugs were administered to 13 cases. The five and 10-year survival rates were 14·6 per cent and 3 per cent respectively. It is only fair to point out that a substantial proportion of cases in this series had locally advanced disease and not distant metastases. Indeed, this was the original finding in all three 10-year survivors in whom radical surgery was carried out.

Although one must stress the wide variation in the biological activity of renal cell cancer and emphasise the care required for the interpretation of treatment results using cytotoxic or hormonal agents, it is clear from the foregoing that in the vast majority of patients the onset of clinical metastases brings death within a year or two.

SPONTANEOUS REGRESSION

The question now is whether the regression of metastases observed in hormone-treated cases is the result of this treatment or due to an unrelated spontaneous event. True spontaneous partial or complete regression of

cancer is a well-recognised but rare event. Everson and Cole (1966) were able to collect 176 cases from the world literature between 1900 and 1965 in which they considered adequate evidence of possible spontaneous regression of malignant disease to exist. Thirty-one cases had carcinoma of the kidney. Two of these, however, had received hormones (testosterone and prednisone) and one, thalidomide. In two further cases the evidence of regression was based solely on pathological changes in the primary tumour, but because of the doubtful significance of such changes it would seem best to consider this type of case separately.

After excluding the two primary and the three treated cases, 26 examples of renal carcinoma remain in Everson and Cole's series. I have found eight further cases in the literature making a total of 34 examples of this phenomenon in relation to the kidney (Bloom, 1971). Although unreported cases have undoubtedly been seen, the incidence of spontaneous regression seems to be remarkably rare. Thus Riches (1963) saw no examples in 130 cases of renal cancer, Von Schreeb (1967) none in 232 cases, and Rafla (1970) none in 244 cases.

In a personal series of some 200 patients with renal carcinoma referred over the past 12 years for radiotherapy or hormone treatment, I have seen two cases in whom spontaneous regression of pulmonary metastases occurred. In one patient, a woman aged 70, spontaneous regression of pulmonary deposits occurred for a period of only three months during which time mediastinal nodes increased and vaginal metastases appeared (Bloom, 1967a). The second case is far more impressive.

Case F.B. male aged 55: A nephrectomy was performed for renal cell carcinoma in the presence of widespread metastases in both lungs. At operation the renal tumour was found to be involving peritoneum. In keeping with a 'wait and see' policy no hormone treatment was undertaken at this stage. Two months after operation the metastases in the left lung were smaller; by five months all metastases were showing signs of regression, and by seven months all but one had disappeared. Ten months after nephrectomy the lungs were clear. The patient remains in excellent health with a clear chest two years after operation (Bloom and Riddle, 1971).

In 36 cases (34 reported in literature and 2 personal cases) showing spontaneous regression, the changes were confined to the

best of my knowledge striking regression of widespread metastases involving the brain, chest, and skeleton, such as occurred in one of our patients (D.W.), and the disappearance of a huge abdominal tumour in another (J.A.D.), have yet to be reported as spontaneous events in cases of advanced renal carcinoma.

In view of the rare occurrence of spontaneous regression of metastatic renal

TABLE 18.13. *Site of spontaneous tumour regression in 34 untreated cases of renal carcinoma reported in the literature (for references see Bloom, 1971) plus 2 personal cases, compared with 11 cases treated with hormones in the present series*

| Series | Cases | Regression: | |
		Site	Cases
Spontaneous	36	Lungs	34
		Skeleton	1
		? Gut	1
Hormone-treated	11	Lungs	5
		Abdomen/scar	6
		Skeleton	1
		Brain	1
		Primary	1

lungs in 34 (Table 18.13): only one example of regression of skeletal metastases has been found in the literature (Mims et al, 1966). In a man, aged 51, a deposit in the humerus and another in the pubic bone recalcified following nephrectomy. The other case of extrapulmonary spontaneous regression seems rather dubious, since recurrent hypernephroma tissue is said to have been passed per rectum (Klimpel, 1957).

In our hormone-treated cases tumour regression was observed in the lungs in 5 cases, in large abdominal masses in 6 cases, in the kidney itself in 1, in the brain in 1, and in the skeleton in 1 (Table 18.13). To the

carcinoma, it would appear that objective improvement lasting 3 to 35 months in 11 cases initially showing signs of tumour advancement, and continued tumour standstill for 20 months in 2 others, in a consecutive series of 80 cases receiving hormone therapy, is more likely to be due to this treatment than the result of a natural event. From the very first, this concept was supported by the short interval between commencing or changing hormone treatment and clinical or radiological signs of improvement. Additional support for hormone dependency of renal cancer is now to be found in reports from other centres (Table 18.8).

Current Status and Prospects for Hormone Therapy of Renal Cancer

SELECTION OF CASES FOR HORMONE TREATMENT

It must be emphasised that hormone administration is not the treatment of choice for patients with strictly limited metastases which are amenable to more radical and possibly curative procedures. Thus, cases with a solitary deposit such as in lung, brain or long bone, should be considered first for surgical excision or amputation. Radiotherapy offers quicker and more certain relief of symptoms for inoperable skeletal or cerebral metastases than does systemic treatment with hormonal or cytotoxic agents. So far, we have restricted hormone therapy in renal cancer to advanced cases in whom local treatment was no longer feasible. Future work, however, may indicate that there is a place for hormone therapy as an adjuvant in the radical treatment of earlier cases. For example, the administration of progestins preoperatively or pre-radiotherapy appears to improve results in primary endometrial cancer (Sherman, 1966; Bonte, Decoster and Ide, 1970).

CHOICE OF HORMONAL AGENT; DOSE AND DURATION OF TREATMENT

At the present time hormonal control of advanced renal cancer, as well as other tumours arising in well-established target organs such as the breast and endometrium, is temporary and largely unpredictable as to frequency and duration. Until a lead can be obtained from further clinical experience, or from organ tissue culture and biochemical studies, the choice of hormone preparation for a particular patient with renal cancer must remain largely empirical.

Although one of our patients enjoyed a remarkable remission lasting three years with testosterone therapy, the evidence, so far, indicates that progestins are more often successful than androgens in producing an objective response in cases of advanced renal cancer.

Based on experience with breast cancer (CCNSC Cooperative Breast Cancer Group, 1964), not all progestins may be equally effective in renal cancer. Synthetic progestins may be divided into two classes: (a) '19-nor' compounds which are characterised by the absence of the C-19 methyl group, for example norethisterone, norenthynodrel, and (b) 'substitution' compounds in which there is a modification of the basic progesterone structure, for example medroxyprogesterone acetate and 17α-hydroxyprogesterone caproate. It is the pure progestational preparations in group (b) which have been used for treating patients with renal cancer. Both medroxyprogesterone acetate and 17α-hydroxyprogesterone caproate have proved capable of inducing regression of carcinoma of the endometrium, breast and kidney. In general, we have used the former agent for renal cancer but have observed a well-marked partial response in 1 case with the latter agent. Talley et al (1969) observed 1 example of regression among 8 cases of renal cancer treated with medroxyprogesterone acetate and 1 of 8 treated with 17α-hydroxyprogesterone caproate.

In our series, once it became clear that the disease was advancing and that neither radiotherapy nor surgery were feasible, treatment was started with medroxyprogesterone acetate 300 mg daily by mouth. If there was no response to this preparation within eight weeks, or less if the patient was

deteriorating, a change to testosterone propionate, 100 mg i.m. daily five times a
week, was made. This approach has resulted
in an occasional additional response in pro-
gestin-resistant cases (Bloom and Wallace,
1964; Samuels et al, 1968). In 15 cases
treated from the start with testosterone,
Jenkin (1967) obtained only one response.

Relatively large doses of progestin appear
necessary to produce significant anti-tumour
effects. It is known that endocrine antagonists in excess are required to inhibit even
normal specific hormone actions. For example,
it requires 1 mg of medroxyprogesterone
acetate to bring about 40 per cent inhibition
of the comb growth in the chick produced by
only 50 μg of testosterone (Lerner, 1964).
In the treatment of endometrial cancer with
medroxyprogesterone acetate, the greater
the total hormone dose during the first
eight weeks of treatment the quicker the
response (Kistner, Griffiths and Craig, 1965).
Favourable responses in cancer of the endometrium have been obtained with 200 to
400 mg of oral medroxyprogesterone acetate
daily, or with intramuscular 17α-hydroxy-
progesterone caproate 250 to 750 mg daily,
or 500 to 1000 mg thrice weekly. Patients
with breast cancer have received 200 to
400 mg of medroxyprogesterone acetate orally
daily.

The lowest effective dose in the treatment
of cancer has not been established and, for
the present, it is recommended that the same
type of high-dose regime be used for renal
carcinoma. Fortunately, the above progestins, even in the high doses mentioned,
are virtually free from serious toxic effects.
Medroxyprogesterone acetate may be given
in daily doses of 200 to 300 mg by mouth or
less frequently as a depot-preparation. Talley
et al (1969) observed that 100 mg of the
depot-preparation intramuscularly daily, or
400 mg intramuscularly once weekly, were
each capable of producing an objective
response.

Since the objective response in two cases
reported by Talley et al (1969) did not appear

until five and eight months had elapsed since
the start of progestin treatment, it may be
advisable to continue with the initial hormone
therapy for longer than the six to eight
weeks which has been our practice. Perhaps
no change in treatment should be made as
long as the patient's general condition remains satisfactory and metastases stationary.
This policy was adopted in the two cases of
tumour 'standstill' referred to in our series
(Table 18.5).

HORMONE COMBINATIONS

Experiments with the transplantable stil-
boestrol-induced renal tumour in the hamster show that a combination of cortisone and
medroxyprogesterone acetate induced complete suppression of tumour growth, whereas
the same dose of cortisone alone achieved
only moderate inhibition (Bloom et al,
1963a). Medroxyprogesterone acetate alone,
in the doses we used, had no effect against
this strain of tumour.

Huggins, Moon and Morii (1962) reported
the extinction of chemically induced mammary carcinoma in rats by a combination
of oestradiol and progesterone, and this type
of treatment (stilboestrol plus 17α-hydroxy-
progesterone caproate) appears to be more
successful in postmenopausal women with
advanced breast cancer than either oestrogen
or progestin alone (Crowley and MacDonald,
1965). An additional 20 per cent of women
with endometrial cancer responded to a
combination of oestrogen and progestin,
compared with progestin alone (Sherman,
1966). Melander et al (1967) reported an
objective response in 4 of 13 patients with
metastatic renal cancer treated with a
combination of testosterone and a depot-
progestin.

We have tried the effects of combining
prednisone and medroxyprogesterone acetate
in a few patients with metastatic renal carcinoma who failed to respond to either hormone alone, but so far without success. On
the other hand, we have observed transient

tumour regression and subjective improvement soon after changing from one gonadal hormone to another, such as testosterone propionate for medroxyprogesterone acetate, or stilboestrol for testosterone propionate. The transient improvement observed in these cases may have been the result of a combination of hormones, a 'hang-over' effect of the first hormone.

COMPARISON WITH RESULTS OBTAINED FOR OTHER HORMONE-DEPENDENT TUMOURS

Collected experience from many sources indicate that some 27 per cent of patients with endometrial cancer (Trelford, 1970), and 25 per cent with breast cancer (Briggs et al, 1967) may show an objective response to various progestins. These overall results are superior to those achieved for renal cancer (16 per cent). In cases of endometrial cancer treated with medroxyprogesterone acetate the objective remission rate was as high as 39 per cent, compared with only 18 per cent for breast cancer (Briggs et al, 1967). Perhaps other progestins may be more successful for renal cancer than medroxyprogesterone acetate.

NEWER HORMONAL AGENTS

The strain of hamster renal tumour transplant used in our laboratory was independent of administered oestrogen but still influenced by the presence of endogenous oestrogen (Bloom et al, 1963b). This tumour was markedly inhibited by oestrogen-antagonists such as U-11, 100A, a diphenyldihydronaphthalene derivative (Bloom et al, 1967). The antitumour effect of this compound can be largely abolished by the simultaneous administration of oestradiol. A few cases of advanced metastatic renal cancer who failed to respond to medroxyprogesterone acetate and to testosterone propionate have been treated with U-11, 100A, but without clinical benefit, although this agent is capable of producing tumour regression in some cases of breast cancer.

ENDOCRINE ABLATION THERAPY

Castration and also adrenalectomy each have an inhibitory effect on the transplanted hamster renal tumour (Bloom et al, 1963b). Could endocrine ablation procedures be of value in selected patients with metastatic renal cancer in whom hormone treatment has either failed from the outset, or is no longer controlling the disease? Orchidectomy has been performed in only two of our patients and pituitary ablation, using radioactive gold grains, in another, but no benefit followed these procedures. Further observations in this field would seem warranted.

TISSUE CULTURE STUDIES

Isolated tumours in tissue culture may create a too-artificial situation to be of much value in the field of cancer investigation. The situation, however, seems to be less unnatural when tumour cells and their stroma are allowed to coexist in organ culture, and some interesting observations with experimental hormone-dependent tumours have already been made using this system. Algard (1960), for example, has shown that the dependent oestrogen-induced renal tumour of the hamster grows well in dispersed cell culture without the addition of oestrogen to the medium. On the other hand, successful organ culture of this tumour can only be accomplished in the presence of oestrogen. As Algard points out, these observations suggest that renal tumour-dependency is at tissue level and that the action of hormones on tumour induction and growth is a direct one, and not indirect through other endocrine organs. It also suggests that hormone dependency is related to the maintenance of normal tissue architecture: with destruction of the tissue the released tumour cells attain hormone independency.

Tchao et al (1968) at this Institute are using organ culture techniques to screen various hormonal preparations against renal carcinoma by measuring the inhibition of tritiated thymidine incorporated into DNA and the degree of degeneration seen in ordinary histological sections. In this way, it is hoped to find the most effective hormonal preparation with which to start treatment in a particular patient. Many technical difficulties have been overcome but there remains, as always, the problem of obtaining a viable piece of tissue with which to attempt in vitro growth from a tumour which so frequently shows areas of spontaneous degeneration.

Of 13 specimens submitted to Dr Tchao, 7 were unsuitable for culture or poorly maintained. In the remaining 6 specimens hydrocortisone appeared to stimulate the culture relative to the controls. Medroxyprogesterone acetate and testosterone each caused inhibition in two cases. It was interesting that stilboestrol inhibited 5 of 6 specimens, recalling the effect of stilboestrol on renal tumour transplants in the hamster. In contrast to the lack of specificity of chemotherapeutic drugs (alkylating agents and antimetabolites) observed in these tissue culture studies, hormones were selective, affecting only a proportion of cases. Furthermore, in these cases no harmful effects were observed with hormones on normal renal tissue controls (Tchao et al, 1968).

To date, there have been too few tissue culture studies from cases treated for metastatic renal cell carcinoma with hormonal agents to permit correlation between in vitro and clinical response. More work needs to be done in this interesting field, especially since hormonal agents appear to act directly on renal tumour cells, while sparing normal kidney tissue.

CONCLUSION

On the basis of our material at the Royal Marsden Hospital and in six other reports from the literature, there seems little doubt that a limited number of renal cell carcinomas can be influenced by hormone therapy, and that this treatment may occasionally offer a new lease of life for a limited period to seriously ill patients, even in old age. Hormone therapy seems to benefit 1 in 5 or 6 patients. In some other cases the degree of regression is not significant, or clinical improvement only transitory. Our experience indicates that striking improvement may occur within four weeks of starting treatment and, with continued high-dose treatment, last for up to three years. A striking response was observed in one of our patients treated with testosterone after exacerbation of the disease occurred during medroxyprogesterone acetate administration. Most responses have been achieved with progestins, chiefly medroxyprogesterone acetate. Other preparations in this class may also be effective. Corticosteroids often improve well-being but produce no significant objective response.

Spontaneous regression is not the explanation for the well-marked objective response seen in 13 of our 80 treated cases, nor in those reported in the literature. If, indeed, this phenomenon was responsible for the changes observed, then its incidence in renal cell cancer must be far greater than is at present generally appreciated. Incidentally, the occurrence of spontaneous regression in renal cancer would seem to favour rather than detract from the concept of hormone dependency in this disease, especially as the process of natural improvement also appears to be sex-related, 80 per cent of such cases being male.

Although the overall response rate in our hormone-treated cases and in those reported in the literature has been limited to about 16 per cent, a higher proportion of cases in selected groups have benefited from therapy. For example, after excluding deaths within six weeks of commencing treatment, the response rate in men was 27 per cent. Perhaps with new progestational preparations, other hormonal compounds or a combination of agents, a greater number of worthwhile responses will be achieved.

ACKNOWLEDGEMENTS

Some illustrations from the author's previous publications have been reproduced by kind permission of Messrs. Livingstone and Co. (Figures 18.2A, B and 18.4A, B), Messrs. Little Brown and Co. (Figure 18.3A), the Editor of the *British Journal of Cancer* (Figure 18.5C) and the Editor of the *British Medical Journal* (Figures 18.6A-D). The author also wishes to thank Mr. K. Morman of the Photographic Department, Royal Marsden Hospital and the Institute of Cancer Research for Plates 18.1 and 18.2.

References

Algard, F. T. (1960) Hormone-induced tumours: Hamster flank organ and kidney tumours in vitro. *Journal of the National Cancer Institute*, **25**, 557.

Bergsjö, P. (1965) Progesterone and progestational compounds in treatment of advanced endometrial carcinoma. *Acta endocrinologica (København)*, **49**, 412.

Bloom, H. J. G. (1964) Hormone treatment of renal tumours: experimental and clinical observations. In *Tumours of the Kidney and Ureter*, p. 311, ed. Riches, E. W. London: Livingstone.

Bloom, H. J. G. (1967a) Treatment of renal cell carcinoma with steroid hormones: observations with transplanted tumours in the hamster and incurable cancer in man. In *Renal Neoplasia*, p. 605, ed. King, J. S. Boston: Little, Brown.

Bloom, H. J. G. (1967b) The kidney. In *Prevention of Cancer*, p. 226, ed. Raven, R. W. and Roe, F. J. C. London: Butterworths.

Bloom, H. J. G. (1970) Unpublished observations.

Bloom, H. J. G. (1971) Medroxyprogesterone (Provera) in treatment of metastatic renal cancer. *British Journal of Cancer*, **25**, 250.

Bloom, H. J. G. & Riddle, P. R. (1971). To be published.

Bloom, H. J. G. & Stephens, E. (1968). Unpublished observations.

Bloom, H. J. G. & Wallace, D. M. (1964) Hormones and the kidney; possible therapeutic role of testosterone in a patient with regression of metastases from renal adenocarcinoma. *British Medical Journal*, **ii**, 476.

Bloom, H. J. G., Dukes, C. E. & Mitchley, B. C. V. (1963a) Hormone-dependent tumours of the kidney. I. The oestrogen-induced renal tumour of the Syrian hamster. Hormone treatment and possible relationship to carcinoma of the kidney in man. *British Journal of Cancer*, **17**, 611.

Bloom, H. J. G., Baker, W. H., Dukes, C. E. & Mitchley, B. C. V. (1963b) Hormone-dependent tumours of the kidney. II. Effect of endocrine ablation procedures on the transplanted oestrogen-induced renal tumour of the Syrian hamster. *British Journal of Cancer*, **17**, 646.

Bloom, H. J. G., Roe, F. J. C. & Mitchley, B. C. V. (1967) Sex hormones and renal neoplasia: inhibition of tumour of hamster kidney by an oestrogen-antagonist, an agent of possible therapeutic value in man. *Cancer*, **20**, 2118.

Bonte, J., Decoster, J. M. & Ide, P. (1970) Radiosensitization of endometrial adenocarcinoma by medroxyprogesterone. *Cancer*, **25**, 907.

Briggs, M. H., Caldwell, A. D. S. & Pitchford, A. G. (1967) The treatment of cancer by progestogens. *Hospital Medicine*, **2**, 63.

C.C.N.S.C. Cooperative Breast Cancer Group (1964) Results of studies 1961–1963. *Cancer Chemotherapy Reports*, **41**, Suppl. 1, 1.

Cobb, L., Bloom, H. J. G., Roe, F. J. C. & MacKenzie, H. M. (1971) Rupture of the aorta produced in the hamster by anti-ovulatory progestogens. *Nature (London)*, **229**, 50.

Crowley, L. G. & MacDonald, I. (1965) Delalutin and oestrogens for treatment of advanced mammary carcinoma in postmenopausal women. *Cancer*, **18**, 346.

Everson, T. C. & Cole, W. M. (1966) *Spontaneous Regression of Cancer*. Philadelphia: W. B., Saunders, p. 11.

Flocks, R. H. & Kadesky, M. C. (1958) Malignant neoplasms of the kidney: analysis of 353 patients followed for five years or more. *Journal of Urology*, **79**, 196.

Ghaleb, H. A. (1961) The metabolism of stilboestrol and the diphosphate ester in relation to treatment of carcinoma of the prostate. Ph.D. Thesis, University of London.

Glenn, J. F. (1967) Speculation on genesis, therapeusis and prognosis of nephrocarcinoma. In *Renal Neoplasia*, p. 535, ed. King, J. S. Boston: Little, Brown.

Hajdu, S. I. & Thomas, A. G. (1967) Renal cell carcinoma at autopsy. *Journal of Urology*, **97**, 978.

Horning, E. (1956) Endocrine factors involved in the induction, prevention and transplantation of kidney tumours in the male Golden Hamster. *Zeitschrift für Krebsforschung*, **61**, 1.

Huggins, C., Moon, R. C. & Morii, S. (1962) Extinction of experimental mammary cancer. I. Oestradiol 17β and progesterone. *Proceedings of the National Academy of Sciences of the USA*, **48**, 379.

Inman, W. H. W., Vessey, M. P., Westerholm, B. & Engelund, A. (1970) Thromboembolic disease and the steroidal content of oral contraceptives. A report to the Committee on Safety of Drugs. *British Medical Journal*, **i**, 203.

Jasmin & Riopelle, J. L. (1970) Nephroblastomas induced in ovariectomised rats by dimethylbenzanthracene. *Cancer Research*, **30**, 321.

Jasmin & Riopelle, J. L. (1964) Facteurs influant sur la production de tumeurs rénales chez le rat par le dimethylnitrosamine. *Review of Canadian Biology*, **23**, 129.

Jelliffe, A. M. (1964) Chemotherapy of renal tumours in the adult. In *Tumours of the Kidney and Ureter*, p. 339, ed. Riches, E. W. London: Livingstone.

Jenkin, R. D. T. (1967) Androgens in metastatic renal adenocarcinoma. *British Medical Journal*, **i**, 361.

Kay, S. (1968) Renal carcinoma, a 10-year study. *American Journal of Clinical Pathology*, **50**, 428.

Kirkman, H. (1959) *Estrogen-induced Tumours of the Kidney*. National Cancer Institute Monograph No. 1. Washington, US: Government Printing Office.

Kistner, R. W., Griffiths, C. T. & Craig, J. M. (1965) Use of progestational agents in management of endometrial cancer. *Cancer*, **18**, 1563.

Klimpel, K. (1957) Spontanheilung eines hypernephroms nach nephrektomie durch mehrfache ausscheidung von geschwulstgeweke aus dem darmkanal. *Zeitschrift für Urologie*, **50**, 201.

Kraicer, J. & Logothetopoulos, J. (1962) Correlation of anterior pituitary morphology with thyroid function after 6α-methyl-17α-hydroxyprogesterone acetate. *Endocrinology*, **71**, 660.

Lerner, L. J. (1964) Hormone antagonists: inhibitors of specific activities of estrogen and androgen. *Recent Progress in Hormone Research*, **20**, 435.

Logothetopoulos, J., Sharma, B. B. & Kraicer, J. (1961) Effects produced in rats by administration of 6α-methyl-17α-hydroxyprogesterone acetate from birth to maturity. *Endocrinology*, **68**, 417.

Macdonald, R. R. (1970) The clinical pharmacology of medroxyprogesterone acetate. *Upjohn Symposium on Provera in Treatment of some Malignancies*. In press.

Matthews, V. S., Kirkman, H. & Bacon, R. L. (1947) Kidney damage in golden hamster following chronic administration of diethylstilboestrol in sesame oil. *Proceedings of the Society for Experimental Biology and Medicine*, **66**, 195.

Melander, O., Notter, G. & Schreeb, T. von (1967) Hormone treatment of metastasizing renal cancer. *Nordisk. Medicin*, **78**, 1309.

Middleton, R. G. (1967) The value of surgery in metastatic renal cell carcinoma. In *Renal Neoplasia*, p. 483, ed. King, J. S. Boston: Little, Brown.

Mims, M. M., Christensen, B., Schlumberger, F. C. & Goodwin, W. E. (1966) A 10-year evaluation of nephrectomy for extensive renal cell carcinoma. *Journal of Urology*, **95**, 10.

Mostofi, F. K. (1967) Pathology and spread of renal cell carcinoma. In *Renal Neoplasia*, p. 41, ed. King, J. S. Boston: Little, Brown.

Paine, C. H., Wright, F. W. & Ellis, F. (1970) The use of progestogen in treatment of metastatic carcinoma of kidney and uterine body. *British Journal of Cancer*, **24**, 277.

Rafla, S. (1970) Renal cell carcinoma. Natural history and results of treatment. *Cancer*, **25**, 26.

Riches, E. W. (1963) On carcinoma of the kidney. *Annals of the Royal College of Surgeons of England*, **32**, 201.

Richardson, F. L. (1957) Incidence of mammary and pituitary tumours in hybrid mice treated with stilboestrol for varying periods. *Journal of the National Cancer Institute*, **18**, 813.

Royce, R. & Tormey, A. (1955) Malignant tumours of the renal parenchyma in adults. *Journal of Urology*, **74**, 23.

Samuels, M. L., Sullivan, P. & Howe, C. D. (1968) Medroxyprogesterone acetate in treatment of renal cell carcinoma. *Cancer*, **22**, 525.

Sherman, A. I. (1966) Progesterone caproate in treatment of endometrial cancer. *Obstetrics and Gynecology*, **28**, 309.

Stoll, B. A., Andrews, J. T. & Motteram, R. (1966) Liver damage from oral contraceptives. *British Medical Journal*, **i**, 960.

Swanson, M. K. & Holmes, F. F. (1970) Renal cell carcinoma: an endocrine-influenced tumour—analysis of 243 cases. *Journal of the Kansas Medical Society*, **71**, 109.

Talley, R. W., Moorhead, E. L., Tucker, W. G., San Diego, E. L. & Brennan, M. J. (1969) Treatment of metastatic hypernephroma. *Journal of the American Medical Association*, **207**, 322.

Tchao, R., Easty, G. C., Ambrose, E. J., Raven, R. W. & Bloom, H. J. G. (1968) Effect of chemotherapeutic agents and hormones on organ cultures of human tumours. *European Journal of Cancer*, **4**, 39.

Trelford, J. D. (1970) A discussion of results of chemotherapy on gynecological cancer and host's immune response. *6th National Cancer Conference Proceedings, Denver, September 1968*, p. 365. Philadelphia: Lippincott.

Von Schreeb, T. (1967) Renal adenocarcinoma: clinical problems with special reference to preoperative evaluation of malignancy. *Acta Chirurgica Scandinavica*, Suppl. 381.

Whisenand, J. M., Kostas, D. & Sommers, S. C. (1962) Some host factors in development of renal cell carcinoma. *Western Journal of Surgery, Obstetrics and Gynecology*, **70**, 284.

Woodruff, M. W., Wagle, D., Gailani, S. D. & Jones, R. (1967) The current status of chemotherapy for advanced renal carcinoma. *Journal of Urology*, **97**, 611.

Chapter 19

Thyroid Cancer

GEORGE CRILE, JR

In 1951 Purves, Griesbach and Kennedy reported the induction of autonomous cancers in the rat's thyroid by feeding thiouracil. The hypothyroidism induced by the thiouracil increased the output of the thyroid-stimulating hormone of the pituitary (TSH) and the rats' thyroids underwent hypertrophy and hyperplasia. Later adenomas began to form, and then well-differentiated metastasising carcinomas. At first these were transplantable only into rats with hypothyroidism, but later they became more anaplastic and could be transplanted into normal rats. In the words of Purves and his associates, 'The existence of hormonal imbalance over a period of years may provide the stimulus to the growth of a primary benign tumour from which a malignant variant is derived, which itself shows no dependence upon hormonal stimulus.'

Furth (1953) reviewed the literature on conditioned or endocrine-dependent neoplasms and concluded that the dependent ones are often but stages in the development of autonomous tumours. Yet these two types of tumours are 'so basically different as to required different approaches for control: one (for dependent neoplasms) to restore the disturbed equilibrium in the host, the other (for autonomous neoplasms) to destroy the altered cell'.

Clinically is has long been known that many goitres regress in response to thyroid feeding (Greer and Astwood, 1953) and that there is little or no relationship between the function of the nodules (as demonstrated by their ability to take up ^{131}I) and their response to thyroid (Zondek and Leszvnsky, 1956).

The first cases in which papillary cancer of the thyroid regressed in response to suppression with thyroid were reported in 1937 by Sir Thomas Dunhill. At that time the concept of the endocrine dependency of cancershadt not been clarified. Dunhill concluded, 'There is much that we do not yet know about cancer of the thyroid and proliferation of thyroid epithelium but I cannot help thinking that hyperplasia in response to demand or

369

stimulation can closely approach the appearances which simulate malignancy.'

In a personal communication, Sir Thomas gave me the history of one of the three patients whose carcinomas regressed in response to thyroid feeding. 'My third patient was sent to me from South Africa 17 years ago. She had had lymph glands removed from the neck and part of the thyroid removed. I removed a gland and had it examined microscopically. It showed papillary carcinoma of thyroid origin. X-ray examination of the chest showed what has been called "snow-flake" deposits throughout both lungs. I have films of these. After treatment with desiccated thyroid the "snow-flake" deposits completely disappeared. The patient has married, has children, and lives an active sporting life.'

The details of the literature on regression of thyroid tumours in man and animals have been summarised in a previous report (Crile, 1957) along with the experience of the Cleveland Clinic prior to 1957. The following material represents an updated report of a now more lengthy and extensive experience with endocrine-dependent tumours of the thyroid.

EXPERIENCE IN THE CONTROL OF PAPILLARY CANCER OF THE THYROID BY THYROID FEEDING

Although we have seen several adenocarcinomas and one medullary carcinoma of the thyroid whose growth appeared to be arrested for a few years by giving three grains of desiccated thyroid (or its equivalent in thyroxine) no permanent control has been obtained in any variety of cancer other than the papillary. The anaplastic carcinomas have shown no response at all, nor have those tall-cell papillary carcinomas that are practically devoid of colloid and which occur almost exclusively in patients beyond mid-life, predominantly in men.

The responses of the usual type of papillary carcinoma and its follicular variants (with or without abundant colloid), are variable but not unpredictable. The best regressions and the most consistent arrests of tumour growth are obtained in females between the age of puberty and 40 years of age. Most of the patients in this age-sex group, which fortunately includes more than half of all patients with papillary carcinoma, have tumours which respond satisfactorily to suppression.

The response, once established, lasts as long as thyroid hormone is given. In patients followed for as long as 27 years, there has been no tendency for the tumour to regain autonomy as occurs in the case of breast cancer. The exception to this observation is the rare case where a totally new tumour arises, and this is almost always in patients who have had previous irradiation, either external, or with [131]I. In patients with multiple cervical node and pulmonary metastases which have remained static for many years, a single node has suddenly developed an undifferentiated appearance histologically, and has progressed to fatal anaplastic cancer.

It is difficult to estimate the efficacy of suppressive therapy when it is given routinely after operation to prevent recurrences, but since 1954, when we began to give suppressive doses of thyroid routinely after operation, the incidence of recurrence in nodes decreased by more than 50 per cent. In the period 1937 through 1954 in which thyroid was not given, 17 of the 76 patients (22 per cent) whose first definitive treatment was given at the Cleveland Clinic developed recurrences and were subjected to a second operation, whereas in the period 1954 through 1964 only 14 of 155 (9 per cent) were reoperated. Likewise the incidence of death from cancer in the entire group of primary and secondary cases fell from 12 of 102 (12 per cent) to 6 of 190 (3 per cent).

The most dramatic proof of the efficacy of suppression by feeding thyroid is found in the patients with the most unfavourable types of cancers; that is, those that were inoperable or had distant metastases. There were 32 such patients, 25 of them with pulmonary metastases. Eighteen of these have responded to treatment with thyroid and are living and well for 5 to 27 years (median 13 years) with regression or no progress of their disease. In the other 14 patients the cancer progressed in spite of adequate suppression. Eleven of the latter died of cancer in 4 to 9 years (median 6 years), and three are still living with advancing disease at 6, 9 and 15 years respectively.

is the difference in the ages of the patients in the two chronological groups and the prevalence of a history of irradiation in the responders. Prior to the 1920s radiation was rarely given to children for benign disorders such as a supposedly enlarged thymus, large tonsils or adenoids, non-specific lymphadenopathy or dermatitis. The median age of the patients with papillary carcinomas seen at the Cleveland Clinic in the decade 1926 through 1935 was 48, a figure similar

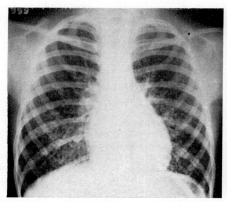 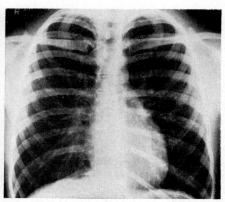

FIGURE 19.1. Chest radiographs of boy aged nine, whose thymus was irradiated in infancy. Showing diffuse snowflake metastases of papillary carcinoma of thyroid which disappeared after treatment with thyroid.

There are differences in the composition of the responders and non-responders in respect to age, sex and a history of irradiation. Twelve of 18 responders were female as compared to 5 of 14 non-responders. The median age of the responders was 23 and that of the non-responders 51. Twelve of the 18 responders gave a definite history of irradiation compared with none of the non-responders. Of the 18 responders 15 had involvement of lungs, and 3 had inoperable cancers in the neck. In 13 of the responders the metastases disappeared or showed striking and sustained regression, while in the other 5 there was no growth of the metastases over long periods of observation (minimum 5 years). Ten of the non-responders had pulmonary metastases, 2 had local recurrences, and 2 had bony metastasis.

The most striking feature of the analysis

to the median ages of patients with other types of cancer. The youngest patient with papillary carcinoma seen in this period was 21 years old. However, in the next 15 years the median age fell to 33 and the youngest patient was only 3 years old. At the same time the incidence of papillary carcinoma, both absolute and in relation to that of other types of thyroid cancer nearly trebled. This was almost certainly the result of irradiation given in childhood which was common in the 1920s and 1930s. The majority of the patients in the second group gave a history of having been irradiated (Figure 19.1).

These observations are important because they enable the physician to select a group of young patients (particularly young women whose disease followed exposure of the thyroid to radiation) whose cancers, although they have already metastasised widely to lymph nodes, will respond well to suppressive doses of thyroid.

The incidence of recurrence in lymph nodes after operation would be considerably less than that here reported if one were to exclude nodes that became palpable as a result of cystic change. In patients who are given thyroid prophylactically more than a third of the nodes that enlarge after neck dissections are found to be cystic and filled with brown fluid rather than cellular. The administration of thyroid does not suppress the tendency to cystic change, a process that is essentially benign.

In summary, the Cleveland Clinic's experience with suppressing the growth of thyroid cancer indicates that it is only the papillary variety occurring in patients under 40 years of age whose growth is likely to be arrested by suppressive doses of thyroid. Women are more apt to react favourably than men and the best results are obtained consistently in the patients whose cancers were induced by irradiation in infancy or childhood. In this group the incidence of recurrence in the cervical nodes and of death from distant spread of cancer is so reduced by thyroid feeding that it seems unwise to employ radical operations that alter the contour of the neck or inflict morbidity. Even if the larynx, trachea or recurrent nerves appear to be invaded by cancer it is better, in this group, to try conservative therapy before sacrificing important structures. Even when pulmonary metastases are present, treatment with thyroid may cause regression which is maintained as long as the thyroid is given, 27 years being the longest period of follow-up in this series.

THE DANGER THAT RADIATION AND HYPOTHYROIDISM MAY RESULT IN DEDIFFERENTIATION OF PAPILLARY INTO ANAPLASTIC CANCER

As Purves and his associates (1951) pointed out 20 years ago, well-differentiated and endocrine-dependent thyroid tumours in rats may progress under the influence of an excess of TSH into autonomous anaplastic cancers. The same seems true of the papillary cancers in human beings, for in a previous communication (Crile, 1957) I have collected 19 patients in whom such transitions took place usually associated with a combination of hypothyroidism and irradiation, either external or as a result of treatment with [131]I. Since this publication, Frazell and Foote (1958) have reported a number of additional patients in whose cancers this transition took place. The results are uniformly fatal.

REPORT OF A CASE

A woman 22 years old stated that she had had two nodules in the side of her neck for the past six years. They had enlarged slowly, and had been thought to be tuberculous nodes. She had been given four roentgen ray treatments to the cervical nodes one month apart, each treatment consisting of 30 per cent of an 'erythema dose'. There had been no change in the size of the nodes. In June 1926 the largest of the nodules was removed, and proved to be papillary tumour of the thyroid. At this time it was classified as an 'aberrant thyroid adenoma'. The patient refused further treatment, and was not seen again for 13 years, at which time she had nodules in both the lobes of the thyroid, the larger 'the size of a plum', and smaller nodules were palpable in both lateral cervical regions. She again refused operation.

In 1953, 34 years after the nodules had first been noticed, the left vocal cord became paralysed. A roentgenogram of the chest showed diffuse nodular metastatic lesions in the base of both lungs. Tracer studies showed that the metastases were concentrating [131]I. Between September 1953 and January 1955 a total of 210 mCi of ^{131}I was given. In April 1955, roentgenograms showed regression of the metastases. The patient became myxoedematous and in February 1955 the patient was given desiccated thyroid in doses of 2 grains daily, later increased to 3 grains daily. In May 1957, roentgenograms of the chest showed no trace of the metastatic lesion, and palpation of the neck revealed only a small round nodule in the isthmus of the thyroid. In November 1957, 35 months after the last treatment with ^{131}I, the patient noticed a mass in the right supraclavicular region. This grew rapidly, more than doubling its size in the course of a month. In January 1958 an attempt was made to remove it, but it was so fixed and invaded surrounding tissues so extensively that it could not be completely removed. The lateral lobes of the thyroid contained no palpable nodules, but a small midline nodule was removed and proved to be a simple adenoma. The pathologist reported that the tumour that had been partially removed was an undifferentiated carcinoma which bore no resemblance to the tissue removed at the original biopsy. The patient was given cobalt-60 teletherapy with no apparent effect on the growth of the tumour. She died on April 4 1958, 39 years after the first nodule was noticed and five months after the appearance of the undifferentiated carcinoma.

In view of Doniach's observations that neither irradiation nor any of a number of carcinogens was able to induce thyroid cancers in rats protected by thyroid feeding, it is safer as the initial treatment for inoperable cancer to suppress the growth of the tumour by thyroid feeding rather than to induce hypothyroidism by the use of ^{131}I. A second and important reason for employing thyroid first is that several patients have developed leukaemia after receiving large doses of ^{131}I (Abbatt, Farran and Greene, 1956; Blom, Querido and Leeksma, 1955; Pochin, Myant and Corbett, 1956; Seidlin et al, 1956) and fatal fibrosis of the lungs from treatment of diffusely metastasising cancers with ^{131}I has also been reported by Frazell and Foote (1958). Finally, a favourable and permanent response of papillary cancers to thyroid is much more common than complete destruction of the tumours by the radiation from ^{131}I. Any cancer that is enough like normal thyroid tissue to be able to concentrate enough ^{131}I to destroy itself is apt to be enough like thyroid to have its growth arrested by thyroid feeding. ^{131}I has been tried in all patients whose cancers contained colloid and were not controlled by thyroid feeding, but there has been no case in the Cleveland Clinic series in which ^{131}I was effective when suppression with thyroid had failed.

PROBLEMS IN THE ENDOCRINE MANAGEMENT OF THYROID CANCER

WHAT DOSE OF THYROID IS REQUIRED?

The dose of desiccated thyroid required to control the growth of tumours of the thyroid is usually the same regardless of the age, sex or size of the patient. Even a small child requires as much thyroid as an adult to suppress the pituitary. For many years we have used Armour brand desiccated thyroid in doses of 3 grains daily (equivalent to 0·3 mg of thyroxine). Thyroxine is just as effective, but in the United States is a little more expensive. It has the advantage, however, of being more uniform and less apt to deteriorate with the passage of time. In general it can be said that 1 grain of thyroid (or its equivalent in thyroxine) has little effect on the growth of thyroid tumours, 2 grains will keep them from enlarging, and 3 grains will cause them to shrink if they are endocrine-dependent. Occasionally thyroid is not well taken up, and 4 grains is required. Side effects from doses up to 3 grains daily are rare, because there is no more circulating thyroxine at this dose level than is normally present. As a result of pituitary suppression the patient stops making thyroid hormone and lives on a normal level of circulating exogenous thyroid.

HOW LONG DOES IT TAKE FOR OBJECTIVE EVIDENCE OF REGRESSION TO APPEAR?

Evidence of regression as shown by shrinkage of pulmonary metastases or cervical nodes may appear in a month or two, but usually it takes three or four months. Sometimes, of course, there is no regression but merely a cessation of growth, and it may take several years to confirm that this is happening. Occasionally the follicular variants of papillary tumours which contain much colloid may function autonomously and serve to suppress the function of the pituitary. Metastases, therefore, may remain the same size for a long time or indefinitely as a result of a self-induced remission in which the amount of thyroid made autonomously by the tumour suppresses the output of TSH.

HOW LONG DO THE REMISSIONS LAST?

Remissions appear to last indefinitely once they are established. In the case of papillary tumours we have never seen a patient with a clear-cut remission who subsequently, in the face of continuing suppressive therapy, had a recrudescence of the tumour's growth (see p. 370).

WHAT EFFECT DOES HYPOTHYROIDISM HAVE ON THE GROWTH OF THE TUMOUR?

Anything that induces hypothyroidism stimulates the output of TSH and may thus stimulate the growth of endocrine-dependent tumours of the thyroid. Usually any growth so induced is reversible, but as a principle it would be unwise to subject a person with a thyroid cancer to a prolonged period of hypothyroidism. This is especially important in patients who have been subjected to irradiation, for the stimulation of the irradiated cells might cause the tumour to be transformed into an anaplastic cancer.

ARE THERE CASES IN WHICH THE TUMOUR FAILS TO TAKE UP ^{131}I BUT RESPONDS TO THYROID FEEDING?

It is not unusual for tumours which take up no significant amount of ^{131}I to respond well to treatment with desiccated thyroid. The reverse situation, in which tumours do not respond to desiccated thyroid but will take up sufficient ^{131}I to destroy themselves, is extraordinarily rare. I have never seen this situation. For this reason, it is better to start treatment of inoperable cancer by thyroid feeding rather than by treatment with ^{131}I.

WHEN SHOULD THYROID SUBSTANCE BE GIVEN POSTOPERATIVELY?

Thyroid should be given after all operations for nodular goitre, for struma lymphomatosa and for differentiated cancers of the thyroid. It should also be considered routinely following thyroidectomy or ^{131}I for Graves' disease, because even many years after the operation hypothyroidism may develop insidiously, just as it does following treatment with ^{131}I. Treatment with thyroid should be a lifetime programme. Usually 2 grains of desiccated thyroid or its equivalent in thyroxine is sufficient to prevent recurrence.

DOES PROLONGED TREATMENT WITH THYROID EVER STIMULATE THE UPTAKE OF RADIOACTIVE IODINE?

Occasionally a patient is seen in whom a papillary carcinoma which did not take up radioactive iodine prior to treatment with thyroid will begin to function autonomously and to take up radioactive iodine. This reaction is rare, but does occur just as the nodules of some patients with multinodular goitre will occasionally begin to take up thyroid for the first time after the institution of thyroid therapy.

WHAT IS THE EFFECT OF PREGNANCY ON A CANCER OF THE THYROID WHICH HAS BEEN UNDER CONTROL BY THYROID FEEDING?

I have never seen pregnancy stimulate the growth of a papillary carcinoma of the thyroid which was being held in control by thyroid feeding.

DOES THE HISTOLOGY OF PAPILLARY CANCER CHANGE AFTER LONG-TERM THYROID FEEDING?

Occasionally nodes that had not been palpable at the time of an operation become cystic. Histologically the tumour around the cyst is still papillary. In most cases there is no significant change in the degree of differentiation with the passage of time.

DOES THE CONCOMITANT PRESENCE OF STRUMA LYMPHOMATOSA (HASHIMOTO'S DISEASE) ALTER THE PROGNOSIS OF THYROID CANCER?

Microcarcinomas are present in about 4 per cent of all thyroids if serial sections of apparently normal thyroids are made. In Hashimoto's disease it has been reported that the incidence of microcarcinoma is slightly higher. This may be because there is some stimulation of the microcarcinomas' growth due to the hypothyroidism. However, the prognosis in the cases of carcinoma associated with struma lymphomatosa is excellent. They are not numerous enough for me to be able to make a valid statistical statement, but I have never seen anyone with a carcinoma arising in struma lymphomatosa die of this disease.

It is interesting that the commonest clinical tumour to arise in patients with struma lymphomatosa is lymphosarcoma. Because of the possibility that the lymphosarcomas that arise in struma lymphomatosa might be endocrine-dependent as is the struma itself, we have been treating them with desiccated thyroid. Nine of the 15 patients treated with various combinations of surgery and irradiation plus desiccated thyroid were living 15 to 150 months after treatment as compared to 14 of 15 not receiving desiccated thyroid who died in less than 14 months.

CONCLUSION

The role of TSH in the aetiology of thyroid cancer and in the progression to anaplastic cancer is outlined.

In patients under 40 years old and particularly in young females whose tumours follow exposure to irradiation, papillary cancers usually stop growing or regress when the output of TSH is suppressed by feeding thyroid.

Patients who are less than 40 years old, female, and with a history of irradiation therapy for benign disease, respond so favourably to suppressive therapy that mutilating operations entailing permanent morbidity should not be performed until conservative therapy has been tried.

Since hypothyroidism and irradiation of papillary cancers may stimulate them to progression into anaplastic cancers, suppressive therapy should be given a trial before resorting to the use of ^{131}I.

Eighteen of 32 patients with inoperable metastatic papillary carcinoma were treated by thyroid feeding and are well for from 5 to 27 years. In 13 of the 18 responders the metastases have decreased in size or disappeared and in 5 they have remained unchanged.

References

Abbatt, J. D., Farran, H. E. A. & Greene, R. (1956) Acute myeloid leukaemia after radioactive-iodine therapy. *Lancet*, **i**, 782–783.

Blom, P. S., Querido, A. & Leeksma, C. H. W. (1955) Acute leukaemia following X-ray and radioiodine treatment of thyroid carcinoma (Case Reports). *British Journal of Radiology*, **28**, 163–166.

Crile, G. Jr (1957) The endocrine dependency of certain thyroid cancers and the danger that hypothyroidism may stimulate their growth. *Cancer*, **10**, 1119–1137.

Frazell, E. L. & Foote, F. W. Jr (1958) Papillary cancer of the thyroid. A review of 25 years of experience. *Cancer*, **11**, 895–922.

Furth, J. (1953) Conditioned and autonomous neoplasms; review. *Cancer Research*, **13**, 477–492.

Greer, M. A. & Astwood, E. B. (1953) Treatment of simple goitre with thyroid. *Journal of Clinical Endocrinology and Metabolism*, **13**, 1312–1331.

Pochin, E. E., Myant, N. B. & Corbett, B. D. (1956) Leukaemia following radioiodine treatment of hyperthyroidism. *British Journal of Radiology*, **29**, 31–35.

Purves, H. D., Griesbach, W. E. & Kennedy, T. H. (1951) Studies in experimental goitre; malignant change in transplantable rat thyroid tumour. *British Journal of Cancer*, **5**, 301–310.

Seidlin, S. M., Siegel, E., Yalow, A. A. & Melamed, S. (1956) Acute myeloid leukaemia following prolonged iodine-131 therapy for metastatic thyroid carcinoma. *Science*, **123**, 800–801.

Zondek, H. & Leszynsky, H. (1956) Genesis of thyroid adenomas. *Lancet*, **i**, 77–78.

Chapter 20

Malignant Melanoma

D. C. BODENHAM and BRENDAN HALE

There is evidence to suggest that hormonal factors may influence the incidence and possibly also the behaviour of at least a small number of malignant melanomas. While remembering that surgery is the treatment of choice in all potentially curable cases and that radiation may influence a small number, this chapter aims at stimulating thought about other, less familiar aspects of the disease. It is not suggested that endocrine therapy is likely to play a major role in its management, but it has been shown to influence the tumour growth in a few patients.

CHILDHOOD AND THE EFFECT OF PUBERTY

The incidence of malignant melanoma in South West England is 3·5 per 100 000 population, the total population being 3 million. Up to the age of 13, only one proven case has been recorded in this area in the 10 years following 1955 and one further

case arose between the ages of 13 and 15. Thus it is apparent that the chance of a child, in this country, developing a malignant melanoma is very remote.

Between the ages of 15 and 20 the number of either sex affected is also very small, but thereafter the incidence for all sites rises to reach a peak between the ages of 40 and 45 years and then decreases. However, in the case of melanoma of the face, a second peak occurs in the 65 to 70 age group.

The occurrence of a peculiar type of melanoma, first described by Spitz in 1948, is of considerable interest. Though these, too, are rare, they are now widely recognised and account for most of the lesions which used to be labelled 'malignant melanoma' in children of either sex. They occur mostly around puberty and although they have many of the clinical and pathological features of the adult type of malignant melanoma, they behave as benign tumours. It is most unusual for any recurrence to follow strictly local excision.

These tumours may be melanotic or amelanotic, and usually show a fairly intense lymphocytic infiltration with a moderate number of giant cells, probably indicating an active host resistance. It has not yet been possible to obtain sufficient material from these childhood tumours to determine the presence, or otherwise, of specific anti-tumour antibodies. In adults, tumours with similar cellular response have been shown to possess such antibodies. There is no obvious explanation as to why these lesions should occur during or shortly after puberty apart from hormonal factors. This type may eventually prove to be a virus-induced tumour, behaving rather like the verruca vulgaris which occurs at the same age, shows a similar reaction and is strongly antigenic.

The rarely occurring true malignant melanoma of childhood appears to have a worse prognosis than its adult counterpart, but there are occasional survivors.

PREGNANCY AND PARTURITION

The highest incidence for malignant melanoma coincides with the childbearing period of a woman's life. It became widely believed that pregnancy influenced both the incidence and course of the disease. Now that many workers (White, 1959, Bodenham, 1968; Lee, 1970) have been able to review larger series, it has been possible to put this aspect of the disease in perspective. There is no evidence from the overall available figures that a pregnant woman carries any added risk of developing a malignant melanoma, but this statement does need further analysis.

Isolated accounts of cases (Allen, 1955) confirm that in rare instances a melanoma developing during pregnancy goes on to spontaneous regression after parturition. In a remarkable case (Boyd, 1957) a melanoma regressed during successive pregnancies and disappeared, but recurred to lead to a fatal issue 10 years after first diagnosis. There are also reports of melanomas moving rapidly to a fatal issue during pregnancy (Conybeare,

1964). In his authoritative paper on 'Marriage and Fatal Malignant Melanomas in Females' (Lee, 1970) states, 'the current observation rules out the possibility that pregnancy is an important influence on the bulk of malignant melanomas. There is room for it to have a major effect on a small fraction of the total cases'.

These unusual cases are not sufficiently numerous to affect the overall survival figures but, because they illustrate that pregnancy can have an effect either way in a small minority, they make it difficult to give advice. In our view, the patient who has had an extensive lesion treated within the previous five years and is progressing well, should be advised not to have a pregnancy. On the other hand, the patient who strongly desires a child and had a slowly growing, small, flat lesion excised more than five years previously and appears recurrence-free, might wish to accept the apparently small risk.

The management of the pregnant patient with melanoma can raise many individual difficulties. The patient who is nearing term, in whom the same operation can be performed as for a non-pregnant patient, presents no great problem. On the other hand, one might feel strongly inclined to advise termination of a three months' pregnancy in a woman whose disease appears to be rapidly progressing. Whenever possible, the surgical management must be the same as for the non-pregnant patient.

CONTRACEPTION

It might be noted that the Family Planning Association (1970) mentions that the contraceptive pill is not advised for patients with carcinoma of the breast and malignant melanoma if a raised level of circulating oestrogens is thought undesirable. Therefore, for the woman who has had this disease apparently successfully treated, it would seem advisable for her to use some other method of contraception and avoid disturbing the hormone balance.

VARIATION IN SURVIVAL RATE ACCORDING TO SEX

The survival of females with malignant melanoma is significantly better than for males as is clearly shown in Figure 20.1 for cases in South West England.

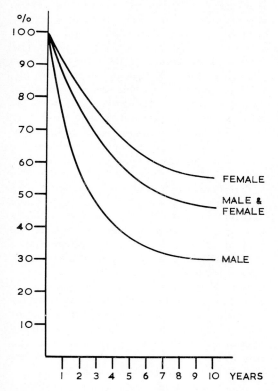

FIGURE 20.1. Ten-year percentage survival curve for 18 patients with malignant melanoma. Male and female survival compared.

Other workers (White, 1959; Olsen, 1966) have made the same observation. While there are wide variations in prognosis between various anatomical sites, the female preserves her advantages over the male in all comparable areas. Olsen (1966) felt that the female advantage was lost once the disease became disseminated, but in our own series most of the long-term survivors even with disseminated disease have been women.

SPONTANEOUS REGRESSION

Spontaneous regression has attracted a great deal of attention in the literature. Undoubtedly malignant melanoma by reason of its appearances and mode of spread makes it a relatively easy lesion to observe in many persons. Spontaneous regression, if it occurs, is likely to be noticed, and there is some evidence that this disease occasionally does regress.

Everson and Cole (1966) have collected all cases in the literature where this is said to have occurred. The incidence of such regression is low and in at least half the cases it is unrelated to any known event in the patient's history. Some cases have been reported where the primary tumour fades as secondaries develop. This is difficult to explain.

In some instances there is recorded a significant event such as an infection which has been followed by regression. Coley, as long ago as 1893, considered the idea of introducing streptococcal and other infections in a deliberate attempt to control the disease. Smallpox vaccination has again been used in the last few years (Milton, 1963) and is reported to lead to necrosis of each successfully vaccinated deposit. It does not however appear to produce regression of deep lesions or of those not locally vaccinated.

Incomplete surgical removal has also been followed by disappearance of the rest of the tumour and an example was a case of one of the authors (Bodenham, 1968). In attempting a radical neck node dissection in a female patient, the growth was found to be deeply fixed and involving vital structures. Removal was known to be incomplete yet she has remained fit and well for 22 years. It seems hardly likely that in every successfully treated case the surgeon has effected a complete removal of all tumour tissue in the body. Defence mechanisms must play their role in many instances unless the rate of tumour growth is remarkably slow.

HORMONE SENSITIVITY ASSESSMENT

The history does occasionally give a guide to hormonal influences on these tumours. Factors such as the rapid change in size of a lesion at the time of the menopause, during pregnancy or at times of menstrual periods should be noted. Bone deposits, or intra-cranial secondaries may cause pain or head-aches particularly at these times.

There is a great need for universally applicable tests to detect hormone sensitivity, and we have had a limited degree of success using a Geiger probe technique as described for breast cancer (Hale, 1961). The technique necessitates the presence of accessible tumour, which is actively growing and of firm con-sistency. The latter is often absent in malig-nant melanoma where friability and necrosis is often present. It is hoped that the develop-ment of solid-state surface counters now under way might broaden the scope of cases to which this technique can be applied.

The probe test has been used only on disseminated cases for fear of spreading the disease but surface counters may well overcome this risk. The lesions will still need to be superficial in order to pick up adequate radiation from the tracer isotope.

GEIGER PROBE TEST

Suitable lesions are selected and also a control point, such as the abdominal wall, in an area clear of growth. The Geiger probes (developed in our department of Medical Physics together with 20th Century Elec-tronics) measure 3 mm in diameter and have an active recording portion of 1 cm length. A coaxial lead is bonded to the thin steel outer case and linked to a small coaxial socket. This leads to a ratemeter and con-tinous recorder.

The technique of insertion is of paramount importance. A local or general anaesthetic is used and a track made in to the tumour, of just sufficient diameter to take the counter. The growth centre must be avoided as it is often necrotic and leads to an unreliable recording. If possible, counters are inserted into more than one lesion and also a control point. They are sutured by 28-day catgut and the leads fixed so as to prevent movement of the probes within the tumours. The counters must not be loose as this will cause false readings due to inverse square law effects. About four hours after insertion a tracer dose of 750 μCi of phosphorus-32 (^{32}P) is given (to adult patients) by mouth. The uptake in the tumour is then recorded con-tinuously. Once a baseline tracing is ob-tained for three or four days, stilboestrol 15 mg is given orally thrice daily and the effect on counter rate noted. A rise indicates that the growth is oestrogen stimulated, and a fall that it is being inhibited by oestrogens possibly acting via the pituitary axis.

A tracing which does not significantly alter (when allowance is made for normal physical and biological decay of the isotope) suggests that the oestrogen has not influenced the tumour growth. It has been shown that a rising curve due to oestrogen administration can be reversed after some days of androgen administration. In general, stimulation of growth is apparent within 24 hours, whereas inhibition by oestrogen may not be apparent for three to four days. If there is no evidence of stimulation then it appears worthwhile to continue the oestrogens for several further days before regarding them as ineffective.

Other hormones, such as norethisterone acetate (SH 420 Schering) 10 mg three times daily have also been employed in a small number of patients. While it must be emphasised that the number of individuals showing response to hormone therapy is very few, the following examples are worthy of note.

CASE NO. 1

A female of 95 years with multiple swellings had one on the left thigh which was ulcerated. Surface counting with an end-window Geiger counter suggested stimula-tion by oestrogens, and therefore in spite of her age, transphenoidal hypophysectomy was performed. For three weeks there appeared no change but then the leg lesions began to regress rapidly. After two months the ulcer had healed and all observable lesions had disappeared. She remained free from any signs of the disease for seven months when she died from heart failure and senility. In order to record response, plaster casts were made of her legs and are reproduced here to illustrate the change after an interval of two months (Figure 20.2).

(phenylalanine mustard) given intravenously at point MEL. At points N.E.A., norethisterone acetate 10 mg (SH 420 Schering) was given orally and followed by a marked decrease in count rate. As oestrogens had stimulated the tumour, he was treated with androgens in the form of testosterone phenylpropionate 100 mg by intramuscular injection three times weekly. This produced marked regression of many visible and palpable masses, but some failed to show any change and he was then maintained on oral androgens.

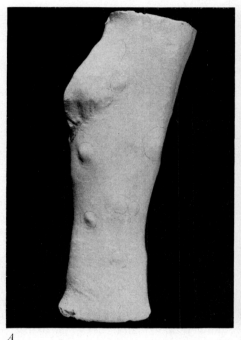 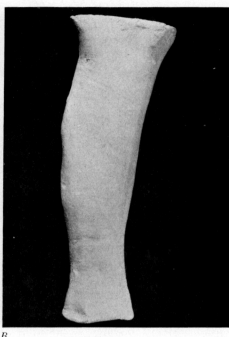

A   *B*

FIGURE 20.2. Plaster cast of left leg in patient with multiple nodules of metastatic malignant melanoma, *A* before hypophysectomy, *B* after hypophysectomy.

CASE NO. 2

A female patient who showed evidence of hormone influence in the tumour during the Geiger probe test, similarly underwent hypophysectomy. After a few weeks, her multiple cutaneous tumours disappeared for a period of nine months but she then developed disseminated disease which rapidly proved fatal.

CASE NO. 3

A male patient aged 39 years, produced the following tracing in the ^{32}P uptake of his tumour (Figure 20.3).

This was interpreted as showing a marked stimulation by oestrogens, given at points marked STB. There had previously been no response to 25 mg melphalan

After three months he was readmitted with active disease and the tumour uptake of ^{32}P was repeated. This again revealed a marked drop in activity after giving testosterone by injection. Again there was marked improvement but a month later he died from haemorrhage into a necrotic cerebral metastasis. This is of course a well-recognised cause of death in this disease.

CASE NO. 4

A female patient aged 64 years, with postsurgical recurrences in the form of multiple cutaneous and gland deposits beyond all forms of radical treatment, was given ethinyloestradiol 1 mg daily. There was dramatic resolution of her deposits after a month and

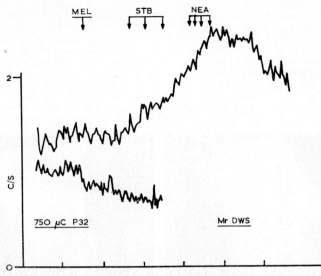

FIGURE 20.3. ^{32}P uptake of tumour in case 3, given melphalan, stilboestrol and norethisterone acetate successively.

she has remained recurrence-free and in good health on this hormone for 10 years, up to this date.

In all, 26 cases were studied by means of the Geiger probe test and four showed evidence of hormone sensitivity in their melanomas. The authors feel certain that this proportion of responsive cases is a falsely high one, as cases were often referred for testing because their histories suggested possible hormonal influences on their tumours.

The number of patients likely to derive benefit from hormone therapy, or hormone-depriving surgery, at present seems to be very few. A more widely applicable test to detect such patients would be helpful. This chapter has been concerned with 'possibilities' and aimed at stimulating thought about the more unusual aspects of this malignancy.

CONCLUSION

Evidence to suggest that endocrine factors influence malignant melanoma includes:

The disease is extremely rare before puberty.

Alteration in growth pattern has been noted at puberty, the menopause, in pregnancy and at times of menstruation.

In the series by Bodenham, females with disseminated disease survive significantly longer than males. These particular females have been found to have active antibody mechanisms.

A small number of male and female patients have responded favourably to alterations in their hormone environment.

References

Allen, E. P. (1955) Spontaneous regression after pregnancy. *British Medical Journal*, **ii**, 1067.

Bodenham, D. C. (1968) A study of 650 observed malignant melanomas. *Annals of the Royal College of Surgeons of England*, **43**, 218.

Boyd, W. (1957) Spontaneous regression of cancer. *Canadian Association of Radiology*, **8**, 45.

Coley, W. B. (1893) Treatment of malignant tumours by repeated innoculation of erysipelas. *American Journal of Medical Sciences*, **105**, 487.

Conybeare, R. C. (1964) Malignant melanoma and pregnancy. *Obstetrics and Gynaecology*, **24**, 451–454.

Everson, T. C. & Cole, W. H. (1966) *Spontaneous Regression of Cancer*, p. 164–220. Philadelphia: Saunders.

Family Planning Association (1970) Medical News Letter No. 32.

Hale, B. T. (1961) A technique for studying human tumour growth in vivo. Preliminary communication. *Lancet*, **ii**, 345.

Lee, J. A. H. (1970) Marriage and fatal malignant melanoma in females. *American Journal of Epidemiology*, **91**, 1, 48.

Milton, G. W. (1963) Some methods used in the management of metastatic melanoma. *Australian Journal of Dermatology*, **7**, 15.

Olsen, G. (1966) The malignant melanoma of the skin. Copenhagen and Aarhuus: Stiftsbogtrykkeries.

Spitz, S. (1948) Melanoma of childhood. *American Journal of Pathology*, **24**, 591–609.

White, L. P. (1959) Sex and survival in human melanoma. *New England Journal of Medicine*, **260**, 16, 789–797.

Chapter 21

Leukaemia and Lymphoma— Corticosteroid Therapy

J. S. MALPAS

The influence of the adrenal cortex on lymphoid tissue was first described by Addison in 1849 when he showed that hyperplasia of lymphoid tissue occurred in adrenal insufficiency. When adrenal cortical hormones and adrenocorticotrophic hormone became available they were shown to produce involution of lymphoid structures and the thymus (Moon, 1937; Wells and Kendall, 1940).

The sequence of events in lymphoid tissue following the administration of adrenal cortical extract, deoxycorticosterone acetate and corticosterone to mice was later described by Dougherty and White (1945). After dosage with ACTH, they showed the rapid development of oedema, followed by a fall in the number of lymphocytes and signs of degenerative change. These changes were not seen in adrenalectomised mice, and this suggested that the changes were due to stimulation of the adrenal cortical hormones.

Marked changes were also noted in the thymus in intact mice treated with ACTH or corticosteroid hormones. The medulla of the thymus became filled with lymphocytes which rapidly began to degenerate. The nuclei became shrunken and there was a marked alteration in chromatin structure. Later the pyknotic nuclei of the degenerate lymphocytes were seen to undergo phagocytosis. The cortex of the thymus became depleted because of a reduction in lymphocyte division which appeared three hours after the steroid administration. This reduction in cell division persisted for up to nine hours after which mitosis again became apparent.

This profound effect on lymphoid tissue was the basis for the introduction of corticosteroids in the treatment of leukaemia and lymphoma. Murphy and Sturm (1944) showed a marked effect on a transplanted leukaemia in rats. Cortieosteroids were introduced later in the decade for the treatment of human acute leukaemia (Pearson et al, 1949), chronic leukaemias and the lymphomas (Rosenthal et al, 1951).

Corticosteroids have three main actions in this group of diseases. Firstly, they have a lympholytic effect which is especially useful since there is no associated bone marrow suppression. Secondly, they are effective

granulocyte pool. Eosinophils and basophils are reduced and the reduction in their numbers comes on quite rapidly following corticosteroid administration and is sustained while the steroid is administered. The changes that occur have been neatly summarised by Videbaek (1969) (Figure 21.1). In addition, corticosteroids may affect

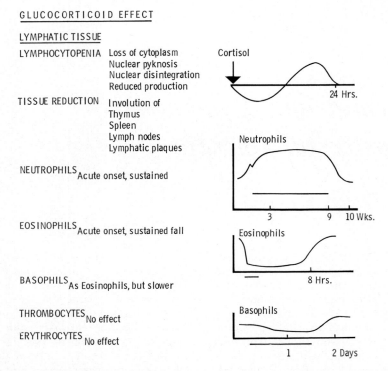

FIGURE 21.1. Effect of glucocorticoids on normal cells in the blood and lymphatic tissues (after Videback, 1969).

against complications such as autoimmune haemolytic anaemia. Thirdly, they have been shown in a number of these diseases to have an additive effect when combined with cytotoxic agents.

These three modes of action will be discussed in detail but, in addition, corticosteroids also affect other cellular components of the blood besides the lymphocyte series. They cause a rise in the neutrophil count as they apparently release cells from the marginal

the immune response in patients with leukaemia or lymphoma, as discussed in another section.

THE MECHANISM OF THE LYMPHOLYTIC EFFECT OF CORTICOSTEROIDS

Although corticosteroids have been used for nearly a quarter of a century in malignant diseases of the blood, their use has been almost entirely empirical and their mode of action is still largely unexplained. The rapid dissolution of large masses of tumour tissue such as may occur in lymphosarcoma implies a direct effect not only on the proliferating cell but also on the non-proliferating cell. How corticosteroids affect this latter type of cell is almost totally unknown, but there is now an increasing amount of evidence of the way in which steroids may affect the cell which is in the process of division.

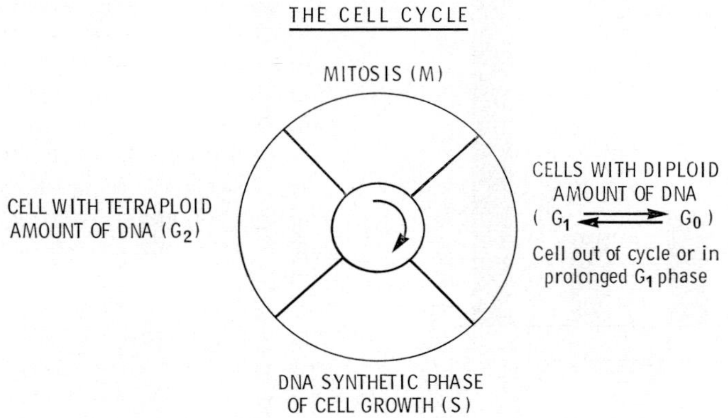

have been seen in human leukaemia cells in culture (Cline and Rosenbaum, 1968; Lampkin, Brubaker and Hartmann, 1969). Steroids have been shown to reduce protein synthesis (Makman, Dvorkin and White, 1968), to depress RNA polymerase (Fox and Gabourel, 1967), but to have no effect on DNA polymerase (Rosen et al, 1970).

Since all these phenomena may be observed in normal cells, it is difficult to identify

THE CELL CYCLE

FIGURE 21.2. The stages of the cell cycle.

Cell division may be represented by a steady progress through a resting phase G, to a synthetic phase S in which DNA is produced, to G_2 where a tetraploid amount of DNA is present, and finally to mitosis M (Figure 21.2). These stages occur in both the normal and malignant cell. The process whereby DNA is synthesised may be studied by the use of tritiated thymidine, while RNA synthesis can be studied by the use of tritiated uridine. The incorporation of the deoxyribose nucleotides has been studied intensively and enzymes involved in synthesis of DNA (DNA polymerase) and RNA (RNA polymerase) have also been studied.

The effect of corticosteroids on mammalian cells in tissue culture (Rosen et al, 1970) or in the intact animal (Frankfurt, 1968) has been to decrease incorporation of nucleotide uptake into nucleic acids. Similar results

the crucial action of steroid on the cell cycle in the malignant cell. Rosen et al (1970), studying the effects of cortisone on DNA metabolism in the sensitive and non-sensitive lines of the mouse lymphoma P1788, showed marked inhibition in the uptake of labelled deoxyribose precursors into tumour DNA in the cortisol-sensitive mouse lymphoma. Cortisol had its greatest effect on thymidine incorporation; deoxycytosine, deoxyguanine, and deoxyadenine were affected less and in that order. They further showed that this was not merely an effect produced by increased breakdown of DNA, with more thymidine made available in a precursor pool or as a result of de novo synthesis.

In a study of human lymphoblastic and myeloblastic leukaemias, Lampkin et al (1969) used tritiated thymidine to label cells from patients with these conditions. They investigated the effects of various cytotoxic drugs, prednisolone and hydrocortisone. They showed a marked effect on the labelling indices (LI) of cells from patients with lymphoblastic leukaemia when steroids were added to the in vitro culture (Figure 21.3). Steroids

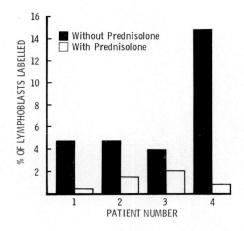

FIGURE 21.3. The effect of prednisolone on the labelling indices obtained using tritiated thymidine on acute lymphoblastic leukaemia cells (after Lampkin, 1968).

had no effect on acute myeloblastic leukaemia cells. Cline and Rosenbaum (1968), using the uptake of tritiated uridine into RNA, also found that corticosteroids inhibited uptake in cells of the lymphoblastic series while the myeloblastic series were unaffected. In some tests Cline showed that steroids actually enhanced the uptake of tritiated uridine by myeloblasts. These studies are consistent with the effect of steroid in these two forms of leukaemia, acute lymphoblastic leukaemia usually responding to steroids while the myeloblastic variety does not.

Evidence is accumulating that steroids act on an early stage of cell proliferation. Lampkin et al (1969) observed a 24-hour delay following the injection of hydrocortisone before the labelling index (LI) was at its lowest, and suggested that steroids decrease the number of cells entering the DNA synthetic phase S. This is supported by Frankfurt (1968) who studied the initiation of DNA synthetic phase in the cells of the forestomach of C311A mice, cells which have the unusual feature that they show a significant diurnal variation in their LI and have been demonstrated as having a high degree of synchrony. The squamous cells enter S phase during a short interval in the late afternoon. The effect of various drugs on the number of cells entering S phase can therefore be studied by injecting them at intervals before S phase. Hydrocortisone in physiological doses has been shown to reduce the number of cells entering S phase if given up to six to nine hours before the onset of S phase.

Evidence that the same effect is at work in human marrow lymphoblasts has been reported by Ernst and Killman (1970). They have used a technique which determines the amount of DNA synthesised in each cell. They have shown that once DNA synthesis has begun in the cell, corticosteroids are unable to affect the DNA content and the cell moves normally through that part of the cycle. Consequently, steroids must be obtaining an effect at an earlier stage. One possible way in which cells could be inhibited from entering the S phase would be if the nuclear RNA polymerase was affected. Fox and Gabourel (1967) showed that nuclear RNA polymerase system, isolated from the thymus of rats treated with cortisol, incorporates tritiated uridine into RNA to a lesser extent than the same system isolated from control animals.

Corticosteroids would appear therefore to affect cell division by a number of actions, but chiefly by inhibiting the number of cells entering the S phase. The way in which they do this is still under investigation. The way in which steroids work on the nonproliferating cell remains obscure.

CLINICAL EFFECT OF CORTICOSTEROIDS IN HUMAN LEUKAEMIA AND LYMPHOMA

CORTICOSTEROID THERAPY IN ACUTE LEUKAEMIA

Since the introduction of corticosteroids on an empirical basis for the treatment of acute lymphoblastic leukaemia (Pearson et al, 1949) ACTH and a variety of corticosteroids have been used for their cytotoxic activity in acute and chronic leukaemias and the reticuloses. While it has been fairly easy to evaluate the role of steroids in inducing remission in leukaemia, the problem has been more difficult in the reticuloses where steroids have been used less often singly than in combination, and frequently only in a late stage of the disease when assessment is difficult.

The main concern in the choice of a suitable corticosteroid has been its freedom from toxic side-effects such as sodium and water retention, hypertension, diabetes, gastrointestinal complications, lowering of resistance to bacterial and fungal infections, osteomalacia and various neuromuscular and psychotic reactions. This wide variety of effects is dealt with in greater detail in another part of this volume. Aspects of pharmacology which are of particular interest to the chemotherapist are the absence of marrow toxicity and the distribution of steroids throughout the total body water including the cerebrospinal fluid. There is also the possibility that corticosteroids may exert a protective effect on the marrow exposed to cytotoxic drugs, though the evidence for this is difficult to evaluate. Prednisone and prednisolone appear to have achieved most favour and are the commonest steroids being used in tumour chemotherapy.

Henderson (1969) presented details of studies where corticosteroids alone had been used to treat children and adults with acute lymphoblastic leukaemia. Table 21.1 is taken from his authoritative monograph on the treatment of acute leukaemia, and shows figures derived from the published series on the use of prednisone and prednisolone in lymphoblastic leukaemia.

It is evident from the response rates seen in Table 21.1 that the frequency with which a complete remission is achieved is not greatly affected by the dose of corticosteroid when it lies between 1 and 4 mg per kilogram per day. With increasing dosage the incidence of remission falls and the incidence of side-effects becomes much greater. Nevertheless, complete remission rates of over 70 per cent from the use of one drug alone compare very favourably with the results of other cytotoxic agents used singly.

Poor results are evident in the treatment of acute myeloblastic leukaemia in both children and adults by corticosteroids (Table 21.2). In acute myeloblastic leukaemia high dose regimes were even less effective than in lymphoblastic leukaemia. Cline and Rosenbaum (1968), studying 10 patients with acute myeloblastic leukaemia, found no evidence of clinical response by the patients or in vitro sensitivity of their cells to prednisolone. In one patient who showed a rise in the peripheral blast count and an increase in the size of the spleen while on prednisolone, in vitro cells were actually shown to be *stimulated* by cortisol.

In acute lymphoblastic leukaemia prednisolone was the obvious choice for a drug to combine with another effective agent in order to induce remission. A very large number of series has now been published using combinations of prednisone or prednisolone with different cytotoxic drugs. The best results reported for the different combinations are given in Figure 21.4.

The dose of drugs given was similar in the various series studied, prednisolone usually being given in a dose of from 40 mg/m² per day to 60 mg/m² per day but more commonly in the lower dosage. The dose of vincristine was between 1·5 and 2 mg/m² per week; 6-mercaptopurine between 70 and 90 mg/m² per day; and methotrexate

TABLE 21.1. *Prednisone in the treatment of acute lymphoblastic leukaemia* (after Henderson, 1969)

		No. of patients	Dose and schedule	% Complete remission	Median length of remission (days)	References
Children						
	1	100	40 mg/day	*71*	—	Boggs, Wintrobe and Cartwright (1962)
	2	72	2 mg/kg/day	*57*	—	Freireich et al (1963)
	3	11	<1 mg/kg/day	*45*	—	Bernard et al (1962)
			<3 mg/kg/day	*64*	—	
			⩾3 mg/kg/day	*74*	—	
	4	333	2 mg/kg/day	*69*	—	Wolff et al (1967)
	5	187	2 mg/kg/day	*76*	—	Leiken, Brubaker and Hartmann (1968)
			4 mg/kg/day	*73*	—	
			8 mg/kg/q2d	*25*	—	
			16 mg/kg/q4d	*19*	—	
	6	15	0·5 mg/kg/day		79	Hyman et al (1959)
		15	No maintenance		75	
	7	72	No maintenance		91	Freireich et al (1968)
Adults						
	1	22	40 mg/day	*36*		Boggs et al (1962)
	2		3 mg/kg/day	*45*		Bernard et al (1962)
	3	10	1000 mg/day	*50*		Shanbrom and Miller (1962)
	4	8	1000 mg/day	*50*		Ranney and Gellhorn (1957)

TABLE 21.2. *Prednisone in the treatment of acute myeloblastic leukaemia* (after Henderson, 1969)

		No. of patients	Dose and schedule	% Complete remissions	References
Children					
	1	20	>3 mg/kg/day	*20*	Bernard et al (1962)
	2	29	2 mg/kg/day	*14*	Wolff et al (1967)
	3	14	2–4 mg/kg/day	*20*	Leiken et al (1968)
		8	8–16 mg/kg/q2–4d	*0*	
	4	3	500 mg/day	*0*	Shanbrom and Miller (1962)
Adults					
	1	39	40 mg/day	*15*	M.R.C. (1966)
	2	27	>3 mg/kg/day	*0*	Bernard et al (1962)
	3	30	500–1000 mg/day	*12*	Ranney and Gellhorn (1957)
					Bouroncle, Doan and Wiseman (1959)
					Shanbrom and Miller (1962)
					Granville et al (1968)

either 3 mg/m² per square per day or 3 mg/kg intravenously every two weeks. It can be seen that the percentage of complete remissions obtained by the combination of prednisolone with vincristine, 6-mercaptopurine and methotrexate was very similar, and the difference in the rates of remission was not statistically significant.

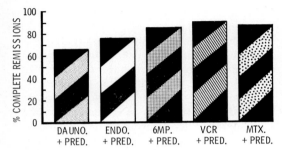

FIGURE 21.4. Combinations of two drugs used in childhood acute lymphoblastic leukaemia, based on data from George et al (1968), Selawry (1965), Holland and Glidewell (1968), Hardisty, McElwain and Darby (1969), Frei et al (1965), Krivit et al (1968), Brubaker et al (1963), Fernback et al (1966) and Holton et al (1969). The drugs used are daunorubicin (DAUNO), 6-mercaptopurine (6MP), vincristine (VCR), methotrexate (MTX) and prednisolone (PRED).

The logical progression is to combine as many active drugs with different major toxicities as possible, and to use them in a cyclical manner in order to achieve the highest rate of remission and the longest possible period of remission. Corticosteroids have played an important part in these regimes, of which some examples are shown diagrammatically (Figure 21.5).

When these treatments are carried out in centres specially equipped to deal with the high incidence of complications such as infections as a result of marrow depression, there has until recently been no greater mortality than experienced in regimes employing two drugs only (Leventhal et al, 1968). Recent experience in these centres, however, suggests that this satisfactory trend is being reversed. It also seems likely that children treated away from major centres

where either pathogen-free rooms, white cells and platelets from an IBM cell separator or simply platelet preparations are not available, have a higher morbidity and mortality. The most suitable regime for inducing remission in acute lymphoblastic leukaemia in children appears to be vincristine and prednisolone in combination.

Although prednisolone has been shown to be effective in combination with methotrexate or 6-mercaptopurine in maintaining remission, the toxic side-effects that develop with long-term administration do not make this drug or any other steroid suitable for long-term maintenance therapy. In patients treated in this way infection, muscle atrophy, and osteoporosis have been very troublesome.

CORTICOSTEROID THERAPY IN CHRONIC LEUKAEMIAS AND LYMPHOMAS

Corticosteroid therapy is sometimes successful in ameliorating the symptoms of patients with chronic lymphocytic leukaemia, Hodgkin's disease, lymphosarcoma and reticulum cell sarcoma. It has no effect on the course of chronic myeloid leukaemia. It may be possible to control chronic lymphatic leukaemia for some time but the length of remission

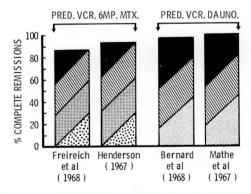

FIGURE 21.5. Multiple drug combinations in childhood acute lymphoblastic leukaemia, using prednisolone (PRED), vincristine (VCR), 6-mercaptopurine (6MP), methotrexate (MTX) and daunorubicin (DAUNO).

in Hodgkin's disease and in reticulum cell sarcoma are short. It does enable the disease to be brought under control when a patient has had radiotherapy and chemotherapy and has depressed marrow function. Corticosteroids may then grant a remission during which marrow recovery takes place.

Corticosteroids were reported as effective in chronic lymphatic leukaemia by Shaw et al (1961) and Galton et al (1961), but both reports noted the increased incidence of infection in patients who had to be kept on prednisolone for any length of time. Galton came to the conclusion that in chronic lymphatic leukaemia corticosteroids should be reserved for a few special situations, namely acute haemolytic anaemia, failure to respond to alkylating agents or radiotherapy, or as a preliminary to both these forms of treatment where patients were showing evidence of bone marrow suppression. Burningham et al (1964), using high-dose intermittent therapy of chronic lymphatic leukaemia, did not find an increased frequency of infection, but in a very extensive survey of the use of corticosteroids in this condition Ezdinli et al (1969) reported the disturbingly high incidence of 25 per cent seriously infected.

One of the major difficulties in assessing the effectiveness of corticosteroids in the reticuloses has been the frequency with which steroids have been combined with other effective agents. Since it is important to know whether any agent has a significant effect against malignancy before it is included in a combination, studies on corticosteroids used alone are of particular importance. Such a study is that by Ezdinli et al (1969). They report the results of steroid therapy alone in 137 patients given 188 courses of therapy; 42 patients had chronic lymphatic leukaemia, 38 had lymphosarcoma, 35 had Hodgkin's disease and 22 reticulum cell sarcoma. Prednisolone was the steroid used in 179 out of the 188 courses. The results of treatment were evaluated as good, fair, or no response, and are shown in Figure 21.6.

The failure of corticosteroids to produce any lasting benefit in reticulum cell sarcoma is noteworthy. The duration of the response for the whole group varied from 0·5 to 96 months with a median duration of 3 months. The median duration of response and the survival from the onset of steroid therapy in the four conditions is shown in Table 21.3.

Complications from steroid therapy necessitated the withdrawal of therapy in only 10 patients. Although infection was a problem in the patients with chronic lymphatic leukaemia the incidence of infection in the other reticuloses was less than 10 per cent.

It may be concluded from this and other studies that corticosteroids do have specific antitumour activity in chronic lymphatic leukaemia and the reticuloses. Used alone, however, there is a tendency for an incomplete response, relatively short remissions and frequent side-effects. They are therefore more suitable for use in combination therapy.

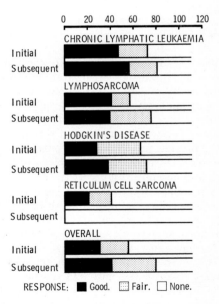

FIGURE 21.6. Response to corticosteroids. Initial and subsequent responses are noted over periods of up to 110 months (after Ezdinli, 1969).

TABLE 21.3. *Median duration of remission and survival from the onset of steroid therapy in 137 patients* (Ezdinli et al, 1969)

	Cases	Median duration of remission (months)	Median duration of survival (months)
Chronic lymphatic leukaemia	42	4·5	26
Lymphosarcoma	38	5·0	19
Hodgkin's disease	35	2·5	6
Reticulum cell sarcoma	22	2·0	2

COMBINATION CHEMOTHERAPY INCLUDING CORTICOSTEROIDS

HODGKIN'S DISEASE

Following the report by Carbone that combinations of alkylating agents, vinca alkaloids, procarbazine and prednisolone were effective in the treatment of Hodgkin's disease (Perry et al, 1967), a number of series confirming the effectiveness of these regimes have been recorded (Nicholson et al, 1970; DeVita, Serpick and Carbone, 1970). In the regime described by Perry et al (1967) vincristine was the alkaloid preferred. Nicholson et al (1970) preferred to use vinblastine. The two regimes are compared in Table 21.4.

DeVita et al (1970) and McElwain (1971) have reported the long-term follow-up on series treated by Perry's and Nicholson's regime respectively. A summary of their findings are compared in Table 21.5.

The results shown in Table 21.5 give impressive figures for the induction of remission and are a considerable advance on the results obtained using any one drug alone. Although there is no evidence yet from properly randomised clinical trials it would also seem that the median survival rates using combination chemotherapy are increased. Median survival time using conventional chemotherapy in Hodgkin's disease is about 20 months (Rapoport, Cole and Mason, 1969). The median survival in the series reported by DeVita was in excess of 42 months. In an analysis of survival of 130 patients with Hodgkin's disease treated by conventional methods and combination chemotherapy, Malpas (1971) has shown a significantly increased survival.

TABLE 21.4. *Combination chemotherapy in Hodgkin's disease*

Perry et al (1967)		Nicholson et al (1970)	
Prednisolone	40 mg/m²/day 0–14	Prednisolone	40 mg/day 0–14
Procarbazine	100 mg/m²/day 0–14	Procarbazine	100 mg/m²/day 0–14
Vincristine	1·4 mg/m²/day 0,7	Vinblastine	10 mg i.v./day 0,7,14
Mustine hydrochloride	6 mg/m²/day 0,7	Mustine hydrochloride	6 mg/m²/day 0,7

Each course lasts two weeks and is repeated in a further two weeks if the blood count permits.

Each course lasts two weeks and is repeated in four weeks if the blood count permits.

TABLE 21.5. *Results of treatment by quadruple chemotherapy in late-stage Hodgkin's disease*

	DeVita et al (1970)	McElwain (1971)
Patients		
Male	23	63
Female	20	47
Total	43	110
Mean age	31	33
Histology		
Lymphocyte depleted	11	10
Nodular sclerosis	14	58
Mixed cellularity	14	18
Lymphocyte proliferation	2	6
Unclassified	2	18
Complete remission achieved at some time	35* (81%)	45† (75%)

* Of 43 patients virtually all were previously untreated
† Of 110 patients 60 had received no therapy or DXR only. Overall complete remission occurred in 72 (65%)

LYMPHOSARCOMA AND RETICULUM CELL SARCOMA

The lympholytic effects of steroids have resulted in their inclusion in a number of regimes for the treatment of lymphosarcoma and also reticulum cell sarcoma. Using a similar regime to that reported by Perry et al (1967) but giving prednisolone only in the first and fourth courses, Serpick, Lowenbraun and DeVita (1969) were able to achieve remissions in 7 out of 15 patients with lymphosarcoma, and 3 out of 8 with reticulum cell sarcoma. The mean duration of unmaintained remission was 13 months in lymphosarcoma, 32 months for reticulum cell sarcoma, although in the latter case the numbers are few and this has not been the general experience.

In conclusion, corticosteroids, and in particular prednisolone, have made a considerable contribution to improved regimes for the management of Hodgkin's disease, lymphosarcoma and reticulum cell sarcoma. While the effect of corticosteroids on the rate of induction of remission in acute lymphoblastic leukaemia would appear to be strictly additive, the complicated therapeutic situation in the new regimes for lymphomas makes it difficult to say how much benefit is contributed by the corticosteroids. An answer could only be obtained by a controlled clinical trial which would not be justifiable ethically.

AUTOIMMUNE HAEMOLYTIC ANAEMIA COMPLICATING LEUKAEMIA AND LYMPHOMA

Corticosteroids have established an important place in the treatment of autoimmune haemolytic anaemia complicating leukaemia and the various reticuloses. Increased red cell destruction due either to haemolysis of

TABLE 21.6. *Autoimmune haemolytic anaemia in leukaemia and lymphoma*

	Dacie (1967)		Pirofsky (1969)	
Total number of patients with AIHA investigated	250		234	
Total number of patients with secondary AIHA	86		190	
Hodgkin's disease, malignant lymphoma, lymphosarcoma, or reticulum cell sarcoma	13	*(15%)*	25	*(13%)*
Chronic lymphatic leukaemia	11	*(13%)*	48	*(25%)*
Chronic granulocytic leukaemia	0	*(0%)*	7*	*(4%)*
Other leukaemias	4	*(5%)*	27	*(14%)*

* Includes both acute and chronic granulocytic leukaemia

autoimmune type or to other causes is not uncommon in these diseases. Chronic lymphatic leukaemia is most commonly associated with the production of warm antibody and a haemolytic state. The incidence of auto-immune haemolytic anaemia (AIHA) in two large series of patients reported by Dacie (1967) and Pirofsky (1969) is given in Table 21.6.

AIHA occurred most frequently in chronic lymphatic leukaemia where it was nearly always due to a warm antibody. Although haemolytic anaemia was not uncommon in Hodgkin's disease, half the patients in Dacie's series, for example, had cold type auto-antibodies. In reports on AIHA complicating Hodgkin's disease there has been considerable variation in the number of patients reported to have a direct antiglobulin test. An incidence of less than 2 per cent is reported by Grob-belaar (1958) while Matthias (1964), also in a series of 50 patients, reported an incidence of 24 per cent. In both chronic lymphatic leukaemia and Hodgkin's disease the development of an AIHA is a bad prognostic sign.

The effect of corticosteroids in AIHA due to a warm antibody is immediate and has been the subject of considerable investigation.

Steroids might act by reducing the mass of malignant tissue, by reducing the production of antibody, or by changing the capillary circulation. Any explanation would have to account for the very rapid improvement that can occur. An example of such an effect is well illustrated by a study by Matthias in 1964 (Figure 21.7). This shows that the excessive loss of red cells was arrested within 24 hours. If the effect had been due to any

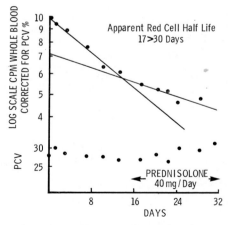

FIGURE 21.7. The effect of prednisolone on red cell survival in chronic lymphatic leukaemia.

reduction in the tumour mass by the direct cytotoxic action of the prednisolone it would have been expected that the response would have been slower. Other studies which included the effect of chemotherapy or radiotherapy were shown to take days and even weeks to produce benefit. Matthias (1964), commenting on these results, suggests that this rapid effect is due to the reduction of capillary fragility and permeability and the arrest of cells being lost from the circulation. In support of this, and indicating that the benefit is not due to any alteration in the cells being released into the circulation, was the finding that labelled transfusion cells also survive a longer time and that the beneficial effects of steroids are not related to such features as the titre of the Coombs test or indeed the strength of these phenomena.

Response to treatment with corticosteroids may vary greatly, being much less satisfactory in Hodgkin's disease than in chronic lymphatic leukaemia. While noting the occasional exception in Hodgkin's disease, Dacie (1967) concluded that they manifest limited benefit at best. Treatment should be started with adequate dosage. This is usually of the order of 60 mg of prednisolone daily. No advantage is gained by a higher dosage.

Following repair of the anaemia, maintenance therapy is required; this will vary with each individual, but doses of between 10 and 30 mg of prednisolone are usual.

The effects of corticosteroids on AIHA, either idiopathic or complicating leukaemia or lymphoma, are presented and compared in Table 21.7.

CONCLUSION

In surveying the role of corticosteroids in disease of the haemopoetic system, their undoubted efficacy both in the treatment of the disease itself or its complications is in contrast with how little is known of the way in which corticosteroids affect fundamental biological processes. Until this information is available it will be difficult to explain the rise in cell counts following steroid administration, the immediate effect on survival of the red cell, or the dramatic suppression of the symptoms of leukaemia and lymphoma. Nevertheless, corticosteroids used in conjunction with cytotoxic agents have established themselves as an integral part of the most successful regimes available for the treatment of leukaemias and lymphomas.

TABLE 21.7. *Corticosteroid response of AIHA either idiopathic or complicating leukaemia or lymphoma* (after Pirofsky, 1969)

Diagnosis	Patients receiving steroids	Therapeutic response:				Percentage success	Percentage failure
		Excellent	Good	Poor	None		
C.L.L.	40	11	9	3	17	50	50
A.L.L.	9	2	1	1	5	33	67
A.G.L.	5	0	1	1	3	20	80
H.D.	10	2	4	2	2	60	40
L.S.A.	4	1	2	0	1	75	25
R.C.S.	3	3	0	0	0	100	0
Idiopathic	33	25	0	2	6	76	24

C.L.L. chronic lymphatic leukaemia. A.L.L. acute lymphoblastic leukaemia. A.G.L. acute granulocytic leukaemia. H.D. Hodgkin's disease. L.S.A. lymphosarcoma. R.C.S. reticulum cell sarcoma.

References

Bernard, J., Boiron, M., Weil, M., Levy, J. P., Seligman, M. & Najean, J. (1962) Etude de la Remission Complet des Leucemies aigues. *Nouvelle Revue Française d'Hematologie*, **2**, 195.

Bernard, J., Boiron, M., Jacquillat, C. & Weil, M. (1968) Rubidomycin in 400 patients with leukaemia and other malignancies. Abstracts of the simultaneous sessions, *XII Congress, International Society of Hematology*, p. 5.

Boggs, D., Wintrobe, M. W. & Cartwright, G. E. (1962) The acute leukaemias. *Medicine*, **41**, 163.

Bouroncle, B. A., Doan, C. A. & Wiseman, B. K. (1968) Evaluation of the effect of massive prednisolone therapy in acute leukaemia. *Acta Haematologica (Basel)*, **22**, 201.

Brubaker, C. A., Wheeler, H. E., Sonley, M. J., Hyman, C. B., Williams, K. O. & Hammond, D. (1963) Cyclic chemotherapy for acute leukaemia in children. *Blood*, **22**, 820.

Burningham, R. A., Restropo, A., Pugh, R. P., Brown, E. B., Schlossman, S. F., Khuri, P. D., Lessner, H. E. & Harrington, W. J. (1964) Weekly high dosage glucocorticosteroid treatment of lymphocytic leukaemias and lymphomas. *New England Journal of Medicine*, **270**, 1160.

Cline, M. J. & Rosenbaum, E. (1968) Prediction of in vivo cytotoxicity of chemotherapeutic agents by their in vitro effect on leukocytes from patients with acute leukaemia. *Cancer Research*, **28**, 2516.

Dacie, J. V. (1967) *The Haemolytic Anaemias, Congenital and Acquired, Part III. Secondary or Symptomatic Haemolytic Anaemias*. London: Churchill, 2nd ed.

DeVita, V. T., Serpick, A. A. & Carbone, P. P. (1970) Combination chemotherapy in the treatment of advanced Hodgkin's disease. *Annals of Internal Medicine*, **73**, 881.

Dougherty, T. F. & White, A. (1945) Functional alterations in lymphoid tissue induced by adrenal cortical secretion. *American Journal of Anatomy*, **77**, 81.

Ernst, P. & Killman, S. A. (1970) Perturbation of generation cycle of human leukaemic blast cells by cytostatic therapy *in vivo*: effect of corticosteroids. *Blood*, **36**, 689.

Ezdinli, E. Z., Stutzman, L., Aungst, C. W. & Firat, D. (1969) Corticosteroid therapy for lymphomas and chronic lymphocytic leukaemia. *Cancer*, **23**, 900.

Fernback, J. D., Griffith, K. M., Haggard, M. E., Holcomb, T. M., Sutow, W. W., Vietti, J. J. & Windmiller, J. (1966) Chemotherapy of acute leukaemia in childhood. Comparison of cyclophosphamide and mercaptopurine. *New England Journal of Medicine*, **275**, 451.

Fox, K. E. & Gabourel, J. D. (1967) Effect of cortisol on the RNA polymerase system of rat thymus. *Molecular Pharmacology*, **3**, 479.

Frankfurt, O. S. (1968) Effect of hydrocortisone, adrenalin and actinomycin D on transition of cells to the DNA synthesis phase. *Experimental Cell Research*, **52**, 222.

Frei, E., Karon, M., Levin, R. H., Freireich, E. J., Taylor, R. J., Hananian, J., Selawry, O., Holland, J. F., Hoogstraten, B., Wolman, I. J., Abir, E., Sawitsky, A., Lee, S., Mills, S. D., Burgert, E. O., Spurr, C. L., Patterson, R. B., Ebaugh, F. G., James, G. W. & Moon, J. H. (1965) The effectiveness of combinations of antileukaemic agents in inducing and maintaining remission in children with acute leukaemia. *Blood*, **26**, 642.

Freireich, E. J., Gehan, E., Frei, E., Schroeder, L. R., Wolman, I. J., Anbari, R., Burgert, E. D., Mills, S. D., Pinkel, D., Selawry, O. S., Moon, J. H., Gendel, B. R., Spurr, C. L., Storrs, R., Haurani, F., Hoogstraten, B. & Lee, S. (1963) The effect of 6-mercaptopurine on the duration of steroid induced remissions in acute leukaemia: A model for evaluation of other potentially useful therapy. *Blood*, **21**, 699.

Freireich, E. J., Henderson, E. S., Karon, M. R. & Frei, E. (1968) The treatment of acute leukaemia considered with respect to cell population kinetics. In *The Proliferation and Spread of Neoplastic Cells*, p. 441. Baltimore: Williams and Wilkins.

Galton, D. A. G., Wiltshaw, E., Szur, L. & Dacie, J. V. (1961) The use of chlorambucil and steroids in the treatment of chronic lymphocytic leukaemia. *British Journal of Haematology*, **7**, 73.

George, P., Hernandez, K., Hustu, O., Borella, L., Holton, C. & Pinkel, D. (1968) A study of "total" therapy of acute lymphocytic leukaemia in children. *Journal of Pediatrics*, **72**, 399.

Granville, N. B., Rubio, F., Unugar, A., Schulman, E. & Dameshek, W. (1968) Treatment of acute leukaemia in adults with massive doses of prednisone and prednisolone. *New England Journal of Medicine*, **259**, 207.

Grobbelaar, B. G. (1958) Haemolytic anaemia and erythrocyte sensitisation in the malignant reticuloses. *South African Medical Journal*, **32**, 271.

Hardisty, R. M., McElwain, T. J. & Darby, C. W. (1969) Vincristine and prednisone for the induction of remissions in acute childhood leukaemia. *British Medical Journal*, **ii**, 662.

Henderson, E. S. (1967) Combination chemotherapy of acute lymphocytic leukaemia of childhood. *Cancer Research*, **27**, 2570.

Henderson, E. S. (1969) Treatment of acute leukaemia. *Seminars in Haematology*, **6**, 271.

Holland, J. F. & Glidewell, O. (1968) Induction, consolidation, intensification, reinduction and maintenance chemotherapy of acute lymphocytic leukaemia. Abstracts of the Simultaneous Sessions, *XII Congress of the International Society of Hematology*, 9.

Holton, C. P., Vietti, T. J., Nora, A. H., Donaldson, M. H., Stuckey, W. J., Watkins, W. L. & Lane, D. M. (1969) Daunomycin and prednisone for induction of remission in advanced leukaemia. *New England Journal of Medicine*, **280**, 171.

Hyman, C. B., Borda, E., Brubaker, C., Hammond, D. & Sturgeon, P. (1959) Prednisone in childhood leukaemia. Comparison of interrupted and continuous therapy. *Paediatrics*, **24**, 1005.

Krivit, W., Brubaker, C., Thatcher, L. G., Pierce, M., Perrin, E. & Hartman, J. R. (1968) Maintenance therapy in acute leukaemia of children. Comparison of cyclic vs. sequential methods. *Cancer*, **21**, 352.

Lampkin, B. C., Nagao, T. & Mauer, A. M. (1969) Drug effect in acute leukaemia. *Journal of Clinical Investigation*, **48**, 1124.

Leiken, S. L., Brubaker, C. & Hartmann, J. R. (1968) Varying prednisone dosage in remission induction of previously untreated childhood leukaemia. *Cancer*, **21**, 346.

Leventhal, B., Henderson, E., Henry, P. & Yankee, R. (1968) Vincristine and prednisone remission induction in childhood acute leukaemia (ALL). Program and Abstracts. *The Society for Paediatric Research, 38th Annual Meeting Atlantic City, May 3–4*, p. 125.

Makman, M. H., Dvorkin, B. & White, P. (1968) Influence of cortisol on the utilisation of precursors of nucleic acids and protein by lymphoid cells *in vitro*. *Journal of Biological Chemistry*, **243**, 1485.

Malpas, J. S. (1971) To be published.

Mathé, G., Hayat, M., Schwarzenberg, L., Amiel, J. L., Schneider, M., Cattan, A., Schlumberger, J. R. & Jasmin, C. (1967) Acute lymphoblastic leukaemia treated with a combination of prednisone, vincristine, and rubidomycin. Value of pathogen-free rooms. *Lancet*, **ii**, 380.

Matthias, J. Q. (1964) The assessment of cancer: the essentially similar nature of the haemolytic anaemias which complicate the different malignant disorders. M.D. Thesis, London University.

McElwain, T. J. (1971) Personal communication.

Moon, H. D. (1937) Inhibition of somatic growth in castrated rats with pituitary extract. *Proceedings of the Society for Experimental Biology and Medicine*, **37**, 34.

M.R.C. Working Party on the evaluation of different methods of therapy in leukaemia; treatment of acute leukaemia in adults. Comparison of steroid and mercaptopurine therapy alone and in conjunction (1966). *British Medical Journal*, **i**, 1383.

Murphy, J. B. & Sturm, E. (1944) Effect of adrenal cortical and pituitary adrenotrophic hormone on transplanted leukaemia in rats. *Science*, **99**, 303.

Nicholson, W. M., Beard, M. E. J., Crowther, D., Stansfield, A. G., Vartan, C. P., Malpas, J. S., Hamilton Fairley, G. & Bodley Scott, R. (1970) Combination chemotherapy in generalised Hodgkin's disease. *British Medical Journal*, **iii**, 7.

Pearson, D. H., Eliel, L. P., Rawson, R. W., Dobriner, K. & Rhoads, C. P. (1949) ACTH and cortisone induced regression of lymphoid tumours in man. *Cancer*, **2**, 943.

Perry, S., Thomas, L. B., Johnson, R. E., Carbone, P. P. & Haynes, H. A. (1967) Hodgkin's disease. Combined Clinical Staff Conference at the National Institutes of Health. *Annals of Internal Medicine*, **67**, 424.

Pirofsky, B. (1969) *Autoimmunisation and the Autoimmune Haemolytic Anaemias*. Baltimore: Williams and Wilkins.

Ranney, H. M. & Gellhorn, A. (1957) The effect of massive prednisone and prednisolone therapy on acute leukaemia and malignant lymphomas. *American Journal of Medicine*, **22**, 405.

Rapoport, A., Cole, P. & Mason, J. (1969) Correlates of survival after initiation of chemotherapy in 142 cases of Hodgkin's disease. *Cancer*, **23**, 377.

Rosen, J. M., Rosen, F., Milholland, R. J. & Nichol, C. A. (1970) Effects of cortisol on DNA metabolism in the sensitive and resistant lines of mouse lymphoma P1788. *Cancer Research*, **30**, 1129.

Rosenthal, M. C., Saunders, R. H., Schwartz, L. I., Zannos, I., Santiago, F. P. & Dameshek, W. (1951) The use of adrenocorticotrophic hormone and cortisone in the treatment of leukaemia and leukosarcoma. *Blood*, **6**, 801.

Selawry, O. S. (1965) New treatment schedule with improved survival in childhood leukaemia: Intermittent parenteral vs. daily oral administration of methotrexate for maintenance of induced remission. *Journal of the American Medical Association*, **194**, 75.

Serpick, A. A., Lowenbraun, S. & DeVita, V. T. (1969) Combination chemotherapy of lymphosarcoma and reticulum cell sarcoma. *Proceedings of the American Association for Cancer Research*, **10**, 78.

Shanbrom, E. & Miller, S. (1962) Critical evaluation of massive steroid therapy of acute leukaemia. *New England Journal of Medicine*, **266**, 1354.

Shaw, R. K., Boogs, D. R., Silberman, H. R. & Frei, E. (1961) A study of prednisone therapy in chronic lymphocytic leukaemia. *Blood*, **17**, 182.

Videbaek, A. (1969) Glucocorticoids in haematology. *Acta Medica Scandinavica supplement*, **500**, 35.

Wells, B. B. & Kendall, E. C. (1940) A qualitative difference in the effect of compounds separated from the adrenal cortex on distribution of electrolytes and on atrophy of the adrenal and thymus glands of rats. *Proceedings of Staff Meetings, Mayo Clinic*, **15**, 133.

Wolff, J. A., Brubaker, C. A., Murphy, M. L., Peirce, M. I. & Severo, N. (1967) Prednisone therapy of acute childhood leukaemia: Prognosis and duration of response in 330 treated patients. *Journal of Pediatrics* **70**, 626

Section V

Prospective Considerations

Chapter 22

An Evaluation of Endocrine Ablation Therapy

THOMAS H. ACKLAND

The problems of managing the advanced stages of cancer require of us the most mature judgment, based not only on scientific knowledge and clinical experience, but also upon human understanding. It is therefore appropriate that, before making an appraisal of the place of endocrine ablation in cancer, we give some consideration to the selection of patients for whom such management may be properly employed.

When a proposed operation for endocrine ablation involves the patient in little discomfort and risk, and when at the same time the likelihood of benefit is considerable, there need be no hesitation in advising such treatment. Such is the case when considering orchidectomy for carcinoma of the male breast or prostate, and, to a lesser degree, oophorectomy for the premenopausal woman with metastatic breast cancer.

When, on the other hand, a choice must be made between such operative procedures as adrenalectomy or hypophysectomy, which may prove formidable and hazardous but have a relatively higher success prospect, and drug or hormone administration which is safer and more easily tolerated but has a relatively lower success prospect, then decision may become very difficult indeed. This is especially so in those cases of advanced breast cancer where the probability of tumour regression after major ablative surgery is small, offering a minimal possibility of advantage over the simpler methods. However, in this particular disease, growing knowledge of the importance of steroid excretion patterns, assisted by proper use of clinical predictors of ablation response, affords promise of considerable and increasing aid in the selection of the patient who is likely to benefit from a major endocrine ablation.

While such operations often result in valuable and even dramatic palliation, care must always be taken that undue enthusiasm does not lead to their indiscriminate use, and that the patient is not regarded merely as a case or a statistic. Unfortunately, it does still happen that patients, already ill and distressed, are subjected, for one reason or another, to the added discomfort of an operation, when the prospect of significant benefit is slender. It is well to remember, moreover, that, should an operation be proposed, a patient hitherto unaware of the nature of his or her disease, must usually be informed of this fact. The consequent emotional trauma is a factor which must be weighed in determining treatment, for it may well be avoided by an alternative method.

Thus the total picture of the patient, both clinical and emotional, must always be taken into account, and the quality of life obtainable must be carefully assessed before an endocrine ablation is advised. Furthermore, difficulty and uncertainty are often associated both with the selection and the timing of the most appropriate procedure for a particular case. The following contribution attempts to elucidate the more important of these dilemmas, considering the following questions:

In advanced breast cancer

(a) Is androgen therapy a suitable alternative to castration?
(b) Should castration be carried out at the time of mastectomy or at the time of recurrence?
(c) Is castration effective after the menopause?
(d) Is radiation menopause as effective as oophorectomy?

In advanced breast and prostatic cancer

(a) What is the cause of immediate pain relief after surgical endocrine ablation?
(b) Should orchidectomy be early and total?
(c) Is major endocrine ablation indicated at the first recurrence?
(d) What determines the choice between adrenalectomy and hypophyseal ablation?
(e) Is there any correlation between the completeness of hypophyseal ablation and the tumour response rate?

Technical aspects

(a) What determines the choice of adrenalectomy technique?
(b) What are the relative advantages of the various methods of hypophyseal ablation?

Dilemmas in Advanced Breast Cancer

ANDROGEN THERAPY AS AN ALTERNATIVE TO THERAPEUTIC CASTRATION

The administration of androgens to premenopausal patients has been commonly recommended as an alternative to surgical or radiation castration. Although amenorrhoea can certainly be achieved in this way, androgen therapy is inferior to castration in breast cancer, since, in addition to its virilising effects, it does not produce either the same proportion of remissions, or remissions of similar duration. Thus, Pearson et al (1955) reported tumour regression in only 13 per cent of premenopausal cases treated with androgens, and Stoll (1969a) was unable to find objective evidence of a favourable response in any of 22 similar cases so treated. Androgen therapy may certainly produce *subjective* beneficial effects such as an increase in weight and appetite and an improved sense of well-being, as a result of a positive nitrogen and phosphorus balance, but these effects are more common in postmenopausal patients.

Some degree of masculinisation can be expected to follow the administration of most androgens currently used if they are administered long enough and at a dose level likely to be effective in bringing about tumour control. Hoarseness, deepening of the voice, hirsutism, and thinning of scalp hair are serious unwanted side effects which cause considerable distress. A woman who has already been subjected to the emotional trauma of mastectomy now finds that her remaining femininity has been further diminished, and added to this, as a 'turn of the screw', an increased libido is often produced.

The writer, after considerable experience in androgen therapy, and with full awareness of its possible effectiveness, especially in relieving pain from bony metastases in approximately 20 per cent of postmenopausal patients, now has reluctance in using this treatment. It must be admitted that many women in the fifth and sixth decades are not unduly disturbed by some degree of masculinisation, but some women so treated silently suffer mental torment. This is especially likely if a younger patient, perhaps between 35 years and 40 years of age, is treated with androgens following therapeutic castration.

There may be sound reasons for Juret (1966a) referring to male hormone as 'a cruel drug'. An alternative method is always available. It is claimed that some of the newer synthetic androgens such as Δ'-testololactone, and drostanolone (2α-methyldihydrotestosterone propionate) have minimal virilising effects; but their therapeutic effectiveness cannot yet be regarded as proven. For this reason, and because of its relative ineffectiveness, androgen therapy cannot be regarded as a justifiable alternative to castration.

THERAPEUTIC CASTRATION FOR BREAST CANCER

It is now generally recognised that a favourable objective response to castration in premenopausal patients with primary inoperable or recurrent breast cancer can be expected in a quarter to a third of operated cases. Therapeutic castration should unquestionably be given priority over all other methods as the first endocrine step in the treatment of such patients.

However, a dilemma often arises in deciding whether to employ oophorectomy alone as the management of an inoperable carcinoma, or whether to combine the ablation with radiotherapy to the breast cancer. Although the latter offers a much greater prospect of causing tumour regression than does castration, this addition of radiation prevents the determining of whether or not the tumour is hormone-sensitive, and thus denies valuable information for subsequent management. On the other hand, the problem may be overcome by excluding from radiation a less prominent lesion from which this information may be obtained; thus, after castration, radiation may be applied to a fungating primary tumour, but withheld from enlarged supraclavicular nodes, at least until such time as the effect of castration is evident.

Although it has been claimed by Wilson, Jessiman and Moore (1958) that aggravation of tumour growth can be caused by castration, it must be remembered that the rate of growth of a tumour in the body is liable to change spontaneously. Of the 70 per cent of cases which will not respond to castration, there will be some in which the biological course of the disease might determine a period of rapid tumour growth after castration, and lead to the fallacious conclusion that a causal relationship exists between what has been done and what has followed. Although there exists a possibility that ACTH production stimulated by operative stress may lead to increased release of adrenal oestrogen, there is little direct evidence that castration can cause significant tumour aggravation.

THE PROBLEM OF 'PROPHYLACTIC' CASTRATION

It is not difficult to understand why it has been hoped that 'prophylactic' castration, performed in the immediate postmastectomy period, might lead to an increased chance of *cure*. In view of the recognised benefits of therapeutic castration, it seemed possible that isolated tumour cells, or small cell groups, which otherwise would grow to form established metastases, might sometimes at least be prevented from so doing.

The first randomised controlled trial of prophylactic castration was carried out by Paterson and Russell in 1959, and, although a study of this by Cole (1964) showed that castrated patients had an improved survival, the difference barely reached statistical significance. However, it should be noted that in this trial, in which irradiation was employed to produce an artificial menopause, the dosage given was only 450 rads; and, in fact, some patients so treated experienced a return of menstruation.

A further controlled trial carried out by Nissen-Meyer (1964) provided evidence that castration of premenopausal and also postmenopausal patients exerted a favourable effect on the recurrence-free period as well as on the survival. From the results of this study Nissen-Meyer advises that all breast cancer patients up to 70 years of age should receive prophylactic ovarian irradiation, but his observations in this regard have not been confirmed, and few have followed this advice in the management of elderly patients.

Kennedy, Mielke and Fortuny (1964) retrospectively analysed cases treated at the University of Minnesota Hospitals, comparing the outcome in cases prophylactically castrated with that in women receiving therapeutic castration for recurrent disease. Although the groups contrasted were not randomised, this study showed that, while prophylactic castration lengthened the 'free interval' from mastectomy to the appearance of metastases, the total survival time from initial surgical treatment to death was not affected, the interval from recurrence to death being shorter. Kennedy stresses that prophylactic castration is not curative, but palliative, and suggests that more desirable than prophylactic castration might be the term 'early therapeutic castration' as opposed to 'late therapeutic castration'.

The most recent information concerning the prophylactic value of castration is provided by the report of Ravdin et al (1970), on a randomised prospective clinical trial initiated in 1961 by the National Surgical Adjuvant Breast Project of the USA. This study, like that of Kennedy, finds no evidence to indicate that prophylactic castration prolongs the interval from mastectomy to death. Contrary to Kennedy's findings, this analysis failed to demonstrate that postmastectomy oophorectomy lengthened the average time from mastectomy to recurrence, except that in patients who were found at operation to have many involved axillary nodes, castration did delay, for one to two years, the manifestation of recurrent disease. It should be remembered that in a previous study (Noer, 1963) the value of administering triethylene thiophosphoramide as an adjunct to surgical treatment was shown to be limited to a similar group of patients, for a similar time, the effect quite possibly being the result of a chemical 'oophorectomy'.

Many may still feel that the place of 'prophylactic' castration has not yet been accurately determined. Yet, even although early therapeutic or prophylactic castration may do no more than delay for a few patients the sad day when recurrent disease becomes evident, this is a strong argument in favour of its performance. Ibsen has written,

'Rob the average man of his life illusion, and you rob him of his happiness at the same stroke'. This philosophy can be adapted to the problem of a cancer sufferer. If a patient's hope of being cured is based on an illusion, it might be held that we should help him or her to live happily in this illusion for as long as possible, before the obvious signs of recurrent disease rob the patient and family of the illusion at the same stroke.

On the other hand, it must be remembered that the potential value of prophylactic castration in lengthening the free interval, applies only to the hormone-sensitive group of patients not cured by mastectomy. Thus, in Stage I disease, where approximately three women will need to be castrated to obtain the possible effect of prolonging the free interval in one, it would seem unjustifiable to urge the procedure. It might be more reasonably employed in the case of a young patient with a Stage II tumour, especially if she already has children.

There are still other factors which should be considered before 'prophylactic' castration is advised. It should be remembered that a woman with a breast already removed is now to be subjected to further deprivation of femininity, adding more psychological trauma. Again, Ansfield (1967) has drawn attention to the fact that early oestrogen deprivation may lead to an increased susceptibility to cardiovascular disease and early osteoporosis. Finally, the observation of a response or lack of response to therapeutic castration is a most useful criterion in selecting patients for adrenalectomy or hypophysectomy. This clinical predictor is lost if castration has been performed prophylactically.

In summary it would seem that, in view of present evidence, castration is to be recommended only for premenopausal patients who are found at operation to have extensive axillary invasion at all levels, and who are likely to have widespread well-established subclinical metastases. Such patients are just as incurable as those with obvious metastatic disease, in which case the castration is in fact

therapeutic. The effect of immediate post-mastectomy castration performed on these occasions is unlikely to be prolongation of survival but it is possible that the recurrence-free period will be lengthened in 30 per cent of patients.

When the procedure is to be employed, the surgeon must decide whether or not to carry out oophorectomy at the same time as he performs the breast operation. Surgically, oophorectomy is only a slight addition to mastectomy. However, with the nature of a breast lump as yet unproven, it will usually be enough for the patient and her husband to be told of the proposed biopsy and possible mastectomy if cancer is found, without proceeding at the same time to discuss simultaneous surgical castration. It is usually preferable to discuss the matter after mastectomy, and ovarian irradiation may perhaps be requested in preference to a second operation. In all of these cases careful weighing of social, psychological, religious, and also legal factors is essential.

THERAPEUTIC CASTRATION FOR POSTMENOPAUSAL PATIENTS

There is difference of opinion concerning the palliative value of castration in postmenopausal patients with breast cancer. Although it is clear, from studies of urinary oestrogen excretion levels, that oestrogen production by the ovaries may sometimes persist for several years after the menopause, it must be remembered that we have no proof that oestrogens play the most important role in favouring the growth of breast cancer. Nevertheless, with present knowledge, it still seems reasonable, in deciding for or against castration for an early postmenopausal woman, to judge ovarian activity from an assessment of oestrogen production.

Vaginal smear examination has been used by many as an indicator of oestrogenic activity, but twice-weekly measurement of urinary oestrogen excretion by Brown's method (Brown, Falconer and Strong, 1959) is a more accurate and sensitive assessment of persisting ovarian activity. In a truly post-menopausal woman with inactive ovaries, the total oestrogens (oestrone, oestradiol-17β and oestriol), adrenal in origin, seldom exceed a level of 10 μg in 24 hours. In such a case there is no laboratory support for ovarian ablation, but, if oestrogen levels are higher, and especially if cyclical fluctuation is found (Brown, 1970) it may be assumed that significant ovarian activity persists, and castration should be performed as for a premenopausal patient.

It sometimes happens that a patient of pre-menopausal age with advanced breast cancer has previously been subjected to hysterectomy, and it may not be known whether or not oophorectomy was performed simultaneously. Under such circumstances urinary oestrogen estimations provide the best method for solving this dilemma.

Published reports of the value of castration performed on postmenopausal patients show conflicting evidence. Thus, in the results of his trial of 'prophylactic' castration, Nissen-Meyer (1964, 1968) sees evidence that castration could benefit patients up to the age of 70 years. On the other hand, Barlow, Emerson and Saxena (1969), after reviewing the world literature, were able to find only 16 cases which responded to castration, and Fracchia et al (1969) found a response in only three of 85 postmenopausal cases. All three were within a year of the menopause. It may be concluded that castration alone is unlikely to assist the postmenopausal patient.

If adrenalectomy is to be performed upon a postmenopausal patient, is oophorectomy an unnecessary addition? Hellstrom and Franksson (1958), comparing the response rate in postmenopausal patients yielded by adrenal-ectomy alone with that obtained by adding castration, found that remission figures for the different procedures were 27·4 per cent and 41·5 per cent respectively. They also observed that a remission of longer duration was associated with the combined ablation.

Another study by Fracchia et al (1959) has yielded similar evidence, from which it may be concluded that oophorectomy should in fact be added to adrenalectomy performed on postmenopausal patients. Although urinary oestrogen excretion levels may be low in such patients it is likely that the ovaries continue to produce small but significant quantities of oestrogens for many years after the menopause.

When a decision has been made to add oophorectomy to adrenalectomy, there should be no rigid policy with regard to whether it should be carried out simultaneously or later. If adrenalectomy is performed by an anterior approach, castration will usually be only a slight additional procedure, no other incision being required. On the other hand, if bi-lateral posterior incisions are employed for adrenalectomy, oophorectomy is usually best performed as a separate operation a few weeks later.

CASTRATION BY SURGERY OR RADIATION

There is no doubt that castration can be accomplished quite successfully by radiation, provided that an adequate dosage is employed. In this regard it has been found that ovaries of younger women are more resistant to radiation than those of women over the age of 40 (Nathanson and Kelley, 1952). It has been found that a fractionated dose of 1500 R is adequate for the latter group, but 2000 to 2500 R is required for young patients (Stoll, 1969b; Stein, 1969). Stoll also reports that radiation achieves a higher tumour remission rate in breast cancer when the dosage is spread over a period of two to three weeks, instead of the customary seven days. It may occasionally happen that even after the use of proper dosage and technique, menses may continue or be resumed. Under such circumstances surgical castration should be performed, certainly if estimations of urinary oestrogen excretion point to persistent ovarian activity.

The frequency of tumour response is generally similar for both methods, but an advantage of radiation is that it avoids the need for hospitalisation and the discomfort of an operation. It should also be remembered that the operative mortality of oophorectomy in patients with advanced disease may, in unsuitably selected patients, be as high as 5 per cent. A further theoretical disadvantage of oophorectomy is that it may temporarily cause an increased adrenal oestrogen release, stimulated by ACTH produced as a result of operative stress (Bulbrook and Greenwood, 1957).

On the other hand, ovarian radiation takes an appreciable time to bring about full reduction of oestrogen production, and the fact that periods have ceased does not necessarily indicate that stromal ovarian secretion has been abolished. Although the maximum radiation effect is usually achieved at the end of six weeks, on some occasions even 130 days may pass before urinary oestrogen excretion falls to a postmenopausal level (Block, Vial and Pullen, 1958). Surgical castration is certainly preferable when rapidly advancing disease, or painful bony metastases, call for speedy control, while radiation should be employed for cases in which the general condition is poor or when operation is refused.

Dilemmas in Both Advanced Breast and Prostatic Cancer

THE PHENOMENON OF IMMEDIATE PAIN RELIEF FOLLOWING ENDOCRINE ABLATION

Pain arising from bone metastases is thought to be due to an increase in tissue tension associated with the presence of expanding tumour within the rigid skeletal framework. Painful stimuli may then be provoked by pressure upon the periosteum, by hyperaemia, by oedema, or perhaps by distortion of arterioles. The term 'paradoxical pain relief' has been rather loosely applied to several different situations where an explanation for relief afforded by endocrine ablation is not immediately apparent. It is necessary to examine this problem as applicable to four groups of patients:

1. In cases of metastatic breast or prostatic cancer dramatic and prompt pain relief may follow castration, adrenalectomy or hypophysectomy, perhaps preceding by many weeks the manifestation of an objective tumour response.

2. The same swift analgesic effect may at times follow the performance of these operations in cases where an objective remission does not follow.

3. Remarkable, and almost immediate pain relief may follow the implantation of yttrium-90 into the pituitary, although tissue destruction of the gland is not obvious before 10 days.

4. Pituitary ablation is sometimes able to relieve pain caused by bone metastases arising from cancers of the colon or cervix uteri, which have no known hormone dependence; and it has even been claimed that pain from osteoarthritis may be alleviated by the same operation (Juret, Hayem and Thomas, 1962).

Unfortunately no one explanation satisfactorily accounts for all of these circumstances.

Reduction in tissue tension, resulting from lowering of oestrogen levels, is the most common reason given for the immediate analgesia which follows castration, adrenalectomy or hypophysectomy in those cases of breast cancer in which an objective response later follows. The fact that stilboestrol administration may aggravate the pain of bone metastases lends support to this argument. When immediate pain relief occurs in a patient not showing subsequent objective evidence of response to endocrine ablation, it is possible that suppression of oestrogens might bring about an immediate, although temporary, decrease in intracellular tension in tumour cells, by lessening of salt and water retention. Thus a quickly produced, but not lasting relief of pain may occur.

As an alternative explanation, it has been suggested that this may be due to the effect of postoperative cortisone maintenance therapy. Dao, Tan and Brooks (1961) have reported that the administration of the usual maintenance dosage of cortisone (37·5 mg daily) does not relieve pain from bone metastases in patients not subjected to adrenalectomy, and denies that the postoperative cortisone therapy given to patients after major endocrine ablations is responsible for immediate pain relief. But these patients upon whom ablation has not been performed cannot be compared with those who have been deprived of endogenous corticosteroids, and who may consequently be more sensitive to the effects of small dosages.

A fall in the level of circulating oestrogens cannot be invoked to account for pain control following immediately upon yttrium-90 implantation when the benefit is sometimes produced in spite of subsequent demonstration that there is no correlation between the reduction in the level of circulating oestrogens and the degree of pain relief (Juret and Hayem, 1960). Nor will depression of oestrogen levels explain the relief at times produced by hypophysectomy in cancers believed to be hormone-independent.

Perhaps on some occasions at least there may occur a placebo effect whereby pain is paradoxically relieved. An exploratory laparotomy for a carcinoma found to be unresectable is sometimes followed by remarkable temporary subjective improvement in spite of the fact that nothing is done which would be expected to bring about immediate pain relief. Indeed, on such occasions one might well anticipate more severe pain to be present during the early postoperative period, merely as a result of surgical interference and wound suturing. But all such patients are properly treated with reasonably heavy sedation; and the immediate relief often experienced may be due to the understandable euphoric effect of 'the operation being over', assisted in large measure by the administration of analgesics.

There may exist other little-understood mechanisms for inhibition of pain appreciation, following upon various types of surgical interference with the pituitary gland. Juret (1966b) suggests that a retrograde degeneration of hypothalamo-hypophyseal centrifugal neurones may follow upon pituitary trauma, and lead to impaired function of the ventrobasal thalamic nuclei, which are certainly concerned with the conduction, if not the appreciation of protopathic pain sensations. But such a degenerative process would take some time to occur, and offers no explanation for immediate pain control. To resolve this problem, Juret points out that some centripetal pathways which pass from the hypophysis to the hypothalamus might be destroyed at attempted hypophysectomy; or alternatively, sympathetic fibres entering the sella turcica from the superior cervical ganglion might be injured, with resultant diencephalic changes affecting pain appreciation.

The precise connections and functions of these pathways are as yet not sufficiently defined for these theories of delayed and immediate pain relief to be satisfactory. Yet it must be acknowledged that operative trauma to the pituitary gland is able to inhibit pain appreciation under some circumstances in which an endocrine effect cannot be invoked as an adequate explanation.

ORCHIDECTOMY—TOTAL OR SUBCAPSULAR

Classical total orchidectomy, in which the whole testis is removed after division of the cord below the external inguinal ring, is not readily accepted by most patients, elderly though they may be, and the obvious emptiness of the scrotum may even lead to serious psychological disturbances. Subcapsular orchidectomy for the most part avoids this problem, and permission for its performance is more likely to be granted. In this operation, after incision of the tunica albuginea through a small scrotal approach, testicular substance is removed by very thorough curettage, and the tunica then resutured. There is always sufficient bleeding to fill the empty space with a haematoma, which later becomes reduced to a small fibrous mass. The patient accepts this as a smaller, but nevertheless present testicle. Testicular replicas made from plastic materials have been inserted into the scrotum, but for the average case their use appears an unnecessary refinement.

A possible objection to subcapsular orchidectomy is that a significant number of androgen secreting Leydig cells may remain, and may perhaps multiply. O'Conor, Chiang and Grayhack (1963), after studying a group of patients treated by subcapsular orchidectomy, report persistent androgen secretion in response to gonadotropin stimulation. This secretion was abolished by total orchidectomy. An autopsy study of patients submitted to subcapsular orchidectomy has been made by McDonald and Canalis (1958), and these workers have in fact demonstrated persistent Leydig cells in almost all of the specimens examined. However, there is no evidence from this study that their numbers were sufficient to be of functional significance.

Castration may lead to impotence, although libido is usually preserved; and gain in weight often follows, with an alteration to the female type of fat distribution, especially in younger patients. Hot flushes, such as occur in menopausal women, are a frequent annoyance, but these respond to small doses of oestrogens.

ORCHIDECTOMY FOR CARCINOMA OF THE PROSTATE

Many surgeons are reluctant to perform orchidectomy for carcinoma of the prostate. This hesitancy undoubtedly stems from the fact that oestrogen therapy relieves the distressing symptoms of the advanced stage of this disease, such as dysuria and pain from bony metastases, in about 90 per cent of cases. It then appears unnecessary to urge an operation to which the patient may well object.

Nesbit and Baum (1951) have reported that the greatest prolongation of life is obtained when castration and oestrogen therapy are used conjointly as primary treatment, and oestrogens are then continued indefinitely. However, the report of The Veterans Administration Co-operative Urological Research Group (1967) did not confirm the superiority of this combined management. Despite varying evidence, some greater use might advantageously be made of orchidectomy, especially when spread beyond the prostate has not occurred.

ORCHIDECTOMY FOR CARCINOMA OF THE MALE BREAST

There is no form of endocrine treatment for any form of cancer which so frequently achieves palliation as does orchidectomy for primary inoperable or metastatic carcinoma of the male breast (Haagensen, 1956). In these cases there is a probability approximating 75 per cent that the ablation will yield a remission lasting for an average period of two-and-a-half years. When relapse occurs, or even if no response has been obtained by castration, subsequent adrenalectomy should be performed, since, although the literature contains reports of few cases so treated, evidence obtained from these indicates that there is a 75 per cent likelihood of a further response which may last up to five years (Li et al, 1970).

These facts have led to a suggestion, which may have some merit, that male sufferers from carcinoma of the breast should be treated primarily by orchidectomy rather than by mastectomy, since it is possible that such a method might be as rewarding as conventional radical mastectomy is for the operable case. However, for a small tumour with no evidence of local or distant metastases, radical mastectomy should be chosen. On the other hand, for an advanced case of doubtful curability, the combination of radiotherapy to the breast tumour and orchidectomy is to be preferred to mastectomy; but if resection is undertaken, the prophylactic addition of orchidectomy will probably delay the appearance of recurrent disease.

EARLY OR DEFERRED MAJOR ENDOCRINE ABLATION

If control of hormone-dependent breast cancer depends upon elimination of oestrogens, it would seem logical to perform hypophysectomy or adrenalectomy as early as possible after the first evidence of disease recurrence. Yet Atkins et al (1966), after conducting a prospective randomised trial, in which adrenalectomy or hypophysectomy without previous hormone treatment was contrasted with performance of these operations after additive hormone therapy, found no difference in the results of the two groups as measured either by length of survival or quality and duration of remission. On the other hand, the response rate to the ablative operations was lower when hormones had been administered first. It would appear that the obtaining of a remission by additive hormone therapy carries the penalty of lessening the likelihood of subsequent response to adrenalectomy or hypophysectomy.

These conclusions are supported by the results of a similar trial carried out by Dao, Nemoto and Bross (1968), and also by the report of a study undertaken by Forrest et al (1968), in which the ablative method employed was yttrium-90 implantation of the pituitary. All reports agree that the early use of hypophysectomy or adrenalectomy confers no benefit in terms of prolonging the total survival period. Moreover, such evidence as is available (Patey, 1960) indicates that the 'prophylactic' use of such ablation does not increase the cure rate. In the making of a decision whether to advise an early major ablative operation or first to employ additive hormone therapy, it must be remembered that the mortality rate associated with both adrenalectomy and the commonly employed techniques of hypophysectomy is far from negligible especially in improperly selected patients. Thus, although the studies quoted above have shown equal *average* survival periods for groups treated by early and late ablations, *individual* patients, whose lives might have been usefully prolonged by conservative initial treatment, will die as a direct result of the operative procedure.

In the case of premenopausal patients with advanced breast cancer, it is the author's opinion that the first method of treatment should be castration alone, rather than immediate hypophysectomy or adrenalectomy with ovariectomy. This policy is strongly supported by the following facts. The likelihood of tumour regression following the performance of a major ablative procedure is not significantly greater than that achieved by castration alone, nor is there any appreciable difference in the duration of remission obtained by either method. Moreover, if castration is followed by a favourable response, there is a 40 to 50 per cent prospect of a further remission being obtained by subsequent adrenalectomy or hypophysectomy (MacDonald, 1962). In such cases it is extremely probable that the total length of the two periods of remission will be greater than that which would have resulted from immediate performance of a major ablation without preliminary castration. A still further advantage of initial castration is that it makes possible the selection of patients unlikely to benefit from major ablative surgery. If no tumour regression follows castration, the probability of a response to subsequent adrenalectomy or hypophysectomy is very low, in the region of 10 per cent, and these procedures should not usually be advised; such patients are best spared the further discomfort and hazards of a major operation.

Most will therefore agree that major endocrine ablation should not be advised before attempting to obtain every possible benefit from surgery, radiotherapy, castration and hormone administration. A possible exception to this general rule is the case of pleural or pulmonary metastases which respond to additive hormone therapy less commonly than do soft tissue recurrences. These are perhaps best treated, as Dao and Libby (1968) suggest, by early adrenalectomy or hypophysectomy. Androgen therapy will also be omitted by those who feel that, at least in the case of some patients, masculinising effects contraindicate its use.

THE CHOICE BETWEEN ADRENALECTOMY AND HYPOPHYSECTOMY IN BREAST CANCER

Although it is now clear that both adrenalectomy and hypophysectomy bring about disease regression in approximately one-third of postmenopausal patients with breast cancer, the relative effectiveness of these operations has not yet been precisely determined. Nevertheless, some information is available. In a retrospective study undertaken in 1959 by the Joint Committee of the American Medical Association, results from 13 institutions were combined. The final report of this analysis, published by MacDonald in 1962, found an overall regression rate of 28·4 per cent in 690 patients after adrenalectomy and 32·6 per cent in 340 patients after hypophysectomy, the difference not being statistically significant. The mortality rates were 13·95 per cent and 12·8 per cent

respectively. Thus, no appreciable difference was demonstrated, and it was concluded that 'the natural history of the disease in the individual patient, and the capacity to respond to hormonal alterations determined the outcome of the ablative measures rather than the type of ablation'.

However, it should be noted that Atkins et al (1960), after conducting a prospective controlled trial of two randomly selected groups, observed that, in their hands, hypophysectomy produced slightly better results, the difference being statistically significant. These same workers have later (1968) recorded that adrenalectomy was less effective in patients who had not previously been submitted to mastectomy. Moreover, the fact that hypophysectomy at times can achieve a further remission when relapse occurs after an adrenalectomy response, might be regarded as indicating that it is a superior procedure.

It may reasonably be concluded that since the results to be expected from these two procedures differ so little, the choice of operation for a particular patient will be made very largely by a consideration of her general condition and the facilities and special skills available. Adrenalectomy can be carried out with reasonable safety by most general surgeons and has an understandable popularity from this point of view; on the other hand, hypophysectomy remains a highly specialised procedure whatever the technique employed. If the results from experienced units are compared, the mortality rates are not significantly different.

The postoperative management of patients submitted to hypophysectomy may be more difficult because of the necessity for treatment of hypothyroidism and diabetes insipidus, in addition to adrenal insufficiency; but, on the other hand, since aldosterone secretion is unaffected, difficulties in controlling postoperative electrolyte balance are less likely to occur. In actual practice it is found that there is little difference in management after either operation. Undoubtedly the future will see further development in techniques of hypophysectomy which will cause minimal disturbance to the patient; when these become generally available it is likely that adrenalectomy will ultimately be abandoned.

Finally, it must be remembered that many patients who are very ill and in poor general condition are best served by heavy sedation and good nursing rather than by any type of operative procedure. But if a major ablation is to be performed on such patients, trans-sphenoidal hypophysectomy or yttrium implantation are at the present time suitable methods.

THE RELATION OF COMPLETENESS OF HYPOPHYSECTOMY TO RESPONSE

As gauged by present methods of estimating pituitary function, complete pituitary ablation does not appear to be necessary for the obtaining of a clinical response, or even of an objective remission of tumour growth. There is considerable disagreement as to the best parameters of completeness of ablation, and some authorities believe that some degree of relationship does exist between the proportion of gland destroyed and the palliation obtained.

Total pituitary ablation presents many practical difficulties. The inaccessible situation of the gland, and its important anatomical relationships, make entire ablation almost an impossibility, and autopsy studies often demonstrate functioning tissue after the most strenuous efforts at its removal or destruction. Moreover, extrasellar collections of adenohypophyseal cells, of appreciable volume, are always present in the wall of the pharynx along the route of development of Rathke's pouch. McGrath (1970) has emphasised the constant anatomical site of this 'pharyngeal hypophysis' in the roof of the nasopharynx, and has suggested that since it is accessible, its destruction should in future be considered an integral part of

hypophysectomy, especially since hypertrophy of these cells follows destruction of the intrasellar gland tissue.

A further problem is that the precise pituitary hormones controlling the growth of breast cancer remain unknown. While the beneficial effect of hypophysectomy may well be by oestrogen depression, resulting from partial or complete elimination of gonadotropin and ACTH, it is also possible that it might derive from removal of other pituitary secretions such as growth hormone and prolactin. We are therefore uncertain as to which hormone is most appropriately measured in assessing residual pituitary function after attempted hypophysectomy.

Most presently available tests have their own inherent inadequacies and the hormonal assay which best reflects the completeness of pituitary ablation is controversial. McCullagh et al (1965) state that a fall in urinary gonadotropin excretion is the most reliable indicator of pituitary destruction; but the validity of this test is undermined by the fact that it is difficult to estimate the follicle-stimulating (FSH) and luteinising (LH) fractions separately. The disappearance of thyrotropic hormone may be demonstrated by a decrease in the serum protein-bound iodine, as well as in the radioactive iodine uptake of the thyroid gland. Beck et al (1966) regard a low ^{131}I uptake occurring in association with a low gonadotropin output as a good indicator of radical pituitary ablation.

Measurement of urinary 17-ketosteroids, and 17-hydroxycorticosteroids before and after operation has also been used to evaluate the degree of pituitary destruction, but this has proved to be an unreliable guide. The estimation of ACTH, or growth hormone may be of greater significance in relation to breast cancer. Landon and Greenwood (1968) have developed a radioimmunoassay for determining plasma concentrations of ACTH in man, and this method, which excels in specificity and sensitivity, is likely to be widely used in the future. Hunter and Greenwood

(1964) have devised a radioimmunoassay for the measurement of growth hormone in human plasma. It has been shown that, although the level of this hormone may fall to zero after hypophysectomy, insulin stimulation will bring about its reappearance in measurable amounts in cases where pituitary ablation has been incomplete. The relative importance of each of these methods awaits further evaluation.

Technical Aspects

SELECTION OF ADRENALECTOMY TECHNIQUE

Although in the past there has been some difference of opinion as to whether adrenalectomy should be a one or two stage operation, there is now almost general agreement that an experienced surgeon should aim to remove both glands at the one operation, whether his preference be for the anterior or posterior approach. Nevertheless, excision of the right gland, which is likely to be the more difficult procedure, should be undertaken first, since, if technical difficulties are encountered here, the left adrenal may be more prudently removed as a second stage procedure, when oophorectomy can be carried out simultaneously if desired.

There is a difference of opinion among surgeons as to the best operative approach. The anterior transperitoneal, and the posterolateral extraperitoneal approaches are those most commonly employed, and other techniques, such as the anterior extraperitoneal, the transthoracic, and the subpleural transdiaphragmatic approaches may, for practical purposes, be disregarded. The obvious advantage of an abdominal approach is that it allows both adrenals, and if necessary both ovaries, to be removed through one incision, without turning of the patient. Many surgeons prefer this method and it must be admitted that in thin subjects it permits an excellent view of the adrenals and their blood supply.

It must be emphasised, however, that the most important step in adrenalectomy is control of the adrenal vein, which is seldom easy to achieve on the right side, where it is a short and often quite wide structure, leaving the middle of the medial border of the gland to enter the inferior vena cava. An error in technique in dealing with this short right adrenal vein may easily lead to its avulsion, bringing about alarming haemorrhage from the vena cava, and the adequate control of such a situation requires skill in vascular suturing. On the left side, whether the abdominal approach to the gland is through the transverse mesocolon, or lateral to the spleen after its mobilisation, there is less difficulty and less hazard in securing the corresponding vein, which may drain either directly into the left renal vein or into the inferior phrenic vein. In obese subjects, and especially those with liver metastases and ascites, the anterior approach is certainly not to be recommended.

The author has found that the posterolateral approach to the adrenals provides the best exposure, with greatest safety in control of the adrenal veins. Turning of the patient during the operation presents no problem. On the other hand, two incisions are required, and oophorectomy must usually be deferred for a second operation. After the 12th rib has been resected, and the lowest part of the pleural reflection mobilised upwards, an incision in the rib bed leads easily to the adrenal gland. The numerous small arteries which supply the gland are readily controlled by coagulation diathermy, and for securing the adrenal veins, Cushing's clips have the advantage that no forceps are applied to these fragile structures.

THE PLACE OF ADRENAL PORTALISATION

A shortcoming of adrenalectomy is the necessity for the patient to rely upon exogenous cortisone administration for the remainder of life. In general, such replacement therapy is easily conducted, although during periods of physiological or pathological stress, cortisone dosage must be increased, and gastrointestinal disturbances may necessitate parenteral administration of the drug. The studies of Israel, Meranze and Johnston (1937), Golden and Sevringhaus (1938) and Biskind and Mark (1939) demonstrated that oestrogens are inactivated by the liver. This information suggested the possibility that oestrogens produced in the adrenals might be eliminated by an operative procedure which would channel their venous blood into the portal system while essential hydrocortisone would remain in circulation.

Various techniques have been devised to bring about the diversion of adrenal-produced oestrogens into the portal system. In all methods the right adrenal gland is removed and the left preserved for portalisation. Dargent's portalisation operation is the method which has been most often used, and Dargent and co-workers have reported their experience with it in 143 cases (Dargent, Mayer and Lombard, 1967; Mayer et al, 1967). Following removal of the right adrenal, the left adrenal is mobilised with preservation of its upper arterial pedicle, and then implanted into the pulp of the spleen after the capsule of the latter has been incised. The implication that splenic haemorrhage is not a serious problem if the splenic capsule is carefully sutured over the implanted gland might well surprise many general surgeons. Only one death from haemorrhage is reported in the above series.

The Lyon group reports that in the 143 patients subjected to this operation the mortality rate was 6·9 per cent and the response rate was the same as that yielded by bilateral adrenalectomy performed in another series of patients. However, permanent cortisone withdrawal proved possible in only 46 patients. This appears to be a disappointing reward for a complicated procedure, especially in view of the fact that serious problems rarely arise in connection with cortisone replacement therapy. A fair assessment would seem to be that adrenal portalisation operations are interesting surgical and physiological exercises, but offer little of practical value.

THE SELECTION OF HYPOPHYSECTOMY TECHNIQUE

Hypophysectomy for advanced breast cancer was originally carried out by Luft and Olivecrona in 1953 by the transfrontal approach. Since then, not only has the trans-sphenoidal approach been introduced, but pituitary ablation has been attempted by interstitial irradiation, ultrasonic waves and cryogenic therapy. It is difficult to estimate the relative merits of different methods of hypophyseal ablation, since results obtained may depend on the skill and experience available rather than on the method itself. Thus, the ideal technique of hypophysectomy remains as yet undecided.

TRANSFRONTAL HYPOPHYSECTOMY

This operation, carried out by a major neurosurgical team through a right frontal craniotomy, is beyond the scope of many hospitals which must deal with cases of cancer. Although the mortality rate of approximately 6 per cent in 345 cases reported by Pearson and Ray (1960), and of 5·6 per cent in 71 cases reported by Kennedy and French (1965) does not differ significantly from that usually associated with adrenalectomy, transfrontal hypophysectomy may be followed by a variety of postoperative complications. The most common of these is diabetes insipidus, being likely to occur in at least 90 per cent of patients, but usually controllable by nasal insufflation of pitressin powder. Other possible sequelae are rhinorrhoea, sinusoturcical fistula, meningitis, impaired vision from optic nerve damage, impaired taste or smell, and personality changes. Although uncommon, in skilled hands, many of these complications are of a very serious nature, and taken together form an unpleasant group of problems, which has no parallel following adrenalectomy. All things considered, the transfrontal technique cannot be recommended as the most desirable method of hypophysectomy for wide use.

The results of pituitary stalk section might theoretically be expected to equal those of total hypophysectomy; but, although a high degree of gland necrosis follows, a considerable amount of viable tissue remains, and present evidence indicates that the procedure does not yield results comparable to those of hypophysectomy. Moreover, the mortality and morbidity rate of stalk section is appreciable (Ehni and Eckles, 1959).

TRANS-SPHENOIDAL HYPOPHYSECTOMY

A combined transnasal transethmosphenoidal surgical approach to the pituitary may well prove to be the most acceptable method of hypophysectomy. The palliative results yielded compare favourably with those of any other method of pituitary ablation. Otolaryngologists should be given more encouragement to develop skill in performing this operation, which can achieve as much as adrenalectomy, with no more hazard, and without causing the corresponding degree of postoperative distress. It has been demonstrated by the Bristol group (Harrold, Cates and James, 1968) which has had the greatest experience with trans-sphenoidal hypophysectomy, that refinements of technique can minimise morbidity from cerebrospinal

rhinorrhoea and meningitis; and these workers report a series of 324 cases in which the operative mortality was 5·8 per cent. Cerebrospinal leakage occurred in 5·6 per cent, meningitis in 5 per cent, and diabetes insipidus in 50 per cent.

YTTRIUM-90 IMPLANTATION

The implantation of yttrium-90 into the pituitary fossa by the screw technique, as described by Forrest, Blair and Valentine (1958), is a comparatively simple and safe alternative to surgical hypophysectomy, and has the advantage that it can be performed by a general surgeon. The operation is usually finished in 30 minutes, and the patient may leave hospital within four or five days, having suffered a minimum of general disturbance. Forrest and Stewart (1967), in a review of 297 cases, reported an immediate mortality of 4·4 per cent, and the following incidence of complications: diabetes insipidus 31 per cent, visual impairment 1·7 per cent, nerve palsies 3·4 per cent, cerebrospinal rhinorrhoea 2 per cent and meningitis 4·7 per cent. Although these figures are at an acceptably low level, evidence has now been produced by the originator of the method (Forrest and Stewart, 1967), that remission of breast cancer does not follow this procedure as frequently as it occurs after surgical hypophysectomy or adrenalectomy.

Destruction of pituitary tissue is often incomplete, autopsy studies in one series revealing that only 71 per cent of patients had more than 95 per cent of the gland destroyed (Forrest, 1967). However, as with other techniques, there is no evidence that the likelihood of a remission being obtained is necessarily related to the completeness of pituitary ablation. It may be concluded that this method should be selected for patients who, by reason of their poor general condition, are unsuitable for adrenalectomy or surgical hypophysectomy. Even so, the very ill patient with visceral metastases is often served best by withholding even this operative procedure, and the securing of pain relief by appropriate sedation.

PITUITARY ABLATION BY EXTERNAL RADIATION

Ablation of pituitary function by external radiation produced with conventional equipment is not practicable. Kelly et al (1951), have reported that in several patients with advanced breast cancer doses up to 10 000 rads delivered to the pituitary, neither resulted in clinical improvement, evidence of hypopituitarism, or even histological changes in the gland. High voltage rays (23 MeV) from a betatron, have been used in doses varying from 6000 to 15 000 rads (Nickson, 1957). Not only was there no clinical response in 12 patients so treated, but severe damage to adjacent brain tissue caused blindness and mental deterioration on several occasions. Only minor histological changes were found in the pituitary cells.

The most effective method of achieving pituitary destruction by high energy external radiation is by use of a proton or alpha-particle beam generated by a synchro-cyclotron, and this technique has been employed by Lawrence and Tobias at the Laboratory of Medical Physics in Berkeley, California. By means of a rotational technique, a dose of 30 000 rads is delivered to the pituitary over a period of five days with a very low skin dose, and Lawrence and his colleagues claim that, by using this method, pituitary function was depressed and microscopic necrosis was produced. These workers, after treating 176 patients with advanced breast cancer, report that more than 90 per cent of the pituitary could be destroyed, producing a remission of disease in 34 per cent of cases, while the only complications were a very low incidence of transient ocular palsies, and mild diabetes insipidus (Lawrence, 1967).

Evaluation of this report is complicated by the fact that a proportion of these patients received other methods of treatment. Unfortunately also, the maximum effect of external irradiation is achieved only after several months. Widespread use of this method of pituitary destruction is at present precluded by the fact that the special apparatus required is not generally available.

CRYOHYPOPHYSECTOMY

Trans-sphenoidal cryohypophysectomy achieves destruction of the gland by freezing with an accurately positioned liquid nitrogen probe; and recent reports, such as those by Rand (1968) and Norrel et al (1970), indicate that this is an effective way of achieving pituitary destruction, associated with minimal discomfort and risk to the patient. Rand claims that the production of five lesions (one centrally and two on each side of the midline) with the cryoprobe tip temperature lowered to —180°C results in 'complete clinical hypophysectomy'. Norrel and his associates have reported a series of 60 cases in which cryohypophysectomy was performed with a 10 per cent incidence of diabetes insipidus, and a similar incidence of cerebrospinal rhinorrhoea. No other complication was encountered, and there were no operative deaths. The most serious potential hazard is freezing of the adjacent 3rd, 4th, 5th and 6th nerves in the cavernous sinus laterally, and of the optic chiasma above. Consequently, local anaesthesia is employed, so that, with the patient cooperative, visual acuity, visual fields, and ocular muscle function can be tested as production of the cryogenic lesion progresses.

Although cryohypophysectomy involves a highly specialised technique, it is likely that it will become widely accepted, since a comparatively safe and near-total gland destruction is possible with neither general anaesthesia nor craniotomy.

ULTRASONIC ABLATION

While pituitary destruction by ultrasonic energy has been reported less than has any other method, it may be used more widely in the future. Ultrasonic ablation of the pituitary shares with external irradiation the considerable advantage that the dural capsule of the pituitary gland is neither opened nor perforated and cerebrospinal rhinorrhoea and meningitis are therefore avoided. Through a transnasal trans-sphenoidal approach, the anterior wall of the sella turcica is removed under microscopic control, and the irradiating ultrasonic probe is then held against the capsule of the pituitary for 15 minutes.

Arslan (1968) has reported using this method without encountering any complications in 28 cases of advanced carcinoma of the breast and prostate, and states that, 'pain from metastases rapidly diminished or disappeared entirely in all patients'—a remarkable claim, difficult to reconcile with the results of other techniques of hypophysectomy. Due to insufficiency of evidence, the true value of ultrasonic pituitary destruction cannot yet be evaluated.

CONCLUSION

The management of the advanced stages of cancer clearly poses many dilemmas, not the least of which is whether or not the statistically small benefits yielded by endocrine ablation, or indeed any method of treatment justify the time, effort and expense required for what so often may be only a brief prolongation of life. Yet, as doctors, we are essentially concerned with the individual human being, and we may well find that it is not only desirable, but enormously important, to extend for as long as possible a life we know to be doomed. This is especially so when the patient still has dependent children or other relatives; then, any extra period of survival is valuable, not only for its own sake, but also for the time allowed in which to organise the future of the family. Further than that, treatment, if successful, may result in dramatic relief of severe pain, and may greatly improve the quality of the remaining months of life. This respite may continue until the final relapse, when death usually comes quickly.

Since such advantages may result, it becomes improper to question the validity of treatment on a purely statistical basis. However, most of us would agree that, if, as in a patient with extensive visceral metastases, the best to be expected from any method of treatment is a slightly prolonged existence of poor quality, it is best to abstain from all therapy, and certainly from a major operative procedure, and to ensure a terminal phase which is free from pain.

But even after the most successful objective remissions achieved by ablative surgery or hormone therapy, inexorable tumour regrowth will begin, finally uncontrolled by any known treatment. At this stage it should be our concern to ensure that, when a life is obviously in its terminal stages, the patient should be allowed peace in which to die with some human dignity. Never in our attempts to prolong life should we forget that compassion may require a cessation of our efforts with drugs, antibiotics, and transfusions. The dying usually accept death more readily than do the living, and inevitably the time will come when we must consider the patient rather than the relatives. At the end, the greatest mercy we can render is to permit the closing of life to be swift and peaceful.

References

Ansfield, D. (1967) Symposium on cancer of the breast. *Cancer*, **20**, 1065.

Arslan, M. A. (1968) Ultrasonic selective hypophysectomy. *Proceedings of the Royal Society of Medicine*, **61**, 7.

Atkins, H. J. B., Falconer, M. A., Hayward, J. L., Maclean, K. S., Schurr, P. H. & Armitage, P. (1960) Adrenalectomy and hypophysectomy for advanced cancer of the breast. *Lancet*, **i**, 1148.

Atkins, H. J. B., Falconer, M. A., Hayward, J. L., Maclean, K. S. & Schurr, P. H. (1966) The timing of adrenalectomy and of hypophysectomy in the treatment of advanced breast cancer. *Lancet*, **i**, 827.

Atkins, H. J. B., Bulbrook, R. D., Falconer, M. A., Hayward, J. L., Maclean, K. S. & Schurr, P. H. (1968) Ten years experience of steroid assays in the management of breast cancer. *Lancet*, **ii**, 1255.

Barlow, J. J., Emerson, K. jun. & Saxena, B. N. (1969) Estradiol production after ovariectomy for carcinoma of the breast. *New England Journal of Medicine*, **280**, 633.

Beck, J. C., Blair, A. J., Griffiths, M. M., Rosenfeld, M. W. & McGarry, E. E. (1966) In search of hormonal factors as an aid in predicting the outcome of breast cancer. *Canadian Cancer Conference*, **6**, 3.

Biskind, G. R. & Mark, J. (1939) The inactivation of testosterone propionate and oestrone in rats. *Bulletin of the Johns Hopkins Hospital*, **65**, 212.

Block, G. E., Vial, A. B. & Pullen, F. W. (1958) Oestrogen excretion following operation and irradiation castration in cases of mammary cancer. *Surgery*, **43**, 415.

Brown, J. B. (1970) Personal communication.

Brown, J. B., Falconer, C. W. A. & Strong, J. A. (1959) Urinary oestrogens of adrenal origin in women with breast cancer. *Journal of Endocrinology*, **19**, 52.

Bulbrook, R. D. & Greenwood, F. C. (1957) Persistence of urinary oestrogen excretion after oophorectomy and adrenalectomy. *British Medical Journal*, **i**, 662.

Cole, M. P. (1964) The place of radiotherapy in the management of early breast cancer. A report of two clinical trials. *British Journal of Surgery*, **51**, 216.

Dao, T. L. & Libby, P. R. (1968) Conjugation of steroid hormones by breast cancer tissue and selection of patients for adrenalectomy. *Journal of Clinical Endocrinology and Metabolism*, **28**, 1431.

Dao, T. L., Nemoto, T. & Bross, I. (1968) Controlled randomized comparative study of early and late adrenalectomy in women with advanced cancer of the breast. In *Prognostic Factors in Breast Cancer*, eds. Forrest, A. P. M. and Kunkler, P. B., p. 177. Edinburgh: Livingstone.

Dao, T. L., Tan, E. & Brooks, V. (1961) A comparative evaluation of adrenalectomy and cortisone in the treatment of advanced mammary carcinoma. *Cancer*, **14**, 1259.

Dargent, M., Mayer, M. & Lombard, R. (1967) Modalités techniques de la chirugie surrénalienne: surrénalectomie bilatérale d'emblée ou en deux temps transplantation surréno-splénique. In *Major Endocrine Surgery for the Treatment of Cancer of the Breast in Advanced Stages*, ed. Dargent, M. and Romieu, Cl., p. 61. Lyon: Simep Éditions.

Ehni, G. & Eckles, N. E. (1959) Interruption of the pituitary stalk in patients with mammary cancer. *Journal of Neurosurgery*, **16**, 628.

Forrest, A. P. M. (1967) Clinical studies in advanced breast cancer. *Journal of the Royal College of Surgeons of Edinburgh*, **12**, 192.

Forrest, A. P. M. & Stewart, H. J. (1967) Technical problems and results of yttrium hypophysectomy. In *Major Endocrine Surgery for the Treatment of Cancer of the Breast in Advanced Stages*, ed. Dargent, M. and Romieu, Cl., p. 89. Lyon: Simep Éditions.

Forrest, A. P. M., Blair, D. W. & Valentine, J. M. (1958) Screw implantation of the pituitary with yttrium-90. *Lancet*, **ii**, 192.

Forrest, A. P. M., Benson, E. A., Ker, H., Jones, V., Kunkler, P. B. & Campbell, H. (1968) Controlled studies in advanced breast cancer. In *Prognostic Factors in Breast Cancer*, ed. Forrest, A. P. M. and Kunkler, P. B., p. 186. Edinburgh: Livingstone.

Fracchia, A. A., Farrow, J. H., De Palo, A. J. & Connolly, D. P. (1969) Castration for primary inoperable or recurrent breast cancer. *Surgery, Gynecology and Obstetrics*, **128**, 1226.

Fracchia, A. A., Holleb, A. I., Farrow, J. H., Treves, N. E., Randall, H. T., Finkbeiner, J. A. & Whitmore, W. F. Jr (1959) Results of bilateral adrenalectomy in the management of incurable breast cancer. *Cancer*, **12**, 58.

Golden, J. B. & Sevringhaus, E. L. (1938) Inactivation of oestrogenic hormone of the ovary by the liver. *Proceedings of the Society for Experimental Biology and Medicine*, **39**, 361.

Haagensen, C. D. (1956) *Diseases of the Breast*, p. 701. Philadelphia and London: Saunders.

Harrold, B. P., Cates, J. E. & James, J. A. (1968) Treatment of advanced breast cancer by trans-sphenoidal hypophysectomy. *British Journal of Cancer*, **22**, 19.

Hellström, J. & Franksson, C. (1958) Adrenalectomy in cancer of the breast. In *Endocrine Aspects of Breast Cancer*, ed. Currie, A. R. and Illingsworth, C. F. W., p. 5. Edinburgh: Livingstone.

Hunter, W. M. & Greenwood, F. C. (1964) A radio-immunoelectrophoretic assay for human growth hormone. *Biochemical Journal*, **91**, 43.

Israel, S. L., Meranze, D. R. & Johnston, C. G. (1937) The inactivation of oestrogens by the liver. *American Journal of the Medical Sciences*, **194**, 835.

Juret, P. (1966a) *Endocrine Surgery in Human Cancers*, p. 269. Springfield: Thomas.

Juret, P. (1966b) *Endocrine Surgery in Human Cancers*, p. 239. Springfield: Thomas.

Juret, P. & Hayem, M. (1960) Implantation de matériel radioactif intra-hypophysaire dans les cancers du sein métastatiques. Bilan clinique et biologique à propos de 75 cas. *Revue Française d'Etudes Cliniques et Biologiques*, **6**, 19.

Juret, P., Hayem, M. & Thomas, M. (1962) Action analgésique de l'hypophysectomie sur les métastases osseuses de cancers non hormono-dépendents. *Presse Médicale*, **70**, 323.

Kelly, K. H., Feldsted, E. T., Brown, R. F., Ortega, P., Bierman, H. R., Low-Beer, B. B. A. & Shimkin, M. B. (1951) Irradiation of the normal human hypophysis in malignancy: report of three cases receiving 8,100–10,000r. tissue dose to the pituitary gland. *Journal of the National Cancer Institute*, **11**, 967.

Kennedy, B. J. & French, L. (1965) Hypophysectomy in advanced breast cancer. *American Journal of Surgery*, **110**, 411.

Kennedy, B. J., Mielke, P. W. Jr & Fortuny, I. E. (1964) Therapeutic castration versus prophylactic castration in breast cancer. *Surgery, Gynecology and Obstetrics*, **118**, 524.

Landon, J. & Greenwood, F. C. (1968) Homologous radioimmunoassay for plasma levels of corticotrophin in man. *Lancet*, **i**, 273.

Lawrence, J. H. (1967) Heavy particle irradiation to the pituitary in metastatic breast cancer. In *Major Endocrine Surgery for the Treatment of Cancer of the Breast in Advanced Stages*, ed. Dargent, M. and Romieu, Cl., p. 89. Lyon: Simep Éditions.

Li, M. C., Janelli, D. E., Kelly, E. J., Kashiwabara, H. & Kim, R. H. (1970) Metastatic carcinoma of the male breast treated with bilateral adrenalectomy and chemotherapy. *Cancer*, **25**, 678.

McCullagh, E. P., Feldstein, M. A., Tweed, D. C. & Dohn, D. F. (1965) A study of pituitary function after intrasellar implantation of ^{90}Yt. *Journal of Clinical Endocrinology and Metabolism*, **25**, 832.

MacDonald, I. (1962) Endocrine ablation in disseminated mammary carcinoma. *Surgery, Gynecology and Obstetrics*, **115**, 215.

McDonald, J. H. & Canalis, J. A. (1958) A histological study of extraparenchymal Leydig-like cells. *Journal of Urology*, **79**, 850.

McGrath, F. (1970) Extrasellar adenohypophyseal tissue in the female. *Australian Journal of Radiology*, **14**, 241.

Mayer, M., Dargent, M., Pommatau, E. & Saez, S. (1967) Résultats de la transplantation surréno-splénique associée à la surrénalectomie droite et à l'ovariectomie dans le traitement du cancer du sein en phase avancée chez la femme. In *Major Endocrine Surgery for the Treatment of Cancer of the Breast in Advanced Stages*, ed. Dargent, M. and Romieu, Cl., p. 67. Lyon: Simep Éditions.

Nathanson, I. T. & Kelley, R. M. (1952) Hormonal treatment of cancer. *New England Journal of Medicine*, **246**, 135.

Nesbit, R. M. & Baum, W. C. (1951) Serum phosphatase determinations in diagnosis of prostatic cancer: a review of 1,150 cases. *Journal of the American Medical Association*, **145**, 1321.

Nickson, J. J. (1957) Radiation hypophysectomy. In *Hypophysectomy*, ed. Pearson, O. H., p. 127. Springfield: Thomas.

Nissen-Meyer, R. (1964) Prophylactic endocrine treatment in carcinoma of the breast. *Clinical Radiology*, **15**, 152.

Nissen-Meyer, R. (1968) Suppression of ovarian function in primary breast cancer. In *Prognostic Factors in Breast Cancer*, ed. Forrest, A. P. M. and Kunkler, P. B., p. 142. Edinburgh: Livingstone.

Noer, R. J. (1963) Adjuvant chemotherapy. Thio-TEPA with radical mastectomy in the treatment of breast cancer. *American Journal of Surgery*, **106**, 405.

Norrell, H., Alves, A. M., Winternitz, W. W. & Maddy, J. (1970) Cryohypophysectomy in patients with advanced cancer. *Cancer*, **25**, 1050.

O'Conor, V. J., Chiang, S. P. & Grayhack, J. T. (1963) Is subcapsular orchidectomy a definitive procedure? Studies of hormone excretion before and after orchidectomy. *Journal of Urology*, **89**, 236.

Patey, D. H. (1960) Early (prophylactic) oophorectomy and adrenalectomy in carcinoma of the breast, an interim report. *British Journal of Cancer*, **14**, 457.

Pearson, O. H. & Ray, B. S. (1960) Hypophysectomy in the treatment of metastatic mammary cancer. *American Journal of Surgery*, **99**, 544.

Pearson, O. H., West, C. D., Li, M. C., McLean, J. P. & Treves, N. (1955) Endocrine therapy of metastatic breast cancer. *Archives of Internal Medicine*, **95**, 357.

Rand, R. W. (1968) Stereotoxic cryohypophysectomy. In *Cryosurgery*, ed. Rand, R. W., Rinfret, A. P. and von Leden, H., p. 226. Springfield: Thomas.

Ravdin, R. G., Lewison, E. F., Slack, N. H., Dao, T. L., Gardner, B., State, D. & Fisher, B. (1970) Results of a clinical trial concerning the worth of prophylactic oophorectomy for breast cancer. *Surgery, Gynecology and Obstetrics*, **131**, 1055.

Stein, J. J. (1969) Surgical or irradiation castration for patients with advanced breast cancer. *Cancer*, **24**, 1350.

Stoll, B. A. (1969a) *Hormonal Management in Breast Cancer*, p. 37. London: Pitman Medical.

Stoll, B. A. (1969b) *Hormonal Management in Breast Cancer*, p. 24. London: Pitman Medical.

The Veterans Administration Co-operative Urological Research Group (1967) Treatment and survival of patients with cancer of the prostate. *Surgery, Gynecology and Obstetrics*, **124**, 1011.

Wilson, R. E., Jessiman, A. G. & Moore, F. D. (1958) Severe exacerbation of cancer of the breast after oophorectomy and adrenalectomy. Report of four cases. *New England Journal of Medicine*, **258**, 312.

Chapter 23

Planning for the Future in Hormonal Therapy

ALBERT SEGALOFF

It appears obvious to me that, as we have learned an increasing amount about the hormonal therapy of breast cancer, the most effective agents have been developed along diverse lines, some of them seemingly contradictory. As yet there are no good grounds for belief that we have arrived at a single biochemical facet, or consistent combination thereof, which we can exploit for designing or finding new hormonal agents for more effective therapy, or if indeed there will be any such thing.

Even though this volume is dedicated to Dr Huggins, I still prefer to use the term *hormone responsive* for human breast cancer rather than *hormone dependent*, since the lesions of breast cancer in women cannot truly be considered hormone dependent, particularly if one tries to generate a unifying theory which can serve as a basis for our future planning.

INTRACELLULAR MECHANISMS

There is a burgeoning knowledge of the mechanics of intercellular transportation of steroids, and a beginning knowledge of the intracellular mechanisms of hormone action in normal target tissue. Therefore we have felt hopeful that this would lead us directly to new series of highly effective hormonal agents, but the path down which we are travelling has more than its share of boulders and detours.

The pioneering work by Jensen (Jensen and Jacobson, 1962; Jensen et al, 1969) on the rat uterine cytoplasmic receptor for estradiol-17β, demonstrated that the estrogen* does not change as it moves into the

*At the author's request, estrogen, estradiol and estriol have been spelt throughout this chapter in accordance with the IUPAC Revised Tentative Rules for Nomenclature of Steroids.

nucleus where it has its effect probably upon the genome, but that the receptor undergoes substantial change. This has not as yet been exploited by finding more effective therapeutic agents, nor have we as yet been able to predict response on the basis of the content of the receptor—possibly because this measurement is still too difficult for wide application, and not micro enough so that the measurement can be applied to small amounts of available human tissues.

Our knowledge of the fate of androgens, much of which we owe to J. D. Wilson and his colleagues (Wilson and Gloyna, 1970) is also growing apace (Williams-Ashman and Reddi, 1971), although the mechanism is in sharp contrast to that for the body's handling of estrogens. In this area more controversy exists. The binding of testosterone to the cytoplasmic receptor seems less firm than the binding of estradiol-17β to its receptor, but for the androgen it appears that the receptor remains the same, while the steroid changes as it migrates into the cell and thence into the nucleus. There is substantial agreement that the first step is for cytoplasmic 5α-reductase to reduce the 4-5 double bond to the 5α configuration. There is the possibility that the receptor is actually the 5α-reductase. Indeed, evidence exists of greater androgenic potency for the resultant 5α-dihydrotestosterone.

However, it seems likely that in many instances, at least, further changes are required before arriving at the ultimate intracellularly active androgen. My own evidence has indicated that the removal of the angular methyl group on the 10 position is necessary (Segaloff, 1963). This has been exploited with the production of androgens of increased androgenic potency which also show evidence of increased activity against advancing clinical breast cancer (Segaloff et al, 1964). Other evidence from organ cultures indicates that further reduction of the molecule (i.e. to the 3β-hydroxyl) is necessary for optimal activity rather than the removal of the angular methyl groups.

However, these may represent independent pathways in various tissues under differing conditions.

These various findings, I believe, point a moral to follow in our present state of knowledge, namely, that there are different routes of inquiry leading to effective agents, and that it is possible that various hormonal agents may be operating on a variety of mechanisms within the host or the tumour itself; and that a final, hopefully effective solution to the problem of breast cancer will be finding a single agent or a combination of agents for interfering successfully in all these areas.

ENDOCRINE CONSEQUENCES OF HORMONAL THERAPY

My own earliest view of a unifying thesis about which we could design hormonal agents, which seemed to be the sole characteristic to tie together the effective androgens and estrogens, was the observation that at that time all the hormonal agents known to be highly effective against advancing human breast cancer inhibited the urinary excretion of gonad-stimulating hormone (Segaloff, 1958). Then came our first exception to this finding, the potent androgen fluoxymesterone (9α-fluoro-17α-methyl-11β, 17β-hydroxy-androst-4-en-3-one), which failed to inhibit gonad-stimulating hormone excretion in the urine yet was effective against advancing breast cancer. This was followed shortly by two other agents effective against advancing breast cancer but which also failed to inhibit urinary gonad-stimulating hormone. One of these was an androgen with preferential anabolic activity, 2α-methyldihydrotestosterone propionate (2α-methyl,17β-hydroxy-5α-androstan-3-one propionate) (Blackburn and Childs, 1959), the other Δ^1-testololactone (17a-oxa-D-homo-1,4-androstadiene-3,17-dione) (Segaloff et al, 1960), which lacks all hormonal properties yet is capable of producing a significant percentage of objective regressions in advancing breast cancer.

Here again we must emphasise that we should continue to look for better gonad-stimulating hormone excretion-inhibiting agents, since despite the fact that we have found compounds which are exceptions to this rule, we have not found compounds which strongly inhibit the excretion of gonad-stimulating hormone and are not also highly effective against advancing breast cancer! So again we must follow each pathway, keeping aware of the knowledge that there are exceptions to our developing rules.

The next correlation which we investigated was that the more androgenic androgens (those more androgenic per milligram of weight) seem to be more effective against advancing breast cancer. Here again the picture is striking in that I am unaware of a highly potent androgen which is not *pari passu* an effective clinical antitumour agent, but there is an increasing number of compounds of lesser androgenic potency active against clinically advancing breast cancer. The most effective agent that we have studied in a large number of patients is a highly androgenic compound, 7α-methyl-19-nortestosterone acetate (7α-methyl-17β-hydroxy-estr-4-en-3-one acetate), which binds tightly to the androgen receptor and substantially inhibits gonad-stimulating hormone excretion in the urine.

However, finding the greatest activity in the more androgenic androgens and the more estrogenic estrogens may be a rather pyrrhic victory. Some patients and physicians are so accustomed to believe in our ability to handle advanced breast cancer without severe physiologic effects, that they feel the objective regressions and increased longevity obtained with these potent agents are not worth the sometimes cruelly rapid induction of such hormonal effects as virilisation for androgens and stress incontinence for estrogens. This may indeed be our fault rather than the patients' since they expect much of us, while those patients with malignancies more commonly treated with cytotoxic agents seem to accept more readily the

equally or even more devastating systemic consequences of these agents.

We may well require the simultaneous use of several hormonal agents, though at the moment it seems that this will probably be less effective than the combinations of cytotoxic agents have been in the treatment of acute leukaemia of children. This is probably because hormones with widely differing biologic activities may create problems in the intracellular handling of each other. It might be necessary to try to combine such activities in various parts of the steroid molecule, even if it requires the production of disteroids. This concept is not really too far-fetched since we do have such agents already, such as 17-methyl-19-nortestosterone (17-methyl-17β-hydroxy-estr-4-en-3-one), which are extremely potent androgens, estrogens and progestogens. Unfortunately this particular agent has hepatotoxic properties in keeping with its 17-methyl-19-nor configuration, but it does point up the fact that such compounds can be made. Indeed, we are aware that it is possible to make highly active hormonal agents which also have cytotoxic properties.

For reasons not entirely clear it has been found that the ability of corticoids to produce objective regression in advanced breast cancer is enhanced quite substantially by the administration of thyroactive substances. This type of study must be pursued further.

PROSPECTS FOR NEW HORMONAL AGENTS

We are, as should be apparent, at the end of our ability to ablate additional endocrine organs. We cannot hope for further improvements in this regard, therefore we must look beyond to the synthesis of new agents. The most hopeful area is that of governing the metabolism of administered hormonal agents, as well as the endogenous ones, through various other drugs. Steroid hydroxylations are carried out by mitochondria. We may be able to exploit for steroids, as well as for other agents, our expanding knowledge of drug interactions through their effects on the hydroxylating systems of mitochondria.

Hopefully we can now also develop means for altering the binding of hormonal agents to plasma proteins, both specific and non-specific, altering the urinary excretion and thereby changing the hormonal milieu offered to the tumour and its host. Hormonal agents rendered less active by either conjugation, binding or excretion, could have their activity altered further by means which are now becoming better understood.

Finally, because of our admitted lack of knowledge of how hormonal agents work *in toto* to produce regression of breast cancer, I hope that, with some restraint, we will continue to test in man some compounds for which our animal hormone assays and our animal tumour systems give us no reasonable hope of activity. Compounds in this category which have been shown to have favourable activity are Δ^1-testololactone and $7\beta,17$-dimethyltestosterone ($7\beta,17$-dimethyl-17β-hydroxyandrost-4-en-3-one). The former is already available commercially and of proved efficacy in advanced breast cancer, while the latter is just now in the early bloom of promise and is currently the subject of intensive study.

The most dramatic application of hormonal therapy in neoplastic disease is undoubtedly the induction of complete remission in childhood acute lymphatic leukaemia by corticoids. Such remissions are unfortunately of limited duration but can be extended in most instances by the use of cytotoxic agents. It is surprising that despite this there has been little, if any, effort to improve on the corticoid results. Most haematologists simply use prednisone.

This reluctance reflects a very parochial view, I believe, because the further improvements in cases of acute leukaemia have depended heavily upon animal models (L 1210 in particular) where corticoids are not effective. There are many corticoids known with greater effect on the lymphatic system in respect to their other physiologic parameters but we still see the inertia about studying them in man. Until we find a model where corticoids work we should try to get more human trials.

The pioneering work of Kelley and Baker (1961) has demonstrated that we can attain substantial regressions in the metastatic deposits from endometrial cancer by the administration of potent progestational agents. Pulmonary metastatic deposits also seem particularly vulnerable to such attack. Various potent progestogens are known to work but I am unaware of well-done comparative trials to determine which might be best. This undoubtedly relates to the relative scarcity of endometrial cancer and the excellent cure rate achieved by hysterectomy and radiation combined.

It seems certain that some clear-cell carcinomas (hypernephroma) of the kidney regress when hormones are administered. The first trials were based on Bloom's studies (1967) of treatment of the estrogen-induced renal cancer in the hamster. I am not aware of any good randomised prospective trial in an effort to reconcile the substantially differing results. What we can say is that progestogens, and in one case testosterone, can produce objective regression of metastatic deposits of renal-cell carcinoma.

References

Blackburn, C. M. & Childs, D. S. Jr (1959) Use of 2α-methyl-androstan-17β-ol-3-one (2-methyl-dihydrotestosterone) in the treatment of advanced cancer of the breast. *Proceedings of the Staff Meetings of the Mayo Clinic*, **34**, 113.

Bloom, H. J. G. (1967) Treatment of renal cell carcinoma with steroid hormones: observations with transplanted tumors in the hamster and incurable cancer in man. In *Renal Neoplasia*, ed. King, J. S. Jr, p. 605. Boston: Little, Brown.

Jensen, E. V. & Jacobson, H. I. (1962) Basic guides to the mechanism of estrogen action. *Recent Progress in Hormone Research*, **18**, 387.

Jensen, E. V., Suzuki, T., Numata, M., Smith, S. & De Sombre, E. R. (1969) Estrogen-binding substances of target tissues. *Steroids*, **13**, 417.

Kelley, R. M. & Baker, W. H. (1961) Progestational agents in the treatment of carcinoma of the endometrium. *New England Journal of Medicine*, **264**, 216.

Segaloff, A. (1958) The therapy of advanced breast cancer with androgens. In *Breast Cancer* (2nd Biennial Louisiana Cancer Conference), p. 203. St. Louis: Mosby.

Segaloff, A., Weeth, J. B., Rongone, E. L., Murison, P. J. & Bowers, C. Y. (1960) Hormonal therapy in cancer of the breast. XVI. Effect of Δ¹-testololactone on clinical course and hormonal excretion. *Cancer*, **13**, 1017.

Segaloff, A. (1963) The enhanced local androgenic activity of 19-nor steroids and stabilization of their structure by 7α- and 17α-methyl substituents to highly potent androgens by any route of administration. *Steroids*, **1**, 299.

Segaloff, A., Weeth, J. B., Cuningham, M. & Meyer, K. K. (1964) Hormonal therapy of cancer of the breast. XXIII. Effect of 7α-methyl-19-nortestosterone acetate (7α-methyl-estr-4-en-3-one, 17β-ol acetate) or testosterone propionate on clinical course and hormonal excretion. *Cancer*, **17**, 1248.

Williams-Ashman, H. G. & Reddi, A. H. (1971) Actions of vertebrate sex hormones. *Annual Review of Physiology*, **33**, 31.

Wilson, J. D. & Gloyna, R. E. (1970) The intranuclear metabolism of testosterone in the accessory organs of reproduction. *Recent Progress in Hormone Research*, **26**, 309.

Index

For ease of reference, details of each treatment are arranged under individual tumour headings.

427